T0384726

DIET IMPACTS ON BRAIN AND MIND

Everybody eats, and what we eat – or do not – affects the brain and mind. There is significant general, applied, academic and industry interest about nutrition and the brain, and yet there is much misinformation and no single reliable guide. *Diet Impacts on Brain and Mind* provides a comprehensive account of this emerging multidisciplinary science, exploring the acute and chronic impacts of human diet on the brain and mind. It has a primarily human focus and is broad in scope, covering wide-ranging topics like brain development, whole diets, specific nutrients, research methodology and food as a drug. It is written in an accessible format and is of interest to undergraduate and graduate students studying nutritional neuroscience and related disciplines, healthcare professionals with an applied interest, industry researchers seeking topic overviews and interested general readers.

RICHARD J. STEVENSON was born in the UK where he completed a degree in biology, and a master's degree and a PhD in experimental psychology. After moving to Australia, he has worked in both applied and academic settings, with a current focus on the impacts of Western-style diets on brain and appetitive behaviour. He is currently Professor of Experimental Psychology at Macquarie University, Australia.

HEATHER M. FRANCIS is a clinical neuropsychologist, whose research has focused on the links between diet and brain function, particularly in young adults. She is Deputy Director of the Master of Clinical Neuropsychology program at Macquarie University, Australia, and works clinically in the Neurology Department at Royal North Shore Hospital, Australia.

DIET IMPACTS ON BRAIN AND MIND

RICHARD J. STEVENSON

Macquarie University

HEATHER M. FRANCIS

Macquarie University

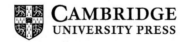

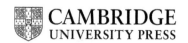

Shaftesbury Road, Cambridge CB2 8EA, United Kingdom

One Liberty Plaza, 20th Floor, New York, NY 10006, USA

477 Williamstown Road, Port Melbourne, VIC 3207, Australia

314–321, 3rd Floor, Plot 3, Splendor Forum, Jasola District Centre, New Delhi – 110025, India

103 Penang Road, #05–06/07, Visioncrest Commercial, Singapore 238467

Cambridge University Press is part of Cambridge University Press & Assessment, a department of the University of Cambridge.

We share the University's mission to contribute to society through the pursuit of education, learning and research at the highest international levels of excellence.

www.cambridge.org

Information on this title: www.cambridge.org/9781108485050

DOI: 10.1017/9781108755399

First published 2023

A catalogue record for this publication is available from the British Library

A Cataloging-in-Publication data record for this book is available from the Library of Congress

ISBN 978-1-108-48505-0 Hardback
ISBN 978-1-108-71915-5 Paperback

Contents

Figures

Tables

Preface and Acknowledgements

This book was born of a simple need. When we first started studying Western-style diets and their impacts, we wanted a general introduction to the broader field of diet, brain and mind. We could find no single source that gave us the overview we desired, and so we decided to write one. Writing a book is always a collaborative endeavour, and many people have helped us in this process. We thank Margaret Allman-Farinelli, Jen Cornish and Deb Mitchison for kindly reading and commenting on some of the chapters; Bob Boakes, Jon Mond, Tuki Attuquayefio, Martin Yeomans and Terry Davidson for many enlightening discussions; and Alysia Robertson, Karina Chan and Fiona Wylie for assistance with the References. We thank the Australian Research Council for their continued support, which assisted with much of our research reported in this book. Dick Stevenson particularly thanks his family for their support – Caroline, Gemma, Lucy, Harry, Chris, Mike, Rosie and Bailey – through good times and bad, and his dear ex-neighbours Charles Kamerman and Jennifer Cheyne for letting him help with Charles's book (in a very small way), which inspired him to work on this one. Heather M. Francis thanks her many supportive colleagues and friends who have provided guidance and wisdom – especially Dick Stevenson, without whom she would never have written this book. She would also like to give a special thanks to her family – Audrey, Gemma and Chris – for being an endless source of joy and inspiration. Finally, both of us thank Stephen Acerra of Cambridge University Press for his unerring support throughout the life of this project.

CHAPTER I

Introduction

1.1 Introduction

The aim of this book is to provide a comprehensive account of the acute and chronic impacts of human diet on the brain and mind. Importantly, this is distinct from the much larger literature studying how the brain and mind affect food intake. It is distinct because in this book, the presumed causal arrow generally points from food → to brain and mind. A further aspect of this book is its emphasis on humans. This is both pragmatic (e.g., for health and policy implications) and reflects our interests in understanding the effects of diet on the human brain and mind. While there is a primary human focus, we have by necessity drawn on the animal literature. Unlike human studies, animal research can get nearly 100% compliance with experimental dietary regimens, and it is possible to undertake studies that are difficult to do with people, especially those concerning mechanism. Inclusion of animal data is also based on the premise that humans and animals share much common biology. In Sir Austin Bradford Hill's consideration of how to establish causality (Hill, 1965), scientific plausibility (i.e., is there a mechanism?) and coherence with known facts were two key criteria. Animal data is very important as they are particularly useful for understanding mechanism (i.e., scientific plausibility), and for experimental demonstrations of dietary effects on brain and mind (i.e., coherence).

As the title implies, the book investigates the impacts of diet on brain *and* mind. It seems important to study both, although the relative emphasis shifts between chapters dependent on what is known and the topic. It is essential to study effects on mind (operationalised as behaviour and cognition) because this level of explanation has great practical utility. If breakfast makes children concentrate better, intermittent hunger makes people immoral, and fruit and vegetables make people happy, it is important to know this *irrespective* of how diet causes these effects in the brain. Notwithstanding, it is also important to determine how diet does these things to the brain. This establishes mechanism, with its implications for the biological plausibility of any observed effect on mind. It can also provide information for human betterment, via say developing nutraceuticals, drugs or other forms of treatment that target the neural mechanism. That aside, the pursuit of knowledge for its own sake is a worthy goal, and it was in this spirit that our book was conceived and written.

There have been many excellent and pioneering books on diet, brain and mind, all of which have appeared as edited volumes (e.g., Lieberman, Kanarek, Nehlig, Dye, Watson). However, these can sometimes lack a consistent approach between chapters, with, for example, greater or lesser emphasis on animal data, epidemiology over experimental work, or whatever. Coverage of the field is also sometimes limited to particular parts, reflecting the interests and expertise of those authors and editors. To date, nobody has tried to pull all of the different strands that make up the field of diet, brain and mind into one volume. Nor has there been a consistent focus on humans, with an interest in both brain and mind. As we have discovered, the field is much larger than we originally thought, it is also very diverse and its parts are often disconnected – but it is endlessly fascinating. The field also faces some significant methodological challenges, both in accurately measuring and manipulating human diet and in measuring brain and behaviour. However, scientists are an ingenious bunch and they have risen to the challenge.

The book proper starts with Chapter 2 on pregnancy, breastfeeding and infancy, followed in Chapter 3 by the acute effects of food intake, looking both at specific meals (e.g., breakfast) and specific nutrients (e.g., particular amino acids). Chapter 4 examines the chronic effects of food intake, with special emphasis on the major dietary pattern found in developed, and now developing, countries: a Western-style diet, rich in saturated fat, salt and added sugar. Chapter 5 explores the acute and chronic effects of dietary neurotoxins, coming both from foods and their contaminants (e.g., fungi, pesticides). Diet can also have an important protective effect on brain and mind, and indeed this is increasingly being recognised as a potential intervention for psychiatric, neurological and neurodegenerative conditions. This is all examined in Chapter 6. In addition, both Chapters 4 and 6 include emerging data on how diet affects the microbial ecology of our large intestine, as these organisms may have an important role in how diet impacts brain and mind. The food and drink we consume are the major routes for ingesting two of the world's most popular drugs, alcohol and caffeine. It has also been suggested that certain foods – ultra-processed items that bear little resemblance to the ingredients from which they are

made – may exert drug-like effects (e.g., dependence, craving) in consumers. Drugs and food form the basis for Chapter 7. Chapter 8 examines
the science of starvation, both its acute and chronic effects in and outside of
the laboratory, and the use of energy-restrictive diets for life extension.
Chapter 9 looks at the impact on brain and mind of specific nutrient
deficiencies (i.e., vitamins, minerals and certain essential macronutrients).
Finally, Chapter 10 provides a reflection on this content, its implications
and where the field might (and perhaps should) be heading.

The remainder of this first chapter has two aims. The first is to provide a
brief overview of the core knowledge and methods that underpin research
into diet, brain and mind, and their limitations. We have included this
because readers coming afresh to this area may have experience in one
domain (e.g., nutrition) but not another (e.g., psychology, brain science),
or indeed no experience at all. The second concerns our focus. We have
already identified that the emphasis is on humans, and brain and mind,
but there is another aspect to our approach that is best discussed with some
understanding of the strengths and weakness of the available methods, as
they relate to measuring diet. Hence, we have left a discussion of this topic
until the end of the chapter, assuming that those unfamiliar with the
nutrition literature will first read the following relevant parts first.

1.2   Basic Nutritional Concepts

The main purpose of eating is to satisfy the body's energy needs (Woods &
Seeley, 2000). In addition, eating provides the materials for growth and/or
maintenance of all bodily systems. In humans, eating and drinking are also
a major source of pleasure – if not an art as gastronomy – and a major
vehicle for intoxication (e.g., alcohol, caffeine). These more uniquely
human aspects of ingestion are of great social and scientific interest. This
is because they contribute in no small part to: (1) overeating and obesity;
(2) drug abuse, with alcohol being one of the most frequently misused; and
(3) to the abuse of other substances which hijack multiple aspects of the
brain's appetite/reward systems that support feeding.

Humans obtain energy from four main constituents of what they eat
and drink – carbohydrates, proteins, fats and alcohol (Eschleman, 1996).
Setting aside alcohol, the three main energy-yielding constituents of food
are termed macronutrients. The amount of energy in a food or a drink is
measured either in the SI unit the joule (and typically in kilojoules (kJ)) –
which is used in this book – or alternatively, and mainly in the United
States, by the calorie (and again typically as the kilocalorie (kcal); to

convert, 1 kcal = 4.18 kJ, and 1 kJ = 0.24 kcal). The formal definition of the calorie is a lot easier to grasp than the formal definitions of the joule. The calorie is defined as the energy required to heat a gram of water by one degree centigrade. The joule is easier to define informally as the energy required to lift a large tomato one metre into the air (or if you prefer more formally – the amount of work done when a force of one Newton is used to move an object one metre in the direction of the applied force (i.e., 1 N·m)).

The energy needs of an individual vary markedly, dependent on age, body composition (muscle vs fat), body weight, pregnancy, lactation, health, activity and climate (Eschleman, 1996). A person's basic energy requirement is the amount of food in kJ they need to eat to maintain their basal metabolic rate. Basal metabolic rate reflects the essential operations of the body necessary to maintain life at rest (i.e., cellular metabolism and maintenance). A man requires around 4.2 kJ per kilogram per hour to maintain basal metabolic rate and a woman around 3.8 kJ. Thus an average US man has a daily energy requirement just to meet basal metabolic rate of around 8,000 kJ and a woman needs around 7,000 kJ. Basal metabolic rates vary markedly over the lifespan, and hence so do energy needs. An infant requires 9.3 kJ per kg per hour, while an elderly woman needs 3.4 kJ per kg per hour. Illness can dramatically increase basal metabolic rate. A change in body temperature from 37 to 41 degrees centigrade due to a fever requires an approximately 60% increase in basal metabolic rate. This is one reason why infection has more lethal effects among starving people.

The other important component in determining energy needs is to establish that spent on moving around and doing things. As activity levels are generally quite low in the developed world, multiplying the adult basal metabolic rate requirement by 1.3 gives a rough guide to typical ideal adult energy intakes (i.e., 10,400 kJ for a man and 9,100 kJ for a woman). For a highly active adult (e.g., a lumberjack), doubling the basal metabolic rate requirement is necessary to satisfy total energy needs.

All of the three macronutrients (and alcohol) can be metabolised to provide energy for the body, and surplus energy from all three sources (and alcohol) can be stored as fat (Eschleman, 1996). Carbohydrates and proteins yield around 17 kJ per gram, while fats provide 38 kJ per gram. Under normal circumstances, carbohydrates provide the main energy source for humans. In our ancestral environment, complex carbohydrates were the principal energy source in the form of starch (e.g., tubers (potatoes, cassava), grass seeds (wheat, rice)), with indigestible complex carbohydrates providing fibre (cellulose, inulin). Starch is composed of multiple glucoses units connected by covalent bonds. This is broken down in the digestive system into glucose. Glucose is a monosaccharide, and is used by the body as an energy source. It is present in blood at around 1,400 mg per litre in a healthy adult, and is stored in small amounts in various bodily depots as glycogen. Glycogen is a polysaccharide, with chains of glucose attached to a glycogenin protein core. Depots of glycogen are found in muscles (about 500 g in total) and the liver (about 100 g). Maintaining adequate supplies of glucose is essential because it is the primary energy source for the brain, where the *only* alternative fuel is ketone bodies (essentially an emergency fuel when all potential sources of glucose are exhausted). Nerve cells are unable to store glucose as glycogen.

In contrast to ancestral diets, a significant source of carbohydrates in modern diets comes from one particular disaccharide – sucrose or sugar. Disaccharides are composed of two monosaccharide units. Glucose is a monosaccharide, and there are two other important monosaccharides. Fructose, which is particularly sweet, and galactose, which is not that sweet – with both of these found in small quantities in certain fruits. The most important dietary sugar is the disaccharide sucrose, which is made of one glucose unit and one fructose unit. In the United States, each person consumes an average of 20 teaspoons (80 g) of sucrose per day (Drewnowski & Rehm, 2014). Other important dietary disaccharides are lactose ('milk' sugar), found in mammalian milk (composed of a glucose and a galactose unit), and maltose, found in beer (composed of two glucose units). Neither lactose nor maltose are particularly sweet.

As noted earlier, glucose is the principal fuel for the brain as well as being a major bodily fuel (Sembulingam & Sembulingam, 2016). In the presence of oxygen (i.e., aerobically) it is converted into pyruvate-liberating energy, and further energy can be released by the conversion of pyruvate into acetyl coenzyme A. All of this takes place in the cytosol (i.e., in the main portion of the cell). Acetyl coenzyme A is then fed into the Krebs cycle, which takes place inside mitochondria (a cellular organelle), liberating yet more energy (see Figure 1.1). Under conditions of high exertion, when the body cannot supply sufficient oxygen to muscle tissues for aerobic respiration (i.e., energy generation), both glucose and pyruvate can be metabolised without oxygen (i.e., anaerobically) in the cytosol, providing a brief burst of energy, but leading to a rapid build-up of lactic acid, which inhibits further anaerobic respiration.

In the absence of adequate supplies of carbohydrate, protein can serve as a good fuel substitute, as approximately half of the protein available in diet

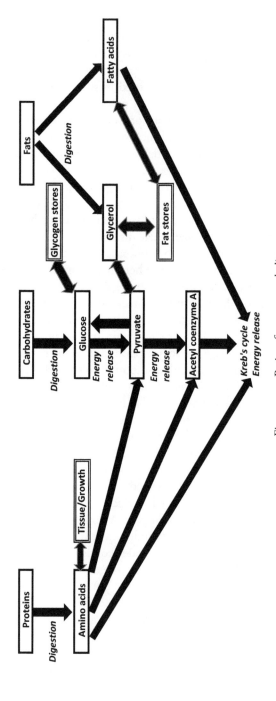

Figure 1.1   Basics of energy metabolism

can be metabolised to pyruvate, which can then be converted back to glucose (Sembulingam & Sembulingam, 2016). The remaining half can be fed directly into the Krebs cycle, the major energy-generation pathway for the body (see Figure 1.1). In the main, dietary protein, which is built from multiple, different amino acids, is essential for tissue maintenance and growth (i.e., creation of new proteins (e.g., enzymes) and biomolecules – like neurotransmitters), and for fluid balance. Humans require 20 different amino acids, some of which have to come from dietary sources as they cannot be synthesised by the body. Meat provides all of the required amino acids. A solely plant-based diet can as well, but care is needed to avoid insufficiency.

While fats are a good source of energy (see Figure 1.1), they are a poor source of glucose and are not used as a fuel by the brain. Fats are composed of a glycerol molecule, which can be converted to glucose, with three fatty acid tails attached, which cannot be converted (Sembulingam & Sembulingam, 2016). The type of fatty acid attached to the glycerol molecule dictates the type of fat – saturated, monounsaturated, polyunsaturated and trans-saturated. Type is based upon the presence/absence and location of carbon double bonds, and subtype by the length of the fatty acid chain. Different types of fats tend to be found in different types of food. Saturated fats, which are solid at room temperature, are generally from animals (e.g., meat, dairy), with the exception of palm and coconut oil. All of these are associated with an unhealthy blood lipid profile and have been linked to coronary arteriosclerosis and heart disease, although this is no longer a universal conclusion (Chowdhury et al., 2014). Monounsaturated fats have plant-based sources (e.g., olive oil, canola oil), and are linked to a beneficial blood lipid profile. With polyunsaturated fats, which are liquid at room temperature (as with monounsaturated fats), one common type is found in nuts and seafood (omega 3) and another in plants (omega 6). Both are linked to beneficial blood lipid profiles. Trans-saturated fats are factory-made from plant-based unsaturated sources. They have very useful properties in that they do not readily oxidise (i.e., go rancid) giving foods made from them a long shelf life. Unfortunately, they seem to have a worse effect on blood lipid profile than saturated fats and they have been banned in several countries. While fats are a major source of energy, they have many other important functions. They form key parts of cell membranes, and nerve fibre myelin sheaths, and they are needed for hormone synthesis, the digestion of certain vitamins, thermal insulation (subcutaneous fat), energy storage and organ padding.

In addition to the macronutrients, the body needs a range of micronutrients, all of which are provided in a typical omnivorous diet (Eschleman, 1996). Micronutrients are divided into vitamins and minerals. Vitamins are a heterogenous collection of organic compounds that the body cannot synthesise, which are necessary for normal function, and so have to come from food. Vitamins are usually grouped into those that are fat-soluble (A, D, E and K) and those that are water soluble (B, C). Dietary insufficiency in particular vitamins is linked to specific deficiency diseases, many of which have a long and tragic history (e.g., beriberi, scurvy, pellagra). In the past, these diseases were not recognised as resulting from a dietary cause (e.g., scurvy was thought to be a manifestation of syphilis). Identifying the cause required use of a scientific method. This was applied to scurvy by English naval physician James Lind in 1797. It revealed scurvy's dietary basis and probably represents the first ever clinical trial (Carpenter, 2003).

Mineral elements (beyond carbon, hydrogen, nitrogen and oxygen) are the other necessary dietary components. These are classified as either macrominerals (requirements greater than 100 mg per day) – calcium, phosphorous, sodium, sulphur, chlorine, potassium and magnesium – or microminerals (<100 mg per day) – iron, iodine, fluorine, selenium, zinc and several others. Deficiencies in these microminerals can produce severe disease (e.g., iodine deficiency, goitre and cretinism) and in some instances either too much or too little can be harmful (e.g., sodium/chlorine (salt); selenium).

1.3   Basics of Digestion and Regulation

The preparation for digestion starts before eating, as a variety of processes are triggered by the thought, sight or smell of food (think Ivan Pavlov, bells, and salivating dogs – the cephalic phase response). Food in the mouth is mechanically broken up by the action of chewing. It is mixed with saliva and formed into a bolus for swallowing (Longenbaker, 2017). Saliva contains the enzyme alpha amylase, which acts rapidly to break down starch into sugars. Whether this is to aid digestion or to promote consumption by making a starchy food taste somewhat sweet is not known.

The swallowed bolus passes down the oesophagus into the upper part of the stomach where it is ground into even small particles by this organ's muscular action. This ground food is then moved into the body of the stomach where it is mixed with acid and enzymes, forming a semi-liquid called chyme which collects in the lower part of the stomach. The chyme is then expelled via the pyloric sphincter into the small intestine, which is the main organ for the absorption and digestion of nutrients in the human body.

The small intestine is a muscular tube 2–3 cm in diameter and 6–7 m in length (but probably less, as these measurements are based on cadavers with 'relaxed' muscles; Longenbaker, 2017). The small intestine has waves of muscular action (peristalsis) so as to move its contents progressively along its length. Because the wall of the small intestine is heavily invaginated and covered with a myriad small projections of tissue (microvilli), it has a large surface area, around 60 m^2 in an adult (a quarter of a tennis court). This assists effective nutrient absorption. The arrival of food into the small intestine triggers the release of cholecystokinin (CCK). This hormone stimulates the production of bile to break down fat, and the release of pancreatic juices to break down protein and carbohydrates. CCK also acts to slow the release of chyme from the stomach. Amino acids, glucose, fatty acids, vitamins and minerals then pass (some actively (i.e., energy driven transporters) and some passively) through the endothelial lining of the gut into cells. In these cells fatty acids are packaged into chylomicrons, which, together with other nutrients, are released into the hepatic portal vein for transport to the liver and other bodily tissues.

The remaining unabsorbed material passes into the large intestine, which is 1–2 m in length, and called 'large' due to its 6–7 cm diameter (Longenbaker, 2017). While digestively of lesser importance than the small intestine, it nonetheless has several functions. The large intestine is home to a vast number of microorganisms, which feed on the undigested produce coming from the small intestine. This microbial ecosystem is increasingly being recognised for its impact on health, as the type of organisms present influences the production of ketones, which serve as both an energy source, but also act to preserve the integrity of the endothelial (i.e., gut–body) barrier (Berding et al., 2021). Leakage of material from the gut, other than nutrients, may initiate a number of disease processes, possibly including dementia, as amyloid beta is produced in abundance by certain types of bacteria, but not by others. Many other factors also influence the integrity of the gut–body barrier, in particular the type of bacteria present. Diet can result in fairly rapid changes in this microbial ecosystem, for the better (plant-based foods) or worse (processed foods). Fermentation by gut microbes is also important in the production of certain B vitamins, and for vitamin K, and these alongside water and ketones are absorbed by this part of the digestive tract. Compactification occurs, followed by temporary storage in the rectum, before defecation ends the digestive process.

The digestive system and the brain are connected in several ways. The brain's sensory systems 'see', 'smell', 'taste' and 'feel' food as it is eaten, providing information to prepare the organism for feeding and to terminate a feeding bout. The vagus nerve links the brain and gut, carrying sensory information (e.g., nutrient sensing, gut fullness) from gut to brain (most traffic) and some signals from brain to gut. Hormonal signals released by digestion, the digestive system and fat stores all impact brain function and regulation (Lowell, 2019). These include grehlin released by the stomach when empty, CCK when the stomach is filling or full, and leptin from fat, indicating the extent of bodily fat stores. All of these hormones affect appetite and exert influences well beyond this domain (e.g., grehlin promotes learning – a good idea if one is to remember a food source). The brain also monitors a range of physiological parameters which provide information about the nutritional status of the body, such as signals of muscle usage and blood glucose, for example. This information feeds into a number of brain areas that are known to be involved in the regulation of appetite (Logue, 2015). The most well-known component is the hypothalamus, particularly the lateral and ventromedial parts, which are early processors of sensory, gut, hormonal and metabolic signals and set up a general brain state either favourable or not for eating. The striatum, frontal cortex, orbitofrontal cortex, insula and hippocampus interact to regulate eating based on both hypothalamic outputs and in many cases via the same sensory, gut, hormonal and metabolic signals as well. These latter structures are the probable basis for the conscious aspects of eating, underpinning sensation, pleasure, feelings of fullness and hunger, thoughts about food, and broader conceptual considerations such as dieting, morality of meat eating or gourmet dining, for example.

While the brain is a major controller of food intake, certain regulatory aspects of digestive/ingestive processes are more peripheral. Glucose and fat are two important examples, reflecting the operation of short-term and long-term energy management systems, respectively. Increases in glucose, typically after eating, are kept in check by the release of insulin from beta cells in the pancreas, which sequesters excess glucose into muscle or liver cells as glycogen. In contrast, falling blood glucose leads to the secretion of glucagon by alpha cells in the pancreas, which liberates glucose from glycogen. For fat stores, which are the body's energy reserve against starvation, fat cells continuously release a hormonal signal leptin, which reflects bodily fat content. As leptin levels fall, indicating a reduction in bodily fat stores, there is a significant stimulatory effect on appetite via the brain, while elevated leptin levels retard appetite. Impairments in sensitivity to the effects of insulin occur in type II diabetes, and insensitivity to the appetite retarding effects of leptin often occur with obesity.

1.4   Measurement

1.4.1   Diet

In the context of this book there are two dietary measurement issues that need to be addressed. The first relates to observing what a person has been eating. The second relates to experimentally manipulating what a person eats. The first is sometimes met with slow headshaking, a sharp intake of breath and warnings about the unreliable nature of dietary self-report data. The reality is not so bleak. It is possible to obtain *fairly* accurate measurements of what a person eats and there are three general methods that have been used to do this.

The most commonly adopted approach involves self-report (Thompson & Byers, 1994). The first form of this appeared in the 1930s, to collect diet information outside of a consultation with a dietician. Participants were asked to keep a diet diary for between 1 and 7 days. The approach is largely unchanged. The diary may be paper or electronic and is used to record everything that is eaten, in terms of when, what it was, and how much of it was consumed (the latter can involve weighing or visually judging portion sizes). Weighing each thing eaten and judging portion size are difficult for participants to do and are prone to a number of inaccuracies (Schoeller, 1995; Smith, 1993). Diary approaches have good short-term reliability, although this varies depending on the specificity of the dietary variable (i.e., being higher for global measures like overall energy intake – correlations of around 0.5–0.8) and they provide good detail about foods eaten. This method's weaknesses are compliance, as it can be burdensome to complete and the high cost of coding (i.e., each diary has to be converted into amounts of food, and then the nutritional value calculated – assuming it is available for that food).

A widely used variant of the diary approach is to interview participants about their previous day's food intake (24-hour recall), typically using a structured approach with probes (e.g., did you have a snack in the morning?). This method is widely used in nutrition research but has an additional *disadvantage* over the diet diary. As the interviewer is a real live human being, the interviewee, who is describing their diet, is likely to err towards reporting foods and behaviours that they think will cast them in the most favourable light (Grimm, 2010). These types of demand effects are often unconscious and affect participant reports of any behaviour which may have negative personal connotations (e.g., unhealthy food, excessive drinking, certain sexual practices, etc.). While demand effects impact all forms of self-report, the presence of an interviewer probably accentuates this problem. This can lead to both under-reporting of nutritionally poor-quality foods (chips, chocolate, etc.) and their quantity consumed and over-reporting of healthy foods. The 24-hour recall method is also time and labour intensive.

For large-scale epidemiological studies, where diet diaries and interviewer-based recall are not practical, the food-frequency questionnaire was developed (Wiehl & Reed, 1960). This is essentially a list of foods, typically grouped by type (e.g., vegetables, fruits, breads) and the respondent indicates how often they consume each food by selecting a frequency of consumption category (e.g., daily, weekly, etc.). This method is usually employed on current diet but has also been applied to a person's historical diet (e.g., as a teenager). It has also been widely adopted outside of nutritional epidemiology, and there are now a number of different standardised food frequency questionnaires, which are often tailored to particular countries (e.g., Australian Eating Survey) or to a particular type of diet (e.g., Western-style diet). This approach often does not collect information about the quantity of food consumed, but there are variants that do.

Dietary data collected by food frequency questionnaires positively correlate with intake data obtained using diet diaries and 24-hour recall (Willett et al., 1985). Participants may also be more accurate at recalling consumption frequencies than the specific details needed for a 24-hour recall (Smith, 1993). Food frequency questionnaires have the major advantage that they are quick, do not intrude on day-to-day life (like diaries), prompt for foods of interest, minimise socially desirable answering (i.e., no interviewer present) and provide a broader timeframe than is available from a detailed study of just a few days.

One of the reasons people are concerned about the validity of all forms of self-report diet data is because of a robust finding indicating under-reporting of food intake (e.g., Fries, Green, & Bowen, 1995; Schoeller, 1995). This has been revealed by the doubly labelled water technique, which allows for an accurate assessment of energy expenditure in people as they go about their normal lives (it requires ingestion of isotopes of hydrogen and oxygen, and measurement of their excretion, so it remains a specialised test). A typical finding is that energy expenditure measured with this technique is higher than energy intake from self-report measures (Livingstone & Black, 2003; Schoeller, 1995). The implication of this discrepancy, often in the order of 20%, is that participants routinely under-report what they eat. A number of studies have examined for systematic variation in under-reporting. The results are not that surprising. Individuals who may feel embarrassed about what or how much they eat tend to under-report the most (e.g., dieters and overweight/obese participants; Tooze et al., 2004). There may also be more systematic reasons, such as memory errors. One example is snacking. Snacking is often not anchored to daily time routines like meals, making recall more problematic, and contributing to under-reporting.

One way to deal with the problem of under-reporting is to mathematically estimate energy requirements based on a person's weight, age, gender, etc. and then exclude their diet data if there is more than a certain level of discrepancy between their reported and expected values. This method is probably necessary if one is interested in individual-level nutrients, especially if comparisons depend on absolute levels of intake or measures relative to overall energy intake. Another approach is to focus on the general dietary pattern, rather than on absolute intake values (Newby & Tucker, 2004; Newby et al., 2006). A lot of studies have started to adopt this approach, either using statistical techniques to identify stable groups of participants with similar dietary patterns a posteriori (e.g., Dekker et al., 2013) or identifying groups based on a priori criteria – typically if it is a healthy diet of one kind or another (e.g., Kant, 1996). The pattern approach has a lot of ecological validity, as people generally eat *whole* diets that share many similarities to others in their culture, country, age and socio-economic group.

A further issue concerns the long-term stability of a person's diet and how it changes across the lifespan. When reliability is measured for a dietary reporting technique, the time span is usually weeks or months, and while there might be some changes over this period (e.g., dieting, illness, travel), one would expect – and typically find – stability. However, many studies are interested in much longer time periods, years or decades. There is a growing amount of data on this. With adult diets over a 10-year period, around 30–40% of people stick with a particular dietary pattern (e.g., Dekker et al., 2013; Pachucki, 2012). Logically, this means that some 60–70% change their dietary pattern, which for epidemiological work is troubling if you want to use diet data at one point in time to predict something at a later point in time (troubling if you *assume* continuity of diet, that is). Across the lifespan, diet changes rapidly during child development, as an infant moves from milk to a growing range of foods and thence to an adult-like diet. There is, however, plenty of evidence that diet can be adequately measured in children (e.g., Lioret et al., 2015).

Two other diet measurement approaches are available, but these are usually used to validate self-reports. The first are observational methods, either covert or overt, where aspects of a person's food habits are observed or recorded. This can include what they buy in a supermarket, shopping receipts, their choices in a canteen, their choices in closed settings (e.g., 1 week in a live-in experiment) or an examination of their kitchen cupboards (e.g., Hise et al., 2002). The second is to use biological markers (biomarkers) of diet. There are several available. The easiest to administer is reflectance spectrophotometry, which involves a device that measurers light reflected by the skin (ideally palms of the hands or inside forearm). The greater the level of carotenoids in the skin, the yellower its colour, which is accurately detected by the spectrophotometer. Diets that increase fruit and vegetable content increase skin yellowness irrespective of skin pigmentation (e.g., Tan et al., 2015), and thus reflectance spectrophotometry provides a rapid means of validating dietary self-reports of fruit and vegetable intake. Other biomarkers involve sampling urine or blood, and less frequently saliva, hair or faeces. Urine can be used to establish dietary protein intake, and the amount of added sugar in a person's diet (Tasevska et al., 2005). It is necessary to determine urine osmolarity and hence dilution, so that samples can be standardised for comparison. Bloods can provide a number of measures of fat intake either in plasma or in erythrocyte membranes. These provide data on fatty acid exposure either immediately (plasma) or over the last week (erythrocyte membrane). Importantly, these fat measures reflect the ratio of different types of fat in a person's diet (Patel et al., 2010) and not the absolute amounts consumed. Vitamin and mineral levels can also be obtained from such samples, but these have been less often used for diet validation.

Measuring diet has its limitations, and so an obvious alternative is to shift from a correlational approach to an experimental one and manipulate diet directly. This is the main-stay of animal models and is one reason why they are of interest to human researchers. In humans, compliance (i.e., are they eating what they are supposed to be?) is the main methodological problem of diet intervention studies. One approach is to feed participants for a set period of time wholly within the laboratory, but this is expensive and typically can only be done with small numbers of participants, as it is time consuming and disruptive for those taking part. A compromise is to have participants eat part of their intervention diet under controlled circumstances, thus ensuring that the key part of the manipulation occurs. Nonetheless, it is still necessary to know what else they ate outside of the lab. For studies that leave it up to the participant to enact changes in 'real life' (e.g., eat more fruit and vegetables), how does one ensure compliance? There are no magic solutions, and the usual approach is to adopt multiple measures. These might include using their smart phone to take photos of meals/snacks, bringing back shopping dockets under the guise of reimbursing them for food, using diet diaries and interviews and spot-contacting participants by text/phone.

Dietary interventions outside the controlled setting of a laboratory often have a bad reputation. This is because they are conflated with self-performed unsupervised *diet* interventions, where the aim is to reduce energy intake and lose weight. Such energy-restricting diets are hard to comply with as it is difficult to forego highly palatable foods, endure cravings and feel hungry. While most participants start well, as weeks pass, compliance becomes a major issue. In contrast, when participants are motivated to make dietary change (e.g., in studies on diet and mental health/cognition), when this occurs as part of a study, when the changes are not excessively restrictive and are for defined periods of time (e.g., a couple of days or weeks), compliance may be no different than for other 'lifestyle' interventions (e.g., therapy, exercise, meditation).

1.4.2 Brain and Mind

As the primary focus of this book is on human data, most of the material outlined in this section relates to people. (For animal studies, relevant methodological issues are dealt with as they arise in subsequent chapters.) The main human approaches involve anecdotal reports, single case designs (one person contrasted to a control group), correlational studies and experimental designs. For anecdotal reports we have included these in a few cases, for two reasons. First, some situations are so extreme that the only available data is anecdotal (e.g., famine). Second, anecdotal information has value for generating hypotheses for more formal study. For single case and correlational designs, it is not possible to establish causality and for this we need experimental studies. One important issue to be aware of with experimental methods here is the shading into the approaches used in psychopharmacology. Some psychopharmacological approaches do not always readily translate into our field, especially utilisation of placebos and blinding, which can be difficult to enact in some circumstances (Lieberman, 2007).

For dependent variables, several types reoccur. Many studies have included systematic behavioural observations, with the Ancel Keys Minnesota Starvation Study being the stand-out example (Keys, 1946). There are many methods that use participant self-report. These may include use of questionnaires (some of which are standardised and highly reliable, such as those of personality dimensions like the 'big 5') and structured interviews. In many cases the dependent variable is of a special sort – neuropsychological tests. These first emerged in the early twentieth century, as a means to reliably and validly measure aspects of general cognitive function. The initial applications were in education, with pioneering work by Sir Cyril Burt in the UK using intelligence tests to identify children with special needs, and in the military in the United States by Lewis Terman, to find recruits suitable for officer training programs. From these beginnings progressively more and more tests of general and specific cognitive function have been developed. Modern test compendium's like Lezak et al. (2012) now feature more than 800 different tests.

The majority of these tests are designed to detect impairments in people with some form of brain injury, by providing a score relative to a healthy and often age, gender and educationally matched normative sample. These tests, especially those that are commercially available, have the benefit of being well designed, reliable (i.e., good test-retest reliability over 1 month, good internal reliability) and valid. Validity may include demonstrable linkages between impaired performance and damage to a particular area of the brain purported to underpin the measured function (e.g., memory-hippocampus; neuroimaging is also important here; Sperling et al., 2003), to functional correlates (e.g., spouse notes person has many memory lapses in day-to-day life – such data is rarely present for many tests) and to other tests that claim to measure similar abilities (this being a common form of validation).

There are several weaknesses of neuropsychological tests as applied to their use in studies examining impacts or correlates of diet and cognitive function (beyond issues of sensitivity *in healthy samples* – more later). The first is that there are so many tests, with many having been used once or twice in the nutrition-behaviour literature (de Jager et al., 2014). Consequently, it can be difficult to know which to select. Some important considerations are: (1) whether the test is in the public domain or whether it has to be purchased; (2) whether it has been employed before in a similar study to good effect; (3) whether it is being used in large-scale scientific enterprises (e.g., UK Biobank); (4) whether it is recommended by experts in the field (e.g., de Jager et al., 2014; Lieberman, 2007); and (5) if it forms part of a broader battery of established tests (e.g., CANTAB). A further issue is whether the test is to be used once or multiple times, as people often improve with practice (Collie et al., 2003). In this respect, some tests have multiple alternate forms; others do not.

Arguably the most critical issue concerns sensitivity to detect a real change in cognitive function. This is important because as described earlier, neuropsychological tests are not generally designed for measuring what *may* be rather subtle changes induced by some nutritional variable. Thus the issue of test sensitivity looms large. As a rule of thumb if the test is to be used in normal participants the mean score needs to be around two-thirds of the maximum score, so as to provide sufficient room for improvement or worsening. This can be gauged by piloting to assess the difficulty of the task in the target population. A control group guards against the effects of practice.

Neuropsychological tests are often organised into particular cognitive domains such as memory, attention, perception, language, motor performance, construction, reasoning, executive function and global cognition – with subdomains for each (e.g., see Lezak et al., 2012). There are many different classifications into domains, and how valid they are is open to question. This is important because when studies are pooled for meta-analyses or for systematic review, such domain groupings are almost universal, and the way that results are grouped can affect whether a significant effect is or is not observed. Part of the problem here is that neuropsychological tests inevitably draw on multiple cognitive abilities even if their *name* suggests they measure just one thing. For example, almost all tests require the participant to attend, and most will utilise some aspect of executive function, namely the ability to coordinate mental activity. Relatedly, because tests often draw on multiple mental abilities, they are not generally sensitive to function in one region of the brain, although this does vary between tests (e.g., certain tests of learning and memory, do seem particularly hippocampal dependent).

Over the last 50 years there has been a major change in the technology available to researchers wanting to link cognitive functions such as those measured by neuropsychological tests, to brain function. At the outset, it is important to note that these technologies generally only have meaning when *they are linked* to cognitive measures or reports. Finding that a dietary variable alters some aspect of brain function in the absence of any cognitive or behavioural correlate is often not very useful (see Coltheart, 2013, for related arguments). That said, these technologies have been beneficial for identifying the neural correlates of cognition and the timing of mental events. Emerging approaches such as multivariate pattern analysis offer a means of testing neural representations of mental content and go beyond these other outcomes.

In terms of technologies, the one most frequently found in this book is functional magnetic resonance imaging (fMRI), where the participant undertakes a cognitive task in the scanner, with contrasts made against a suitable control task. The aim is to identify areas of the brain that are experiencing altered blood flow and which are correlated just to task performance. fMRI has excellent spatial resolution but is not so good for temporal resolution, which is where electro-encephalography (EEG) and magnetic encephalography (MEG) have their advantage. These techniques measure electrical currents and magnetic fields on the brain's surface, respectively, but are poor at localising effects in space, but good at determining the temporal ordering of mental processes. Another approach is fDG PET, but this is less often used in healthy populations as it requires exposure to radioisotopes. Newer techniques using infrared and ultrasound are not yet established in our literature.

1.5   What to Include and What Not to Include

In reading thousands of papers on diet, brain and behaviour, it becomes apparent that the literature can be crudely split into studies dealing with single dietary agents (e.g., glucose, a vitamin, a particular food (say grapes)) versus those dealing with dietary patterns (e.g., a Mediterranean diet, a Western-style diet). This divide appears in both correlational studies and in experimental designs (e.g., manipulating exposure to a particular dietary agent vs a dietary pattern). In this book we have given *somewhat* greater emphasis to dietary pattern data than to single dietary agents. There are several reasons for this. As others have noted before, studies of single foods/ nutrients are problematic because the normal human diet contains hundreds of chemicals, resulting in multiple complex interactions amongst these constituents (Newby & Tucker, 2004; Newby et al., 2006). Thus, a finding of an effect related to or caused by one dietary agent, when so many other correlated and interacting agents are present, can be hard to interpret (although there are some very important exceptions, especially relating to vitamins and micronutrients).

As we described earlier in this chapter, the accuracy with which we can measure a person's diet is good, but it is also limited. The question we pose is this: Which is likely to be more accurate (i.e., closer to what is objectively consumed): to characterise adherence to a particular dietary pattern or to determine intake of a particular dietary agent? We suggest *in general* dietary patterns can be assessed more accurately because: (1) they are less reliant on quantification of the amount of each food that a person eats – something that is known to be difficult to measure accurately (Schoeller, 1995; Smith, 1993), and (2) pattern data is more likely to utilise all of a person's nutritional data points, thereby increasing the internal reliability of the measure. The 'in general' was italicised as there are some important caveats surrounding the claimed superiority of dietary pattern data over single dietary agent data.

The first concerns single dietary agent studies that include biomarkers relevant to that agent. These biomarkers are likely to be either an indirect correlate of the target dietary agent (e.g., a metabolite) or a direct measure of it (e.g., vitamin, mineral). Assuming that the biomarker is lawfully related to ingestion of the particular dietary agent, and that non-dietary influences are minimal/understood (e.g., it is possible to have a micronutrient deficiency even with adequate intake because the body may miss an enzyme needed to utilise it), then these types of single dietary agent studies are methodologically robust.

If there is no biomarker data, then additional considerations come into play (noting that these apply generally). The first concerns the quality of the dietary measures, and the extent to which they provide an accurate guide to consumption of the target agent (i.e., do they conform with the sort of measurement approaches outlined earlier in this chapter and an *awareness* of their limitations?). The second issue concerns adequate sample size, a particular problem in the field of psychology and neuroscience generally, and hence here too (Szucs & Ioannidis, 2017). While large sample sizes cannot compensate for poor methodology, good methodology cannot compensate for unduly small sample size, especially when dealing with the type of effect sizes that are typical in our field (i.e., small to moderate effects, with Cohen's d's between 0.2–0.5). Third, study funding source needs to be actively considered. The medical literature has amply illustrated the consistently positive relationship between funding source, and findings favourable to that funding source (e.g., Lundh et al., 2018). Fourth, there should be reasonable grounds to expect an effect, or in Hill's (1965) terminology there should be coherence. In particular, is the finding convergent with: (1) data from animal studies, (2) how the agent could affect the brain, and (3) its other known effects in humans.

If the study of a particular dietary agent has no biomarker data and is solely reliant on a dietary report, then good diet collection methodology, a suitably large sample size, the absence of a biasing funding source and a suitable a priori expectation for obtaining the effect are factors favourable to its validity, and hence for its inclusion in this book. If it is an experimental design using a particular dietary agent, then largely the same considerations apply, plus two additional ones. First, with regards to methodology, a key issue becomes compliance (did the participant consume the dietary agent?), and again whether any biomarker data was available to confirm this. Second, whether adequate blinding (if needed) and control conditions (e.g., placebo) were instigated to ensure that attribution of an effect to the dietary agent is the correct conclusion (Lieberman, 2007).

With dietary pattern data, we suggest that because it is possible to measure this more accurately, there is likely to be less error variance with this measure. This makes studies using dietary pattern data *somewhat* less susceptible to the biases identified before. However, it will not rescue a poorly designed, low-powered study with little a priori scientific expectation of finding a particular effect (and noting the subjectivities that are involved in data-driven dietary pattern analyses, see Newby & Tucker, 2004). Dietary pattern data is not an invitation to abandon scientific standards, it just offers a somewhat more accurate indication of what a person is consuming, as well as better reflecting what people actually do – eat combinations of foods with all their complex interactions (Kant, 1996; Newby & Tucker, 2004; Newby et al., 2006). It is for this reason that we treat dietary pattern data somewhat more favourably.

CHAPTER 2

Pregnancy, Infancy and Development

2.1 Introduction

Nutrition during early life is important because it affects neurodevelopment not just acutely, but with potentially long-term consequences into childhood and adulthood. The majority of brain development occurs during the perinatal period (see Figure 2.1). The brain begins to form approximately 2 weeks from fertilisation, and reaches 80% of its adult size by 2 years of age (Lagercrantz, 2016). The growth rate of the neonatal brain is among the highest during the lifespan, with a rapid rate of neuronal and glial growth, and establishment of complex structural connections (Lagercrantz, 2016). The brain has high energy demands during this period, consuming 60% of the body's oxygen (Kuzawa, 1998).

The perinatal period begins from fertilisation, and lasts through gestation and lactation until weaning. In utero during gestation, the foetus receives vital nutrients through the placenta, which regulates their exchange and that of oxygen, as well as serving as a barrier to control which maternal endocrine and immune factors reach the foetus. After birth during lactation, the infant receives breast milk from the mother or supplementation with formula as a primary form of nutrition. During weaning, the infant transitions to solid food, and gradually adopts a more adult-like dietary pattern through childhood. Diet, supplying both energy and nutrients, is therefore an important environmental factor on brain and cognitive development. In this chapter we discuss the effects of breastfeeding, weaning, maternal starvation, starvation during infancy and early childhood, its remediation, maternal and child overnutrition, and specific nutrient and micronutrient deficiencies and their supplementation on brain and cognitive development.

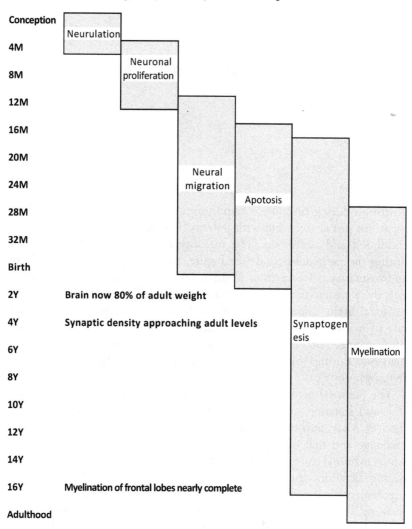

Figure 2.1   Development of the human brain

2.2   Breastfeeding

2.2.1   *The Neurobiology of Breastfeeding*

Breastfeeding is argued to have many benefits, including improved neuro-development. There are several mechanisms through which breastfeeding could improve brain function of the child. It provides the infant with a nutritionally complete diet, which also includes proteins that assist the development of immunity to respiratory infections. There are also several constituents of breast milk that are thought to confer benefit, such as essential long-chain polyunsaturated fatty acids (lcPUFAs). In this regard, docosahexaenoic acid (DHA) and arachidonic acid (AA) have been of particular interest as they are essential for the development of the central nervous system and are found in greater concentrations in human breast milk than in infant formula (Koletzko et al., 2001). Breastfed infants have higher concentrations of these fatty acids that are positively associated with brain development (Farquharson et al., 1992; Isaacs et al., 2010).

Rather than nutritional factors, however, the intimacy of breastfeeding may facilitate the development of the infant–mother bond, and provide a soothing environment in which the infant can feed. Breastfeeding promotes release of oxytocin for the mother, can benefit mother's mood and helps mothers bond with their child, therefore indirectly affect the child's neurodevelopment through environmental enrichment.

Breastfeeding is now strongly promoted both by the American Pediatrics Association and by the World Health Organization. Although some of this drive to get women breastfeeding comes from the clear benefit in not exposing infants to formula mixed with pathogen-laden water, a significant component of the argument in favour of breastfeeding, especially in the developed world, comes from the putative long-term benefits that it confers. These benefits appear to be extensive, spanning lower body mass index in adulthood, reduced rates of asthma and eczema, and improved neurodevelopment, including academic performance, intelligence quotient (IQ), mental health outcomes and neuroanatomical differences. The evidence for impact on neurodevelopmental outcomes is discussed next.

2.2.2   *Breastfeeding and Cognition*

2.2.2.1   *Observational Studies of the Relationship between Breastfeeding and Cognition*

Numerous studies report that breastfeeding is associated with improved cognitive outcomes in childhood. The majority of studies undertaken on this subject are observational.

A meta-analysis of articles published between 2007 and 2013 identified 17 studies investigating the relationship between breastfeeding and performance on intelligence tests. All studies showed a beneficial effect of breastfeeding on intelligence tests, with breastfed children showing a mean of 3.44 points higher on intelligence tests (95% confidence interval: 2.30; 4.58). The authors note, however, that studies that controlled for maternal IQ showed a smaller effect of 2.62 points.

Since that meta-analysis, a few additional studies have been conducted. We have reported here only those that control for relevant confounding factors such as parental education or maternal intelligence quotient in their analysis. Julvez et al. (2014) examined exclusive breastfeeding compared to no breastfeeding, for differing durations (<4 months, 4–6 months and >6 months). After controlling for maternal IQ, as well as for other socio-demographic factors, strong positive associations were observed with neuropsychological development in children at 4 years of age, particularly amongst the group who was breastfed for >6 months. Belfort et al. (2016) followed 1,037 participants from birth to 7–10 years of age. Executive functions and social-emotional functions were assessed using self-report measures completed by parents and teachers. Neither were found to differ according to either breastfeeding duration or exclusive breastfeeding duration. Breastfeeding duration in 926 Korean children predicted cognitive development, as well as internalising (e.g., worry) and externalising (e.g., aggression) problems at 5-years of age (Kang, 2017). A further report suggests the effects of breastfeeding persist into old age, with a study of 931 men born in 1934–1944 in Finland showing that breastfed men had higher cognitive ability. Longer duration of breast-feeding predicted cognitive ability scores, when tested at both 20.2 years and 67.9 years (on average) of age.

Overall, most of these observational studies show that breastfeeding is associated with higher scores on cognitive tests. However, these findings do not demonstrate causality as they are confounded by sociodemographic factors that are simultaneously related to infant feeding practices, as well as long-term child outcomes. Studies show that compared with bottle-fed infants, infants that are breast fed tend to (1) be born into families with higher socioeconomic status; (2) have higher parental educational attainment; (3) have easier access to healthcare services; (4) live in areas with less exposure to environmental toxins; (5) have mothers that are less likely to have smoked during pregnancy; and (6) have carers with parenting attitudes or styles more favourable to successful development (Rothstein, 2013; Singh, Kogan, & Dee, 2007; van Rossem et al., 2009). Duration of breastfeeding is also associated with these factors, as well as a mother's psychological state 4 years postnatally (Julvez et al., 2014). While observational studies typically attempt to statistically control for some of these factors, it is difficult to control for all heterogeneity, particularly unobserved heterogeneity. As such, comparison of breast- and formula-fed infants is likely to observe outcomes more favourable to those who have been breastfed.

2.2.2.2 *Experimental Studies Investigating the Effect of Breastfeeding on Cognition*

Though it is difficult ethically to conduct an experimental design assigning mothers to breastfeed or formula, a few studies have employed naturalistic experiments or experimental manipulations. Four studies have used sibling comparisons to separate the impact on cognition and behaviour of factors that predict a mother's selection to breastfeed from the actual consequences of breastfeeding. By comparing outcomes of siblings who were fed differently in infancy, it is possible to estimate what the bottle-fed sibling's outcomes might have been.

Der, Batty, and Deary (2006) compared the academic achievement of differently fed siblings and found no impact of breastfeeding status (yes vs no) or duration of breastfeeding. Evenhouse and Reilly (2005) examined the relationship between breastfeeding and 15 different outcomes related to physical health, emotional health and cognitive abilities. Using the typical between-family model, all 15 correlations were significant. However, when using a within-family model to determine if the differences in outcomes between siblings were correlated with different breastfeeding histories, all but one correlation became non-significant. The one remaining significant correlation was with the Peabody Picture Vocabulary Test, a measure of verbal intelligence. However, it is notable that the children did not differ on other cognitive measures – grade point average across maths, science, social studies, language and arts; history of repeating a grade; or whether the child reported being "highly likely" to go to college. In terms of mental health, there was no significant relationship between depression symptoms, mother or child report of closeness, how strongly the child agreed that the mother is usually warm and loving, or the range of activities in which child and mother participate each month.

Using a similar design, Colen and Ramey (2014) examined 11 different outcomes in children who were aged 4–14 years old, including body mass index, obesity, asthma, hyperactivity, parental attachment, behavioural compliance, reading comprehension, vocabulary, math ability, working memory and academic skills. When the full sample was analysed, findings suggested that children who were breastfed during their first year of life had better outcomes on all variables except asthma. However, when limiting comparisons to within, rather than across families, none of the effects remained significant. Again, with a similar design, Rothstein (2013) showed that breastfeeding for 6 months or more was associated with better cognitive outcomes in children aged 5–6 years. However, when comparing within families, there was no statistically significant effect. Thus, overall, the sibling studies show that the observational findings are overestimating breastfeeding benefits, and, with the exception of one significant relationship between verbal intelligence and breastfeeding, a large number of correlations between physical, emotional and cognitive outcomes appeared to be due to unobserved variation between families that leads to bias in selection to breastfeeding, rather than a causal outcome of breastfeeding itself.

While sibling comparisons are a powerful method for reducing between-family selection bias, they do not control for difference that might occur within families. That is, there are some factors that contribute to why one sibling might be breast fed, whereas another is bottle fed. Two studies have been conducted that have performed experimental manipulations that have increased the amount of breast milk in the infant diet. The first, conducted by Isaacs et al. (2010), included mothers who elected to breastfeed, but for varying reasons were unsuccessful in doing so and therefore their infants were bottle fed. Study infants were randomised to receive either preterm formula (PTF; n = 28), standard infant formula (SIF; n = 13) or banked breast milk (BBM; n = 9). Percent exclusive breast milk (%EBM) in the infant diet was found to be positively correlated with verbal IQ in adolescence (average age 15 years, 9 months). In turn, verbal IQ was associated with white matter volume, whereas no association was seen with grey matter volume. Notably, this study was performed in mothers who had chosen to breastfeed and there was no relationship between either social class or maternal education and %EBM. Furthermore, maternal IQ was no different between those mothers who tried to provide breast milk but failed and those who did not try to provide breast milk. This does seem to suggest that there is a difference in cognitive function in those infants who actually received the breast milk, rather than pre-existing differences in those who chose to breastfeed.

There is only one randomised controlled trial (RCT) in this area. Kramer et al. (2008) compared two groups: one that received breastfeeding promotion and education, the other receiving no education. The educational program increased the rates of exclusive breastfeeding at 3 months in the experimental group (43.4%) compared to the control group (6.4%). When children were tested at age 6.5 years, a higher overall intelligence quotient (IQ) of about 5.9 IQ points was observed for the Education group compared to the Control group. Note, however, that this is only 0.6 of a standard deviation of the population IQ distribution. Subsample analyses showed that the advantage of breastfeeding was around three IQ points for children born at term and about five IQ points for children born pre-term. While these are moderate effects in population terms, at the individual level a difference of three IQ points is unlikely to make a large difference over and above other environmental factors. Furthermore, the paediatricians who administered the neuropsychological tasks were not blinded to the condition of the subjects, and some of the scales' scoring criteria can be subjective. In particular, the verbal subscales are more subjective in scoring than non-verbal, and there was a greater effect found for the verbal than non-verbal subscales. To compensate for the non-blinding of the paediatricians, an audit was undertaken whereby one in five of the participants underwent repeat testing by a clinician who was blind. While a significant effect was still obtained in this smaller sample, it was of a smaller magnitude, of about three IQ points. Furthermore, teacher ratings of academic achievement were obtained for 75% of the children, and showed that across four domains (reading, writing, mathematics, other), although ratings were slightly higher in the experimental group, the 95% confidence intervals included 0, indicating non-significance. It should be noted, however, that the nature of the experimental design would likely underestimate the causal effect of breastfeeding due to the substantial overlap in rates of breastfeeding in the educated versus control groups (although maternal IQ might be predictive of a greater response to the educational manipulation). Therefore, the study does provide some evidence of a causal relationship between breastfeeding and IQ; however, the magnitude of the true effect remains unknown.

What does seem to be clear from this body of research is that the risks associated with a failure to breastfeed appear to be overestimated in the observational literature. This is an important point because there is often significant pressure for mothers to breastfeed, and it can also be a stigmatising decision to switch to formula feeding if breastfeeding is unsuccessful. This can alienate mothers and can result in stress and anxiety, which in turn have an effect on developmental outcomes of the child. Based on the available evidence, mothers should be encouraged to breastfeed, and supported in their ability to do so. However, they should also be reassured that should they be unable to do so, that the adverse consequences are likely to be minimal in terms of cognitive development.

2.2.2.3   Breastfeeding and Cognition in Preterm Infants
As with the literature examining breastfeeding and cognition in term infants, most of the studies on preterm infants have been observational. Of those that are of adequate methodological quality and control for confounding factors such as maternal IQ, none found any difference between breastfeeding and formula feeding (Elgen, Sommerfelt, & Ellertsen, 2003; Pinelli, Saigal, & Atkinson, 2003). Furthermore, a re-analysis of data from a randomised controlled trial comparing breastfeeding with a formula enriched with arachidonic acid and docosahexaenoic acid showed no differences in cognitive development between the groups. A Cochrane review of formula feeding compared to breast milk feeding in preterm infants identified four trials that have assessed neurodevelopmental outcomes in children aged at least 12 months, measured using validated assessment tools, and overall found no evidence for effects on neurodevelopmental outcomes (Quigley, Embleton, & McGuire, 2018).

2.2.3   Breastfeeding and Mental Health Outcomes

Mental health outcomes in this section refer specifically to the child. While there is a substantial literature regarding the relationship between breastfeeding and mental health of the mother, this is not related to nutritional intake per se. Overall, while there are some studies that have observed that breastfeeding is associated with fewer psychosocial difficulties in childhood and adolescence (Heikkila et al., 2011; Julvez et al., 2007; Liu, Leung, & Yang, 2014; Oddy et al., 2010), most others have observed that these associations are no longer significant after adjusting for the many potential confounding factors that were identified earlier in this chapter (e.g., Lind et al., 2014; Waylen et al., 2009). Importantly, in the one RCT of a breastfeeding promotion intervention (as described in Section 2.2.2.2), no difference between experimental groups was found for psychosocial measures.

2.2.4   Breastfeeding and Brain Development

The cognitive findings described so far are complemented by neuroimaging and psychophysiological findings, although these too are affected by exactly the same confounds that dog interpretation of the cognitive data. Analysis of evoked potentials in 1-year-olds (as a measure of neural maturation) showed greater wave latencies in the visual and auditory pathways of formula-fed infants, suggesting delayed myelination of these pathways compared to breastfed infants (Khedr et al., 2004). In 133 healthy children aged 10 months through to 4 years, those who were exclusively breastfed (n = 85) exhibited increased white matter volume in late maturing white matter regions, compared to the formula-fed (n = 38) and mixed breast- and formula-fed (n = 51) groups (Deoni et al., 2013). Longer breastfeeding duration was also associated with a more intact white matter microstructure. Notably, there were no significant differences between breastfed, formula-fed and mixed feeding groups on potential confounding variables (age, gender, birth weight, gestation duration or maternal age, education or socioeconomic status). In 571 adolescents aged 12–18 years, breastfeeding was a significant predictor of cortical thickness in the parietal lobe, controlling for other relevant predictors such as parental education (Kafouri et al., 2013). In the randomised feeding trial described (Isaacs et al., 2010), brain imaging demonstrated that higher percentage expressed breast milk consumption was associated with greater total brain volume and white matter volume in adolescents (average age 15 years, 9 months). Furthermore, white matter volume was correlated with both verbal and full-scale intelligence quotients, suggesting that white matter development may underlie the effect of breastfeeding on cognition. This is turn may be linked back to differences between formula and breast milk in lcPUFAs, which are important to myelination.

2.3   Weaning and Consequences of Lack of Exposure to Solid Food

All mammals move from suckling to the separate processes of drinking fluids and eating solid foods (Bond et al., 2020). Humans are unique amongst mammals in that weaning occurs before the offspring is capable of independently obtaining their own food. In pre-industrial cultures, mothers start introducing solid foods at around 4–6 months, with breast milk consumption faded out over a 30-month period (Borowitz, 2021). While there is considerable cultural variation, this general pattern tends to hold true in developed countries too. There also appears to be a window, less than 12 months and greater than 3 months, in which the infant is particularly receptive to new flavours and textures. Missing this window by delaying the introduction of solid foods beyond 12 months is reportedly associated with a greater likelihood of feeding problems into childhood, and with less tolerance for textural variety – vegetables and fruit in particular (Borowitz, 2021).

Several authors have observed that once a baby has been tube fed – perhaps because they were preterm or failed to thrive – and when the tube feeding stops, a large proportion (over two-thirds) seem to have major problems transitioning to oral feeding with either milk (from breast or bottle) or to solid food (Avitzur & Courtney-Martin, 2016; Miller, 2009; Wilken et al., 2018). The suggestion is that infants in general have to: (1) learn that the sensations of food in the mouth and swallowing are associated with the cessation of hunger and the rewarding development of satiety; (2) become familiar with the unusual sensations of fluids and foods in the mouth and oesophagus; and (3) learn how to swallow, and practice this repeatedly so that appropriate aerodigestive coordination develops (Miller, 2009). It seems that if this process is delayed, as occurs with tube-fed babies, the more difficult it becomes to get the infant to feed orally.

2.4   Malnutrition: Impacts on Foetal and Child Development

2.4.1   Introduction

In infants, malnutrition may result from either an energy-deficient (manifesting as Marasmus) or protein-deficient (manifesting as Kwashiorkor) diet – or more commonly both (protein-energy malnutrition, or PEM). The effects on development of all forms of malnutrition are profound. Its most evident physical manifestation is stunting, namely a reduced height for age, formally defined as a height for age more than 2 standard deviations below the norm. Stunting affects around *150 million children under the age of 5* (World Health Organization, 2020). Moreover, malnutrition is responsible for between 3 and 5 million deaths in children under 5 each year (i.e., conservatively 1 child dying every 10 s), with most stunting and associated mortality concentrated in sub-Saharan Africa and Asia (Black et al., 2008; Collinge et al., 2006). This section examines the impacts of malnutrition during pregnancy on the foetus in animal models and humans, the effects of stunting on child development, and its remediation. As many authors regard overnutrition and poor diet quality as also being aspects of malnutrition, we also examine the impact of these during pregnancy and on the developing child in this section.

2.4.2   *Foetal Development and Models of Dietary Impact*

Nutrition during the perinatal period is thought to impact brain structure and function throughout the lifespan, well beyond any periods of deficiency. There are two basic models proposed to account for why early nutrition may have such long-term consequences (see Georgieff, 2017, for review). The first is the critical period hypothesis. A critical period can be defined either as the point of maximal brain growth or the point(s) at which fundamental organisation of brain structure is taking place – this distinction can be important because in rats maximal brain growth occurs *postnatally* (Levitsky & Strupp, 1995). The critical period hypothesis proposes that at these point(s) the brain has high nutritional requirements (Rice & Barone, 2000). Deficiencies during a critical period result in structural brain changes that may not be reversible by remediation of the deficiency after the critical period has passed. This theory is supported by findings that early deficiencies in several nutrients (long-chain polyunsaturated fatty acids (lcPUFAs), iron, zinc, iodine) can result in long-term dysfunction into childhood and adulthood (Georgieff, Brunette, & Tran, 2015).

The second model is the altered-regulation hypothesis, which suggests that early nutrient deficiency results in epigenetic changes. That is nutrient status is an environmental factor that can alter gene expression with long-term consequences on the central nervous system (Moody, Chen, & Pan, 2017). These two models are not mutually exclusive and both are likely to represent pathways by which dietary deficiencies can cause long-term impacts on the brain.

2.4.3   *Maternal Starvation: Animal Data*

Animal models have been used extensively to examine the impacts of maternal malnutrition on foetal and infant development, but less frequently so into adulthood (Levitsky & Strupp, 1995). Findings can be organised into the general effects of malnutrition, where an inadequate diet is provided, and more specific studies that separately model protein- and energy-deficient diets. The most general effect of malnutrition during pregnancy on the foetus is reduced brain size. This is accompanied by increased cortical cell packing, a reduction in brain myelin, greater numbers of mitochondria in cortical cells, alterations in brain metabolism and in the production and turnover of neurotransmitters and their receptors, and extensive abnormalities in the hippocampus and cerebellum. Some of these effects seem reversible (Levitsky & Strupp, 1995), while others seem to persist into adulthood, although their functional consequences are not always apparent on behavioural testing at that point in time (e.g., could these abnormalities confer vulnerability in old age for neurodegenerative disease?).

For protein-deficient diets, a normal rat chow will deliver approximately 15–20% protein by weight, and restricted diets for pregnant dams may reduce this to as little as 6%. The consequences for foetal brain development are significant, and while a lot of parameters vary between studies (e.g., duration of maternal low-protein diet, protein concentration) the basic effects are well understood (Barra et al., 2018). Abnormalities to the hippocampus, cerebellum, cortex and basal ganglia are usually observed, along with alterations in neurotransmitter levels in particular structures, such as dopamine reduction in the pre-frontal cortex, and an increased propensity for oxidative stress in the hippocampus and cerebellum (Alamy & Bengelloun, 2012; Morgane, Mokler, & Galler, 2002). In the developing rat, these brain deficits manifest in abnormal behaviour (Barra et al., 2018). There are changes to exploratory, social and emotional activity; abnormal sleep-wake cycles; impairments to hippocampal-dependent learning and memory (HDLM); and inhibition. Just as gross structural deficits do not seem evident in adult rats following maternal protein deprivation, behavioural deficits do not seem to continue either (Alamy & Bengelloun, 2012). This may often reflect the impact of normal levels of nutrition postnatally, suggesting some degree of recovery.

Models of calorie restriction during pregnancy cut the pregnant dams energy intake anywhere from 25–75% of what it would normally be. The effects seem more specific, with notable impacts again on the hippocampus, a smaller corpus callosum (suggesting abnormal myelination) and increased hypothalamic–pituitary–adrenal axis activity, stress reactivity and elevated levels of corticosterone (Barra et al., 2018). Behaviourally, there are abnormalities on some tests of HDLM, as well as increased impulsivity, greater reward sensitivity and socialisation deficits. The neuroanatomical effects do not seem to persist into adulthood, and the evidence for behavioural persistence is mixed (Alamy & Bengelloun, 2012). Again, this may reflect study designs favouring normal postnatal diet, thereby allowing some recovery. In many situations where human maternal malnutrition occurs (i.e., in extreme poverty), adequate postnatal diet, and hence recovery, may not be possible.

Malnutrition during pregnancy has a further legacy for the offspring (Smith & Reyes, 2017). They are at greater risk for obesity and type II diabetes than those raised in a healthy foetal environment. They also prefer and more readily consume foods rich in fat and sugar, which is probably due to dopaminergic hypofunction in brain reward areas. That is these animals seek our more potent rewards to compensate for reduced dopamine release. One way of interpreting this pattern of biobehavioural changes is the thrifty phenotype model (Hales & Barker, 1992), in which malnutrition in the foetal environment shapes the organism, probably via epigenetic changes, towards a postnatal environment in which food is scarce. In this scarcity environment, storing excess fat, eating whenever food is available, and especially so if it is indicative of energy (i.e., sweet and fatty), and maintaining a higher resting blood glucose level are arguably adaptive. The problems emerge, however, if the foetal environment does not match the actual postnatal environment, in which case the thrifty phenotype lends itself to overeating and metabolic syndrome.

A further and related question is whether malnutrition produces any adaptive shift in behaviour paralleling the thrifty phenotype – namely foraging, exploring and risk-taking so as to maximise the chance of obtaining food – in contrast to a more risk-averse, less active and more anxious phenotype, which might be associated with a well-fed foetal and postnatal environment. Besson et al. (2016) undertook a meta-analysis of relevant rodent pregnancy malnutrition studies, but found no evidence favourable to this hypothesis. The only consistent finding was a tendency for *reduced* activity in the offspring of calorie-restricted dams.

Finally, animal studies have explored possible mechanisms by which maternal malnutrition can affect brain function. Proinflammatory factors have been shown to mediate the increased risk for models of neurodevelopmental disorders in the offspring of rat dams with 50% reduced caloric intake during pregnancy (Shen et al., 2008). In an animal model of foetal malnutrition – intrauterine growth restriction – epigenetic changes have been observed (i.e., consistent with the altered-regulation hypothesis), such as disrupted hippocampal histone methylation (Ke et al., 2014) and brain-derived neurotrophic factor (BDNF) DNA methylation (Ke et al., 2010). Maternal malnutrition may also affect the developing foetal brain through lack of specific nutrients that are critical for growth and development, including glucose, fatty acids, iron, zinc, folate, choline and several other vitamins and minerals, which are discussed later in the chapter.

2.4.4 Maternal Starvation: Human Data

Post mortem studies of severely malnourished babies, born to mothers who were malnourished during pregnancy, versus well-nourished controls show multiple brain impairments including fewer cortical neurons, shorter dendrites and abnormal dendritic spines (Benitez-Bribiesca, De la Rosa-Alvarez, & Mansilla-Olivares, 1999). Not surprisingly then, and given the animal data, one might expect significant sequelae to foetal malnutrition.

In epidemiological studies, which form all of the human data, maternal malnutrition can occur due to internal causes, such as disease (e.g., eating disorder), or from external causes, such as famine. We look at both here.

Several studies have examined internal causes, all based in developed countries. Infants born to mothers with anorexia nervosa or bulimia nervosa have reduced head circumference at birth and delayed expressive language skills when assessed at age 5. However, it is not possible to rule out confounding factors such as maternal stress during pregnancy as a cause for these developmental problems. A number of medical conditions can lead to intra-uterine growth restriction, such as hypertension in the mother, which serves to restrict blood flow to the placenta and thus to the foetus. Such restricted blood flow can result in a small for gestational age foetus, with increased risk of developmental delay, learning difficulties and lower IQ (Nyaradi et al., 2013). Maternal diabetes, with unstable blood sugar, and thus periods of hypoglycaemia (and hyperglycaemia), is linked to lower child IQ and poorer performance on several cognitive domains at age 7–11 years (Rizzo et al., 1997) – this correlated with the degree of metabolic abnormality in the mother.

Studies of underweight mothers (i.e., BMI <18) suggest that they have children who are more likely to have some form of cognitive impairment (Veena et al., 2016). Significant maternal weight loss can occur with hyperemesis gravidarum (*severe* nausea in pregnancy). Fejzo et al. (2009) selected mothers with this condition who had experienced significant weight loss during pregnancy (15% of their *pre-pregnancy* body weight). Most of these mothers, and the control mothers, were surveyed around 1–2 years post-pregnancy. Even though there was no difference in the weight of the newborn, there was a trend ($p = 0.07$) for increased rates of behavioural disorders in the extreme weight loss group (9.3% of initial body weight (IBW)), relative to controls (5.5% IBW; Fejzo et al., 2009). This may be a conservative test as many children would not have yet reached an age where behavioural disorders would be most apparent.

There are two series of studies examining the effects of famine on neurodevelopmental outcomes. The Dutch Famine Study documented the effects of a severe famine which occurred during the 'hunger winter' of 1944–1945. The German army imposed an embargo on transport to several regions in the Netherlands, with the daily ration of mainly bread, potatoes and sugar beet yielding less than 4,200 kJ. The comprehensive health records kept over this time meant that the effects on birth cohorts exposed to the famine at specific times during gestation could be compared to those who were not exposed. The offspring of mothers who had reduced caloric intake during the third trimester of gestation had lower birth weight, placental weight, length at birth, and head circumference. There was also a higher rate of congenital abnormalities of the central nervous system, including spina bifida, hydrocephalus and cerebral palsy, and from birth to age 17 there was a higher rate of deaths from congenital neural defects (Stein & Susser, 1975). The cohort conceived during the famine had a two-fold increased rate of schizophrenia at age 18 (Susser et al., 1996). There are, however, some confounding factors such as the effects of consuming toxic food, notably tulip bulbs; exposure to an exceptionally cold winter; and significant maternal stress. However, the findings of a second series of studies based on the Chinese famine of 1959–1961 are consistent with the Dutch famine findings, suggesting that toxic foods and intense cold are unlikely causes. Rates of adult schizophrenia were two-fold higher in individuals who were conceived or in early gestation during the Chinese famine compared to those conceived before or after the famine years (St Clair et al., 2005; Xu et al., 2009).

2.4.5 Stunting

As described at the start of this section, stunting refers to abnormally reduced height for age, which affects around 150 million children aged under 5 worldwide (WHO, 2021). A major driver of stunting is poor nutrition; however, many other factors contribute both to stunting per se (e.g., chronic illness) and co-occur with it (e.g., poverty; Grantham-McGregor et al., 2007). A major motivation for understanding the causes and correlates of stunting, and hence to design effective means of remediation, is its association with negative developmental outcomes. Stunted children are apathetic, they are emotionally detached from their surroundings, they have various cognitive deficits, and as they pass through schooling into adulthood they have much poorer educational outcomes, and ultimately reduced economic prospects relative to their non-stunted peers (Perkins et al., 2017). Moreover, they are likely to have children who are at increased risk of stunting, thereby perpetuating the cycle of poverty.

Remediating the developmental consequences of stunting may not be as simple as providing additional food, because stunting itself has so many adverse correlates (Sarkar, Patro & Patro, 2019). Parents of stunted children may be malnourished, they may abuse licit or illicit drugs, and they may have chronic infectious diseases (HIV, tuberculosis). During pregnancy any or all of these factors can affect foetal development, and postnatally it will affect the parent's capacity to effectively nurture their child. The child themself may have had a difficult birth exposing them to a period of anoxia, they may have suffered frequent gastrointestinal infections, lived in unhygienic conditions, have a neurodevelopmental disorder, experienced abuse, trauma, parental separation and violence. Any or all of these correlates of stunting would have significant negative developmental consequences.

Not surprisingly then, and as many authors have pointed out, there is a complex relationship between malnutrition and its potential remedy in appropriate nutrition, stunting, behaviour and development (Grantham-McGregor et al., 2007; Laus et al., 2011; Sarkar et al., 2019). Three examples should suffice to illustrate this complexity. First, Laus et al. (2011) reported that Mexican children fed dietary supplements became more physically active and thus interacted more with family members. This in turn prompted greater adult attention directed back towards the child. Thus, here, the actual developmental/cognitive benefits of the dietary supplementation may be indirect, and perhaps result from the additional social interaction and stimulation provided by greater activity levels. Second, the apathy and withdrawal in stunted children may lead parents to treat them as they would younger children, robbing them of age-appropriate stimulation (Perkins et al., 2017). Again, it may be the reduced psychosocial stimulation that impairs development, with this being an indirect consequence of malnutrition. Third, parents may opt to carry stunted children as they may be slow walkers or be reluctant to move. This in turn reduces the child's opportunity for psychomotor development and independent exploration – again an indirect consequence of malnutrition (Perkins et al., 2017). Stunting then exerts complex effects on the child's interaction with people and the environment. This makes it difficult to ascertain whether the primary cause of stunting (i.e., malnutrition) is *sufficient* to impair development by its effects on the brain, or whether its effects are primarily interactive as the above examples would seem to suggest.

Perkins et al. (2017) attempted to address this question, by systematically examining the evidence for whether stunting per se causes developmental problems. Longitudinal studies do suggest that stunting precedes developmental problems, but the issue here is whether there is adequate control for all of the correlates of stunting identified above, that are also known to impair development. Three types of experimental interventions have also been studied: (1) families are provided money to buy additional food, (2) the child is given some form/duration of nutritional supplementation and (3) dietary supplementation is provided along with environmental enrichment.

The outcomes for all three study types have been mixed, suggesting – not surprisingly – no simple linkage between stunting (i.e., malnutrition) and developmental problems. Perkins et al. (2017) draws three conclusions from this literature: (1) stunting and its correlates all contribute to developmental problems; (2) the most successful interventions, especially involving nutrition, *probably* need to be early, that is in the first 2 years of life; and (3) if there are better circumstances in the child's mid and later years, catch-up growth and development can occur.

2.4.6 Remediation

An adequate supply of protein and energy is critical to support normal growth and development of the foetus and young infant. In this section, we examine the putative cognitive/developmental benefits from nutritional remediation, looking first at the immediate and then at longer-term outcomes from studies in developing countries, and then at supplementation for low-birth-weight (LBW) babies in studies from developed countries.

There has been one meta-analysis examining the benefits of any type of nutritional intervention on the cognitive development of malnourished infants (and pregnant mothers) or those at risk of malnourishment, in developing countries (Larson & Yousafzai, 2015). The two primary analyses examined the impact of prenatal (i.e., administered to the mother during pregnancy) and postnatal interventions, pooling across different forms of supplementation (zinc, iron/folic acid, vitamin A, multiple micronutrients, and macronutrient combinations) and cognitive/developmental measures. There were 10 prenatal interventions, with assessment of their impact on development generally being made in the first 2 years of the child's life. These exerted no significant effect ($d = 0.042$). The postnatal intervention analysis, composed of 23 studies, adopted the same pooling approach, with interventions ranging from 2–24 months in length, and all children tested and supplemented within the first 5 years of life. There was a small significant effect of supplementation ($d = 0.076$). However, as there was a larger body of postnatal studies, they followed up this analysis, with sub-analyses, examining multiple micronutrients in one (6 studies); zinc, iron and folic acid in a second (19 studies), and those using macronutrients alone (primarily energy supplementation) or in combination with micronutrients (7 studies). The only significant impact was for macronutrient supplementation, which had a small effect size ($d = 0.14$) – but noting the considerable heterogeneity of intervention length and form of supplementation. Perhaps these modest results are less surprising when the broader context in which malnutrition occurs is considered (i.e., see Section 2.4.5 on stunting).

There have been at least five studies examining the longer-term impacts of nutritional supplementation (protein and energy here) of pregnant mothers and/or infants and young children (Prado & Dewey, 2014; Veena et al., 2016). One study conducted in Taiwan focussed on maternal supplementation through pregnancy and breastfeeding, and while this aided motor development at 8 months of age, it had no effect on IQ when children were tested aged 5. Another study conducted in Guatemala, provided nutritional support to the pregnant mother and then the child until 7 years of age. This study reported positive impacts on reading ability, IQ, and earnings, when participants were tested in adulthood. A further study, conducted in Indonesia, involved a 3-month dietary intervention during infancy. When these children were tested aged 5–8 years, there were some limited cognitive benefits, which were restricted to working memory. A Jamaican study undertook a 2-year nutritional intervention in stunted children, but found no long-term benefit when assessed on multiple cognitive tests into adulthood. Finally, a study in the Gambia, which provided maternal supplementation, testing the offspring when they were adults, also found no effect on cognitive measures or upon school achievement.

Out of these five longer-term studies, the Guatemala one is by far the most remarkable, because of its long-term impacts into adulthood (Hoddinott et al., 2008). It was also the longest intervention, but as with any study conducted in a real-world setting it has its limitations. There was no baseline evaluation of child/maternal nutrition, and assignment to supplementation was not random as allocation was by village. Thus, the observed beneficial effects *could* have resulted from extraneous causes (e.g., pre-existing differences between villages).

Protein supplementation in LBW, preterm infants has been studied in developed countries. A Cochrane review and meta-analysis including 6 RCTs involving 204 preterm infants found that there was low-quality evidence (largely due to small sample sizes) that protein supplementation of human milk increased growth rates and head circumference, but insufficient data to draw conclusions about neurodevelopmental outcomes (Amissah, Brown, & Harding, 2018). Of particular interest here was one study that was not included in the that review, presumably as there was no zero-protein control group. It did find different neurodevelopmental outcomes with increased levels of protein intake. For extremely-low-birthweight (580–1,250 g), preterm (23–32 week) infants, a group ($n = 34$) receiving higher-protein (4.8 g/kg/day) fortified human milk not only had higher growth rate, but also had better Griffith Development Mental Scores at 3 and 6 months compared to a group (n = 27) receiving lower-protein (3.5 g/kg/day) fortified human milk (Biasini et al., 2012). It is not clear whether these benefits are restricted to only extremely-low-birth-weight infants, and whether the neurodevelopmental outcomes are sustained beyond 12 months.

2.5 Overnutrition

Maternal obesity in humans has been associated with an increased risk in the offspring for cerebral palsy, ADHD, schizophrenia, anxiety, depression and autism spectrum disorder (ASD; Edlow, 2017; Smith & Reyes, 2017). For ASD and ADHD, the severity of these conditions has been correlated with the severity of maternal obesity. These relationships between maternal obesity and mental health and neurodevelopmental disorders generally survive control for confounders such as maternal age and socio-economic status, but noting that diet quality is rarely included as a covariate (Edlow, 2017). In addition to these observations, there is also evidence that maternal obesity adversely affects the cognitive and scholastic capacity of the child. Some studies find evidence of poorer academic performance, intelligence and visuospatial skills, while others do not (Veena et al., 2016). This heterogeneity raises concerns about adequate control of confounding variables, as obesity in developed countries is linked to lower educational, social and economic status, and whether these can be adequately controlled by 'covarying out' a measure of socioeconomic status is questionable. However, animal models do suggest that maternal obesity results in abnormal hippocampal development, indicating socio-economic status at least cannot account for all of the relationship between maternal obesity and neurocognitive development in humans (Nyaradi et al., 2013). Mechanistically, there are plenty of ways that maternal obesity (and/or poor diet quality) might impact the developing foetal brain, via increased neuroinflammation and oxidative stress, and through dysregulation of energy-related hormones and neurotransmitter systems (Edlow, 2017).

As we noted earlier, consumption of highly palatable processed foods that are rich in salt, saturated fat and added sugar – nutritionally poor-quality foods – are strongly linked to excess weight gain and obesity. Not surprisingly then, there has been some interest in whether maternal diet might impact foetal development. Borge et al. (2017) undertook a systematic review and meta-analysis of this question. They identified 18 correlational studies, which measured a range of dietary variables that were taken as proxies for maternal diet quality (e.g., fish exposure, S3/S6 fatty-acid ratio, saturated fat intake, fruit intake, fibre intake). Each study also measured a developmental outcome. Socio-economic status was the only confounder controlled in all 18 studies, while, importantly, maternal BMI was rarely controlled. Developmental outcomes were classified into four categories. There were small but significant effect size relationships between diet quality and cognition, externalising behaviour (aggressiveness, impulsivity, etc.) and socioemotional development. In all cases poorer diet quality was linked to more adverse developmental outcomes. There was no relationship between diet quality and internalising behaviour. A major concern with these findings is that they may result from maternal adiposity rather than from maternal diet. Equally, though, the reverse caveat applies to the maternal obesity studies discussed, as these rarely controlled for differences in maternal diet quality.

A number of studies have also examined if diet quality during childhood is linked to developmental outcomes (Nyaradi et al., 2013). At least three studies report that better diet quality is linked to higher IQ during early childhood, with these controlling for differences in socio-economic status. A further review included six studies on diet quality and executive functioning in children/adolescents, with all reporting that better diet quality was linked to better executive function (Cohen et al., 2016). However, it was unclear what confounders had or had not been controlled for, and thus the same interpretive problems arise here as with other studies in this section. Namely, where socioeconomic status is controlled, is this adjustment adequate? And to what extent does child adiposity from consuming a poor-quality diet cause the reported deficits, relative to the effect of diet quality per se (or the two in combination). While these issues remain unresolved, it does seem likely that overnutrition (i.e., poor diet and/or excess adiposity) *probably* exerts an adverse impact on foetal and child development.

2.6 Specific Deficiencies and Supplementation

2.6.1   Introduction

Many individual nutrients and micronutrients have significant effects on neurodevelopment, including specific amino acids, glucose, long-chain polyunsaturated fatty acids (lcPUFAs), iron, folate, iodine, zinc and vitamin B12 – and several others. Each is discussed below, separately addressing (where evidence is available) the effects of deficiency and supplementation, as they pertain to neurodevelopment. A final section examines the impact of multi-micronutrient supplementation, as in many cases individual deficiencies do not occur alone.

2.6.2 Aminoacidopathies

Deficiencies in the supply of specific amino acid (the building blocks of proteins) can arise. These usually occur for the amino acids that the body cannot synthesise – termed indispensable amino acids. These happen as a consequence of inborn errors of metabolism – termed aminoacidopathies – with each type of error being individually rare (the commonest has a prevalence of between 1 in 10,000 to 1 in 25,000 and the rarest around 1 in 4 million). However, because there are so many potential points at which indispensable amino acid metabolism can be disrupted, overall, they occur with a prevalence of 2–3% (Wasim, Awan, & Khan, 2018). Table 2.1 presents some of the most well studied examples (Aliu, Kanungo, & Arnold, 2018).

There are three main ways aminoacidopathies affect metabolism. Some cause a deficit of a particular amino acid, others result in an excess, and nearly all cause a build-up of toxic metabolites (see Table 2.1). They do, however, all have similar effects. The infant is generally healthy at birth (unless the mother is also suffering from a poorly controlled aminoacidopathy), mainly due to the placenta serving to normalise these metabolic abnormalities in the foetus. If the aminoacidopathy is not detected by routine genetic screening (for the commoner ones), the effects start to become apparent as the infant develops. Typical consequences are developmental delays, specific learning difficulties, general intellectual

Table 2.1. *Aminoacidopathies affecting indispensable and conditionally indispensable amino acids*

Disorder	Primary metabolic impact	Neurological impact
Phenylketonuria (PKU)	Phenylalanine deficiency	Intellectual disability (ID)
Maple Syrup Urine Disease	Leucine, isoleucine and valine build-up	ID, seizures
Tyrosinemia	Tyrosine build-up	ID
Argininosuccinic acidosis acronym (ASUD)	Argino-succinic acid build-up	ID, appetite loss
Argininemia	Arginine build-up	ID, seizures, tremor
N-acetylglutamate synthesase deficiency	Ammonia build-up	Fatal brain damage

impairment and seizures, with some aminoacidopathies being fatal if left untreated. While genetic therapies offer a potential form of treatment in the future (to remedy the missing enzyme), dietary therapy is the current mainstay treatment. For the commonest aminoacidopathy, phenylketonuria (PKU), this involves avoiding soybeans, egg whites, seafood, chicken, nuts and legumes – foods rich in phenylalanine, which builds up in this condition unless intake is restricted. This type of dietary restriction may be difficult to maintain in the longer term, but at least for PKU, most of the benefits from adhering to this diet seem to occur during childhood (Aliu et al., 2018). Later detection of PKU, as with the other aminoacidopathies, is associated with poorer outcome and a greater degree of brain damage, presumably due to the build-up of neurotoxic metabolites.

2.6.3   Hypoglycaemia

During the first 24–48 hours of life, it is normal for neonates to experience low plasma glucose concentrations as they transition from intrauterine to extrauterine life. However, episodes of hypoglycaemia that persist or occur repeatedly can have adverse long-term consequences to developmental outcomes. In preterm infants, repeated moderate episodes of hypoglycaemia are associated with reduced Bayley psychomotor developmental scores at 18 months of age (Lucas, Morley, & Cole, 1988). In 85 preterm infants that were small-for-gestational-age, those with repeated episodes of hypoglycaemia had significantly reduced head circumference at 12, 18 months and 5 years of age, compared to euglycaemic infants, despite having normal head circumference at birth (Duvanel et al., 1999). Furthermore, the infants with repeated hypoglycaemic episodes had lower scores on the perceptive performance and motricity subscales of the McCarthy test at 3.5 and 5 years of age. These effects can occur even with asymptomatic hypoglycaemia. For instance, a blood glucose level of <47 mg/dL was associated with abnormal evoked potentials (Koh et al., 1988). Based on such findings, but also considering that transient hypoglycaemia is considered a normal adaptation to postnatal life, guidelines to manage hypoglycaemia consider not only plasma glucose level, but also physiologic age and additional clinical risk factors and signs (Wight, Marinelli, & Med, 2014).

2.6.4   Long-Chain Polyunsaturated Fatty Acids

Long-chain polyunsaturated fatty acids (lcPUFAs) acids are prominent in neural tissue and are essential for the developing brain. Docosahexaenoic acid (DHA) is the predominant structural omega-3 PUFA in the brain and is an important component of the neuronal membrane. DHA is essential for normal CNS development and is vital to brain structure and function. Eicosapentaenoic acid (EPA) is detected as a trace component in the brain and is used to synthesize DHA (Moore et al., 1991). The brain is unable to efficiently synthesize these PUFAs by itself, therefore; they must be obtained through dietary sources.

There are four recent systematic reviews of the outcomes of lcPUFA supplementation on neurodevelopmental outcome. The first two were in term infants, the third compared maternal supplementation during pregnancy with preterm and term infant supplementation, and the fourth examined only preterm infants. A Cochrane review examined the effect of lcPUFA supplementation in infants born at term on neurodevelopmental outcomes prior to 2 years of age (Jasani et al., 2017). Of 11 identified studies, 9 used the Bayley Scales of Infant Development (BSID) and only 2 reported beneficial effects of supplementation. Meta-analysis revealed no significant difference between lcPUFA and supplementation groups for BSID mental development index or psychomotor development index at 1 year, 18 months or 2 years.

The second systematic review, published in 2018, evaluated the long-term outcomes of cognitive function in children who have participated in RCTs of lcPUFA supplementation in the first few months of life (Lien, Richard, & Hoffman, 2018). The authors reported that the results of trials conducted in this field are quite variable, and seem to depend in particular on: (1) how old the infants were at testing; (2) the dose of linoleic acid (LA) and alpha-linolenic acid (ALA) in the formula and (3) the tests administered, with particular cognitive domains appearing to be more affected. Supplementation with DHA at varying doses (0.32–0.96%) compared to a 0% DHA formula resulted in better sustained attention when tested at 4, 6 and 9 months (Colombo et al., 2011), better global intellectual functioning at 1.5 years of age (Mental Development Index) and better language functioning at age 2 (Drover et al., 2012), and better verbal and global intellectual quotients at age 6 (Colombo et al., 2013). None of these studies found a dose-response curve, suggesting any level of DHA supplementation confers benefit. In this same cohort, at 2.5 and 3.5 years of age, no effect of DHA supplementation was found for global school readiness or language function.

When outcomes were evaluated in slightly older children, global intelligence (measured by the WPPSI) was not significantly different between 4-year-olds who, as infants, were randomised to receive either 0.35% DHA,

0.36% DHA + 0.72% ARA or unsupplemented formula for 17 weeks (Birch et al., 2007). When tested at age 6, infants randomised to receive 0.21% DHA + 0.36% ARA for 4 months had better scores on processing speed measures compared to controls receiving unsupplemented formula, but there were no significant differences in full-scale, verbal and non-verbal intelligence quotient of the WPPSI-R. Neurological outcomes (using the Touwen examination) at 9 years of age did not differ between an lcPUFA-supplemented group compared to a control formula group.

Thus, lcPUFA supplementation may result in improvements in selected cognitive domains such as verbal intelligence, executive functions and processing speed, though the effect seems more robust when outcomes are evaluated in younger children compared to older children.

The third systematic review was also conducted in 2018, and evaluated the effects of maternal, preterm infant and term infant n-3 supplementation (i.e., DHA and/or EPA) (Shulkin et al., 2018). The effect of n-3 supplementation on BSID Mental Development Index pooled across all supplementation periods was significant, though reliable differences were observed between intervention periods, with stronger results for supplementation in preterm infants compared to maternal supplementation. The effect of n-3 supplementation on IQ in later childhood was not significant in the pooled analysis, nor when each supplementation period was analysed separately.

Another systematic review was conducted to evaluate the effect of lcPUFA supplementation in preterm infants. Meta-analysis showed no significant effect of supplementation on the BSID at 12 months (four studies), nor at 18 months (three studies). In a study that was excluded from this systematic review, Almaas et al. (2015) tested the effects on cognition of supplementation with the lcPUFA, DHA and arachidonic acid (AA), in very low birth weight (VLBW) infants fed human milk. Ninety-eight children were randomly assigned to receive the supplement or placebo and were tested at 8 years of age. There were no differences between the placebo or intervention group on any of the cognitive measures, nor any neuroanatomical differences on MRI.

2.6.5 Choline

Choline is especially important during growth and development, not surprisingly when considering that it constitutes 25% by weight of the grey matter of the human brain, and around 10% for myelin (McCann, Hudes & Ames, 2006). In animals, a fairly extensive literature indicates that depriving the mother of choline results in offspring that have an impaired capacity for HDLM (e.g., Niculescu, Craciunescu, & Zeisel, 2006). In addition, choline supplementation of the mother during pregnancy results in offspring that show reduced age-related decline in learning and memory (McCann et al., 2006). Choline supplementation also seems to protect the developing foetal brain from the impact of neurotoxins such as alcohol.

Maternal choline intake has three main consequences for foetal development (Korsmo, Jiang, & Caudill, 2019; Zeisel, 2006). The first concerns the viability of the placenta, where choline derivatives are important in angiogenesis. The second relates to epigenetic programming, where animal data indicates that later stress responsivity is adversely affected if choline is restricted during pregnancy, because of its impact on the hypothalamic–pituitary–adrenal axis. The third is for foetal brain development. Animal studies show that piglets born to choline-deficient sows have an overall lower brain mass, reduced brain volume and less white and grey matter, relative to controls. These effects arise because choline is necessary for the development of cell membranes, appropriate lipid metabolism, myelination, cholinergic metabolism and cell differentiation.

There is far less work on choline deficiency during human development. The most relevant data concerns mutations to one or other of the choline transporters, resulting in reductions in cellular uptake. Fagerberg, Taylor, and Distelmaier (2020) described four cases with a mutation in one of the five forms of the intermediate affinity choline transporter. Children born with this mutation are developmentally normal until between 2–8 years of age. The disease starts with tremor and motor abnormalities, affecting walking, swallowing and eye movements. The condition is degenerative, first impairing mobility and self-care, and finally affecting cognition and ending in coma and death. It is unclear if the condition is responsive to choline supplementation, because by the time it is identified, significant brain damage has already occurred. MRI reveals extensive white matter abnormalities, and at the cellular level, there are reductions in the capacity of cells to take up choline and impaired cell membranes. Why this disease only manifests some years after birth is unclear, but one possibility is that it may reflect accumulated brain damage from long-term impaired choline utilisation.

2.6.6   Vitamin A (Retinoic Acid)

Functionally, vitamin A (retinoic acid) is involved in embryonic development, vision, immune function, skin health and with an overarching role in regulating gene transcription (Olson & Mello, 2010; Shearer et al., 2012). Vitamin A deficiency is a major cause of blindness (estimated to be 0.25–0.5 M cases per year) and mortality (estimated around 0.7 M deaths) in children. Retinoic acid exerts potent effects on the developing brain and so its presence is highly regulated. During embryonic development, retinoic acid assists in neuronal patterning via concentration gradients and in the induction of neurogenesis (Shearer et al., 2012). Consistent with its known functions, infant and child deficiency results in visual impairment (and ultimately blindness) and increased susceptibility to disease (with this contributing to infant mortality via malaria), while maternal deficiency can cause foetal loss (abnormal embryonic development) and LBW babies (Shearer et al., 2012).

2.6.7   Vitamin B1 (Thiamine)

White rice is often a dietary staple, but unfortunately it offers little thiamine. If a child's diet is heavily dependent on this food, then the thiamine necessary for the body to metabolise it may be greater than the thiamine it provides. This is one reason why the nutritional diseases caused by thiamine deficiency – variant forms of beriberi – are so prevalent in South and Southeast Asia (15–58% of children and 27–78% of mothers; ; Nazir, Lone, & Charoo, 2019; Whitfield, Bourassa, & Adamolekun, 2018). Some African countries also face high levels of thiamine deficiency, with many people reliant on the carbohydrate-rich cassava, which also needs more thiamine to metabolise than it offers. Two further factors are important here: (1) the presence of cyanogenic glycosides, which can worsen thiamine deficiency, and (2) the process of removing cyanogenic glycosides from the cassava, by cycles of mashing and washing, which depletes thiamine content due to its solubility in water. There is also an additional factor, common to both Africa and Asia – childhood gut infections. These cause an increase in metabolism (using more thiamine) and decrease the capacity of the body to take up thiamine from food (impaired gut absorption). This is why children admitted to hospitals in these regions tend to have higher rates of thiamine deficiency than children in the community (Hiffler et al., 2016).

The impact of thiamine deficiency on foetal development has been studied using animal models. Here foetal deficiency produces a range of deficits at the cellular, system and behavioural levels of analysis. Nerve conduction velocities are reduced alongside impaired myelination and altered cell membrane conductance. During the earliest phases of brain development, cell proliferation and migration do not occur in the normal sequence and so there is large loss of neuronal tissue – equivalent to that seen in a foetus of a starved mother (Kloss, Eskin, & Suh, 2018). At the systems level, reduced brain weight and spinal-cord abnormalities occur, and the animal has significant behavioural impairments, notably in learning, motor and sensory functions.

In human infants, the consequences of thiamine deficiency are usually described as belonging to one of three distinct forms. The most classic is wet beriberi (from the Sinhalese word for weakness), which is characterised by cardiovascular abnormalities, oedema and weight loss. It has a rapid onset and can lead to heart failure, coma and death (Nazir, Lone, & Charoo, 2019). A variant of wet beriberi is the aphonic form, in which the presenting symptom is vocal paralysis. This then develops into the wet form. The final type is dry beriberi, which is principally neurological in presentation. In children, it is often called the pseudomeningetic form and is classically described as having a triad of symptoms – visual problems, confusion and delirium – although all three may not be present.

Whether these conditions actually represent three distinct disease patterns is hard to tell. Some have suggested that each pattern reflects different interactions with other nutritional deficiencies, genes and concurrent illness (Whitfield et al., 2018). However, an Israeli study on otherwise healthy infants who were just deficient in thiamine observed symptoms associated with all forms of beriberi, but without any obvious segregation into the three different patterns. The study focussed on the 600–1,000 Israeli infants who were accidentally fed a soy milk formula that contained no thiamine. Medical and public health officials were alerted to this problem after a series of 20 infants had presented with a mixture of cardiac and neurological symptoms, the latter including opthalmoplaegia, lethargy and coma. Neuroimaging revealed bilateral hyperintense signals in the mammillary bodies, basal ganglia and periaqueductal grey. Together, this suggested thiamine deficiency, and while supplementation ameliorated these symptoms, ten children were left with significant residual disability (e.g., cardiac problems, ataxia, hearing loss, epilepsy). Children exposed to at least 1 month of this formula, but who were asymptomatic at the time, were followed up 5 years later. Nearly all of this sample had language impairments, and 10% had impairments in understanding concepts (Fattal, Friedmann, & Fattal-Valevski, 2011) – suggesting a far broader impact on development than was originally recognised.

2.6.8   Vitamin B6 (Pyridoxal 5'-Phosphate)

Vitamin B6 has several developmental functions. Animal models suggest that maternal deficiency produces structural abnormalities in the off-spring's hippocampus, affecting the number and functionality of the NMDA-type glutamate receptor, and lowering glutamate and glycine levels (Guilarte, 1993). In addition, deficiency leads to less axon and dendritic branching in the neocortex and cerebellum, impairs myelination, degrades synaptic efficiency and lowers dopamine levels in the striatum and the number of D2 dopamine receptors (Prado & Dewey, 2014). The impact of deficiency on human infants is not well studied, but a longitu-dinal study found that vitamin B6 levels (and those of folate (B9)) were predictive of improved cognitive development over the first 2 years of life, even when taking account of other key developmental influences (MAL-ED network, 2018).

2.6.9   Vitamin B7 (Biotin)

Hypovitaminosis B7 is potentially important in pregnant women as animal data suggest that a similar state can be teratogenic. The profound effects of biotin deficiency are most evident in infants born with defective biotini-dase (necessary to convert the vitamin into its active form) and holocar-boxylase (one of the main groups of enzymes where biotin is used) enzymes. Both conditions share common symptoms and outcomes (Leon-Del-Rio, 2019). These mutations are relatively rare in the West, but more common in cultures that sanction consanguineous marriages (Canda, Ucar, & Coker, 2020). Neurological signs appear within months of birth, and where the capacity to metabolise biotin is not completely lost, failure to treat results in significant developmental delays, movement problems, blindness and deafness. Biotin treatment is able to ameliorate these symptoms if it is applied promptly; otherwise the effects are irrevers-ible, and result from persistent ketoacidosis, alongside a build-up of other metabolites (Wolf, 2011).

2.6.10   Vitamin B9 (Folate)

In the brain, folate is involved in various physiological pathways and is particularly important for foetal growth and development due to its role in DNA synthesis, methylation and cell replication. During pregnancy, maternal folate concentrations can decline by approximately 50%, partly due to the increased folate requirements for rapid growth of the placenta and foetus (McNulty et al., 2011). Folate deficiency during pregnancy is a well-known risk factor for neural tube defects (NTDs), and it has been conclusively shown that supplementation with folic acid prior to and in the first trimester of pregnancy can dramatically lower this risk (Czeizel & Dudas, 1992; MRC Vitamin Study Research Group, 1991). This protective effect in early pregnancy relates to the closure of the neural tube, which occurs around 21–28 days post-conception. There is now additional literature exploring whether folic acid supplementation confers additional benefit against other areas of atypical neurodevelopment.

The most recent systematic review in the area found 22 eligible studies looking at the association between folic acid supplementation in pregnancy and neurodevelopmental outcomes (Gao et al., 2016). Of the two RCTs, one found no benefit to mental developmental of children followed to age 6 of multivitamins containing 0.8 mg folic acid daily taken from before conception to the second month of pregnancy compared to placebo (Dobo & Czeizel, 1998). The other showed a benefit of folic acid together with either iron, iron and zinc, or a multivitamin on tests of working memory and executive function at age 7–9 (Christian et al., 2010). However, again the effects of folic acid alone were not tested.

Epidemiological studies have observed an increased rate of autism spectrum disorders (ASD) in children whose mothers took folic acid compared to those who did not (Suren et al., 2013), and that greater folic acid intake during the first month of pregnancy was associated with lower risk of ASD (Schmidt et al., 2011, 2012). Other studies have found that folic acid supplements in first trimester had a protective effect from internalising and externalising behaviours at 18 months (Roza et al., 2010), and from emotional problems at 3 years old (Steenweg-de Graaff et al., 2012).

A number of studies have shown improved cognitive function associated with folic acid supplementation during the first trimester of pregnancy, including higher receptive and expressive language scores on the BSID at 18 months (Chatzi et al., 2012), better vocabulary at 3 years (Villamor et al., 2012) and a lower risk of severe language delay at 3 years (Roth et al., 2011). Folic acid supplementation in pregnancy was associated with higher scores on verbal, motor, executive function and social competence in children age 4, after adjusting for a number of sociodemographic and behavioural factors (Julvez et al., 2009).

While neuronal proliferation and myelination also occur in later pregnancy, and brain areas such as the hippocampus and striatum undergo rapid growth (Georgieff et al., 2015), fewer studies have examined the role of folate in the second and third trimester on the child's subsequent neurodevelopment. Higher maternal blood folate levels at 30 weeks gestation predicted better cognitive performance in children age 9–10 (Veena et al., 2010). A pilot RCT in a small sample (n = 39) examined folic acid supplementation in the second and third trimester, demonstrating better performance on the cognitive domain of the BSID at 3 years (Pentieva et al., 2012).

While attempts are made to control for confounding variables, much of the observational evidence is based on self-reported folic acid usage, without measurement of dietary intake or blood levels of folate. Furthermore, it is difficult to separate out the effects of multi-nutrient supplementation. Nevertheless, the animal evidence does seem to be supportive for a role of folate in neurodevelopment of the offspring. The offspring of rodents fed a folic-acid-deficient diet have been shown to be less viable, with lower brain weight (Middaugh et al., 1976), a net reduction in brain cells (Xiao et al., 2005) and a reduction in progenitor cells in the neocortex (Craciunescu et al., 2004). Similarly, the offspring of rats with gestational B-vitamin deficiency had increased homocysteine, a cytotoxic amino acid, with corresponding apoptosis in the cerebellum, striatum and hippocampus, and alterations in learning and memory (Blaise et al., 2007). Increased anxiety-related behaviours have also been observed in the offspring of mice with gestational dietary folate deficiency (Ferguson et al., 2005).

2.6.11   Vitamin B12 (Cobalamin)

Not surprisingly, given that B12 is necessary for the methionine cycle – as is vitamin B9 (folic acid) – vitamin B12 deficiency in pregnancy also leads to neural tube defects (Prado & Dewey, 2014). Maternal hypovitaminosis B12 may also predispose the foetus to other developmental risks. Children born to mothers with low levels of B12 perform more poorly on tests of cognitive development at 1 year, have poorer memory and frontal functioning at 9 years, and poorer scores on a broad range of neuropsychological tests towards the end of primary school – relative to those born to mothers with adequate B12 levels (Van de Rest, Van Hooijdonk, & Doets, 2012; noting that some studies have also observed an inverse association with B12 levels in childhood and cognition). Infants fed a vegan diet, which can be deficient in B12, demonstrate lower fluid intelligence as adolescents, and infants with B12 deficiency are irritable, poor feeders and have abnormal development of their frontal and parietal lobes. These effects seem at least partially reversible via supplementation (Van de Rest et al., 2012).

2.6.12   Vitamin C (Ascorbic Acid)

Vitamin C is important for foetal brain development, notably for neuronal differentiation, and neuron and myelin growth (Travica, Ried, & Sali, 2017). The complete absence of vitamin C is fatal during development, and so there have only been limited studies on the effects of hypovitaminosis on foetal brain development in animals. These studies show persistent reductions in hippocampal volume, which, while not accompanied by behavioural changes (e.g., poorer spatial memory), may set the stage for more rapid cognitive decline during aging (Hansen, Tveden-Nyborg, & Lykkesfeldt, 2014). In humans, the closest analogy to these animal studies is intrauterine growth restriction, which can deplete the foetus of a range of nutrients including vitamin C. Here, the brain is significantly affected, with reduction in hippocampal volume, and the size of certain white matter tracts, and ventricular enlargement, alongside lifelong behavioural impacts on learning and memory (Hansen et al., 2014).

While the effects of deficiency in human infants cannot be studied experimentally, week-old guinea pigs subjected to around 6 weeks of low vitamin C diet showed impairment of spatial memory and changes to neurotransmitter levels and synaptogenesis in the hippocampus (Hansen et al., 2018; Tveden-Nyborg, Johansen, & Raida, 2009). Similar effects on the hippocampus have been observed in juvenile mice who lack the capacity to move vitamin C into the brain (Kurihara, Homma, & Kobayashi, 2019).

2.6.13   Vitamin D (Ergocalciferol, Cholecalciferol, Calcitriol)

Vitamin D deficiency has been studied in developmental animal models – but noting that rodents are nocturnal and seemingly for this reason have some capacity to generate Vitamin D unlike humans. Notwithstanding, the functional consequences of foetal deprivation are a unique set of behavioural changes, characterised in rats by hyperlocomotion in novel environments, increased sensitivity to stimulants in this context, increased impulsivity, impaired latent inhibition and enhanced memory for aversive events (Overeem et al., 2016). The profile for mice is different and milder, with hyperlocomotion a more general feature and with more restricted memory deficits. There are some difficulties in drawing any inferences for humans from these results, partly because of the lack of consistency across these two rodent species and because the gestational period for a rat or mouse is really only equivalent to the first and second trimester of the human pregnancy – a more general consideration for any such developmental comparison (Cui, Gooch, & Groves, 2015). There do not seem to have been any studies on whether children with rickets (the classic manifestation of vitamin D deficiency) – many of whom will have experienced some degree of foetal deficiency – have a related abnormal neurodevelopmental profile.

There has also been interest in whether two neurodevelopmental conditions may relate to vitamin D metabolism. Both schizophrenia and ASD have been linked to reduced exposure to UV light, and hence to hypovitaminosis during foetal development. In the Northern hemisphere, winter births, dark skin color and more northerly births are independently and interactively risk factors for later developing schizophrenia (Chiang, Natarajan, & Fan, 2016). This has led to the suggestion that reduced vitamin D during pregnancy may be a factor in shaping a brain more disposed to this condition – but currently the evidence is largely restricted to these findings. A similar argument has also been made for ASD, the claim being that the increase in cases over the last 30 years is a result of telling people to avoid sun exposure (Cannell, 2008). While this is speculative, there is consistent evidence of hypovitaminosis for vitamin D in people with ASD (Modabbernia, Velthorst, & Reichenberg, 2017). The effects of intervention with vitamin D are not currently clear.

2.6.14   Vitamin E (α-Tocopherol)

In animals, significant maternal vitamin E deficiency leads to spontaneous abortion, suggesting a critical role in early embryonic development. Young animals exposed to a deficient vitamin E diet, demonstrate heightened anxiety (Desrumaux, Mansuy, & Lemaire, 2018) and impaired HDLM, with evidence suggesting that oxidative brain damage accounts for the latter effect (Fukui, Nakamura, & Shirai, 2015). A more total loss of vitamin E can be engendered in animal models that knockout the α-tocopherol transporter protein (TTP; this moves vitamin E from liver cells into lipoprotein packages to transport around the body). In this case the animals develop a fatal neurological degenerative disease, characterised by cerebellar ataxia. An almost identical syndrome has been observed in humans. In this case it can occur from a defect in TTP (e.g., Bonello &

Ray, 2016), from a disruption in the formation of lipoproteins that carry vitamin E (abetalipopoteinemia) and from other causes that nearly totally impair gut absorption or hepatic cell processing of vitamin E (Muller, 2010). The resulting syndrome, termed AVED (ataxic vitamin E deficiency) is clinically similar to Friedreich's ataxia. It results in loss of reflexes, balance, position and vibration sense, retinal damage, muscular weakness and foot and spinal abnormalities – all of this impairs movement, and results in progressive degeneration unless high-dose vitamin E supplementation is started. This treatment can present further loss of function and if applied early in the disease course, it halts all neurological signs. It is generally agreed that this disorder develops gradually during childhood, because of the accumulating damage caused by lipid peroxidation to the brain.

2.6.15   Iron

Iron deficiency (ID) is reportedly the most common nutritional insufficiency worldwide (Yip, 2002). Iron is an essential element in the production of haemoglobin, and therefore iron deficiency anaemia (IDA) is a major consequence of ID. Iron is also an essential co-factor for many enzymes, proteins and lipids that are vital for normal cell functions. It is essential for neurodevelopment through effects on dendritic growth, synapse formation and myelination (Greminger et al., 2014; Lozoff, 2007; Siddappa et al., 2007). Many animal and human studies have demonstrated a crucial role for iron in brain development, which is broken down below into the period of exposure during pregnancy and infancy.

2.6.15.1   Iron Deficiency and Supplementation during Pregnancy
In pregnancy, the mother has a rapid expansion of blood volume, and thus the body consumes iron stores in order to make haemoglobin. The World Health Organisation estimates that ID affects between 30% and 50% of pregnancies worldwide (McLean et al., 2009). Low reported maternal iron during pregnancy has been shown to alter normal development of brain white matter pathways and tissue organisation of the grey matter of the frontal lobe (Monk et al., 2016). In male rats, foetal-neonatal IDA altered mRNA and protein levels in the hippocampus (Callahan et al., 2013).

A systematic review in 2019 identified 27 articles on gestational iron and offspring neurodevelopmental outcomes. Of the 19 observational studies, the quality varied greatly. Based on just high-quality studies, the authors concluded there was some evidence to suggest that low iron during pregnancy, particularly during the third trimester, is associated with off-spring neurodevelopment. Behavioural and cognitive changes were most commonly observed in infancy, including a higher rate of abnormal reflexes in premature infants at 37 weeks gestational age (Armony-Sivan et al., 2004), abnormal auditory neural maturation within 48 hours after birth (Amin et al., 2010), poor recognition memory of mother's voice in the immediate neonatal period and at 2 months of age (Geng et al., 2015; Siddappa et al., 2004) and poorer psychomotor development at 1 year of age (Siddappa et al., 2004).

There were few studies assessing outcomes in childhood and adolescence. The only high-quality study in this age group found that haemoglobin levels during the third trimester (but not first or second) were associated with lower offspring school outcomes at 14 and 16 years of age.

Two of the RCTs, in the same cohort, found no benefits of iron supplementation over placebo on offspring intelligence or behaviour assessed at 4 years (Zhou et al., 2006) and 6–8 years (Parsons et al., 2008), but both found a higher incidence of abnormal behaviour problems. Another RCT found no benefit of iron and folic acid supplementation compared to folic acid alone on IQ at 7 years (Li et al., 2015). When motor or mental development outcomes were assessed prior to 12 months, there was no benefit to iron supplementation compared to placebo (Angulo-Barroso et al., 2016) or to combined iron and folic acid supplementation (Chang et al., 2013; Li et al., 2009; Nguyen et al., 2017).

2.6.15.2   Iron Deficiency and Supplementation during Infancy
Early ID has been shown to affect development of specific brain regions, including the hippocampus, basal ganglia and prefrontal cortex (Beard, Erikson, & Jones, 2003; Fretham, Carlson, & Georgieff, 2011). ID anaemia in infancy has been examined using fMRI and is associated with alterations in the default mode network – involved in memory, social cognition and attention, specifically finding changes in connectivity to the left posterior cingulate cortex and medial frontal gyrus (Algarin et al., 2017). As with ID during pregnancy, ID in rat pups appears to particularly affect the hippocampus, leading to molecular, metabolic, structural, and synaptic changes, as well as altered expression of genes critical for hippocampal development and function (Carlson et al., 2007; Jorgenson et al., 2005; McEchron et al., 2008).

Behavioural and cognitive developmental delays have been reported in infants with iron deficiencies. Several studies have found an association between lower iron levels and lower cognitive and motor scores on the

Bayley Scales of Infant Development (BSID; Lozoff, 1989; Walter, Kovalskys, & Stekel, 1983). Furthermore, BSID scores improve with iron therapy administered either orally (4 months) or via intramuscular injection (1 week; Idjradinata & Pollitt, 1993; Lozoff et al., 1982). Poorer object permanence and memory encoding and retrieval were observed in infants with ID anaemia at 9 months of age (Carter et al., 2010). ID in infancy has been associated with poorer inhibitory control and attentional deficits at 10 years of age (Algarin et al., 2013) and risky behaviour in adolescence (East et al., 2018). In a double-blind, placebo-controlled RCT in Papua New Guinea, infants who were given an iron injection at 2 months of age had longer attention spans at 1 year of age when compared to controls (Heywood et al., 1989).

LBW infants are at particular risk for ID. Berglund et al. (2018) randomised 285 LBW infants (2–2.5 kg) to receive 0, 1 or 2 mg/kg/day of iron supplements from 6 weeks to 6 months of age. When children were tested at age 7, there were no differences in cognition (using the Wechsler Intelligence Scale for Children version IV); however, both supplemented groups had fewer externalising behaviour problems (using the Child Behavior Checklist).

Socio-emotional deficits have also been observed, including increased shyness, and decreased positive affect and soothability at 9–12 months in infants with ID and ID anaemia compared to iron-sufficient infants (Lozoff et al., 2008). ID is also associated with dulled affect, and social reticence at age 5, which was linked to social isolation at age 10 (East et al., 2017). These cognitive and social deficits persisted into adulthood. One study showed that teens who were iron deficient during infancy had poorer executive functioning and recognition memory at 19 years of age when compared to teens who were iron sufficient during infancy (Lukowski et al., 2010). The same cohort when followed up at 25 years had poorer functional social outcomes, such as being less likely to complete secondary school and having fewer long-term relationships (Lozoff et al., 2013).

2.6.16   Iodine

Iodine is absorbed by the thyroid gland to be converted into the thyroid hormones thyroxine (T4) and triiodothyronine (T3). Thyroid hormones are involved in various neurodevelopmental processes, including neurogenesis, axon and dendrite formation, neuronal migration, myelination, synaptogenesis and neuronal transmission (de Escobar, Obregon, & del

Rey, 2004a, 2004b). More than 1.9 billion individuals worldwide are estimated to have inadequate iodine intake (de Benoist et al., 2003). The consequences of iodine deficiency on brain development during pregnancy, infancy and childhood are discussed here.

The effects of iodine deficiency are most profound if they are experienced in utero, with this causing the most prevalent, but preventable form of developmental disability (Bunevičius & Prange, 2010). The mother provides the foetus with T3 and T4 for at least the first half of the pregnancy, until the foetal thyroid gland is functional (Bernal, 2007). Where iodine is deficient, the mother is not able to supply these hormones in the necessary quantity to the foetus, during the early stages of development. In addition, even when foetal thyroid production starts, reduced or absent dietary iodine will result in minimal in vivo T3/T4 production. If the degree of iodine deficiency is very severe, the foetus is likely to die. Severe deficiency exerts major adverse impacts on the foetus, which differ depending upon when during development the deficiency is experienced. If it is during early foetal development, and especially between weeks 10–20, this results in a developmental disorder traditionally called neurological cretinism (or more preferred *neurological iodine deficiency disorder* (NIDD)). If the deficiency is most profound later in development, typically past week 35, this results in a developmental disorder traditionally termed myxedematous cretinism (now *myxedematous iodine deficiency disorder* (MIDD)). These two disorders shade into each other, dependent upon the timing and severity of the iodine deficiency during foetal development (Bernal, 2007).

The typical characteristics of NIDD are mental retardation, hearing and speech problems and disorders of stance and gait (Delange, 1994). For MIDD (see Figure 2.2), the usual features are less severe mental retardation, restricted growth, delayed sexual maturation, thick dry skin, with some stance and gait problems (Zimmerman, 2009). The extent of disability from foetal iodine deficiency is exacerbated if it continues through infancy and childhood. However, historically, areas with severe iodine deficiency only reported NIDD and MIDD in 5–15% of the population, suggesting that apart from dietary variation, genetics may also play an important role in why some children are more severely affected than others (Bunevičius & Prange, 2010). Nonetheless, even children born seemingly intact in iodine-deficient areas appear to have some degree of cognitive impairment, manifesting as lower IQ and poorer motor skills. Some of these effects seem to be ameliorated by iodine supplementation. Indeed, meta-analyses on supplementation benefits reveal an increase in child IQ

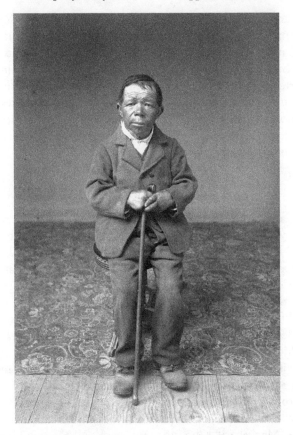

Figure 2.2   A person with myxedematous iodine deficiency disorder

of between 7–10 points (which is quite substantial), and a major reduction in risk of 72–76% for low IQ (i.e., < 70; Zimmerman & Boelaert, 2015).

As we noted earlier, thyroid hormones have a number of significant roles in neurodevelopment (Chen & Xue, 2020; Ghassabian & Trasande, 2018; Moog, Entringer, & Heim, 2017; Leach & Gould, 2015). Peak neuronal proliferation and migration during brain development occurs in weeks 5–20. T3/T4 are important here as they turn on and off genes that control these processes. The size of the pool of proliferating neurons is much smaller if T3/T4 concentrations are reduced, which results in a thinner cortical layer. Reduced T3/T4 also causes migration errors via, for example, impacts on reelin, such that neurons go to the wrong destination, resulting in dysfunctional connectivity between brain regions. Thyroid hormones are also necessary for the differentiation of oligodendrocytes that undertake myelination, and for the development of GABAergic interneurons in the neocortex, hippocampus and cerebellum. Brain areas that seem to be especially affected by these major neurodevelopmental impacts are the neocortex, striatum, cerebellum and cochlea, which, not surprisingly, parallel their functional consequences in NIDD. Later neurodevelopmental disruption by low thyroid hormone levels impacts the hippocampus and its capacity for learning and memory, myelination, synapse formation, and axon and dendritic sprouting.

2.6.17   Zinc

Zinc is essential for normal foetal development. In humans, severe zinc deficiency will result in foetal death or, if the foetus lasts to term, ancephaly – with no cerebral cortex (Sandstead, 2003). The primary reason for the severity of zinc deficiency during the earliest stages of foetal development is that zinc is necessary for the first steps in the formation of the brain. The brain develops out of neural stem cells, which proliferate, migrate and then differentiate into neurons, astrocytes and oligodendrocytes. This whole process is directed by transcription factors, which serve to switch genes on and off at the right time, in the right place in the right cell and for the right length of time. Zinc forms a major part of the largest family of transcription factors (Zinc fingers), and so, not surprisingly, disrupting this regulatory process has severe consequences on early brain development – notably in the first trimester (Al-Naama, Mackeh, & Kino, 2020).

Animal data indicate that even mild zinc deficiency during the first trimester produces adverse effects, rendering the offspring seizure prone, and subject to growth and developmental delays, as well as immunological complications. Deficiencies during later stages of pregnancy does not have as severe consequences. It produces learning and memory deficits, and impaired social behaviour, all of these being evident into adulthood in rodent and primate animal models (Hagmeyer, Haderspeck, & Grabrucker, 2015). At the neural level, these deficits seem to be associated with lower overall number of cells in the brain, alongside slower brain growth – effects that seem difficult to reverse after birth. Postnatal zinc deficiency produces a spectrum of dysfunction, including stress intolerance, depression and anxiety. In this case, anatomical correlates include impaired dendritic arborization, and neuronal growth. Into childhood, periods of zinc deficiency impact learning and memory, and produce lethargy and apathy. The later the age of onset, the more reversible these deficits appear to be (Sandstead, 2003).

The effects of zinc supplementation have been studied quite extensively in infants and children. In infants, studies of LBW babies, and children in countries where dietary deficiency is more frequent – India, Brazil and Guatemala – all suggest positive but limited benefits to child development (Penland, 2000). For older children, the effects are also positive, but even more limited, as indicated by a systematic review and meta-analysis of this literature (Warthon-Medina, Moran, & Stammers, 2015). Zinc supplementation had no effect on child IQ, but produced small improvements in motor and executive function. In adolescents, there is only one cross-sectional study examining for zinc–cognition links in a cohort of Iranian schoolgirls (Amani, Tabmasebi, & Nazari, 2019). They found that IQ and scores on the Weschler Memory Scale were poorer in the girls with lower levels of plasma and dietary zinc. It seems likely that the maximum benefit of zinc supplementation would probably be in women of child-bearing age in populations that are known to be zinc deficient (Penland, 2000).

2.6.18 Copper

An adequate supply of copper is necessary for normal foetal development. Most of the evidence for this comes from animal studies. Rat dams put on a restricted copper diet during pregnancy give birth to pups that have specific abnormalities of the hippocampus and especially the dentate gyrus, as well as having smaller brains (Hunt & Idso, 1995). More severe deficiency results in foetal death, and outside of the laboratory, restricted copper intake in pregnant ruminants results in offspring with cortical lesions, impaired myelination and limited white matter, with neuronal degeneration. The afflicted animals have trouble walking, hence the name neonatal ataxia. It has been suggested that copper is particularly important for myelination during the later stages of gestation (Zatta & Frank, 2007).

In humans, knowledge about the effects of copper deficiency have been gained from studying several genetic conditions that impair copper utilisation by the body. The most common is Menkes disease, a less severe variant is called occipital horn syndrome, and there is also ATP7a related distal motor neuropathy (Prasad et al., 2011). ATP7a is the transporter necessary for moving copper out of cells, including those of the gut wall. If this transporter is abnormal, as in Menkes disease, then copper cannot pass through the gut and into the body. Menkes disease is a lethal infantile neurodegenerative disease, which usually results in death before the age of 1 (Vairo, Chwal, & Perini, 2019). It is widely suspected that Menkes disease results in abnormal brain development, especially of the cerebellum and its purkinje cells, and more generally for axonal growth and synaptogenesis (Madsen & Gitlin, 2007; Olivares & Uauy, 1996). Infants with Menkes disease have been brain-imaged using MRI from shortly after birth and as the condition progresses. The earliest observable abnormality in the infant is arterial tortuosity, followed by changes to white matter tracts (Manara, D'Agata, & Rocco, 2017a). Abnormalities in the basal ganglia, cerebellar and cerebral atrophy all emerge more clearly as the disease progresses (Manara, Rocco, & D'Agata, 2017b). Although an inability to get copper into the brain and its cells is at the heart of this disorder (and copper-based treatment is of limited utility), the disease course is worsened by the frequent seizures that afflict these infants (producing additional brain damage) and by their proneness to frequent infection.

2.6.19   Multiple Micronutrient Supplementation

As Benton (2008, 2012) and several other authors have remarked (e.g., Liu, Zhao, & Reyes,2015), it is uncommon for specific nutritional deficiencies to occur alone. The norm is inadequate supply of multiple nutrients. Not surprisingly then, there has been some research examining the effects of multiple supplementation on various aspects of cognitive development. These studies are grouped by supplementation of the mother during pregnancy, infant supplementation, and supplementation during childhood and into adolescence.

Taylor et al. (2017) undertook a systematic review and meta-analysis of maternal supplementation during pregnancy. The paper drew upon 8 multi-micronutrient studies, conducted in a range of countries (low, medium and high income), and using various periods of dosing covering before, during and after pregnancy. Across the studies, all provided vitamin A and C, and B-group vitamins, including folate and thiamine, and several minerals (zinc and iron especially). Cognitive outcomes from these multi-micronutrient studies were examined in children aged under 10 when tested, with a median age of 3 or 4 years. Four cognitive domains were explored – motor skills (5 studies), global cognition (5 studies), fluid and crystallised intelligence (2 studies each). There were no significant effects on child cognitive outcomes from maternal multi-micronutrient supplementation.

The impact of multiple micronutrient supplementation on infant development has been examined in a systematic review and meta-analysis conducted by Larson and Yousafzai (2016). They reported six studies of varying length, that all provided at least B-group vitamins (often folate and thiamine), zinc and iron, to children aged under 2 years. All of these studies were conducted in developing countries. They found no overall effect on cognitive development of multiple micronutrient supplementation in their meta-analysis.

Eilander et al. (2010) undertook another meta-analysis this time of multiple micronutrient supplementation in later childhood, covering a total of 20 studies, from various countries (developing and developed). The minimal common set of supplements across all of the studies were B-group vitamins (generally folate and thiamine), zinc and iron, although over half the studies offered all vitamin groups and many mineral supplements. The meta-analysis revealed a marginally significant effect of supplementation on fluid intelligence (with a small effect size, $d = 0.14$), no effect on crystalised intelligences and no effect on any specific cognitive domain (memory, speed of processing, etc.). The only significant effect was obtained for a measure of school achievement $(d = 0.3)$, and these four studies were all conducted in developing countries.

In addition to this work in children, it is also interesting to mention the studies that have examined the effects of multiple micronutrient supplementation on juvenile delinquency. Benton (2008, 2012) provides an overview of these reports. At least two prison-based studies have been conducted using a double-blind placebo-controlled approach, contrasting multiple micronutrients with a placebo capsule. This led in one study to a 28% reduction in aggressive behaviour, and in the other to a reduction in violent offending. In the former case, the extent of behavioural improvement was correlated with micronutrient changes in the blood, suggesting a biological basis for this effect. In addition to these findings, a further well-conducted study undertaken in a school setting, and using disciplinary records as the dependent variable, found a reduction in impulsive conduct in supplemented children. In sum, while the effects of multiple micronutrient supplementation seem disappointing in the maternal and early infancy context, older children and adolescents may obtain some benefit. While this benefit has been attributed to the poor nutritional quality of their diet, this seems an unsatisfying explanation because many of the maternal and infant studies were also conducted in settings where poor-quality diet was also present.

2.7 Conclusion

Breastfeeding seems to confer at best only a small benefit to brain development, as indexed by IQ. There do not appear to be any beneficial effects of breastfeeding on child mental health during development. One positive consequence of these findings should be to reduce pressure on mothers – in high-income countries – to breastfeed. The literature on malnutrition – including overnutrition and poor diet quality – indicates adverse neurodevelopmental consequences. However, in the particular case of stunting, the extent to which its relationship with impaired development is solely due to the effects of malnutrition on the brain is questionable. This is due to the complex interaction between the behavioural consequences of malnutrition and environmental and social factors, which together act to impair normal development. It may be for this reason that nutritional supplementation seems to have only a weak positive impact on remediating development in malnourished – stunted – children. Finally, a lot is now understood about the role of specific micronutrients in development, and in some cases the effects of maternal supplementation are clearly effective (e.g., folate, iodine).

CHAPTER 3

Acute Effects of Food Intake

3.1 Introduction

There has been considerable interest in whether specific meals (e.g., breakfast) and individual macronutrients (e.g., glucose) can acutely affect brain and behaviour. Apart from the practical ramifications of this research (e.g., post-meal drowsiness and accidents, breakfast improving scholastic performance, glucose boosting cognition in the elderly), it has opened up important methods to investigate links between cognition and energy utilisation in the brain (i.e., glucose) and the manipulation of monoamine neurotransmitter systems. This chapter examines these various topics, focussing in the first part on the effects of specific meals, and meal timing, and in the second part on specific macronutrients, especially glucose and the amino acid precursors of the monoamine neurotransmitters.

3.2 Meal Times

3.2.1 Breakfast

Breakfast has been called the most important meal of the day (Spence, 2017). This claim is based on several correlational findings, which suggest that missing breakfast is associated with a greater risk of workplace injuries, a generally poorer-quality diet (e.g., more snacking, less fibre), poorer mental health and more cognitive failures (e.g., Chaplin & Smith, 2011). Research in this area has also been driven by concerns over the number of individuals who miss this meal, with somewhere around a third of US adolescents and a quarter of adults reportedly skipping breakfast (Siega-Riz, Popkin, & Carson, 1998; Spence, 2017). Moreover, the effects of missing breakfast in children and adolescents has attracted a lot of research attention, as several studies have found that school breakfast programs can improve academic outcomes (Hasz & Lamport, 2012).

Studying the acute effects of breakfast typically involves comparing a no-breakfast condition to a breakfast condition, with assessment taking place before and at some point after breakfast (or after when breakfast would normally be). More recent studies have tended to use a cross-over design (i.e., each participant completes all cells of the design in counter-balanced order), which is superior in so much as it equates for individual differences in diet and other factors (Kanarek, 1997). However, this approach is not without its problems, especially managing the consequences of repeating the same neuropsychological tests (e.g., using alternate forms).

The breakfast literature, including both adult and child studies, is composed of around 40 individual experiments (see Table 3.1). There are several reviews both narrative (Kanarek, 1997) and systematic (Adolphus et al., 2016; Edefonti, Bravi, & Ferraroni, 2017; Edefonti, Rosato, & Parpinel, 2014; Galioto & Spitznagel, 2016; Hoyland, Dye, & Lawton, 2009), but no meta-analyses. Across this body of work there is no obvious difference in study outcome among children, adolescents and adults, nor does it appear that the type of breakfast (i.e., macronutrient profile) has much impact either (Williams, 2014; Zilberter & Zilberter, 2013). The key question then is whether having breakfast exerts some systematic and replicable acute effect (especially a benefit) to cognition, mood or alertness (arousal). As all of the systematic reviews conclude, it is difficult to find any consistent effect on cognition, at least among well-nourished participants. To the extent that there are *any* benefits, these may lie with improvement in memory following breakfast – in adults (Galioto & Spitznagel, 2016) – and perhaps also in those children at risk of malnourishment (Hoyland et al., 2009). For mood and arousal, there are also no consistent benefits, although some studies find that participants report increased feelings of alertness after breakfast (e.g., Defeyter & Russo, 2013; Smith et al., 1994) and better mood (e.g., Benton & Brock, 2010), but even these effects do not seem to translate into cognitive performance benefits.

The inconsistency across studies has led a number of authors to question the basic claim that having breakfast confers cognitive benefits (Rogers et al., 2016; Zilberter & Zilberter, 2013). As these authors note, breakfast can sometimes exert *deleterious* effects on cognition (albeit uncommonly), and they also question why skipping breakfast would somehow adversely affect brain function – after all, the body has sufficient energy available to maintain brain function in the absence of one meal (Rogers et al., 2016). Two final points are also important to consider. The first is that routine

Table 3.1. *Summary findings for the impact of specific meals on different cognitive domains*
(units are studies testing a cognitive effect/s)

Meal type and comparison details	Effect on cognition				
	Executive function	Language	Motor	Memory	Attention/processing speed
Breakfast (B)					
	B better, B no effect, B worse				
B vs no B (adults)[1]	10, 9, 2	0, 4, 0	1, 1, 0	22†, 11, 0	8, 13, 2
B vs no B (children)[2]	7, 8, 1	2, 1, 1	2, 2, 1	8, 9, 3	13, 14, 3
Lunch (L)					
	L better, L no effect, L worse				
L vs no L (adults)[3]	0, 2, 0	1, 1, 0	No data	No data	0, 2, 2
L vs no L (children)[4]	0, 2, 0	No data	No data	0, 1, 0	0, 2, 0
Dinner (D)					
	D better, D no effect, D worse				
D vs no D (adults)[5]	0, 1, 0	1, 0, 0	0, 1, 0	0, 0, 1	0, 1, 0
Snacks (S)					
	S better, S no effect, S worse				
S vs no S (adults and children)[6]	1, 0, 0	1, 0, 0	No data	2, 0, 0	2, 1, 0

[1] 34 studies from Galioto and Spitznagel (2016), systematic review.
[2] 24 studies from Adolphus et al. (2016), systematic review.
[3] 4 studies from Muller et al. (2013), systematic review.
[4] 3 studies from Schroder et al. (2015, 2016), Muller et al. (2013).
[5] 1 study from Smith, Maben, and Brockman (1994).
[6] 3 studies from Kanarek and Swinney (1990), Benton, Slater, and Donohoe (2001), Mahoney, Taylor, and Kanarek (2007).
† Note that many of these effects were for long-term memory.

breakfast eating may be a powerful and indirect marker of above-average socio-economic status; thus, to the extent that breakfast skipping has *any* adverse consequence, these may result from more fundamental causes such as poverty (Hopkins et al., 2017). The second is to note the heterogeneity of neuropsychological tests used to assess cognitive function (a problem that dogs almost all of the research in this book), making across-study comparison (and meta-analysis) difficult. In addition, as some neuropsychological tests are more sensitive than others, it is conceivable that breakfast effects may only be found in those using such tests. This would imply that the effects of breakfast are at best likely to be subtle.

3.2.2   Lunch

That a dip in alertness and increased drowsiness follow lunch has been noted by researchers for many years (e.g., Kanarek, 1997; Laird et al., 1936). More contemporary studies have confirmed this effect (e.g., Craig, Baer, & Diekmann, 1981; Craig & Richardson, 1989), which does not appear to depend on either the size of the meal or its macronutrient composition (Smith et al., 1988). One potential confound is that lunchtime occurs during a particular part of the day, and so it may be that as morning passes into the afternoon, this happens to coincide with circadian changes that predispose to drowsiness. This possibility seems unlikely. First, the effect of lunch on alertness can be detected by comparing reports of drowsiness on a day when lunch is eaten versus a day when it is not – crucially at the same time of day (Craig et al., 1981). Second, changes in cortisol, which are in part dependent on circadian rhythms, appear unrelated to post-lunch drowsiness (at least in adolescents; Schroder et al., 2015). Third, when a person is sleep deprived, a meal (vs no meal) acts to exacerbate sleepiness (Gupta, Dorrian, & Grant, 2017), suggesting that it is some aspect of ingesting food at this time that induces sleep rather than the time-of-day itself.

One explanation for post-lunch drops in alertness and increased drowsiness is an increase in the cytokine IL1 following lunch. Reducing IL1 (α and ß) levels post-lunch has a small but significant effect in reducing drowsiness, suggesting that IL1 may play a role in the post-lunch drop in alertness (Lehrskov, Dorph, & Widmer, 2018). There are also other explanations for why eating lunch might increase drowsiness. These include dietary effects on plasma tryptophan levels (noting that such impacts are likely to be modest at best (Benton & Donohoe, 1999)), and hence on serotonin and melatonin levels in the brain, and the effects of intestinal (e.g., CCK) and other bioactive (e.g., α-s1-casien hydrolysate) peptides (Peuhkuri, Sihvola, & Korpela, 2012). None of these accounts have any substantial evidence base as yet and they would presumably apply to all meals, not just lunch, suggesting some interaction with circadian rhythm is also required.

As lunch can make you drowsy and less alert, one would think this would impair cognitive performance (see Table 3.1). Müller et al.'s (2013) systematic review identified 11 reports in adults exploring different facets of this issue. Four studies compared the effects of lunch versus no lunch, finding either no effect, improvements (Kanarek & Swinney, 1990) or deleterious effects on measures of attention and executive function (Craig et al., 1981; Smith & Miles, 1986). A larger lunch size increased attention-related errors (Craig & Richardson, 1989; Smith, Ralph, & McNeill, 1991). For macronutrient composition, lunches high in carbohydrates seemed to slow visual search performance (Smith et al., 1988), while across all six such studies, high-fat meals seemed to slow performance but increased accuracy (Müller et al., 2013). Müller et al. (2013) noted that '...effects were mostly very small, inconsistent and restricted to certain tasks or sub-groups...' – which parallels the findings from the smaller literature in teenagers and children (e.g., Schroder et al., 2015, 2016). In sum, while lunch may increase reports of drowsiness, there is no consensus on its effects on cognitive performance.

3.2.3 Snacks

Even through snacking is common, relatively few studies have explored its effect on cognition, mood and arousal (Miller et al., 2013; see Table 3.1). Organised by time of day, this small literature suggests: (1) At mid-morning, a milk and cereal snack in adults can improve mood and memory (Benton et al., 2001). (2) A mid to late afternoon energy-dense snack, in adults and children, is associated with improved memory in two studies, but with inconsistent effects on attention (Kanarek & Swinney, 1990; Mahoney et al., 2007). (3) Providing four snacks (milkshakes) versus two over the course of the day is associated with improved verbal reasoning in adults (Hewlett, Smith, & Lucas, 2009). (4) In assessments of momentary well-being in adults throughout the day, having a snack is associated with lower levels of fatigue (Strahler & Nater, 2018). (5) Milk with high melatonin content (from night milking) may be efficacious in promoting sleep, but the evidence base for other night-time snacks is inconclusive in this regard (Peuhkuri et al., 2012).

Studying the impact of snacks on behaviour is difficult, unless full control over food intake is undertaken to ensure that only the presence or absence of the snack is the differentiating factor (e.g., see Mahoney et al., 2007). In addition, the range of potential times for snack delivery and the range of potential macronutrient profiles makes determining the impact of snacks on cognition, mood and arousal a tricky endeavour.

3.2.4   Dinner

Only one study has examined the impact of an evening meal on cognition and mood. Smith et al. (1994) used a between-subject design, with participants receiving either a three-course meal or no meal in the evening (see Table 3.1). Testing conducted before and after the meal time revealed little impact of dinner on cognition or mood.

A second strand of research has looked at the impact of an evening meal on sleep. The majority of studies in this area tend to manipulate diet for either several days or across a day (e.g., Phillips, Chen, & Crisp, 1975), and only two studies have focussed on just manipulating the evening meal. In adults, Driver et al. (1999), using a cross-over design, examined the impact on sleep of a high-energy, normal-sized and no-meal condition. They found no effect of evening meal type on sleep on either self-report or polysomnographic measures. In toddlers, Diethelm et al. (2011), in a cross-sectional study, observed that higher energy intakes in the evening meal were associated with longer sleep duration (an additional 1.4 s/kJ). Finally, many people report that the foods they eat before going to bed can influence their dreams (Nielsen & Powell, 2015). In an exploratory survey in 396 undergraduates, 18% reported disturbing or bizarre dreams following particular foods, with dairy products identified most frequently as the suspected culprit (Nielsen & Powell, 2015), which may reflect popular beliefs linking cheese and vivid dreaming.

3.3   Preparing to Eat

While having or missing certain meals may affect cognition, two other literatures have looked at a different but related problem, namely the effect of being prepared (or not) for food intake. While it could be argued that this is not an acute effect of food intake, it seems relevant to consider it here, as the same meal eaten at different times *could* exert quite different effects on the brain, and thus potentially on behaviour. One literature that has explored this concerns the health impacts of shift work, where a person either changes work patterns to include some periods of night work, or works routinely at night. It has been known for some time that shift work results in increased risk for obesity and type II diabetes (e.g., Lowden et al., 2010). It was originally suspected that shift work exerted this effect by alterations in nutrient intake, but a large number of studies suggest that diet patterns (i.e., how much is eaten and the number of meals) and quality (i.e., nutritious vs processed food) are similar between shift workers and controls, suggesting that the cause may lie elsewhere (e.g., McHill, Melanson, & Higgins, 2014). Indeed, it seems that the adverse effects of shift work are a metabolic phenomenon, associated with decreased energy expenditure during the night period (McHill et al., 2014). In this case the clock time the meal is eaten does not seem to be that important, and there is little evidence that the effects on cognition and performance of food intake differ between night and day (e.g., Grant, Dorrian, & Coates, 2017).

The second place these issues have been considered is in relation to the cephalic phase response, which occurs both as a learned response to food cues (e.g., time of day, sight of food; Power & Schulkin, 2008; Smeets, Erkner, & de Graaf, 2010) and as a consequence of food stuffs stimulating oral taste and tactile receptors. The extent of these preparatory responses is large (Zafra, Molina, & Puerto, 2006), covering the mouth (e.g., enhanced salivation), stomach and gut (e.g., acid secretion, CCK release) and pancreas (e.g., insulin). The question here is whether an unexpected bout of food intake might result in a different consequence (for brain or mind) than an expected eating bout, due to differences in preparatory responses. Routinely, this situation is unlikely to occur, as while a surprise eating bout might minimise learned preparatory responses, innate effects from food contacting taste and tactile receptors in the mouth would still result in an effective preparatory response before food entered the stomach. However, it is interesting to note that under circumstances where no preparatory response is likely to be mounted, such as in feeding parenterally (intravenous) or enterally (via a tube into the gut or stomach), significant adverse metabolic consequences have been documented in both clinical settings (especially parenteral nutrition) and in animal models (e.g., impaired glucose control; Power & Schulkin, 2008; Zafra et al., 2006). However, in general, expecting (vs not expecting) a meal or the time it is eaten does not seem to influence the way brain and mind react to it.

3.4 Acute Effects of Macronutrients

3.4.1 Carbohydrates

This section examines the effects of carbohydrates on cognition. It starts with the effects of glucose, which have been extensively studied in animals and humans. This is followed by sections on other carbohydrates, glycaemic index, and disorders of carbohydrate metabolism (i.e., diabetes). This last mentioned section is relevant because both forms of diabetes are associated with particular patterns of cognitive impairment, which have a bearing on the issue of how glucose may affect cognition. Both the location of the glucose effect in the brain and its potential mechanisms are examined.

3.4.1.1 Glucose

The carbohydrate glucose is a key energy source for the body's metabolic system and the primary energy source used by the brain (Siesjo, 1978). Animals and humans find the taste of glucose pleasant, and it can enhance various aspects of cognition, especially learning and memory (White, 1989). These various responses to glucose are presumably highly functional. First, its oro-sensory properties facilitate consumption of an energy-containing substrate. Second, its cognitive enhancement properties may increase the likelihood of future consumption by augmenting attention to, and memory of, events surrounding the ingestive episode (Messier, 2004).

It has been suggested that oro-sensory and cognitive responses are dissociable, and indeed this is why energy-free artificial sweeteners are typically used as control conditions in human studies of the cognition-enhancing properties of glucose (e.g., Boyle, Lawton, & Dye, 2018; Smith et al., 2011). However, it is important to note that the oro-sensory properties of artificial sweeteners (i.e., their sweet taste alone), may have some limited memory-enhancing properties in animals (e.g., Messier & White, 1984; Stefurak & van der Kooy, 1992) and that *just* the sweet taste of glucose (swilling in the mouth) may enhance certain types of cognitive performance in humans (e.g., Molden, Hui, & Scholer, 2012). So, while the focus here is on the cognitive-enhancing properties of glucose *controlling* for its sweet taste, it is worth bearing in mind that sweet taste alone may have cognitive-enhancing properties, something that has not been well explored.

Animal and human research on the cognitive-enhancing properties of glucose is extensive. Credit for the earliest human publication in this area goes to a German study by Hafermann (1955), who administered glucose to school children reporting that this benefitted their capacity to concentrate, and their mathematical ability in a classroom setting. A further study by Lapp (1981), seems to have been the next published attempt to explore the benefits of glucose on cognition, again in children, and it is this paper – published in English – that seems to have stimulated contemporary interest in this topic. The animal literature was a surprising latecomer. Two separate groups started working on this, Gold and colleagues in the United States (Gold, 1986) and Messier and colleagues in Canada (Messier & White, 1984). While nobody appears to have done a recent systematic review of findings in the animal domain (Gold, 2014, is closest), the effect of glucose on cognition seems to be well supported, with findings observed across a range of different species, including rodents (Gold, 1986), pigeons (Parkes & White, 2000) and chickens (Gibbs & Summers, 2002). These findings in animals have mainly been observed in the area of learning and memory, and the effect is sufficiently robust to partially reverse deficits in performance generated by drugs known to affect this domain (e.g., scopolamine; see Messier, 2004).

Effects of Glucose on Neuropsychological Tests of Human Performance The most recent systematic review of glucose's effect on cognition was completed by Boyle et al. (2018). They identified 64 studies, covering a large range of cognitive performance tests, as well as mood, including data from participants across the lifespan. In addition to this, there is a related but distinct literature – and one that does not have an obvious animal counterpart – that has emerged on self-control, self-regulation and decision-making. In a review of this literature, Orquin and Kurzban (2016) identified 17 studies with a few more having been published since. We start by examining the literature on cognitive performance tests, which is better developed and less controversial.

In a prototypical glucose-enhancement paradigm, young adults are either randomised into a treatment or control arm using a between-groups design or serve in counterbalanced order in both conditions using a cross-over (repeated-measures) design. In the treatment arm they receive 25 g of glucose dissolved in water and in the control arm an equivalently sweet-tasting solution of aspartame or saccharin (e.g., Brandt, 2015; Foster, Lidder, & Sunram, 1998; Sünram-Lea et al., 2001). Testing usually occurs between 10–30 min following administration when blood glucose levels peak (e.g., Scholey et al., 2009, 2013). In tests of learning and memory, variants of this procedure have been used to explore the locus of any

Table 3.2. *Summary findings (units are studies testing a cognitive/mood effect/s) for the impact of glucose on different cognitive domains, with data extracted from Boyle et al. (2018)*

	Effect on cognition				
Studies and outcomes	Episodic memory	All HDLM[1]	Executive function	Mood	Attention/ miscellaneous
Total studies (%)	53 (100)	60 (100)	35 (100)	11 (100)	33 (100)
Enhancing/positive effect (%)	32 (60)	36 (60)	15 (43)	2 (18)	18 (55)
Impairing/negative effect (%)	1 (2)	1 (2)	3 (9)	0 (0)	1 (3)
No effect (%)	20 (38)	23 (38)	17 (48)	9 (82)	14 (42)

[1]HDLM stands for Hippocampal dependent learning and memory

benefit. A learning phase can occur either following glucose administration to examine effects on encoding (e.g., Stollery & Christian, 2013) or before glucose administration to determine effects on consolidation (e.g., Stollery & Christian, 2015). Glucose can also be given before a recall or recognition phase, to determine effects on the retrieval process (e.g., Stollery & Christian, 2015). These design basics are common for the majority of studies described below.

Tests of episodic memory, and more broadly tests of hippocampal-dependent learning and memory (HDLM) dominate this literature (see Table 3.2). Sixty percent of both the episodic memory tests and those more generally of HDLM (i.e., including episodic memory, visuospatial memory and miscellaneous tests) returned positive effects following glucose ingestion (Boyle et al, 2018). Making some modest assumptions about these data (i.e., that significant enhancement effects have a $Z = 1.96$, non-significant effects a $Z = 0$ and impairment effects a $Z = -1.96$) yields a highly significant overall outcome using Stouffer's meta-analytic Z formula ($Z \approx 9$). Nonetheless, while glucose enhancement of learning and memory appears a robust phenomenon, it is still clearly a heterogenous one (and as with the other effects discussed later), with around 40% of published studies reporting null results.

A large range of other non-HDLM cognitive tests have also been used, including of reaction time (e.g., Owens & Benton, 1994), executive function (e.g., Martin & Benton, 1999), facial recognition (e.g., Metzger, 2000), mental arithmetic and attention (e.g., Giles et al., 2018). Grouping these various findings in such a way as to preserve some degree of uniqueness for the cognitive function under test, but with sufficient studies to get some sense of glucose's enhancing performance, yields three further categories (see Table 3.2). These are tests of executive function (including subcategories of visuospatial functioning, working memory and problem solving (used in Boyle et al.'s, 2018 review)), tests of mood and tests of other cognitive domains, with these being principally tests of attention.

Of the 35 tests of executive function, 15 (43%) returned a significant enhancement effect and three (9%) an impairment effect – fractionation into more specific test subcategories did not reveal any different pattern. Using the effect estimation procedure described earlier and Stouffer's formula reveals a highly significant overall outcome for the effects of glucose on executive function ($Z \approx 4$). For mood, of the 11 studies, 9 (82%) found no effect, and of the remaining 2 (18%), 1 observed enhanced alertness and the other increased fatigue. Changes in mood/alertness do not seem to be a consequence of glucose ingestion. For other domains (mainly attention), of the 33 studies, 18 (55%) returned a positive effect, with 1 negative effect – suggesting an overall positive impact using our effect estimation technique and Stouffer's formula ($Z \approx 6$). Based on these counts of glucose effects across cognitive domains, it would seem that those on memory are most robust, followed by those on attention and executive function. This conclusion echoes that of the major reviews of this field (Hoyland, Lawton, & Dye, 2008; Smith et al., 2011).

As glucose can remediate drug-induced learning and memory deficits in animal models and so appears to have 'drug-like' effects (see Messier, 2004), there has been interest in whether it has a dose-response curve. Animal data (e.g., Gold, 1986) suggests an inverted U response to glucose, with an optimal dose for memory enhancement in rats being 100 mg/kg (so approximately equivalent to about 7 g for a 70 kg adult human), with lower doses having no effect and higher doses either no effect or impairment. Three human studies have examined for dose-response effects with glucose and memory: (1) Parsons and Gold (1992) found that 25 g (range 0–50 g) was the optimal dose for memory enhancement (logical memory) in elderly subjects; (2) Messier et al. (1998) reported that both 300 mg/kg (so equivalent to about 21 g for a 70 kg adult) and 800 mg/kg (approximately 56 g in an adult) doses were enhancing, but not 10, 100, 500 or 1,000 mg/kg doses; and (3) Sünram-Lea et al. (2011) found a marginally significant effect of 25 g of glucose on both a verbal delayed memory task (but no effect of 15, 50 or 60 g doses) and significant effects on working and recognition memory tasks. Outside of the memory domain Flint and Turek (2003) failed to obtain any evidence of a dose-response effect for an attention task. Finally, drawing on the data provided in Table 2 of Boyle

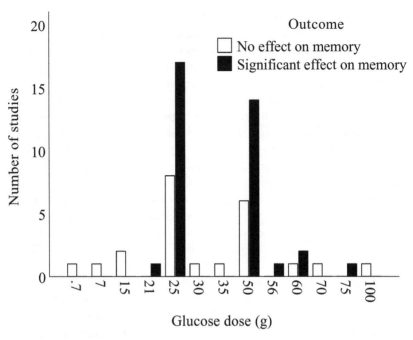

Figure 3.1 Dose-response graph for the effects of glucose on learning and memory

et al. (2018) we calculated whether there was a linear or quadratic relationship between study outcome (episodic memory effect, yes/no) and glucose dose used in the study – collapsing across different study designs, age groups and tests of episodic memory. This analysis revealed a weak quadratic effect (p = 0.035; 1-tailed; with no linear effect), with the optimal dose for an enhancement effect being around 40 g (see Figure 3.1 for an overview of the dose-outcome relationship). In sum, the human and animal data suggest there is an inverted U response to glucose for its effects on learning and memory, although there is no convincing evidence in humans for active impairment at low or high concentrations, rather just no effect.

A significant issue in this literature has been whether glucose enhancement effects are more likely when the task is especially demanding. One reason why this may be relevant is, as discussed later, that brain glucose usage may increase with task demand and so the benefits of additional circulating glucose may not become apparent until local glucose usage outstrips supply. Task demand has been manipulated in two ways, first, by varying task difficulty (e.g., inclusion of a distractor task) and, second, by using the same task on participants who should differ in how taxing they find it to be (e.g., by age, neurological impairment; but noting in both these examples there may be adverse changes in the brains capacity to metabolise glucose, thereby confounding task difficulty).

The outcomes of these approaches *tend* to favour the idea that under more difficult conditions glucose enhancement effects are more consistently evident (Boyle et al., 2018; Smith et al., 2011). With enhancing cognitive load, most of these experiments have been undertaken with undergraduates, either using divided attention at encoding (e.g., Sünram-Lea et al., 2001) or by increasing the length of the word lists that participants are asked to learn (e.g., Kennedy & Scholey, 2000). The benefits of making tasks more difficult seem to be evident irrespective of whether it is of learning and memory (the bulk of studies) or some other aspect of cognitive performance (Smith et al., 2011). One obvious caveat here is that this approach may be removing ceiling effects, but the literature does not show any overt sign of this.

With varying participant type, age has been the principal independent variable. There have been at least 14 studies using tests of verbal learning and memory in elderly participants, of which 9 recorded a positive effect (64%) – a slighter higher overall rate than observed for studies of *just* younger participants (56%) – and recalling that several of these studies in younger adults used more demanding tasks (Boyle et al., 2018; van der Zwaluw et al., 2015). Some studies have directly contrasted younger and older participants. Hall et al. (1989) and Manning et al. (1997) both found evidence of improved episodic memory performance in older samples, but not in younger samples, when using the same task following glucose. Macpherson et al. (2015) in a two-by-two design (age by task difficulty) found a benefit for glucose only in older participants with the harder task – not perhaps what would be expected, as the predicted outcome would be beneficial in young participants on the hard task and on both tasks in older participants. But of course, this depends on an objective assessment of what constitutes a hard task, of which there is no formal measure. In addition to looking at older participants, four studies have examined task difficulty in children. While some find positive effects for glucose, others do not and no clear picture emerges here (see Smith et al., 2011 for further discussion).

Apart from studies in older populations, there have also been efforts to see if glucose can be beneficial in participants who have a demonstrable cognitive impairment. Many of these studies have focussed on episodic memory, as its decline is a prominent feature of many neurological and psychiatric conditions. In Alzheimer's disease (AD) and mild cognitive impairment (MCI), there is evidence of cognitive enhancement on tests of episodic memory in patients administered glucose (e.g., Manning, Ragozzino, & Gold, 1993), but the size of the benefit to AD and MCI participants is either similar or in some cases less than observed in controls (van der Zwaluw et al., 2015). Three studies have examined the use of glucose to enhance episodic memory performance in schizophrenia, a disease in which there is a known performance deficit in this cognitive domain. All three studies found evidence of a glucose enhancement effect, with data from one study indicating that older schizophrenic participants may gain the most (Smith et al., 2011). In sum, these various findings relating to task difficulty, age and cognitive impairment suggest that glucose's enhancing effects on cognition, and in particular on memory, are *somewhat* more likely to occur when task demand increases (or as we noted earlier, perhaps they supplement impaired glucose metabolism – see discussion later).

Before the close of this section there are a number of residual issues that require mention. In any design involving a psychological variable, participant expectancy effects are always a potential concern, and one that is usually well managed in glucose studies by using a non-nutritive sweetener control. The importance of using such a control is evident from the research that has taken place on expectancy bias with glucose. Expectations over what has been drunk can independently improve memory performance (Stollery & Christian, 2013), vigilance (Green et al., 2001), self-control and decision-making (Job et al., 2013). In most reports, participants are not told what they are drinking until the end of the study. Green et al. (2001) demonstrated that glucose enhancement on a vigilance task did not occur if participants were told, falsely, that the glucose they were about to drink was aspartame. Relatedly, Stollery and Christian (2013), found that believing that glucose had been drunk (even if it was saccharin) improved delayed recall. These findings imply that participants do have positive expectations about the impact of glucose on performance, and they stress the importance of the non-nutritive sweetener control.

A number of studies have also examined whether a participant's glucoregulatory control is a factor in whether glucose will enhance cognitive performance. This is an important consideration and one that is examined further here in the context of diseases of glucose metabolism. The same load of glucose will exert different effects on a person's blood glucose profile across time, dependent on their normal regulatory ability. This baseline ability is itself dependent upon genetic variation, fat mass, time since last meal, age and so forth. As Boyle et al. (2018) point out, this may account for much variance in outcome between experiments. However, as described below, studies that have attempted to take individual-level glucose responses into account do not present an obviously clearer picture.

Looking first at older participants, glucoregulatory capacity seems to have no bearing on study outcome (e.g., Parsons & Gold, 1992). Glucose enhancement of cognition works as well in poor glucoregulators (Kaplan et al., 2000; Messier et al., 2003) as it does in good glucoregulators (Craft, Murphy, & Wemstrom, 1994; Messier, Gagnon, & Knott, 1997). A similarly inconclusive picture emerges with young adults. In these studies participants have blood glucose profiles that all fall within the normal range, but are split into 'better' or 'worse' glucoregulators with responses contrasted between these groups (Boyle et al., 2018; Lamport et al., 2009). Two points need to be made about these types of studies, beyond the *presumed* reliability of these measurements (i.e., would the same assignment be made on a repeat measurement?). First, Smith et al. (2011) suggest that a major confound is the way in which 'better' and 'worse' glucoregulators are identified. Not only are there several potential measures that can be used to classify, the classification itself is typically achieved by median split. Consequently, what may be regarded as poor glucoregulation in one study may count as good glucoregulation in another. A second issue that needs to be considered is the length of fast, which varies markedly between experiments. Using the 55 studies identified with fast length data from Boyle et al.'s (2018) review, we could find no association between a successful glucose enhancement effect and length of fast (p = .23). In sum, while differences in glucoregulatory ability appear a promising source of inter-study and inter-participant variability, the evidence so far has not been supportive.

Diseases of Glucose Metabolism and Cognition As that discussion suggests, variation in glucoregulation in largely normal (i.e., euglycemic) populations has not revealed much about variability in the outcome of glucose enhancement studies. However, the diabetes and cognition literature has some interesting and relevant findings. The first concerns the cognitive effects of episodes of hypoglycaemia (i.e., acute decreases in blood sugar), which is to some extent the reverse of what has been examined so far (i.e., acute increases in blood glucose). The second concerns the neural and cognitive consequences of impaired control of blood glucose. Although this material pertains to chronic conditions, it can be revealing because chronic effects are to some degree the sum of multiple acute impacts. Thus, their study has the potential to offer insights into the brain areas affected under acute glucose manipulations – something we will return to when considering mechanism.

The first issue concerns the effects of episodes of hypoglycaemia. These usually occur in patients who are insulin dependent, and so these cases tend to have Type I (i.e., childhood onset and typically not lifestyle related) diabetes rather than Type II (i.e., late onset and lifestyle related), where use of insulin is less common. A number of early studies with Type I (Brands et al., 2005) and type II diabetics (Reijmer et al., 2010) found no evidence that single or multiple hypoglycaemic episodes were connected with any impact on cognitive function (or abnormality on neuroimaging; Moulton et al., 2015). However, a more recent meta-analysis, combining studies of type I and II diabetics, with and without hypoglycaemic episodes, suggests that experience of prior hypoglcaemic episodes is associated solely with a small impairment in learning and memory (Chen et al., 2017). Although a weak effect, this suggests that out of all cognitive domains, it is learning and memory that is sensitive to the effects of very low blood glucose.

A second issue concerns the pattern of cognitive and neural impairment associated with poor blood glucose control. Interestingly, type I diabetes has a cognitive impairment and neuroimaging profile that is somewhat different from type II diabetes. Meta-analysis suggests that the cognitive impairment profile for type I diabetes impacts IQ, attention, cognitive flexibility and speed of processing, but with no consistent deficits in learning and memory (Brands et al., 2005). For type II diabetes, deficits in verbal learning and memory, executive function, attention and speed of processing are prominent features (Reijmer et al., 2010). On imaging, type I diabetes is associated with significant reductions in thalamic volume, while type II diabetes is linked to reductions in the hippocampus, orbitofrontal cortices and basal ganglia, with younger age associated with especially prominent volume loss in the hippocampus (Moulton et al., 2015). What is interesting about these findings is that it is type II diabetes that is associated with prominent impairments in HDLM, and hippocampal volume loss, and it is HDLM that seems most responsive to the acute administration of glucose. What this may imply is that chronic exposure to diets rich in added sugar and saturated fat – a feature of the Western lifestyle linked to type II diabetes – seem to impair the same brain structure and related functions that *benefit* from acute administration of glucose. This seems an interesting symmetry.

Effects of Glucose on Decision-Making   With very limited overlap with the literature on the effect of glucose on neuropsychological test performance, another body of work has emerged over the last 20 years studying what are termed the effects of 'glucose' on human decision-making (glucose is in quotes for reasons that will become apparent). Much of this work (depending on how you categorise it), concerns self-control, and because of the major practical ramifications that flow from self-control failures – drug abuse, gambling, etc. – this literature has attracted much scientific and popular attention. For example, one of the key theoretical papers in this area, Muraven and Baumeister (2000), has been cited more than 1,800 times. The basic idea advanced by Muraven and Baumeister (2000) is that self-control is a limited resource. This is illustrated by a particular type of experimental outcome called the ego-depletion effect. Participants are randomly assigned to two groups – Depletion or Control. Depletion participants undertake either a self-control task, or a task that requires considerable motivation to complete successfully (e.g., a boring vigilance task). Control participants complete a task that has neither of these features (i.e., one *not* requiring high motivation/self-control). Following a short break, all participants are then asked to undertake a self-control task (typically unrelated to the one completed by the Depletion group). Performance is usually poorer in the Depletion group, although in line with the general high-level of disagreement in this area, there is now a dispute over whether this effect is actually 'real'. One widely influential meta-analysis finds a moderate-to-large effect size (Hagger et al., 2010), while another using a different approach concludes there is no effect at all (Carter et al., 2015). Could anyone claim that meta-analysis can settle scientific debates? It all depends on the assumptions that you make or your 'priors' in Bayesian terms.

Building on the idea of self-control as a limited resource, Gailliot and Baumeister (2007), suggested a simple but testable metabolic model: (1) self-control is a limited resource; (2) the physical manifestation of this resource is blood glucose; and (3) self-control tasks draw down blood glucose, because the brain requires additional energy in the form of glucose to exercise willpower. Three testable consequences flow from this model. First, self-control tasks should lead to reductions in blood glucose. Second, the further blood glucose falls following a self-control task, the poorer one should perform on a subsequent self-control task. And finally, and most importantly here, ingesting glucose should improve self-control, by boosting the availability of this limited fuel resource. Meta-analysis has cast some doubt on the validity of the first and second testable consequence

(Dang, 2016), but our focus is on the impact of glucose on self-control, even if the 'whole brain' glucose-depletion model is unlikely to be correct (more later; and see Messier, 2004).

There are five sets of findings relating to self-control, where 'glucose' has been manipulated. Importantly, and as our use of quotes suggests, rather than directly manipulating glucose, many of the studies in this literature use other carbohydrates, from the disaccharide sucrose (e.g., Gailliot, Baumeister, & DeWall, 2007; Molden et al., 2012) right through to whole foods like bread (e.g., Tom & Rucker, 1975) and tomato soup (e.g., Forzano et al., 2010). While all of these provide glucose following digestion, they also involve other carbohydrates and macronutrients (amongst other differences), clouding our attempt to discern glucose-specific effects. For example, take the simplest case of sucrose, which has been used in several key studies. Upon digestion, sucrose yields both glucose and fructose. Fructose does not appear to affect blood glucose levels (Sánchez-Lozada, Le, Segal, & Johnson, 2008), however it has been hypothesised to exert effects on cognition via other pathways (vagal afferents), something considered later in this section. So, while these self-control studies are far from being 'pure' tests of Gailliot and Baumeister's (2007) glucose-based model, the reported studies will all impact blood glucose. Moreover, because Gailliot and Baumeister's (2007) theory explicitly concerns acute changes in blood glucose, it seems appropriate to include them all here.

The five domains of self-control where the effects of manipulating blood glucose have been explored are: ego depletion; decision style; willingness to pay; willingness to work; and time discounting. Starting with ego depletion, Dang (2016) conducted a meta-analysis of such studies that had utilised a glucose manipulation (i.e., some form of carbohydrate) versus placebo; that is, following the depleting task participants received a sucrose drink (glucose-generating energy source) before undertaking the key outcome self-control task (or a non-nutritive sweetener in the placebo control). The conclusion from these studies is not clear-cut and depends on how one categorises the depletion and outcome tasks. If definitions are based on 'self-control' in its narrowest sense, then there is no overall effect on the meta-analysis, but if *all* studies using a depletion design are included there is a significant effect. To complicate matters further, taking into account publication bias using the trim and fit procedure renders this last-mentioned significant effect non-significant, but whether such statistical adjustments are appropriate is also open to debate.

A further issue has been the finding that simply rinsing the mouth with glucose (or sucrose) can confer the same benefits as ingesting it, with the rinse having to be an energy source to be effective; rinsing with a non-nutritive sweetener is not effective (Molden et al., 2012). However, these effects have also proved difficult to replicate (Boyle et al., 2016). In sum, and setting aside the wider concerns over whether ego-depletion itself is a reliable effect (Carter et al., 2015), there is at best only weak support for the idea that glucose (or glucose-generating energy sources) can improve self-control.

Decision style refers to whether a more automatic and intuitive approach to problem solving is adopted versus a more effortful and deliberative approach. In Orquin and Kurzban's (2016) review, four studies examined whether providing a glucose-generating energy source would facilitate more effortful and deliberative reasoning style. All four reported effects consistent with this outcome. For willingness to pay and work, and time discounting, the outcome depends on the type of target (Orquin & Kurzban, 2016). For willingness to pay (i.e., decisions whether or not to spend money) and willingness to work (i.e., decisions about whether to expend effort on working or not), a glucose-generating energy source reduced willingness to work and pay when the target object was food (all six studies consistent with this outcome). In contrast, when the target object was not food related, consuming a glucose-generating energy source encouraged thrift and harder work to obtain the goal (all four studies consistent with this outcome). Finally, for time discounting (immediate smaller reward now or a bigger reward later), there is no clear effect for either non-food or food-based outcomes (Orquin & Kurzban, 2016). For food-based outcomes, some studies find enhanced self-control following a glucose-generating energy source (e.g., Forzano et al., 2010) and others find reduced self-control (e.g., Kirk & Logue, 1997).

In sum, glucose-generating energy sources facilitate more effortful and deliberative decision-making. Consuming glucose-generating energy sources lowers the amount of effort that people are prepared to expend on obtaining food, while increasing it for obtaining non-food goals. For the more directly self-control-relevant paradigms of ego depletion and time discounting, the evidence for a glucose effect was not well supported.

3.4.1.2 Other Carbohydrates

Apart from the studies on self-control, which used a variety of glucose-generating energy sources, there are two additional bodies of research that have examined the acute effects of other classes of carbohydrate. These can be divided into studies examining specific chemicals, namely sucrose, fructose and isomaltulose, and those exploring the impacts on cognition of the blood glucose response profiles (notably the glycaemic index) to different carbohydrate-containing foods. The specific chemicals are dealt with first.

Starting with the disaccharide sucrose, six studies have examined its acute cognitive effects (Boyle et al., 2018) – setting aside those in the self-control literature. Two studies in children found no cognitive benefits. In younger adults, one study found beneficial effects on attention, another on visuospatial skills and a third found no specific benefits. In elderly participants, one study examined people with mild memory impairments, and found several cognitive improvements following a larger (100 g) but not a smaller (50 g) sucrose dose. For the disaccharide isomaltulose (Boyle et al., 2018), which has the same constituents as sucrose (i.e., glucose and fructose) but connected at different points (α-1,6), the literature on its acute cognitive impacts is as diverse as sucrose. In adults, two studies suggest it may benefit attention, another indicates no effects on cognition, while in children it may enable longer study time if used as a sweetener at breakfast. Finally, one study has examined fructose, observing that it enhanced problem solving. As noted earlier, fructose does not affect blood glucose levels and in addition it neither crosses the blood-brain barrier nor does it directly affect cellular metabolism. This implies that any cognitive effects are either motivational (i.e., from its oro-sensory properties) or from peripheral metabolic detection in the liver, transmitted to the brain via vagal afferents (Boyle et al., 2018).

The remainder of the carbohydrate literature has focussed on comparing the cognitive effects of low versus high glycaemic index meals. Glycaemic index (GI) refers to the 2-hour post-ingestion blood glucose profile (measured as the area under the curve – see Figure 3.2) of a food/meal relative to the profile from consuming glucose or white bread. Glycaemic load (GL) is an additional measure which takes into account variation in the quantity of carbohydrate consumed. So, while GI is fundamentally a measure of carbohydrate quality, GL is a measure of both quantity and quality. The literature has, however, focussed almost exclusively on GI.

Lower-GI foods (e.g., beans) are those that have a smaller blood glucose response profile (i.e., 2 h area under the curve) than higher-GI foods (e.g., corn flakes). This smaller blood glucose response profile has been associated with a number of health benefits when looking at chronic exposure to high- or low-GI diets, with low-GI diets especially linked to better

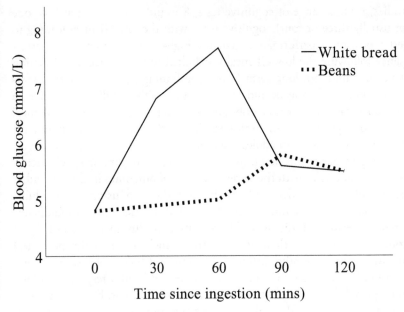

Figure 3.2   Blood-glucose response across time following consumption of white bread and beans

metabolic and cardiovascular parameters as people age (Chiu, Liu, & Willett, 2011). In the context of this general idea that low-GI foods may be healthier, and knowing that low-GI foods result in a slower and more sustained release of glucose into the bloodstream, several investigators have explored whether acute exposure to low-GI foods is associated with a *better* set of cognitive outcomes. However, in the context of all of these findings for the cognitive benefits associated with the acute consumption of glucose, one might reasonably presume the *opposite* outcome, namely that high-GI foods should enhance cognition relative to low-GI foods!

Most studies in this area contrast a high-GI meal, typically breakfast, with a low-GI meal, usually employing a within-subject (cross-over) design. Cognitive tests are administered before the meal, and then at varying time intervals afterwards (up to 3–4 hours). An early review by Blaak, Antoine, and Benton (2012) was inconclusive in terms of the benefits of low-GI versus high-GI meals. A more recent systematic review (Philippou & Constantinou, 2014), alongside a search for new studies since this review was undertaken (i.e., Bragg et al., 2017; Cooper et al., 2015), suggests a similarly inconclusive picture. Across the 13 identified studies, using a range of cognitive tests, 8 found evidence on at least one (of usually three or four) cognitive tests, with the low-GI meal leading to better post-meal performance than the high-GI meal. Enhanced performance following the low-GI meal was linked to better executive function (1 positive finding), long-term (2 positive findings) and short-term memory (3 positive findings), and attention (3 positive findings), relative to high-GI meals. In contrast, only one study reported that a high-GI meal enhanced cognition, with Smith et al. (1988) finding better long-term memory performance in adolescents following a high-GI breakfast.

Trying to clarify this literature by stratifying it by participant characteristics does not help, with the same mixed set of outcomes in the six studies using children, the five with adults and the two using older adults. Philippou and Constantinou (2014) note that the many procedural inconsistencies between studies probably contribute to this mixed picture. Apart from participant age, these inconsistencies include when the post-meal cognitive tests were administered, the neuropsychological tests used and variation in individual blood glucose profile and insulin responses to low- and high-GI foods. Two further issues are also pertinent. First, contrasting a high- with a low-GI meal makes interpreting the cognitive outcomes difficult, as it is unclear if high-GI meals lower performance or low-GI meals enhance it (or vice versa). Second, if glucose administration – effectively a high GI manipulation – tends to acutely improve cognition, it is surprising that the preponderance of findings favour low GI manipulations. This relates to the issue of test timing, as tests closer to the meal may favour high-GI foods (more immediate boost in blood glucose), while perhaps ones further out from the meal may favour lower-GI foods (more sustained release). Moreover, there may be demand characteristics that are inherent in presenting participants with actual foods rather than cups of sweetened fluid, with negative expectations surrounding some foods and positive ones surrounding others. In sum, it is currently unclear whether low-GI meals offer any cognitive benefit over high-GI meals.

3.4.1.3   *The Basis of the Glucose Enhancement Effect*
This section focuses on both the location and mechanism by which glucose may enhance cognition, and especially learning and memory.

Location of the Effect   Several workers have pinpointed the hippocampus as the location for glucose's effects on learning and memory (Messier, 2004; Riby, 2004; Smith et al., 2011). Smith et al. (2011) identified two basic sources of evidence for this claim. First, and as noted earlier, tests of

HDLM, episodic memory and related hippocampal-dependent tasks (e.g., remember-know paradigm) seem to be more responsive to the effects of glucose administration than tests from other cognitive domains (Boyle et al., 2018). This impression is buttressed by findings from the animal literature, which also suggests a preponderance of hippocampal-based effects (e.g., Gold, 1995; Messier, 2004). Second, a variety of imaging findings indicate hippocampal involvement.

For functional magnetic resonance imaging (fMRI), there are three studies of interest. First, Stone et al. (2005) scanned schizophrenic participants with poor verbal learning ability, on a word-encoding task undertaken either following a placebo or glucose. While novel word encoding led to hippocampal activation, there was greater parahippo-campal activation when contrasting placebo and glucose conditions (plus activation in occipital, frontal and temporal lobe structures on this key contrast). How specifically this relates to learning and memory is harder to evaluate, as there was no difference in learning and memory perfor-mance between the glucose and placebo conditions – probably due to low power (n = 7). Thus, while some differences in brain activation in the region of interest were identified, this occurred in the absence of a performance benefit and alongside glucose-related activation across sev-eral unanticipated brain areas.

The most extensive investigation of glucose's acute effect on brain and cognition was conducted by Parent et al. (2011) who examined the impact of glucose versus saccharin on memory for negative (i.e., unpleasant) and neutral pictures. Using a within-subject design, participants consumed either the glucose or saccharin-containing fluid, and then were exposed to neutral and negative images while being scanned. Immediately on removal from the scanner participants were asked to verbally recall in detail each of the images they had seen. As blood glucose levels would still be elevated at this stage, in those administered glucose, this tests the effects of glucose on encoding and retrieval. The following day participants were given the same free recall test, but here any beneficial effects of glucose must pertain to encoding, as blood glucose levels cannot differ *here* between the glucose and saccharin recall conditions.

As with the Stone et al. (2005) study, Parent et al. (2011) found no beneficial effect of glucose on memory performance, which may again be attributable to low power. However, two other findings are of interest. First, using all picture-learning trials, the contrast of 'with versus without glucose', revealed just one activity difference in the superior parietal gyrus. When examining this *same* contrast, but now for negative versus neutral

pictures, greater frontal, parietal and insula activity was observed, suggesting that glucose enhances activity across multiple cortical sites during
learning. Second, the authors then examined whether brain processing,
in the glucose versus saccharin condition, differed for successfully retrieved
items versus unsuccessfully retrieved items. Looking at the 5 min recall
test, successful recalls following glucose, were associated with enhanced
activity within several areas of the parietal lobe, while successful recalls the
following day were linked to heightened activity in the hippocampus, and
the frontal and parietal cortices. The key finding here then is evidence of
hippocampal involvement, suggesting that the presence of glucose facilitated hippocampal encoding of images that were later recalled.

While this study highlights hippocampal involvement, it also clearly
demonstrates that many other brain structures are more active following
glucose consumption. Indeed, Parent et al. (2011) also examined for
increases in functional connectivity, and glucose was linked to substantial
enhancements of connectivity (versus saccharin) when using the hippocampus as the seed (connections propagating from this source), but also
when using the amygdala as the seed. Animal studies suggest that glucose
applied directly to the amygdala (and striatum) can enhance performance
on tasks that are presumed to rely upon these areas – including memory
tasks – (Gold, 2014; Schroeder & Packard, 2003), suggesting a more
general brain enhancement effect beyond the hippocampus.

A number of studies have examined the impact on the brain of administering a dose of glucose, but without any imposed cognitive task. Most of
these resting fMRI studies have focussed on specific regions of interest,
finding reduced activity in the hypothalamus following glucose administration and enhanced connectivity between the hypothalamus and other
sub-cortical structures. Only one study has examined whole brain activity
following glucose administration (Al-Zubaidi et al., 2018). They measured
a variety of resting state connectivity parameters (local and regional), while
participants just lay in the scanner. Enhanced connectivity between neigh-
bouring areas within the hippocampus and parahippocampus were identified following glucose administration. However, glucose also impacted a
range of other brain structures, including those in the frontal, parietal and
insular cortices.

Smith et al. (2011) describe evoked potential data, which they suggest
supports a hippocampal origin for glucose's effects on learning and memory. However, spatial localization is not a strong point of electroencepha-
lography (EEG) and there are frequent debates about the neuroanatomical
loci of specific types of evoked potential, and so the relevance of these data

to this particular debate is limited. This leaves the MRI and cognitive data as the two main sources of evidence, and while both indicate hippocampal activation, they also clearly show the involvement of many other brain areas. The MRI data suggests that ingesting glucose affects several cortical and sub-cortical locations, which is consistent with glucose benefitting cognitive functions beyond learning and memory.

A final location-related issue is whether the faciliatory effects of glucose partially or fully originate in the periphery, and thus exert their effects on the brain via some indirect mechanism (Sünram-Lea & Owen, 2017). One route involves peripheral detection of glucose in the liver. Alterations in cell membrane transport of glucose in the liver would offer one means of detecting its presence, and consistent with this is the finding that meta-bolically inactive forms of glucose can have a facilitative effect on memory performance (Messier, 2004). Detection is then followed by a signal to the brain indicating the presence of glucose, with this likely being performed by vagal afferents. Lesions of afferent nerve fibres from the liver stop the facilitative effect of glucose on memory performance in animals (White, 1991), and vagal nerve stimulation can significantly affect (positively and negatively) human cognition (Messier, 2004). Vagal nerve stimulation results in the activation of a wide range of brain structures (Chae, Nahas, & Lomarev, 2003), including much of the neocortex (frontal, parietal, temporal, insula and occipital), and many sub-cortical regions (e.g., thalamus, hypothalamus, hippocampus). It is conceivable then, that glucose exerts its effects – partly or in whole – via the vagus, and so the activations reported in the imaging studies above could be vagally driven. In the absence of further data, it is probably best to assume that glucose has both peripheral impact via the vagus, as well as direct effects on the brain and cognition.

Glucose as the Primary Cause   Glucose is the primary energy source of the brain, except under conditions of starvation when ketone bodies are oxidised for energy (Siesjo, 1978). Glucose is also necessary for the synthesis of acetylcholine. Given the brain's metabolic reliance on glucose, completing a task might temporarily deplete supplies. Consequently, providing additional glucose should either prevent this shortfall occurring or rapidly replace the deficit, thereby enhancing performance. One prob-lem with this account is that the energy supply system to the brain is *very* carefully choreographed (Benarroch, 2014). Glucose is transported across the blood-brain barrier by the GLUT1 glucose transporter. Some of the transported glucose remains in the extracellular space directly available for neurons to take up, but the greater proportion seems to be moved into astrocytes and then transported directly into neurons as either glucose or lactate. Variations in local brain metabolism cause the capillaries *in that specific area* to expand, increasing available glucose and the uptake process just described. This rapid haemodynamic response to local energy needs driven by cognition, forms the basis for much neuroimaging, but more importantly suggests that the brain is generally well able to coordinate delivery of glucose (and oxygen) to where it is needed.

Having said this, a number of findings suggest that there may be rate-limiting steps in the processes described, and that providing additional glucose may sidestep these. Gold and colleagues have been the most prominent advocates of this idea, and claim that neuronal uptake of glucose, especially from the extracellular fluid, is a rate-limiting factor on neuronal function (e.g., McNay, & Gold, 2002). A different perspective is that of Convit (2005) who claims that the rate-limiting factor is the movement of glucose via GLUT1 across the blood-brain barrier (i.e., through capillary endothelial cells). However, the number of GLUT1 transporters available for moving glucose into the brain can be rapidly increased following local depletion of glucose (Lee & Klip, 2012), and so it is possible that this becomes more of an issue if the ability to up-regulate GLUT1 is impaired – something that may happen in elderly people and elderly animals.

Gold's model is based on the premise of specific local need, which assumes – quite reasonably (and think neuroimaging) – that neuronal activity and energy requirements in one brain area are relatively discrete from another (McNay & Gold, 2002). According to this model, greater task demand increases neuronal activity within the area (areas) of the brain engaged in solving the problem. As task demand increases, neuronal glucose usage increases, depleting extracellular reserves (see Figure 3.3). McNay, Fries, and Gold (2000) demonstrated this phenomenon in rats, by monitoring hippocampal blood glucose levels in response to tasks of varying difficulty, and which were reliant upon this brain area for perfor-mance. Three key findings emerged from this study. First, as task difficulty increased, extracellular glucose levels in the hippocampus fell. Second, providing systemic glucose about 10 min before testing eliminated these task-difficulty-related differences in glucose. Third, performance on the more difficult task was facilitated by the administration of systemic glucose. Together, these findings suggest that: (1) more demanding cognitive tasks deplete local extracellular glucose, (2) augmenting this supply by increasing blood glucose levels results in task-stable hippocampal extracellular glucose

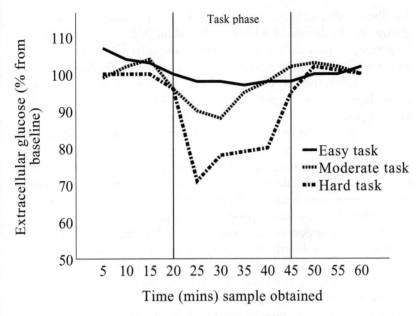

Figure 3.3   Neuronal glucose usage.
Source: Adapted from data presented in McNay et al. (2000)

levels and (3) this causes better task performance (Gold, 2014). One additional mechanism here is that astrocytes may also accumulate greater glucose reserves following the elevation in blood glucose and can thus also better buffer against a period of enhanced neuronal metabolic activity. Irrespective of the specifics, the idea that systemic administration of glucose exerts its beneficial effects on cognition by leading to increases in the local availability of glucose to task-relevant neurons seems well-supported (Gold, 2014). While there are additional pathways (below) that can also facilitate cognition, these are in many cases independent of what we are discussing here.

Glucose as the Secondary Cause   Elevating blood glucose levels has a number of secondary consequences that could affect cognition. One consequence of ingesting glucose is that it will result in peripheral insulin release. Insulin is actively transported into the rat and human brain (Pomytkin, Costa-Nunes, & Kasatkin, 2018). The rat and human brain both contain insulin receptors in multiple sites (including the hippocampus), and at a cellular level they are especially abundant on astrocytes. As described earlier, astrocytes play a central role in managing the supply of glucose in the brain. In addition, the brain, and again including the hippocampus, contains a further glucose transporter GLUT4 that is insulin sensitive (i.e., insulin activates glucose transport). The GLUT4 transporter is found especially on neurons, and very densely on pyramidal cells in the hippocampus. Exposure to insulin, which occurs after a meal or ingesting glucose, acts then to enhance glucose uptake into neurons, and especially neurons in the hippocampus involved in learning and memory (Pearson-Leary et al., 2018).

While there is growing support for the idea that the human brain may itself generate insulin de novo, the role of this in the brain's system of energy management is unclear (Pomytkin et al., 2018). However, what is abundantly clear and well supported is that insulin in animals can act to improve cognitive performance, and especially learning and memory, both when it is injected directly into brain areas like the hippocampus (holding glucose constant) and when administered peripherally (holding glucose constant; Convit, 2005; Heni et al., 2015; Pomytkin et al., 2018). Insulin can also be administered intranasally in humans, and this too has been shown to improve cognition in healthy adults, in the elderly and in people with Alzheimer's disease (Heni et al., 2015; Pomytkin et al., 2018). A key issue here is the difficulty in teasing apart any effects of insulin from those of glucose, and vice versa. Should this seem to be contradicted by glucose clamp studies (i.e., holding glucose constant while insulin level is manipulated), it should be remembered that this technique involves actively infusing glucose to keep its levels stable. In other words, it is not really possible to manipulate one without altering the other, and thus any effects of glucose could be mediated via insulin or vice versa (Messier, 2004).

Glucose ingestion can also influence the production of the neurotransmitter acetylcholine, which is involved in learning and memory (Messier, 2004). The most telling demonstration of this phenomenon is a rat experiment conducted by Ragozzino, Unick, and Gold (1996). Only a moderate dose of glucose, administered peripherally via injection, resulted in enhanced (over saline injection) acute production of acetylcholine in the hippocampus, during a maze-learning task. Similarly, only the moderate dose of glucose enhanced learning on this task, suggesting that the effects of glucose may be exerted through its effect on acetylcholine production. This conclusion is further strengthened by the finding that the effects of the anticholinergic agent scopolamine can be ameliorated by the administration of glucose, and that subthreshold doses of glucose and choline (precursors to acetylcholine) act synergistically to enhance memory in mice (e.g., Kopf et al., 2001). However, as Messier (2004) notes, one problem with this explanation of glucose's effects is that the cellular reservoir of acetylcholine is likely to be large, and so additional glucose might not be expected to impact this. Nonetheless, animal data suggest that acetylcholine production is enhanced by glucose, and this may be an additional route by which it effects cognition, and especially learning and memory.

A further suggestion has been the impact that ingested glucose has on a particular form of inwardly rectifying potassium channel – the K_{atp} channel. Many cell types, and especially neurons, possess K_{atp} channels. These channels are metabolically sensitive, such that increases in ATP abundance (generated by the degradation of glucose) result in channel blockade. This channel blockade seems to enhance learning and memory, at least in animal models, and the effect can be obtained without using glucose, by employing a K_{atp} channel blocking agent (Stefani, Nicholson, & Gold, 1999). Two questions remain. First, does this also occur in humans, and second, how does blocking the K_{atp} channel facilitate learning and memory? Functionally, channel blockade may alter the stability of the neuron, leading to a more concerted response across many neurons during a learning event (i.e., a larger number of depolarisation events due to a greater number of unstable neurons). Whether this occurs in humans is not known.

A number of authors have suggested what has become known as the emotional memory hypothesis (Gold, 2014; Smith et al., 2011). According to this account, stressful events or arousing stimuli lead to the release of epinephrine, both peripherally, from the adrenal medulla of the kidney, and centrally. One consequence of epinephrine release is an increase in blood glucose (Rizza, Haymond, Cryer, & Gerich, 1979). One consequence of experiencing stressful and arousing events is that they often form robust memories (LaBar & Cabeza, 2006) – as functionally it may be beneficial to learn the antecedents and consequences of emotionally arousing situations (e.g., nearly getting run over by a car while looking at your phone *should* change behaviour). The emotional memory hypothesis links these two consequences, with the claim that glucose is the, or one of the, mechanisms that generates a more robust memory. The principal problem here is not scientific (indeed the animal data is consistent – see Gold, 2014, for review), but whether it can ever be appropriately tested in humans. That is, can an ethically *and* scientifically sound test be undertaken? The Parent, Varnhagen, and Gold (1999) neuroimaging study included a test of part of this hypothesis by using unpleasantly arousing pictures, and while they found increased activity in the amygdala (a brain structure that may facilitate arousal-related memories) during viewing of these images, they found no evidence of selectively better memory performance. The obvious interpretive problem here is whether the stimuli were of sufficient emotional potency, and using more potently arousing stimuli can generate ethical concerns.

Finally, Messier (2004), makes the interesting point that any energy source will act as a memory enhancer. In some sense this has to be true, because if an event is followed by a reward that yields energy, this will lead to a change in behaviour, which will be underpinned by a change in neural connectivity between the representation of the event and its consequent – a memory. Psychologists normally think of this type of situation as a logical consequence of organisms acting to maximise biologically important goals (feeding, drinking, sex) and minimising dangerous outcomes (disease, pain) with such reward or punishment triggering the brain to encode a memory. However, Messier's (2004) analysis (and see White, 1989) suggests something additional, namely that energetic food rewards (e.g., glucose) serve an active *pharmacological role* in encoding memory.

3.4.1.4 Carbohydrates: Conclusions

Glucose seems to facilitate learning and memory in animals and humans, and cognition more generally. The self-control literature offers a less convincing picture. How glucose exerts its enhancing effects, especially on memory, has provoked substantial interest. Several brain areas show enhanced activity after peripheral administration of glucose, and the idea that its local availability, especially in the hippocampus, may be a rate-limiting factor for certain tasks seems well supported in animal models. A number of other hypotheses have also been advanced to explain glucose's enhancement effects, including its effects on acetylcholine synthesis and the hard-to-disentangle role of insulin. At a more functional level of explanation, glucose's capacity to facilitate cognition, and especially learning and memory, may be part of the system that generates strong emotional memories, and/or as the primary energy source of the brain, glucose may serve to consolidate memories linked to obtaining itself – energy.

3.4.2 Proteins and Fats

3.4.2.1 General Effects

Around 13 studies have examined the acute impact of protein and fat on cognition (see Table 3.3). These studies have generally been conducted in young people (Kaplan et al., 2000, being the exception and using elderly

Table 3.3. *Summary of studies testing acute macronutrient effects beyond just carbohydrates*

Study	Tests	Compares	Mood	Fatigue	Attention	RT	Memory	Executive
Lloyd et al., '94	F[1]C[2]	L[3]FH[4]C, M[5]FMC, HFLC	No effect	HFLC most	No effect	MFMC best	No effect	Not tested
Uijtdehaage et al., '94	CP[6]	C, P, Con[7]	No effect	No effect	No effect	Not tested	Not tested	No effect
Lloyd et al., '96	FC	LFHC, MFMC, HFLC, Con	No effect	MF/HF most	No effect	No effect	No effect	Not tested
Wells and Read, '96	FC	HFLC, LFHC	No effect	HFLC most	No effect	No effect	Not tested	Not tested
Cuncliffe et al., '97	FC	C, F, Con	No effect	C most	No effect	No effect	No effect	Not tested
Kaplan et al., '01	FCP	C, F, P, Con	Not tested	Not tested	No effect	Not tested	CFP all+	Not tested
Fischer et al., '01	FCP	C, F, P	No effect	No effect	F weak+	F weak+	Not tested	Not tested
Fischer et al., '02	CP	C, P, CPmix[8]	No effect	No effect	No effect	P+	Not tested	Not tested
Nabb and Benton, '06[9]	FCP	HC, LC, HF, LF, HP, LP	Not tested	Not tested	No effect	No effect	No effect	Not tested
Jones et al., '12	FCP	C, F, P, Con	No effect	No effect	C weak+	No effect	P+	CFP all+
Silvola et al., '13	CP	C, P, Con	No effect	C most	No effect	Not tested	Not tested	No effect
Bachlechner et al., '17	FCP	C, F, P, Con	FP mood-	P most	No effect	Not tested	Not tested	No effect
Miller et al., '18	F	F_{sat}[10], F_{cla}[11], Con	Not tested	Not tested	Not tested	Not tested	F_{cla} learn+	Not tested

[1]Fat, [2]carbohydrate, [3]low, [4]high, [5]medium, [6]protein, [7]control (sometimes zero energy), [8]mixture, [9]Note that Nabb and Benton (2006) found that blood glucose profile moderated responses to most test domains, but as there were no main effects of macronutrients, we just report these as null effects, [10]saturated fat, [11]conjugated linoleic acid.

participants), and usually contrast either two or three macronutrients (generally including a carbohydrate), determining their effects on mood, fatigue, attention, reaction time, learning, memory and executive function. There are no clear outcomes, and the reasons for this are likely to reside, as noted earlier, in the many procedural differences between studies, in addition to some systemic problems. The procedural differences relate to the specific nature of the fats and proteins under study (i.e., are they in a food matrix, alone and what specific fat or protein is used?), the large array of neuropsychological tests used, some of which are hard to classify, and the varying length of time from ingestion to test. More systemic problems include a lack of clarity over the theoretical basis for predicted outcomes, and low sample size and attendant lack of power.

As a casual glance at Table 3.3 will suggest, there is no consensus across the various test domains. For fatigue, examples where fat, protein and carbohydrate ingestion result in greater tiredness can be found. Attention and reaction time tests also reveal examples of facilitation by fats, proteins and carbohydrates, as with memory and executive function testing. Looking at more specific studies, three warrant comment. First, Kaplan et al (2000) is the only study in the elderly, and used a very delimited range of test domains, finding strong evidence that all three macronutrient types could affect immediate and delayed memory, relative to a sweet non-nutritive control condition. Second, Jones, Sunram-Lea, and Wesnes (2012) made a much more specific and defined choice of macronutrient stimuli (i.e., using *just* fats in the fat condition) and equated presentation across stimulus types to minimise expectancy effects. Third, Miller et al. (2018) contrasted two fat types (saturated vs conjugated linoleic acid (CLA)) with a vehicle control, and was unusual in having clearly developed and specific hypotheses about the acute effects of these agents – at least some of which were confirmed (i.e., CLA facilitates extinction of a conditioned fear response). In sum, there is no clear picture of what acute effects follow from protein and fat ingestion.

Finally, it is useful to ask what effects might be expected. Based on Messier's (2004) hypothesis that energy-containing nutrients should serve as memory enhancers, one would expect fats to be especially potent enhancers as they contain more energy per gram than carbohydrates and proteins. Of course, this macronutrient is not directly available for neural metabolism like glucose, but it seems odd that this would rule out what might be a highly functional action, namely rapid and interference-resistant learning about sources of fat (and also protein). Kaplan et al. (2001), Jones et al. (2012) and Miller et al. (2018) all test this idea more or less directly, but only Kaplan et al. (2001) provide support, and then again, there is no data as yet to suggest that fat is superior to carbohydrates and protein in facilitating learning and memory.

3.4.2.2 Specific Effects Derived from Protein I: Tryptophan, Tyrosine, Phenylalanine, Histidine

Before turning to the effects of using diet to alter certain neurotransmitter systems, it is important to outline rather specifically how this might occur. One reason for approaching this topic with mechanism first is that for tryptophan in particular, claims surrounding its effects on brain serotonin have been quite controversial. Consequently, it is useful to understand first what manipulating diet can theoretically achieve in terms of altering particular neurotransmitter systems, before turning to see if such manipulations have any impact on the mind.

Three groups of monoamine neurotransmitters, the catecholamines (dopamine, epinephrine and norepinephrine), the indolamines (serotonin) and the imidazoleamines (histamine), are all subject to precursor control (van Ruitenbeek et al., 2009; Wurtman, Hefti, & Melamed, 1980). The amino acid precursor in each case is a digestive product of protein breakdown, namely tyrosine and phenylalanine for catecholamines, tryptophan for serotonin and histidine for histamine. Turning first to tryptophan, this essential (i.e., not synthesisable by the body) amino acid tends to be scarce in dietary protein. Following digestion, tryptophan enters the bloodstream, where its levels are not modulated by any feedback loop (Bank, Own, & Erickson, 2012). This means that if more tryptophan is consumed (e.g., via injection, supplementation), then levels in the blood can increase. Tryptophan, which is a large neutral amino acid (LNAA) is moved across the blood-brain barrier by the same transporter (system L) that also moves the other LNAAs (e.g., tyrosine, threonine), thus there is competition for this transporter. The LNAA with the highest ratio to the remaining LNAAs will enter the brain at the highest rate – a key observation for manipulating entry of tryptophan into the brain.

Tryptophan is unusual in binding to albumin when in the bloodstream. One consequence of this is that when insulin is secreted, which also serves to increase the uptake of LNAAs into muscle, tryptophan is not taken up by this tissue, meaning that the tryptophan to LNAA ratio increases. As tryptophan appears to be released from albumin when in proximity to the blood brain barrier, this then allows the passage of tryptophan into the brain driven by the favourable LNAA ratio (Fernstrom, 2013). It was thought at one time that significantly increasing carbohydrate intake, combined with a low protein intake, would be sufficient to lead to a more favourable tryptophan:LNAA ratio, thus enhancing uptake. While this does seem to occur, the ratio increase is not dramatic (14–34% above normal; Lyons & Truswell, 1988; Wurtman et al., 2003), and even this is unlikely to be obtained using 'natural' foods due to their need to be high in carbohydrate whilst being very low in protein (i.e., <5%; Soh & Walter, 2011). A far more successful means of elevating the tryptophan:LNAA ratio comes from using protein sources that are unusually rich in tryptophan, notably alpha-lactalbumin or, more potently still, by intravenous injection of tryptophan (Hulsken et al., 2013).

When tryptophan is transported into the brain, to have any impact on serotonin levels, the steps involved in its synthesis must be amenable to increased production. Serotonin requires a two-step synthesis, with both steps utilising a different enzyme to catalyse each step. Importantly, neither of these enzymes are fully saturated – including the rate-limiting one tryptophan hydroxylase – meaning that greater bioavailability of tryptophan will increase serotonin synthesis (Fernstrom, 2013; Hulsken et al., 2013). That manipulation of tryptophan levels results in lawful and measurable changes in serotonin in the brain has been confirmed in animal models (e.g., Fernstrom & Wurtman, 1971; Sharp, Bramwell, & Grahame-Smith, 1992), and although there is unanimous agreement that this is likely to also occur in humans, there does not appear to be any direct evidence (i.e., beyond measurements of plasma tryptophan:LNAA ratio).

A further and very extensively used approach for modifying the tryptophan:LNAA ratio is to use depletion, which can involve either a high protein (with minimal tryptophan) low carbohydrate diet for a day, followed by a 12 h fast, or loading with LNAAs (i.e., consuming a mix of amino acids – noting that these are highly unpleasant to drink) in the absence of tryptophan. Loading with LNAAs appears to activate protein synthesis in the liver, which draws down peripheral tryptophan. Over several hours this has the effect of depleting central stores of tryptophan, which are not replaced from the periphery (Young, 2013). The consequences of this process have been studied quite extensively in rats and humans. In humans, using radiolabelled tryptophan and positron emission tomography indicates a major reduction in serotonin synthesis in the brain following acute tryptophan depletion (Nishizawa, Benkelfat, & Young, 1997). Relatedly, human levels of the serotonin metabolite 5HIAA in the cerebrospinal fluid, which is used to estimate brain levels of serotonin, are significantly reduced following tryptophan depletion protocols (e.g., Moreno, Parkinson, & Palmer, 2010). While there is consensus that tryptophan depletion drives down brain serotonin levels, there is some controversy over whether any effects of this on behaviour are a sole consequence of serotonin depletion. van Donkelaar et al. (2011) has detailed a variety of other actual or suspected consequences of tryptophan depletion, including its effects on nitrous oxide, neurotophins, the kynurenine pathway and melatonin, amongst other things. More troubling is the notion that serotonin depletion is probably not uniform across the brain and that the size of the serotonin reservoir in particular synapses may sometimes buffer against depletion. As more stressful tasks or procedures are likely to lead to greater serotonin release at synapses, behavioural effects may not be uniformly evident.

Unlike tryptophan, which cannot be synthesised by the body, tyrosine is both more abundant in dietary sources of protein and can be obtained by biosynthesis from phenylalanine. Increasing oral intake of tyrosine from food or by dosing acts to increase the amount of tyrosine in the blood – again there being no modulation of plasma tyrosine levels as with tryptophan (Banks et al., 2012). Increasing plasma tyrosine relative to other LNAAs results in greater transport of it into the brain. Once in the brain, tyrosine is transformed into dopamine in a two-stage synthesis and then in further steps into norepinephrine and epinephrine (Fernstrom, 2013; Wurtman et al., 1980). The rate-limiting process in the synthesis of these catecholamines is the first enzymatic step with tyrosine hydroxylase, and as this is not fully saturated – as with the remaining steps – greater bioavailability of the precursor tyrosine should result in increased production of catecholamines. However, animal data suggests that this process only occurs in actively firing neurons, implying that it may be only under more extreme conditions (e.g., stress, fatigue, task load) that any beneficial effects of tyrosine loading occur (Jongkees et al., 2015). In addition, dopamine levels seem to be rigorously subject to feedback control, such that beyond a certain level tyrosine hydroxylase is inhibited, shutting down further production until dopamine levels again start to fall. It is also unclear what downstream effects tyrosine has on norepinephrine and epinephrine, again with animal data suggesting it may also elevate the latter (e.g., Lehnert et al., 1984), but with little information on the former. This implies that tyrosine dosing may have unintended downstream impacts on norepinephrine. Finally, there is both animal and human (in patients with Parkinson's disease) evidence that tyrosine administration (via dosing, diet and injection) results in central up-regulation of dopamine production in the brain (e.g., Growdon et al., 1982; Scally, Ulus, & Wurtman, 1977). These effects peak 1–2 h post-administration, and last for up to 8 h.

Paralleling the acute tryptophan depletion literature, it is also possible to deplete peripheral and central tyrosine levels, with flow on impacts that seem principally limited to dopamine production (Biggio, Porceddu, & Gessa, 1976; noting this apparent selectivity has not been confirmed in humans). Animal and human studies have utilised mixtures of LNAA's, with no tyrosine and phenylalanine included, which when consumed following an overnight fast have the effect of lowering plasma tyrosine and brain tyrosine, dopamine and its metabolites (e.g., Biggio et al., 1976; McLean et al., 2004; Nagano-Saito, Cisek, & Perna, 2012). The consequences of this have been measured in humans in several different ways. First, using PET, there is a modest increase in (^{11}C) Raclopride (a dopamine receptor antagonist (blocker)) binding following tyrosine depletion, indicating a 10–20% reduction in extracellular striatal dopamine concentration (Montgomery et al., 2003). Second, tyrosine depletion produces a general reduction of activity (using fMRI) in the striatum (e.g., Frank, Veit, & Sauer, 2016) and nucleus accumbens (e.g., Bjork et al., 2014), both areas rich in dopaminergic cells. Third, as dopaminergic neurons in the arcuate nucleus exert a controlling effect over hypothalamic regulation of prolactin release from the pituitary gland, depressing dopamine levels should lead to increases in prolactin levels, which has been observed in several studies (e.g., McTavish et al., 2005; Sevy, Hassoun, & Bechara, 2006). There are also some reports that tyrosine depletion exerts a more potent effect on dopamine in females, than in males (see Frank et al., 2016).

Manipulation of brain histamine via dietary means is the least studied. The only approach to manipulation has been acute histidine depletion, by presenting participants with a mixture of amino acids, but lacking the essential amino acid histidine (van Ruitenbeek et al., 2009). This procedure lowers the histidine to LNAA ratio. This should serve to deplete brain histamine levels by limiting its production. Histamine is synthesised in the brain in a one-step process, by the non-fully-saturated rate-limiting enzyme histidine decarboxylase. The same interpretive caveats apply here as with tyrosine, phenylalanine and tryptophan depletion studies.

The Effects of Manipulating Tryptophan on the Serotonergic System   Tryptophan dosing and depletion have been used extensively to explore the function of the brain's serotonergic system. The central serotonergic system consists of anatomically discrete neurons originating from the raphe nucleus in the brain stem, which project to multiple brain areas. Principal projections from the dorsal and median raphe nuclei are to motor function areas (e.g., cerebellum, substantia nigra), emotion-related areas (e.g., amygdala), stress and homeostatic regulation (e.g., hypothalamus), learning and memory (hippocampus) and to most of the cerebral cortex. Mendelsohn, Riedel, and Sambeth (2009) suggest that the widespread penetration of serotonergic neurons within the brain indicates some form of tonic modulatory role. More specifically, a wide range of functional roles have been suggested, including roles in stress and coping, general inhibition, reward processing, processing aversive stimuli and managing conflicts between the need to act versus the need to restrain.

In addition, the serotonergic system is involved in mood and anxiety disorders, as suggested by the effectiveness of drugs such as selective serotonin reuptake inhibitors, which increase the amount of serotonin left in the synaptic cleft. Given the broad range of anatomical projections and the breadth of hypothesised functional roles, it would seem likely that manipulations of brain serotonin levels would have multiple effects on cognition, emotion processing, and arousal – and all of these areas have been investigated.

Since the 1970s, nearly 50 studies have examined the effects of trypto-phan dosing on cognition, emotion processing, mood, aggression, impul-sivity, fatigue and sleep (Silber & Schmitt, 2010; Steenbergen et al., 2016). Silber and Schmitt (2010) have provided a detailed overview of many of these areas, which we have updated for this section. A number of conclusions emerge from this literature. First, there is little clear evidence for effects of tryptophan dosing on execution function (seven null effects, two enhancement effects, one impairment effect), but slightly more evidence favouring attention (two null effects, three enhancement effects, one impairment effect). Second, there seems to be some evidence for the effects of tryptophan loading on long-term memory, and while there is no agreement over the type of memory stimulus that may benefit (e.g., verbal, visual, abstract), the general trend is consistent (six studies, all with positive effects), and especially so for vulnerable (e.g., stressed), recovering or recovered depressed participants. Third, there seems to be a clear effect of tryptophan loading on psychomotor performance (seven impairment effects, one null effect, one enhancement effect), with this generally worsening after receiving this amino acid. Fourth, effects of tryptophan loading on mood and emotional processing tasks present a very mixed picture and no conclusion is evident (even when taking participant type (stressed, patient, etc.) into account). Fifth, fatigue generally increases following tryptophan loading (7/9 studies), sleep latency is decreased (6/9 studies), especially in those with poor sleep, and objective sleep parameters are altered and reports of sleep improved. It seems likely that this propensity for fatigue following tryptophan dosing, may explain poorer psychomotor performance. Finally, tryptophan dosing does not seem to systematically improve impulsivity or reduce aggression, although relatedly, two studies suggest it improves trust and generosity (Colzato et al., 2013; Steenbergen, Sellaro, & Colzato, 2014). In sum, two general conclusions emerge: long-term memory is improved and fatigue increased.

The literature on acute tryptophan depletion (ATD) is more extensive still, with nearly 300 papers including both human and animal studies. Interest in this procedure developed around understanding serotonin's role in depression, and at least some early studies reported that ATD in people recovering or recovered from depression led to temporary relapse, with the re-emergence of their depressive symptoms (Young, 2013). Indeed, this initial finding echoes the more general picture that emerges on the effects of ATD on mood. In animals, it is difficult to detect any systematic effect of ATD on affective behaviour, and perhaps the reason for this is that there needs to be some pre-existing or latent psychopathology for ATD to exert an effect (Jenkins et al., 2016). In humans, people who have recovered from depression, people who are recovered and on drugs for depression, and people with a family history of depression are susceptible to low mood following ATD, but this does not routinely occur in otherwise healthy people without these risk factors (Ruhé, Mason, & Scheene, 2007).

The impact of ATD on cognition has also been examined. There is little evidence for any consistent effect of ATD on executive function, attention (except perhaps in elderly participants) and psychomotor performance (Mendelsohn et al., 2009). The effects of ATD on memory are complex, with a seemingly selective impairment on long-term verbal memory that involves a visual learning component, in contrast to an auditory learning component. Effects on other forms of episodic memory are inconsistent, with this heterogeneity not readily explained by methodological or participant characteristics (Mendelsohn et al., 2009). There are no consistent findings for ATD effects on measures relating to impulsivity. In contrast, emotion-related processing deficits do seem to emerge in the same population groups who are vulnerable to ATDs effect on mood (Jenkins et al., 2016). fMRI data suggests that these effects may be mediated by increased amygdala activation – the most consistent activation effect observed in ATD neuroimaging studies examining emotion processing (Raab, Kirsch, & Mier, 2016).

Another body of research that has utilised the ATD technique is that exploring the role of serotonin in aggression. The basic hypothesis is that lower levels of serotonin in the brain are associated with higher levels of aggression; thus, as ATD lowers serotonin levels it should act to increase aggression. In a meta-analysis of 38 studies examining this proposition, Duke et al. (2013) reported a small but significant overall effect. As hypothesised, lowering serotonin levels resulted in an increase in aggression. This effect was significantly heterogenous, and this variability across studies was not explained by either methodological variables or sample characteristics. Thus, patient populations were as likely to show increased aggression as those without any identified vulnerabilities. Related to aggression, researchers have also explored the impact of ATD on punishment and reward. It is apparent from this literature that ATD has little effect on reward processing, but does alter perception of punishment (Faulkner & Deakin, 2014). Amidst a number of contradictory findings, ATD punishment studies suggest that serotonin may improve resilience to aversive stimuli.

The most convincing effects to emerge from the tryptophan dosing studies concern its fatigue-enhancing effects, with related findings on more rapid sleep onset latencies and poorer psychomotor performance. The obvious corollary of this would then be increased arousal and poorer sleep following ATD. Indeed, animal data suggest that drug-based inhibition of serotonin or destruction of the raphe nucleus serotonergic neurons leads to a protracted period of insomnia. However, monitoring of animal brains suggests that raphe activation is highest during wakefulness and suppressed during sleep (Jenkins et al., 2016). One way of reconciling these results is that high serotonin levels during wakefulness may be a necessary state for later effective sleep (Arnulf, Quintin, & Alvarez, 2002). On this basis, then, ATD given prior to sleep (i.e., during the day/evening) should impair sleep by lowering serotonin levels during wakefulness, and thus interfering with the appropriate pattern of release. In healthy participants this seems to be the case, with the most notable impacts on REM sleep, and impaired sleep quality (Jenkins et al., 2016). In participants with existing vulnerabilities (see earlier), ATD tends to worsen sleep quality, noting that many of these individuals already had sleep-related problems.

The Effects of Manipulating Tyrosine on the Dopaminergic System Most of the focus of tyrosine dosing and depletion studies have been on its impact upon the dopaminergic system. In addition to the regulatory control of the pituitary gland (see earlier), there are two main sources of brain dopaminergic projections, that are relevant to function. The first source is the ventral tegmental area of the midbrain, with two major projections – the mesocortical and mesolimbic pathways. The mesolimbic pathway is involved in reward and aversion, and projects to the amygdala, hippocampus, nucleus accumbens and olfactory tubercle. The mesocortical pathway, involved in working memory, attention, inhibitory control and cognitive flexibility, projects to the entire cortex, but especially densely to the prefrontal, motor/perirhinal and cingulate cortices. The second source is the substantia nigra of the midbrain, which projects dopaminergic neurons to the caudate nucleus and putamen. As damage to these dopaminergic cells results in the abnormalities of movement associated with Parkinson's disease, functionally these set of projections are important in initiating and inhibiting voluntary movements. Abnormalities of the dopaminergic system have featured in theories of schizophrenia, depression, and attention deficit disorder. Not only has there been clinical interest in the effects of manipulating tyrosine in these disorders, but more generally in exploring its effects on reward, impulsivity and executive function.

There are around 40 studies examining the effects of tyrosine dosing on cognition, mood and motor performance in healthy and patient participants (Hase, Jung, & aan het Rot, 2015; Jongkees et al., 2015). In the two major reviews of this literature (Hase et al., 2015; Jongkees et al., 2015), which have been updated here, several conclusions emerge out of what is a varied set of outcomes (i.e., non-replications, variation in supplementing tyrosine dose, variation in interval between dosing and testing). First, and consistent with the way in which dopamine turnover is boosted by tyrosine dosing (i.e., active firing neurons), effects seem more likely under conditions of challenge. This might involve task difficulty, physical or mental fatigue, older age, heat and especially the effects of cold (Baker, Nuccio, & Jeukendrup, 2014; Jongkees et al., 2015). Under such challenge conditions, the most consistent effect has been observed on tests of working memory, such as the N-back task (e.g., Colzato et al., 2013) – with at least nine successful demonstrations (i.e., enhanced performance). However, it is important to reiterate that several studies that meet these challenge conditions have not obtained effects on working memory (e.g., Bloemendaal, Fröböse, & Wegman, 2018), and in some cases have found that tyrosine dosing worsens performance (e.g., van de Rest et al., 2017). Second, tyrosine dosing does not appear to facilitate physical performance or fatigue tolerance, and its effects on mood are unclear (Hase et al., 2015; Jongkees et al., 2015). Third, while effects on vigilance, attention and response inhibition are often positive, there are too few studies and too varied methods to draw any firm conclusion. Fourth, acute studies in patient populations (notably ADHD, schizophrenia, depression and Parkinson's disease) have generally been disappointing (i.e., few benefits; Jongkees et al., 2015). Fifth, one additional source of variation, which might turn out to be important, relates to individual differences in the D2 dopamine receptor. Colzato et al. (2016) have demonstrated that young healthy participants with a particular allelic variation associated with lower striatal dopamine, are significantly more susceptible to tyrosine loading on the N-back and stop signal tasks – measures of working memory and response inhibition – than participants with allelic variations associated with higher levels of striatal dopamine.

The acute tyrosine depletion literature sits at around 30 papers, covering some of the same ground as the dosing literature. For executive function, tyrosine depletion had little effect on either patient or healthy populations (e.g., McLean et al., 2004; McTavish et al., 2005). In their meta-analysis of mood data, Ruhé et al. (2007) found a significant effect of tyrosine depletion on people with a family history of depression, but no effect of this manipulation on people who were in remission from a previous bout of depression. For impulsivity, this literature can be divided into that dealing with impulsive choice (i.e., thoughtless choice) and that dealing with impulsive action (i.e., thoughtless action). For impulsive choice, the results are supportive of a general tendency to: (a) choose short-term large gains at the cost of long-term losses, (b) expend less effort to get a delayed reward and (c) misinterpret the probability of less frequent events (D'Amour-Horvat & Leyton, 2014). For impulsive action, the picture is less clear, with two favourable studies suggesting that tyrosine depletion impairs the capacity to inhibit responses and two studies failing to find such effects (D'Amour-Horvat & Leyton, 2014).

A final set of studies have examined reward processing. The behavioural data is unconvincing, with a number of studies not finding much evidence, apart from a trend for more rapid learning from negative outcomes (Martins, Mehta, & Prata, 2017). Three studies combined behavioural testing with neuroimaging. In two cases, while tyrosine depletion decreased activations in brain areas known to process reward (Bjork et al., 2014; Frank et al., 2016), this was not accompanied by or correlated with abnormalities in reward processing when contrasted with placebo. A further study by Nagano-Saito et al. (2012) observed that reward anticipation on the behavioural task was uncorrelated with striatal activation in the depletion condition, while significantly associated in the placebo condition. So, while tyrosine depletion clearly impacts dopaminergic processing in brain areas associated with reward processing, this does not consistently translate into behaviour.

The Effects of Manipulating Histidine on Brain Histamine Histamine is synthesised in the brain from the essential amino acid histidine, in a one-step process. Animal data suggest that histamine levels can be altered by precursor availability to a greater extent than any other catecholamine (Young, 1996), suggesting that the levels of this neurotransmitter are amenable to dietary manipulation. Histaminergic neurons originate in one location, in the tuberomamillary nucleus of the hypothalamus, and project widely within the brain (Blandina et al., 2012). Histamine seems to exert broad modulatory functions, and it has been suggested that when released from its synapses it behaves more like a local hormone, affecting surrounding neurons, glia and blood vessels, than as a synaptic neurotransmitter (Blandina et al., 2012). Pharmacological studies suggest that increasing histamine levels is associated with improvements in alertness and cognition, and that decreasing histamine levels are linked to impaired performance, fatigue and sleep (van Ruitenbeek, Vermeeren, & Riedel, 2010). Only one study has attempted to manipulate histamine levels through dietary means. In this experiment, participants fasted the night before and were then provided with an amino acid mixture deficient in histidine (van Ruitenbeek et al., 2009). This procedure significantly lowered the histidine/LNAA ratio (59% decrease 2 h following the drink). While the procedure had no effect on behavioural measures of psychomotor performance and reaction time, nor on subjective reports of alertness, it did produce some alterations in electroencephalogram data, relating to response complexity.

3.4.2.3 Specific Effects Derived from Protein II: Excitatory and Inhibitory Amino Acids
The brain employs several amino acids as either excitatory (L-glutamate, L-aspartate, L-cysteine, L-homocysteine) or inhibitory (gamma-aminobutyric acid (GABA), glycine, beta-alanine, taurine) neurotransmitters. Influencing these transmitter systems is clinically significant, particularly because of the ubiquity of GABA and glutamate receptors in the brain, and their involvement in many health conditions (e.g., excitotoxicity associated with glutamate following brain injury, epilepsy, ADHD, etc.). Consequently, there has been a lot of interest in whether dietary supplementation might affect levels of these amino acid neurotransmitters in the brain. However, a key issue is whether any alteration in blood

plasma levels of these amino acids results in changes in brain levels, that is do these amino acids cross the blood-brain barrier?

The answer would appear to be *probably not* (Boonstra et al., 2015; Hawkins et al., 2006; Pardridge, 2007). As with all of the excitatory and inhibitory amino acids, with the exception of cysteine, these can be synthesised by the brain, and as a general rule it is principally essential amino acids (with the exception of cysteine) that are readily transported by facilitative carriers across the blood-brain barrier (Hawkins et al., 2006). With many of these amino acids, and especially with glutamate, their toxicity requires very careful control of brain extracellular levels. Consequently, all of the amino acid neurotransmitters possess sodium dependent transporter systems, which remove these agents from the brain and transport them into endothelial cells that constitute the capillary wall (Hawkins et al., 2006). Here they are either recycled, degraded or shunted into blood plasma.

Based on this perspective, one would not expect consumption of supplements or diets rich in these amino acid neurotransmitters to have much influence on cognition, mood or sleep. There are though several papers claiming they do affect cognition, and especially for GABA (see Boonstra et al., 2015, for discussion of this issue). However, it is plausible that such effects may be mediated by changes to peripheral systems, which then affect the brain via the vagus. A further consideration are amino acids that do pass the blood-brain barrier and that structurally resemble amino acid neurotransmitters. The most well studied example is theanine, which is structurally similar to glutamate (Lardner, 2014). Theanine has been examined in animals and to a lesser extent in humans. It has effects on multiple amino acid transmitter systems (glutamate, glycine, GABA, aspartate) and beyond (affecting catecholamines too), and there is some very limited evidence of acute anxiolytic effects in animals and humans (Lardner, 2014).

3.4.2.4 Specific Effects Derived from Fat: Choline

Choline (and see Chapter 9 for material on deficiency) is classified as an essential nutrient and is derived from phosphatidylcholine, a commonly occurring lipid in foods such as eggs and soya beans (Young, 1996). It has been claimed that dietary increases in choline can result in greater release of acetylcholine in rat brains (Blusztajn & Wurtman, 1983). Choline readily passes through the blood-brain barrier, and increased plasma levels correspond with increased levels in the brain (Amenta & Tayebati, 2008). As a significant proportion of choline is not recycled into acetylcholine production, greater extracellular choline in the brain could in theory result in enhanced choline synthesis. Choline and acetyl coenzyme-A are the two chemicals that form this neurotransmitter, in a single step catalysed by choline acetyltransferase. While there is less controversy about the longer-term effects of choline supplementation on cholinergic neurotransmission in rodents, and agreement that longer-term doses during pregnancy may enhance the foetal cholinergic system, acute effects remain controversial (Tayebati & Amenta, 2013). Moreover, in humans, chronic supplementation in Alzheimer's disease appears to have little benefit in enhancing cognition (in contrast to supplementation of the dopamine precursor L-DOPA in Parkinson's disease), and there is no evidence favouring acute effects on cognition in healthy participants at this time.

3.5 Conclusion

A great deal of effort has been expended on studying the acute effects of food intake. We can say with some certainty that missing breakfast probably does not affect cognition, and that lunch makes you drowsy, although we do not know why. It is also apparent that consuming small quantities of glucose is immediately beneficial for a range of cognitive operations, and that several different mechanisms have been identified that could explain this effect. The monoamine neurotransmitters can be affected by dietary manipulations that serve to increase or deplete their amino acid precursors. Interestingly, their effect on behaviour tends to be complex, and does not resolve into a neat matching of neurotransmitter and function (e.g., serotonin 'the feel good chemical'), although some broad effects come through (e.g., tryptophan dosing and fatigue, tyrosine dosing and enhanced working memory). What perhaps is more surprising is that these potentially powerful techniques to explore neurotransmitter systems have not been adopted by researchers in other areas of psychology and behavioural neuroscience – to explore, for example, distinctions between wanting and liking. Finally, this chapter underscores the benefit of linking well-crafted animal studies to suggest mechanisms for effects observed in human participants, with the glucose literature providing an excellent example of how well this can work.

CHAPTER 4

Chronic Effects of Food Intake
Western-Style Diets

4.1 Introduction

Prior to the Industrial Revolution, diet was largely comprised of wild foods obtained through hunting and gathering (Cordain et al., 2005). However, with rapid technological advances in food processing and preservation over the past 200 years, there has been a shift to highly processed foods that have a markedly different macronutrient composition. As a result, the typical diet consumed in most Western countries today is rich in saturated fats, refined sugars, cholesterol and salt, and with lower content of omega-3 fatty acids and complex carbohydrates (Cordain et al., 2005).

It is well-known that excessive consumption of this diet is associated with weight gain and metabolic dysfunction including diabetes, cardiovascular disease and hypertension (Haslam & James, 2005). There is now evidence that overweight and obesity are associated with cognitive impairment. An evolving body of work shows that there are also effects of Western-style diet (WS-diet) on brain function, independent of obesity and its associated metabolic impairments. This chapter explores the evidence that WS-diet can alter cognition and mood, and is a risk factor for several psychiatric, neurological and neurodegenerative conditions, and explores the putative underlying mechanisms.

4.2 WS-Diet Models

To model the modern food environment, rodent studies typically involve giving rats access to either a cafeteria diet, where rats are provided with energy-dense processed human foods such as pies, cakes and cookies, or a specialised rat chow (with either high saturated fat, high sugar, or both). A rodent 'high-fat' diet typically involves increasing the amount of fat to between 45–60% of total kilojoules, compared to the standard low-fat, high-carbohydrate rodent chow. A 'high-sugar' diet typically involves higher amounts of monosaccharides (glucose or fructose) and/or disaccharides (sucrose) as opposed to the complex carbohydrates in standard chow. Following a period of time on the experimental diet, which can be a short as 5 days, but typically ranges from 2–3 months, various behavioural tasks are used to measure different aspects of cognition.

4.3   WS-Diet and Cognition

4.3.1   Hippocampal-Dependent Learning and Memory (HDLM)

The hippocampus, a brain region crucial for learning and memory processes, appears particularly vulnerable to the adverse effects of WS-diet. Animal data have shown that in rats WS-diet consumption impairs performance on HDLM tasks such as Morris Water Maze and Novel Object Recognition (e.g., Kanoski & Davidson, 2010). A meta-analysis of 41 rodent studies showed that WS-diet exposure impaired HDLM across a range of exposure durations from as little as 1 week up to 2 months, and across a range of tasks assessing learning and memory (Abbott et al., 2019). The greatest effect was seen with exposure to a combined high-fat, high-sugar diet.

The effects of WS-diet consumption during development are similar to what is observed in adult rats. Rats born to dams who consumed a WS-diet during gestation and/or lactation show poorer object-based episodic memory (Moreton et al., 2019) and poorer ability to learn and extinguish a conditioned odour aversion (Janthakhin et al., 2017; Rincel et al., 2018) when they reach adolescence. This occurs despite being maintained on a standard low-fat, complex carbohydrate chow after weaning. When rats who are initially raised on healthy rat chow are switched to high-fat and/or high-sugar diet during adolescence, the same pattern emerges. This is concerning, considering the highest sources of energy for 2–18-year-olds in the United States are processed foods, grains, desserts, pizza and sugar-sweetened beverages (Reedy & Krebs-Smith, 2010). Children aged 1–18 obtain approximately 11–12% and 11–17% of total kilojoules from saturated fat and added sugar, respectively (health.gov, 2015), exceeding the WHO recommendations of less than 10% for these nutrients.

Consistent with the animal work, human studies have demonstrated that habitual consumption of WS-diet (assessed using food frequency questionnaires) is associated with poorer performance on HDLM in adolescents (Kendig, Leigh, & Morris, 2021) and young adults (Attuquayefio et al., 2016; Francis & Stevenson, 2011), and with decreased volume of the left hippocampus in 60–64-year-olds (Jacka et al., 2015). Furthermore, brief experimental exposure to a WS-diet for 4 days and 7 days resulted in poorer performance on a HDLM task in otherwise healthy young adults (Attuquayefio et al., 2017; Stevenson et al., 2020).

4.3.2   Prefrontal Cortex and Executive Functions

Animal work has additionally demonstrated adverse effects of WS-diet on the prefrontal cortex (PFC) and related cognitive functions. The PFC is involved in a range of cognitive processes, including attention, emotion regulation, mental flexibility and inhibitory control of behaviour, which together are referred to as executive functions. Rats fed WS-diets show reduced levels of BDNF, decreased serotonin expression and elevated numbers of microglial cells in the PFC (Kanoski et al., 2007; Veniaminova et al., 2020). Several studies have shown rats fed a WS-diet show altered emotionality, impulsivity, hyperactivity and antisocial behaviours (Takase et al., 2016; ; Veniaminova et al., 2016, 2017).

Human studies support the animal literature, demonstrating that from children through to older adults, there are associations between WS-diet patterns and executive functioning. A systematic review of 21 studies showed that poorer executive function in children and adolescents was associated with higher dietary intake of red meat and sugary beverages (Cohen et al., 2016). In a large-scale study of 8,914 adults aged 70–90 without dementia, WS-diet was associated with poorer overall cognitive function and poorer specifically executive function (Chen et al., 2021).

4.4   Effects of Individual Nutrients on Cognition

4.4.1   Saturated Fat

Cross-sectional studies have shown that higher saturated fat (SF) intake is associated with poorer memory, processing speed and cognitive flexibility in middle age (Kalmijn et al., 2004), and poorer memory, working memory and verbal fluency in women with type II diabetes (Devore et al., 2009). Prospective studies have also shown that high SF intake at baseline was associated with greater cognitive decline across multiple cognitive domains after 4 years (Okereke et al., 2012) and 6 years (Morris et al., 2004). Some experimental human work has shown that short-term exposure to 75% high-fat diet for 5 days (Holloway et al., 2011) and 7 days (Edwards et al., 2011) impaired attention and reaction times in sedentary young men. Longer-term exposure to a 45% high-fat diet over the course of 6 weeks resulted in poorer verbal learning compared to a low-fat, high-carbohydrate diet (Schuler et al., 2018). The animal literature supports these findings, with a wealth of studies since 1990 demonstrating that rats maintained on high-fat diets show impaired performance on tasks assessing memory and inhibitory control, and with corresponding neurological changes in the hippocampus and prefrontal cortex (Granholm et al., 2008; Greenwood & Winocur, 1990, 1996; Kanoski et al., 2007).

4.4.2   Sugar

High-sugar foods and drinks are readily available, cheap and highly palatable. Sugar consumption per capita in the United States rose from 5 to 70 kg per year between 1800 and 2006, and similar rises in sugar consumption have been observed in both developed and developing nations (Basu et al., 2013; Lustig, Schmidt, & Brindis, 2012; Tappy, 2012). Perhaps the most popular theory surrounding the effect of sugar on behaviour is the notion that sugar increases hyperactivity in children. While early cross-sectional studies supported this view (Crook, 1974; Prinz, Roberts, & Hantman, 1980), a meta-analysis of 23 intervention studies conducted in 1995 and a more recent review in 2008 both concluded there was no evidence for a negative effect of sugar on behaviour (Benton, 2008b; Wolraich, Wilson, & White, 1995). The inconsistent results from cross-sectional studies are thought to be due to children who are hyperactive or with behavioural difficulties being predisposed to consume excess sugar.

Although there is no evidence to support a causal relationship between sugar consumption and hyperactivity, the animal literature certainly demonstrates that high sugar diets impair cognition. As with the WS-diet literature, hippocampal functions appear to be the most consistently affected. A review of animal studies that experimentally increased sucrose intake and assessed learning and memory found impairment in 9 of 10 included studies (Kendig, 2014). Since the time of that review, additional studies have shown that impairment in HDLM can occur within a very short duration such as only one week, and in the absence of weight gain and related metabolic perturbances (Beilharz et al., 2016a; Beilharz, Maniam, & Morris, 2016b). The effect of high sugar intake on other aspects of cognition is not as consistent. Longer-term exposure to sucrose in adolescent rats that was sufficient to impair HDLM also impaired performance on a PFC-dependent executive function task in adulthood (Reichelt et al., 2015). Whereas, no adverse effects of sucrose were found across three studies assessing instrumental learning (Kanoski et al., 2007; Kendig et al., 2014; Messier et al., 2007).

The differing effect of various forms of sugar remains to be clarified. While these findings regarding sucrose were somewhat consistent, the animal literature on the cognitive effects of fructose is more variable. Studies have shown adverse effects (Agrawal & Gomez-Pinilla, 2012), positive effects (Messier et al., 2007) and no significant difference to standard chow (Kanoski et al., 2007). There is also some human literature to suggest that glucose can improve cognitive performance, in particular attention and working memory, though these are typically acute effects and results are inconsistent (Giles et al., 2018; Smith et al., 2011).

4.4.3   Salt

Salt (i.e., sodium chloride) is commonly used to enhance the flavour of or preserve food. While it is well known as a table condiment, the majority (approximately 75%) of the salt we consume is already in the food we buy (European Food Safety Authority, 2010). Consumption of salt exceeds the WHO's recommended maximum daily intake of 5 g (or 2 g sodium) per day for many countries, including Australia (9.6 g/day, Land et al., 2018), China (9.1 g/day, Hipgrave et al., 2016), India (9.45–10.41 g/day, Johnson et al., 2017)) and the United States (3.4 g sodium/day, Cogswell et al., 2018). High salt intake is associated with hypertension and cardiovascular disease, increasing the risk of stroke and cerebral small vessel disease (Hucke, Wiendl, & Klotz, 2016; Strazzullo et al., 2009). Animal studies consistently show adverse effects of high salt intake on cognition (e.g., see Kendig & Morris, 2019 for a review). The typical high-salt diet administered in these studies is 7–8%, compared to 0.2–0.4% salt in controls. Impairments are most commonly observed on spatial memory tasks, and with corresponding increased oxidative stress, and reduced cerebral blood flow and synaptogenesis in the hippocampus (Chugh et al., 2013; Ge et al., 2017; Guo et al., 2017; Liu, Leung, & Yang, 2014). The human literature is more varied. A systematic review of human studies examining sodium intake and cognitive outcomes found that of 15 identified studies, only 4 were rated as good quality (Mohan et al., 2020). Of those, two assessed cognition using a basic screening measure. One found no relationship between sodium intake and cognition, but did find that a higher sodium:potassium ratio was associated with poorer cognition (Nowak et al., 2018). The other found that higher sodium was associated with greater cognitive decline over years, but only for those with low physical activity (Fiocco et al., 2012). In a prospective study with follow-up over 9.1 years, for women with the highest level of sodium intake only, hypertension was associated with greater risk of mild cognitive impairment or probable dementia (Haring et al., 2016). The difficulty with using cognitive screening measures or clinical diagnosis is that they may not be sensitive enough to detect subtle cognitive deficits. The only good-quality study to use a composite score of a range of cognitive tests found that lower sodium intake was a randomised controlled trial (Blumenthal et al., 2019). While the authors showed that lower sodium intake during the intervention resulted in improved cognitive performance after 6 months, the diet administered was the DASH diet, which emphasizes low fat dairy and increased fruit and vegetables. Therefore, it is difficult to attribute the improvement in cognition to reduced salt intake alone.

4.4.4   *Cholesterol*

Cholesterol is another diet component that has been identified as being detrimental to cognition. In animals, a diet high in cholesterol has been shown to impair performance on spatial memory and passive avoidance tasks (Granholm et al., 2008; Mogi et al., 2007). These cognitive changes are accompanied by increased amyloid beta production, deleterious effects to the cerebrovasculature, activation of microglial cells and increased oxidative stress (Hooijmans et al., 2009; Shie et al., 2002). Discrepant results have been produced in human studies. Higher total cholesterol has been associated with both worse cognitive function (Stough et al., 2019) and better general cognition and processing speed (van den Kommer et al., 2009). Similarly low-density lipoprotein (LDL) cholesterol has been associated with worse cognitive function in some studies (McFarlane et al., 2020; Stough et al., 2019), but has a protective effect against cognitive decline and dementia in others (Lv et al., 2016). It is particularly difficult to isolate the effects of cholesterol on cognition, as diets that are high in cholesterol are by default high in other nutrients shown to affect cognition, such as saturated fat and salt. However, treatment with Olmesartan, an angiotensin receptor blocker, decreased serum cholesterol levels and prevented cognitive impairment in rats fed a high salt and cholesterol diet (Mogi et al., 2007). This does suggest a causal role for cholesterol.

4.4.5 Summary

It is generally quite difficult in human studies to isolate the effects of individual components of WS-diet, as saturated fat, sugar, cholesterol and salt tend to co-occur in high amounts in processed foods. Similarly, there are a vast range of dietary approaches in animal studies (e.g., high sucrose, high saturated fat, highly palatable, cafeteria diets). Note that it may also be the case that the adverse effects of WS-diet are in fact due to a lack of certain nutrients, for example lower vitamins and minerals obtained from fruit and vegetables or lower omega-3 fatty acid intake. We discuss these in the next chapter. Regardless, considering the literature overall, the general finding is that consumption of these diets consistently leads to cognitive impairments, with hippocampal-dependent functions being the most vulnerable to insult.

4.5 Potential Mechanisms

To investigate the physiological mechanisms by which WS-diet can affect the brain, we turn primarily to animal models. Several pathways have been established, and they are likely linked: (i) neuroinflammation, (ii) oxidative stress, (iii) reductions in brain-derived neurotrophic factor (BDNF), (iv) blood-brain barrier (BBB) integrity and (v) dysregulation of the gut microbiome. These are discussed next, and summarised in Figure 4.1 alongside their consequences for health.

4.5.1 Brain-Derived Neurotrophic Factor

Brain-derived neurotrophic factor (BDNF) plays a crucial role in the processes underlying learning and memory such as synaptic plasticity and neurogenesis (Bergami et al., 2008; Danzer et al., 2008). BDNF levels are altered in many neuropsychiatric conditions – including depression, anxiety and schizophrenia – and neurodegenerative conditions such as Alzheimer's disease. Reductions in BDNF caused by WS-diet have been proposed as a mechanism underlying the effects to cognition. In support of this, several studies have demonstrated reductions of BDNF in the hippocampus of rats maintained on high saturated fat and sugar (HFS) diets, and these are associated with impaired performance on hippocampal-dependent tasks of learning and memory (Molteni et al., 2002; Stranahan et al., 2008; Wu, Ying, & Gomez-Pinilla, 2004; Yu, Wang, & Huang, 2009). BDNF has also been shown to be reduced in the medial

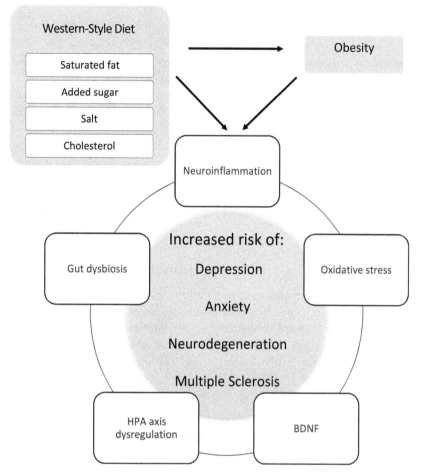

Figure 4.1   Consequences of a WS-diet and its associated health conditions

PFC in rats fed a high-fat, high-sugar diet, and this was associated with impaired performance on a reversal discrimination task (Kanoski et al., 2007).

4.5.2   Neuroinflammation

It is now understood that brain function is adversely affected by inflammatory pathways and mediators. For instance, increased cytokine production can disrupt synaptic plasticity required for learning and memory

(Bellinger et al., 1995; Jankowsky & Patterson, 1999). Performance on HDLM tasks is impaired by peripheral infections (Barrientos et al., 2006), and neurodegenerative conditions such as Alzheimer's disease are thought to be mediated by neuroinflammation (Combs, 2009). Numerous studies have now shown that WS-diet-fed animals show increased markers of neuroinflammation. The diets range from high fat to high fat, high sucrose to cafeteria diet, and the durations on the diet range from 3 days to 18 months. (See Wieckowska-Gacek et al., 2021 for a review of this literature.) In one study, neuroinflammation and impaired memory performance were associated with a reduction in BDNF levels, suggesting an interaction between these two factors in producing diet-induced cognitive impairment (Pistell et al., 2010).

4.5.3 Oxidative Stress

Oxidative stress occurs when there is an imbalance between reactive oxygen species and the ability of the body to repair or remove their harmful effects. Animal models have shown that oxidative stress causes cognitive decline, both in young and aging rats (Fukui et al., 2002). Oxidative stress is also thought to play a causal role in many psychiatric disorders such as depression, anxiety and schizophrenia (Ng et al., 2008), as well as neurodegenerative conditions (Lin & Beal, 2006). Several studies have demonstrated that WS-diets result in an increase in various markers of oxidative stress, including increased reactive oxygen species generation (Zhang et al., 2005), oxidative modifications (White et al., 2009) and protein oxidation (Souza et al., 2007; Wu et al., 2004). Wu et al. (2004) additionally showed a strong negative correlation between levels of oxidised protein and memory deficits in rats fed a high-fat diet, whereas supplementation with the antioxidant vitamin E significantly attenuated the oxidative damage and also normalised levels of BDNF. These findings strongly suggest that oxidative stress contributes to cognitive impairment due to high HFS intake, perhaps by interacting with BDNF to modulate neuronal plasticity.

4.5.4 The Hypothalamic–Pituitary–Adrenal (HPA) Axis

The HPA axis is involved in regulating the stress response. In the face of threat, the fight or flight response is activated, including release of corticotrophin-releasing hormones (CRH) from the hypothalamus, inducing the release of adrenocorticotropic hormone (ACTH) by the pituitary

(Herman et al., 2016). ACTH then triggers the release of glucocorticoids, such as cortisol, from the adrenal gland. These hormones are detected by glucocorticoid receptors, many of which are located in the hippocampus and PFC, with both of these regions being implicated in the inhibition of CRH neurons (Herman et al., 2005).

As it has been established that WS-diets exert adverse effects on hippo-campal and PFC function, it is evident that there may be subsequent effects on the HPA axis. Indeed, mice maintained on a high-fat diet for 12 weeks showed complex changes to the diurnal regulation of HPA axis activity (Auvinen et al., 2012). WS-diet-induced HDLM impairments have been shown to be mediated by decreased hippocampal glucocorticoid receptor levels (Soares et al., 2013). Studies also suggest the effects of WS-diet on the HPA-axis are also evident during the developmental period. Rats fed a high-fat diet from weaning to adolescence (3 months) had higher corticosterone and lower glucocorticoid receptor levels in the hypothalamus and hippocampus at puberty onset compared to controls (Boukouvalas, Gerozissis, & Kitraki, 2010). This persisted in adult rats who continued to consume the high-fat diet, but was reversed in rats that switched to normal chow at puberty onset. Similarly, WS-diet was associated with dysregulated diurnal cortisol profile in young adults aged 18–22 (Heaney, Phillips, & Carroll, 2012). These alterations to the stress response may underlie the increased vulnerability to neuropsychi-atric disorders associated with WS-diet, such as depression and anxiety (reviewed below).

4.5.5   Blood-Brain Barrier

The brain is encased in a highly specialised BBB, which is a system of endothelial cells that protect the brain by limiting the entry of toxic substances, whilst allowing the passage of nutrients and endocrine signals into the CNS. Increased permeability of the BBB and reduction of tight junctions between endothelial cells allows passage of toxic substances into the brain, resulting in inflammation and oxidative stress.

Exposure to HFHS diet for between 28 and 90 days has been shown to increase BBB permeability, as demonstrated by increased transport of sodium fluorescein (NaFl) into the brain. The increased BBB permeability was associated with impaired performance on hippocampal-dependent tasks (Davidson et al., 2012, 2013;Hargrave et al., 2016a; Kanoski et al., 2010; Rutkowsky et al., 2018). The increased NaFl fluorescence was observed selectively in the hippocampus for most studies, and also in the dorsal striatum for one study, whereas other studies did not find NaFl leakage in the striatum or prefrontal cortex. These findings may help to explain why hippocampal-dependent cognitive functions appear particularly vulnerable to disruption from HFHS-diets. However, there are several rodent studies that have reported impairments in cognition following shorter diet exposures in the absence of BBB changes (Hargrave et al., 2016a; Rijnsburger et al., 2019), suggesting BBB dysfunction may not account for the entire picture.

4.5.6 Gut–Brain Axis

Another potential mechanism involves WS-diet changes to the gut microbiota, and subsequent impact to the bidirectional gut–brain axis. The human gastrointestinal tract is populated by a diverse population of microorganisms, mostly comprised of bacteria, but also including archaea, viruses, fungi and protozoa, known as the gut microbiome. These microbes are involved in the metabolism of dietary compounds, immune defence and regulation, and maintenance of the intestinal barrier. And they also play a role in cognition and behaviour, via the gut–brain axis. The gut–brain axis is a complex communication network whereby neural signals (via the vagus nerve), endocrine signals (via gut hormones) and immune signals (via cytokines) transmit information between the gut and the brain.

Alterations in gut microbiota composition are associated with changes in cognition and behaviour, and with mood-related and neurodegenerative disorders. There is a growing literature on the role of the gut microbiome in human disease and brain health; much of this relationship has been demonstrated through experimental manipulations of the gut microbiota such as in germ-free mice, exposing animals to bacterial infections, microbiota transfers, and probiotic and antibiotic treatments (Sandhu et al., 2017). Generally, it is accepted that markers of a healthy microbiota include microbial diversity, an abundance of beneficial bacteria such as bifidobacterial and lactobacilli, and a lower ratio of *Firmicutes* to *Bacteroidetes* (Tojo et al., 2014; Valdes et al., 2018). There are numerous factors that are known to influence the gut microbiota, such as age, environment, genetics and diet composition (Berding et al., 2021; Sandhu et al., 2017). These are largely outside the scope of the current chapter, with the exception of the latter. Here we aim to summarise the literature demonstrating diet composition alters the gut microbiota, with subsequent associations with cognition and behaviour.

Diet plays a key role in the regulation of the gut microbiota composition. WS-diet causes a reduction in gut microbiota diversity, as well as reductions in beneficial microbes, such as Bifidobacteria, and a shift in the relative abundance of species, with an increased *Firmicutes:Bacteroidetes* ratio (Brown et al., 2012; Sonnenburg et al., 2016). Switching from a plant-based diet to a WS-diet has been shown to shift the gut microbiota of mice within as little as 24 hours (Turnbaugh et al., 2009). In humans, 4 days of WS-diet increased bile-tolerant microbes and decreased fibre-fermenting bacteria, compared to 4 days of Mediterranean diet (Zhu et al., 2020). Similar to WS-diets, high-fat diets in animals decrease microbial diversity and beneficial bacteria, and increase the *Firmicutes:Bacteroidetes* ratio (Bisanz et al., 2019; Hildebrandt et al., 2009). High SFA intake has been shown to increase inflammation in mice by activating toll-like receptors (TLRs), which leads to the synthesis and release of proinflammatory cytokines, and by increasing gut permeability, promoting leakage of LPS into the bloodstream (Devkota et al., 2012). High SFA consumption was associated with reduced bacterial abundance in pregnant women (Roytio et al., 2017).

Animal studies have linked WS-diet-induced changes in gut microbiota to cognition and/or behaviour. Exposure to a WS-diet for 28 days during the adolescent period led to a reduction in the relative abundance of several species, and microbiota profiles predicted changes in social behaviours and memory performance (Reichelt et al., 2020). Rats exposed to a WS-diet for 25 days showed both drastically reduced gut microbial diversity and impaired hippocampal-dependent memory performance (Beilharz et al., 2018). A WS-diet that caused memory deficits, also reduced abundance of *Bacteroidetes* and induced gut-barrier dysfunction, including reduced thickness of the colonic mucus and tight-junction proteins (Shi et al., 2020). A high-fat diet (60% fat) for 9 weeks led to memory impairment and increased anxiety-like behaviours in mice, and also increased *Proteobacteria* in the gut microbiota (Jeong, Jang, & Kim, 2019). Similarly, a high-fat diet (60% fat) for 8 weeks increased depression-like behaviours, decreased relative abundance of *Bacteroidetes* and increased abundance of *Firmicutes* and *Cyanobacteria* (Hassan et al., 2019).

Most of these studies also investigated the mechanisms by which diet-induced changes to the gut microbiota may impact cognition. Altered cognition was associated with reduced BDNF in the PFC (Reichelt et al., 2020) and hippocampus (Jeong et al., 2019), hippocampal gene and serotonin receptor expression (Beilharz et al., 2018; Leigh et al., 2020; Shi et al., 2020), and markers of inflammation such as higher faecal and blood LPS and colonic TNFα expression (Jeong et al., 2019); altered energy metabolism (e.g., lactate) and neuronal signalling (e.g., γ-aminobutyric acid) in the PFC and striatum; and decreased expression of neuropeptide Y in the hippocampus and hypothalamus (Hassan et al., 2019).

To our knowledge, there are no human WS-diet intervention studies that have linked gut microbiota data to cognitive or behavioural changes. Though there are cross-sectional studies showing associations between gut microbiota composition and age-related cognitive decline (Manderino et al., 2017), as well as neurological conditions that affect cognition such as Alzheimer's disease, Parkinson's disease, autism spectrum disorder and multiple sclerosis (e.g., see Cryan et al., 2020 for a review).

4.6 WS-Diet and Risk of Psychiatric, Neurological and Neurodegenerative Conditions

4.6.1 Mental Health

A growing literature demonstrates a role for diet quality in highly prevalent mental health conditions such as depression and anxiety. A WS-diet pattern was associated with higher likelihood of psychological symptoms and disorders in 1,046 women aged 20–93 years, after adjusting for age, socioeconomic status, education and health behaviours (Jacka et al., 2010). This relationship appears to hold true across the lifespan, with systematic reviews showing significant relationships between unhealthy diet patterns and depression and anxiety in children and adolescents (O'Neil et al., 2014), young adults (aged between 18–29 years) (Collins et al., 2020) and older adults (>50 years) (Masana et al., 2019).

While these reviews showed a consistent relationship in cross-sectional studies, animal studies are able to demonstrate that diet plays a causal role. Chronic consumption of high fat diets and highly palatable diets have been shown to increase both depression and anxiety behaviours in rats (Hassan et al., 2019; Jeong et al., 2019; Souza et al., 2007). Furthermore, maternal diet consumption can affect outcomes in offspring, with high-fat diet consumption during the early stages of gestation causing increased depression symptoms in male rodents during the adolescent phase (Giriko et al., 2013).

Notably, we have addressed both depression and anxiety together under the umbrella of mental health. The rationale for doing so is that there are many associations between depression and anxiety. There is high comorbidity between depression and anxiety (Kessler et al., 2005), family and twin studies indicate there is high heredity for both conditions (Kendler, 1996), and the same brain regions and pathways appear to be implicated, in particular the hippocampus, amygdala and the HPA axis (Frodl & O'Keane, 2013). The physiological mechanisms underlying WS-diet effects on mental health are likely the same as those described before – inflammation, oxidative stress, BDNF and the gut–brain axis have all been implicated in the association between WS-diet and mental health (Marx et al., 2017).

4.6.2   Multiple Sclerosis

Multiple sclerosis (MS) is an autoimmune condition which causes inflammation and demyelination in the optic nerves, brain and spinal cord. Symptoms include loss of vision, numbness, weakness and gait changes, as well as more global symptoms such as fatigue, depression and cognitive difficulties. The pathogenesis of MS is complex, but is likely a combination of genetic and epigenetic factors. Environmental factors such as smoking, sun exposure and vitamin D status are well-known risk factors for MS. The higher prevalence of MS in Western countries has led to investigation of whether the typical diet characteristic of these areas plays a role.

In 1950, Swank observed geographic variations in MS incidence in regions with higher consumption of dairy fats and red meat (Swank et al., 1952), leading to the suggestion that saturated fat intake is linked to increased risk of MS. A prospective study in paediatric MS showed that energy intake from saturated fat had a strong association with relapse rate over 2 years (Azary et al., 2018). Studies in experimental autoimmune encephalitis (EAE), an animal model of MS, have demonstrated that mice fed a high-fat diet showed increased T cell and macrophage infiltration, as well as higher spinal cord expression of pro-inflammatory cytokines IL-1B, IL-6 and IFN γ (Timmermans et al., 2014).

T_H17 cells have been identified as playing a pivotal role in the development of autoimmune diseases, and are critical for the development of EAE (Korn et al., 2009). Dietary salt intake can dramatically increase the induction of T_H17 cells, and mice fed a high-salt diet develop a more severe form of EAE (Kleinewietfeld et al., 2013). Higher dietary salt intake has also been linked to higher clinical relapse rates in people with relapsing-remitting MS, as well as a greater chance of developing new lesions on MRI (Farez et al., 2015).

While these studies have linked individual components of WS-diet to MS, few studies have examined overall dietary patterns. In more than 185,000 women in the Nurse's Health Study (NHS) I and II, a WS-diet pattern was not associated with MS risk (Rotstein et al., 2019). However, studies examining diet quality in people with MS have shown that overall poorer diet quality was associated with higher disability level, more severe depressive symptoms, and poorer physical and mental health quality of life (Fitzgerald et al., 2018; Hadgkiss et al., 2015). Thus, although there is no epidemiological evidence that WS-diet increases risk of developing MS, there is some evidence that it affects disability and symptom severity in people with MS.

4.6.3 Neurodegenerative Diseases

Chronic consumption of WS-diet is now a widely recognised risk factor for the development of two common neurodegenerative disorders, Alzheimer's disease (AD) and Parkinson's disease (PD). AD is the most common cause of dementia, accounting for approximately 70% of the global incidence of dementia (Reitz & Mayeux, 2014). The pathophysiological mechanisms include extracellular amyloid plaques and intraneuronal hyperphosphorylated tau in the form of tangles (Reitz & Mayeux, 2014). It is characterised by atrophy of the temporal lobes, particularly the hippocampus, and the most marked cognitive impairment is to HDLM. The considerable evidence discussed earlier regarding WS-diet effects on HDLM provide a background for how WS-diet may predispose to AD. Other underlying mechanisms discussed have also been linked to AD development. A comprehensive recent review paints a consistent picture whereby WS-diet triggers gut dysbiosis, leading to chronic inflammation and subsequent BBB permeability, which increases transmission of pro-inflammatory molecules into the brain, damaging the microglial and glymphatic systems, which are critical for amyloid clearance (Wieckowska-Gacek et al., 2021). Supporting this, animal models of AD have shown WS-diet increases the main AD neuropathological features, including accumulation of AB and tau pathology (see Wieckowska-Gacek et al., 2021 for a review).

A growing body of epidemiological research has investigated the association between WS-diet consumption and AD in humans. Several studies show that, in older adults without dementia, higher adherence to a WS-diet pattern is associated with greater decline in cognition over time (Shakersain et al., 2016). But these findings are not specific to AD. In the Australian Imaging, Biomarkers and Lifestyle (AIBL) study, WS-diet was associated with greater decline in visuospatial abilities. This was only true for APOE ε4 allele carriers, perhaps reflecting that WS-diet is only a significant factor for those without a significant genetic risk. In the Washington Heights-Inwood Columbia Aging Project (WHICAP) study, a diet pattern with higher intakes of salad dressing, nuts, fish, tomatoes, poultry, cruciferous vegetables, fruits and dark and green leafy vegetables and a lower intake of high-fat dairy products, red meat, organ meat and butter, was associated with lower risk of developing AD after 4 years (Gu et al., 2010). Longitudinal studies have also shown increased risk for AD in adults with high saturated fat intake (Kalmijn et al., 1997; Morris et al., 2003). A randomised controlled trial demonstrated that consumption of a high saturated fat/high-GI meal for 4 weeks resulted in increased cerebrospinal fluid levels of a marker for AD compared to a low saturated fat/low-GI diet (Bayer-Carter et al., 2011).

Parkinson's disease is the second most common neurodegenerative disease after AD, and is characterised by degeneration of dopaminergic neurons in the substantia nigra, causing a primarily movement disorder of rigidity, slowed motor movements and tremor (Gratwicke, Jahanshahi, & Foltynie, 2015). Subsequent cognitive decline and dementia may occur, and is characterised by slowed processing speed and attention deficits. WS-diet has also been proposed to play a role in the development of PD. Consumption of higher quantities of saturated fat is associated with greater risk of developing PD (Anderson, Checkoway, & Franklin, 1999; Johnson et al., 1999; Logroscino et al., 1996). In PD patients, higher intake of sweets, cookies, chocolate, desserts, sweetened beverages and candy was reported prior to disease onset (Hellenbrand et al., 1996). Higher caloric intake correlates with worse PD-related symptoms (Barichella et al., 2017). Furthermore, for people with PD, consumption of WS-diet is associated with more rapid PD progression (Mischley, Lau, & Bennett, 2017). Similar mechanisms are implicated as with AD, including gut dysbiosis, leading to systemic and neuroinflammation, and impacting on mitochondrial function and BDNF production (Jackson et al., 2019).

4.6.4 Summary

We have reviewed the literature pertaining to how WS-diet may predispose to several psychological, neurological and neurodegenerative diseases. We have elected to cover those conditions with the largest supporting literature. These, however, do not constitute all of the possible conditions affecting the brain, and we acknowledge there is a vast literature we have not been able to cover here. Nevertheless, the literature we have covered paints a somewhat consistent picture overall, of WS-diet increasing risk of developing conditions that affect the brain and that these tend to have overlapping underlying mechanisms.

4.7 Obesity: Weight and Metabolic Effects on Cognition – Diet or Brain, or Both, as Cause?

4.7.1   Weight and Metabolic Effects on Cognition

Obesity and overweight are associated with impaired cognition (Attuquayefio & Stevenson, 2015), and are also risk factors for the disorders mentioned earlier, particularly depression, anxiety and AD (Dye et al., 2017; Luppino et al., 2010; O'Brien et al., 2017). But the evidence from rodent models suggests that the effects of diet are independent of overweight and obesity. For example, rats and mice consuming high-fat and high-sugar diets demonstrate cognitive impairments within only a few days, prior to any weight gain (Beilharz et al., 2016a, 2016b; Kanoski & Davidson, 2010). Furthermore, diet-induced cognitive deficits can be reversed within a week of removing access to the diet, again suggesting that the cognitive changes are due to the shifts in diet rather than change in body weight (Tran & Westbrook, 2017).

4.7.2   Cognitive Processes in Appetite Regulation

It is a generally held view that excess consumption of food – particularly highly processed, energy-dense food – results in an imbalance between kilojoules consumed versus energy expended. However, it may be the case that the relationship is bi-directional; obesity not only leads to impaired cognitive function, but deficits in reward processes, memory and executive functions may predispose to obesity by impairing appetite regulation. We have earlier described the evidence that WS-diet can affect reward processes and possibly induce addiction-like eating behaviours. Here, we present complementary evidence that WS-diet consumption causes impairments in hippocampal-dependent cognitive functions. While it is well known that the hippocampus is involved in learning and memory, it is now becoming more apparent that it is also involved in appetite regulation.

The idea that HDLM was important for appetite regulation stemmed from observations that patient HM, who had a bilateral temporal lobectomy (i.e., entorhinal cortex, hippocampus and amygdala), rarely mentioned being hungry (Hebben et al., 1985). HM's ratings of hunger did not change from before and after a meal, and if a second meal was presented to him shortly after eating the first, he would eat it. Following on from this, Rozin et al. completed a series of studies on two patients with medial temporal lobe damage (Rozin et al., 1998). They, too, could not remember what they had just eaten, and so would accept and eat a second lunch shortly after the first, with no reported change in hunger across the meals. This relationship between memory and appetite regulation also holds true in healthy adults. When asked to recall a previously consumed meal, people will reliably eat less than controls asked to recall non-food related information (Higgs & Donohoe, 2011; Higgs, Williamson, & Attwood, 2008). Further, recall of intake is impaired when eating under distraction, and people consume more when distracted (Robinson et al., 2013).

The hippocampus is critical for another process with implications for appetite regulation – interoception. Interoception is the detection of internal bodily signals. Importantly, patient HM, in addition to rarely reporting hunger, also rarely reported being thirsty or tired, and had reduced pain perception (Hebben et al., 1985). Animal studies show that selective lesions of the hippocampus impair interoception of hunger and fullness, with a subsequent propensity to eat more and gain weight (Davidson et al., 2009; Davidson & Jarrard, 1993).

4.7.3   The Vicious Cycle Model of Obesity

Taken together, the information provided here suggests that the hippo-campus plays a key role in appetite regulation. Considering habitual consumption of WS-diet impairs hippocampal function, thus eroding appetite regulation, this then causes increased consumption of this very same diet, with further hippocampal impairment. This argument is known as the vicious cycle model (VCM – see Figure 4.2) of obesity, developed by Davidson and colleagues (Hargrave, Jones, & Davidson, 2016b). The model is supported by animal studies showing that WS-diet reduced utilisation of interoceptive hunger and fullness signals (Sample et al., 2016). Paralleling the animal literature, otherwise healthy young adults who are given an intervention to increase WS-diet for 4 and 7 days (in two studies, respectively), show reductions in HDLM and poorer interoceptive sensitivity (Attuquayefio et al., 2017).

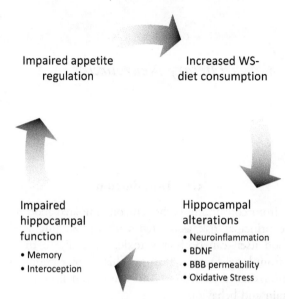

Figure 4.2 The vicious cycle model of obesity, originally proposed by Davidson and colleagues (Hargrave et al., 2016b), suggests that a WS-diet causes physiological changes to the hippocampus, affecting hippocampal-dependent cognitive functions that are involved in energy intake regulation and subsequently causing increased consumption of this same diet

4.8 Conclusions

Overall, this chapter has reviewed the scientific literature showing that WS-diet and its individual components can impair cognition and increase risk of a range of conditions affecting the brain. These findings raise the question as to whether the converse is true – does diet have the potential to improve cognition or treat neurological conditions? This literature will be reviewed in the subsequent chapter.

CHAPTER 5

Dietary Neurotoxins

5.1 Introduction

Getting sick from consuming pathogen-contaminated food may come to mind as the principal risk associated with eating, but as this chapter illustrates, food itself can be highly toxic, especially to the brain, both acutely and from longer-term exposure. This chapter examines acute and chronic neurotoxins, their history and cause, and how they exert their effects on brain and behaviour.

5.2 Acute Dietary Neurotoxins

This section examines acute dietary neurotoxins. The following inclusion and exclusion criteria apply: (1) the neurotoxin has to act rapidly after a single dose; (2) ethanol is excluded as it is examined in Chapter 7; (3) neurotoxins from non-food plants, animals and fungi are generally excluded (e.g., accidental poisoning form eating *Laburnum* 'peas'), except where they serve as contaminants or adulterants; (4) the toxin needs to act primarily on the central nervous system; and (5) medicinal herbs, such as St. John's wort, for example, which may at higher levels be neurotoxic, are not considered as they are non-foods.

Applying these criteria results in six main groups of acute neurotoxins: (1) plant and fungal alkaloids; (2) marine neurotoxins; (3) neurotoxins from plants that are used as flavour additives; (4) neurotoxins that result from food processing, storage and ripening; (5) plant fodder neurotoxins that can concentrate in grazing animals; and (6) acute chemical neurotoxins from food adulteration or miscellaneous sources. Each is considered in turn and they are summarised in Table 5.1.

Table 5.1. *Acute dietary neurotoxins*

Agent	Food	Name	Neurotoxicity Primary mechanism	Primary effect	Acute lethality
Glycoalkaloids	Potatoes	–	Acetylcholinesterase inhibitor	Hallucinations/confusion	Yes
Ergot alkaloids	Bread	Ergotism	Effects on biogenic amines	Hallucinations/seizures	Yes
Tropane alkaloids	Beans, honey	–	Muscarinic antagonists	Hallucinations/confusion	Yes
Quinolizidine alkaloids	Lupin beans	–	Muscarinic/nicotinic antagonists	Confusion	No
Isoquinoline alkaloids	Poppy seed	–	Opioid agonist	Opiate intoxication	No
Saxitoxin	Shellfish	PSP[1]	Voltage-dependent Na channel	Muscular paralysis	Yes
Brevetoxins	Shellfish	NSP[2]	Voltage-dependent Na channel	Motor control loss/seizures	No
Ciguatoxins	Apex fish	CRFP[3]	As above + increase NMDA activity	Paralysis/Cognitive damage	No
Domoic acid	Shellfish/sardines	ASP[4]	Glutamate agonist	Amnesia/dementia	Yes
Tetrodotoxin	Puffer fish	–	Voltage-dependent Na channel	Muscular paralysis	Yes
Scombrotoxin (histamine)	Tuna	Scomberism	Histamine receptors	Allergic reaction	No
Tetramine	Whelks	–	Muscarinic/nicotinic antagonists	Confusion	No
Acrylamide	Cooked meat/bread	–	Neural membrane disruptor	–	No
3-Nitroproprionic acid	Mildewed sugarcane	TD[5]	Metabolic disruptor	Status epilepticus	Yes
Hypoglycin-A	Lychee/ackee fruit		Glucogenesis disruptor	Coma	Yes

Table 5.1. (*cont.*)

Agent	Food	Name	Neurotoxicity Primary mechanism	Primary effect	Acute lethality
β-Thujone	Absinthe	Absinthism	Multiple neurotransmitter systems	Anxiety, impaired attention	No
Myristicin	Nutmeg	–	Main active metabolite is MDMA	Mood	No
Anisatin	Japanese star anise	–	GABA antagonist	Hyperexcitability/ seizures	No
Trematol	Milk	Milk sickness	Multiple pathways	Trembling, anorexia, coma	Yes
Grayanotoxins	Honey	–	Voltage-dependent Na channel	Confusion	Yes
Methanol (formic acid)	Alcoholic drinks	–	Cytochrome oxidase inhibitor	Blindness, extrapyramidal	Yes
Polychlorobiphenyls	Oil/fish	–	Multiple toxic pathways	Cognitive impairments	Yes
Thiaminases	Silk worm larvae	ASA[6]	Acute thiamine deficiency	Wernicke's encephalopathy	Yes

[1]Paralytic shellfish poisoning.
[2]Neurotoxic shellfish poisoning.
[3]Ciguatera reef fish poisoning.
[4]Amnestic shellfish poisoning.
[5]Toxic dystonia.
[6]African seasonal ataxia.

5.2.1 Plant and Fungal Alkaloids

5.2.1.1 Glycoalkaloids

Several glycoalkaloids occur in the genus *Solanum*, which includes potatoes, tomatoes and aubergines (Milner, Brunton, & Jones, 2011). Glycoalkaloids function as plant chemical defences against pests and pathogens, and consist of an aglycone unit attached to a carbohydrate side chain. While tomatoes and aubergines contain glycoalkaloids (respectively, tomatine, and solasonine and solamargine), which do not appear toxic to humans, potatoes harbour two neurotoxic glycoalkaloids, solanine and chaconine. Levels of solanine and chaconine vary greatly between potato tubers, but are always elevated following high temperatures, light exposure and mechanical and pest damage (Pariera Dinkins, & Peterson, 2008). Higher levels of these two glycoalkaloids are evident through green colouration (caused by chlorophyll, a marker of light exposure), the presence of sprouts, and a notably bitter taste. Mild poisoning is probably quite common and may be mislabelled as bacterial or viral in origin. This is because the symptoms resemble 'food poisoning' (i.e., nausea, vomiting, diarrhoea). Episodes of more severe poisoning have been reported, including deaths. In this case the symptom profile has a significant neurological component, with apathy, restlessness, confusion, hallucinations and trembling (Milner et al., 2011). These neurotoxic effects result from at least two causal pathways. First, both chaconine, and especially solanine – like organophosphate pesticides – inhibit acteylcholinesterase, the enzyme that normally terminates binding of acetylcholine to its dendritic receptors (a potent means of killing insect pests). Second, chaconine disrupts lipid membranes, by forming complexes with sterols, thus damaging their integrity.

5.2.1.2 Ergot Alkaloids

The fungus *Claviceps purpurea* parasitises the seed heads of grain crops, most notably rye and barley (Krska & Crews, 2008). The fungi grows a sclerotia (or ergot), which looks like a black claw coming out of the seed head (see Figure 5.1). When the sclerotia is fully grown, it drops off the plant and lays dormant until appropriate environmental conditions occur. Mushroom bodies then develop on the sclerotia, drawing on its abundant store of energy. The need to protect this store of energy from pests and pathogens has resulted in the same selection pressure on fungi as on plants, leading to the emergence of chemicals – ergot alkaloids here – to repel predators. The range of ergot alkaloids is large and can vary significantly

Figure 5.1   A sclerotia (black claw) growing out of the seed head of Rye grass

(hence ergot poisoning can come in different forms), but they are all based around an ergoline structure attached to an amino acid ring system (Klotz, 2015).

Ergot poisoning was a major problem in medieval Europe. There have, however, been more recent outbreaks, such as the mass poisoning in 1951 of several hundred residents of the French town of Pont-Saint-Esprit (Gabbai, Lisbonne, & Pourquier, 1951) and more recently, the Ethiopian outbreak of gangrenous ergotism in 2002. Ergotism is a significant contemporary veterinary problem, with many grazing animals affected by grasses contaminated by *Claviceps* species (Klotz, 2015). Two main sets of symptoms result from consuming food – most notably rye bread – contaminated by ergot. Peripheral blood circulation is reduced, leading to tissue death of toes and fingers, feet and hands, which then develop gangrene. The intense pain associated with this constriction of blood flow was known as *St Anthony's fire* in the middle ages. The second set of symptoms relate to the brain, and are characterised by visual hallucinations, insomnia, mania, psychosis and intense fear. While both of these types of symptoms can occur together, some ergot poisoning outbreaks seem more characterised by the peripheral effects while others are more dominated by central effects. A case in point was the poisoning at Pont-Saint-Esprit. Here contaminated rye bread was consumed, and while hundreds of people were affected, only one developed gangrenous ergotism, while many more demonstrated its neural effects. This commonly included incoherent talkativeness, absolute insomnia (often lasting several days), terrifying visual hallucinations of flames and animals, followed by delirium and violent seizures (Gabbai, Lisbonne, & Pourquier, 1951). Symptoms gradually remitted in most individuals, with only four deaths recorded.

Ergot alkaloids exert multiple effects on the peripheral and central nervous system because of the close resemblance of the ergotamine ring structure to the biogenic amine neurotransmitters, dopamine, serotonin and adrenaline (Liu & Jia, 2017). Although various ergot alkaloids act as biogenic amine neurotransmitter receptor agonists/antagonists – meaning they impact many bodily systems – three more distinct forms of biological effect are known. First, one means of identifying whether ergot poisoning has taken place is to examine for decreased serum prolactin levels (Klotz, 2015), as ergot alkaloids activate the D2 receptor in the pituitary gland inhibiting prolactin secretion. Second, the peripheral effects on the circulatory system appear to be mediated by adrenergic blockade by ergot alkaloids. Third, the effects on biogenic amine receptors in the brain, and especially the serotonin receptor 5HT2A, probably account for the neurotoxic impacts of ergot alkaloids, most notably the hallucinations and psychiatric effects (Liu & Jia, 2017). Indeed, ergot alkaloids were the starting point for the synthesis of LSD, which shares a close structural similarity to the ergoline ring structure, and which also targets the 5HT2A receptor.

5.2.1.3 *Tropane Alkaloids*
The two psychoactive tropane alkaloids that have resulted in acute poisoning from contaminated food are hyoscyamine and scopolamine, which are chemically characterised by their bicyclic tropane ring system (Adamse et al., 2014). These tropane alkaloids occur in many members of the *Solanaceae* family, but are in especially high concentrations in the genus *Datura*. Buds from *Datura* that have become mixed with green beans (in France in 2010; Finland in 2013), buckwheat flour and millet (Austria in 2006), and honey derived from bees feeding on *Datura* (Venezuela in 1999). All of these have resulted in outbreaks of acute tropane poisoning, exemplified by dizziness, blurred vision, dry mouth, muscle spasms, hallucinations and delirium, which can prove fatal if not treated (Adamse et al., 2014). Both the peripheral (inhibition of the parasympathetic nervous system) and central effects are mediated by hyoscyamine and scopolamine's capacity to non-selectively serve as muscarinic receptor antagonists, thereby preventing the binding of acetylcholine to its post-synaptic receptors (Kohnen-Johannsen & Kayser, 2019). These tropane alkaloids have long histories in traditional medicine and as hallucinogens (e.g., as an ointment rubbed onto the vaginal mucosa using a broomstick, creating the sensation of flying), and in the case of medicine continuing into the current day (e.g., scopolamine is used to prevent motion sickness, and other tropane alkaloids such as cocaine have important medical uses).

5.2.1.4   Quinolizidine Alkaloids

Lupin beans (and derivative products made from lupin flour) are widely consumed in Southern Europe (Koleva et al., 2012). Lupin beans contain high levels of the acute neurotoxins sparteine and lupanine, which are usually safely removed from this product by soaking and washing the beans prior to consumption. There have been several documented cases of people consuming lupin beans and their products where the pre-processing has been inadequate, resulting in a variety of peripheral and central nervous system symptoms. These include dry mouth, weakness, dizziness, anxiety, confusion, loss of coordination and visual disturbances. Both the peripheral and central nervous system symptoms result from two effects of these quinolizidine alkaloids, namely blocking nicotinic and, to a lesser extent, muscarinic cholinergic receptors (Koleva et al., 2012). Finally, lupins can also be eaten by livestock with the toxic quinolizidine alkaloids expressed in their milk at concentrations sufficient to cause poisoning in consumers (Panter & James, 1990).

5.2.1.5   Isoquinoline Alkaloids

The tyrosine-derived isoquinoline alkaloids, codeine and morphine, are widely used analgesics that bind to brain opioid receptors. Acute dietary neurotoxic effects from consumption of these isoquinoline alkaloids are rare, but do occur. Seeds from *Papapaver somniforum* (also known as the opium or bread seed poppy) are employed as a garnish in baking, with much larger quantities being used to make certain sweets and desserts, and in the manufacture of poppy oil. Poppy seeds contain appreciable amounts of codeine and morphine, certainly sufficient for someone consuming a slice of poppy seed cake to fail a urinary or blood test for opiates (Meadway, George, & Braithwaite, 1998). Moreover, there have been cases of people reporting mild opiate symptoms (e.g., sleepiness, respiratory depression) after consuming poppy seed products, and at least one case of severe intoxication and near death in an infant fed a milk drink infused with poppy seeds as a 'sleep aid' (Meadway et al., 1998).

5.2.2   Marine Neurotoxins

5.2.2.1   Marine Neurotoxins Originating from Dinoflagellates and Diatoms

In the United States, around 10% of all episodes of food-borne illnesses result from eating fresh or salt-water-based seafood that has ingested and accumulated toxins from marine dinoflagellates and diatoms (Van Dolah, 2000). Worldwide, these toxins may be responsible for between 50,000 and 500,000 poisoning episodes per year, with a mortality rate of 1.5% (Wang, 2008). Several different groups of neurotoxins have been identified as detailed below, and new discoveries continue to be made (e.g., Azaspiracid shellfish poisoning, and palytoxin poisoning – both resulting from dinoflagellate species not previously associated with generation of neurotoxins; see Wang, 2008).

Saxitoxin (Paralytic Shellfish Poisoning)   Saxitoxins cover a range of related heterocyclic guanidines, which are ingested by shellfish consuming various dinoflagellates (species of *Alexandrium*, *Gymnadinium*, *Pyrodinium*) that synthesise these toxins. The first documented case was probably an outbreak in San Francisco in 1927, which made 102 people sick and left 6 dead (Wang, 2008). Current estimates suggest there are around 2,000 cases worldwide each year, with a 15% mortality rate. Symptoms are primarily peripheral, becoming central in cases exposed to higher concentrations of this toxin. Initial presentation is with nausea, perioral tingling and numbness, followed by progressive loss of motor control, drowsiness, delirium and death from respiratory failure. Saxitoxins exert their effects on site 1 of voltage-dependent sodium channels, which results in the blockade of neural activity (Van Dolah, 2000).

Brevetoxins (Neurotoxic Shellfish Poisoning)   The nine identified brevetoxins are structurally related ladder-like polycyclic ethers, which cause illness either by direct ingestion of contaminated water or, more commonly, through shellfish that have fed on the dinoflagellate *Kerenia brevis* and accumulated these toxins (Nicolas et al., 2014). Poisoning by brevetoxins is not usually fatal, and it involves both peripheral and central features. The symptoms start with nausea, perioral tingling and numbness, loss of motor control and muscle pain, followed by seizures and unconsciousness. Its mechanism of action is understood, with the toxin binding to site 5 of voltage-dependent sodium channels. The toxin causes the channels to open, and also inhibits their inactivation, leading to the loss of motor control and seizures (Wang, 2008).

Ciguatoxins (Ciguatera Reef Fish Poisoning)   Ciguatoxins are structurally similar to brevetoxins, but enter the food chain in a quite different manner. Herbivorous fish graze on macro-algal species that *sometimes* (and the factors dictating this 'sometimes' are not well understood) include extensive microscopic colonies of the dinoflagellate *Gambierdiscus toxicus* (Dickey & Plakas, 2010). Larger predatory fish then consume these herbivorous fish, with the ciguatoxins progressively accumulating in the tissue and especially organs, and becoming highly concentrated in apex predators such as barracuda, grouper and snapper. The apex predators are highly prized for eating, and so perhaps not surprisingly instances of ciguatera poisoning are common, with conservative estimates of between 25,000 and 50,000 cases worldwide per year. Early onset symptoms are nausea, vomiting and diarrhoea, followed by numbness of the perioral region and extremities, reversal of temperature sensation, muscular pain, blurred vision and paralysis. While recovery from peripheral symptoms is typically rapid, a proportion of people continue to suffer neuro-cognitive deficits (notably of memory and attention) for weeks or even months after all other symptoms have resolved (Dickey & Plakas, 2010). Ciguatoxins exert an immediate effect as an agonist on site 5 of the voltage-dependent sodium channel. The prolonged sodium channel opening results in excessive N-methyl-D-aspartate (NMDA) activity, which in turn leads to oxidative stress and damage to neurons and glia (Nicolas et al., 2014). It may be this damage that causes the more prolonged neuro-cognitive deficits that can be observed following episodes of ciguatera poisoning.

Domoic Acid (Amnestic Shellfish Poisoning)   Domoic acid accumulates in shellfish, sardines and anchovies that have fed on phytoplankton that contain diatoms of the *Pseudo-nitzchia* species. This neurotoxin rose to prominence in November 1987, when more than 100 people fell ill on Prince Edward Island, Canada, after eating blue mussels (Stewart et al., 1990). Seven of these people died, and post mortem examination of their brains revealed extensive lesions to the hippocampus, amygdala, thalamus and various areas of the cerebral cortex. Initial symptoms included dizziness, lethargy, nausea and vomiting, followed by severe seizures. As these symptoms abated, some of the survivors (and especially elderly ones), continued to display profound neurological deficits, notably disorientation and amnesia, which resembled dementia (Stewart et al., 1990). An examination of the cause suggested domoic acid as the agent. It is a potent agonist of the kainate and α-amino-3-hydroxy-5-methyl-4-isoxazolepropionic acid (AMPA) glutamate receptors (Van Dolah, 2000). Exposure to domoic acid results in a significant increase in intracellular calcium ions, causing cell death in brain areas that have these receptors – notably those areas identified in the post mortem analysis of the Prince Edward Island poisoning, and especially in the CA1 and CA3 fields of the hippocampus. This pattern of damage is very likely the cause of the dementia-like amnestic symptoms evident in certain survivors of this poisoning event.

5.2.2.2 Marine Toxins Originating from Other Sources

Toxins from marine sources other than dinoflagellates and diatoms can be more lethal (tetrodotoxin), are just as common (scombrotoxin poisoning) and are often far less studied (e.g., tetramine poisoning).

Tetrodotoxin   Tetrodotoxin is present at high concentrations in the liver, ovaries, intestines and skin of most species of puffer fish, including the muscle (i.e., edible flesh) in a few chemical forms (FDA, 2012). Consumption of puffer fish species is uncommon outside of Asian countries, with Japan, Korea and China being the main consumers. In Japan, consumption of this fish is highly regulated, with it unavailable for sale to the general public, and since 1958 only licensed chefs have been able to prepare puffer fish dishes (fugu) for consumption. This caution is well placed, because between 1965 and 2007, there were 211 fatalities in Japan from consumption of fugu, and all of these occurred following preparation and cooking of puffer fish in private homes (FDA, 2012).

The origins of this neurotoxin are poorly understood. Some argue that it arises as a consequence of endogenous bacteria in the puffer fish, while others suggest that it has an environmental origin. Indeed, some studies suggest that raising puffer fish in aquaria can lead to species *typically known* to contain tetrodotoxin having no poison at all, but this is disputed by other authorities (FDA, 2012). What is not questioned is tetrodotoxin's toxicity. The poisoning process unfolds in a particular way. First, a numbness develops in the hands and feet, along with restlessness, feeling tired and floaty (flying sensation), and an unsteady gait (e.g., Kiernan et al., 2005). This then progresses within 1–2 hours – assuming sufficient toxin has been ingested – to a progressive paralysis, with death occurring from respiratory failure. While some people appear to slip into a coma, others have been reported to be lucid in this final stage (FDA, 2012; Kiernan et al., 2005). The cause of the muscular paralysis is well understood, with tetrodotoxin acting in a similar manner to saxitoxin, and targeting neuronal-voltage-dependent sodium channels, preventing membrane depolarisation and the transmission of action potentials (Nicolas et al., 2014). Although tetrodotoxin has effects on the central nervous system, or at least people report symptoms which strongly suggest central involvement, it is not believed to cross the blood-brain barrier, so how its central effects arise is currently unknown. It has also been suggested that it effects other receptor systems, including preventing the opening of NMDA receptors and blocking neuronal voltage-gated calcium channels (Nicolas et al., 2014). If mechanical ventilation is available, most people recover from this form of poisoning with no residual aftereffects.

Scombrotoxin Scombrotoxins are a decomposition product of fish, which have been caught but *not* stored at a suitably cool temperature. Bacteria in the fish decompose biogenic amines producing the three main components of scombrotoxin – histamine, putrescine and cadaverine (Al Bulushi et al., 2009). Certain fish species seem particularly susceptible to this form of degradation, notably tuna, bluefish, sardines and anchovies. If fish with appreciable levels of scombrotoxins are consumed (and it may have no obvious visible or olfactory signs of decay), symptoms appear rapidly. These include peri-oral tingling and burning, nausea, vomiting, diarrhoea, asthma-like symptoms and pruritis, alongside some central symptoms such as dizziness and headache. Most of these effects are exerted peripherally, by histamine acting on its receptors and producing symptoms of an allergic response. These effects seem to be potentiated by the presence of putrescine and cadaverine (FDA, 2012). Most people recover within a few hours and there are no recorded fatalities from this form of poisoning. As with tetro-dotoxin it is currently unclear how scombrotoxins exert their central effects.

Tetramine (Tetramethylammonium)   Tetramine (or more formally tetra-methylammonium) poisoning occurs after consuming improperly pre-pared Whelks (*Neptunea* species). Whelks manufacture tetramine in their salivary glands (possibly using it as a form of venom), so consumption of Whelks with intact salivary glands significantly increases the odds of poisoning (Kim, Lee, & Suzuki, 2009). After consumption of tetramine, symptoms appear within 30–60 minutes, including headache, dizziness, abdominal pain, nausea, diplopia, wobbling gait, sleepiness, feeling intox-icated and paralysis of the hands and feet (Kim et al., 2009). Tetramine exerts these effects by first stimulating both nicotinic and muscarinic acetylcholine receptors, and then rapidly blocking their action (Power, Kegan, & Nolan, 2002). Tetramine does not appear to cross the blood-brain barrier, so again it is unclear how its central effects arise. Most people recover from tetramine poisoning within 1–2 days.

5.2.3   *Food Storage, Processing and Ripening*

5.2.3.1   *Acrylamide*
Acrylamide occurs in a wide variety of food products and is generated by heating carbohydrate-rich foods (e.g., breads, potatoes) to temperatures

between 140°C and 170°C. This leads to Maillard reactions in which reducing sugars such as glucose and fructose react with amino acids to generate both the visible brown colouration of chips and bread, alongside a large range of chemical compounds – including acrylamide – that give these foods their characteristic flavour (Koszucka et al., 2019). Acrylamide gained notoriety via an unusual set of events. During the construction of a railway tunnel in south-west Sweden, several workers fell ill with an unknown neurological disorder that presented with peripheral and central neuropathy, gait abnormality and tiredness. Preliminary detective work revealed that employees who had been using a sealant to waterproof the tunnel walls were the most affected group. One ingredient of the sealant was acrylamide, this being a very widely used chemical ingredient as a binder and filler. Blood assays revealed acrylamide as a potential culprit, but to the investigators surprise often significant levels were also observed in control tests conducted on people not exposed to the sealant. This led to a set of investigations into the neurotoxicity of acrylamide in animals and studies determining how people outside of industrial exposure settings could be accumulating acrylamide. It turns out, as we now know, that preparation of certain foods (e.g., burnt toast, potato chips) can yield high levels of acrylamide (Exon, 2006).

Acrylamide exerts its neurotoxic effects in several ways. First, it inhibits kinesin-related axoplasmic transport motor proteins, which normally shuttle large molecules along microtubules. Impairment of this macromolecular transport system has a particularly adverse effect on peripheral nerves resulting in neuropathies, and as the kinesins are also involved in cell division it may account for some of the carcinogenic properties of acrylamide. Second, it interferes with trans-axonal nerve growth factors. Third, it prevents normal membrane fusion processes at synapses. Both these second and third effects result in neuronal death. While these effects are exerted both peripherally and centrally – especially in the cerebellum in animal models – there has been some concern as to whether neurotoxic effects may also be evident in humans as a consequence of dietary exposure. To generate minimal neurotoxic effects in rats requires doses at or above 0.2 mg of acrylamide per kg of body weight, whilst dietary exposure at the highest concentrations is unlikely to exceed 0.001 mg/kg per day (Exon, 2006). There is no *current* evidence to suggest that acrylamide is a dietary neurotoxin, but nobody has examined this question in detail because most attention has been on its carcinogenic properties. Ironically, while it is a carcinogen in rats and mice, the balance of epidemiological evidence suggests it is not a carcinogen in humans. However, it is a human neurotoxin, but whether it is a human dietary neurotoxin remains uncertain.

5.2.3.2   Toxic Dystonia

The mycotoxin 3-nitroproprionic acid (3-NPA) is found in many foods that involve fermentation. It also occurs when there has been fungal invasion or from sub-optimal storage (*Arthrinium* sp.). It is unusual to encounter 3-NPA at a concentration in food sufficient to induce its neurotoxic effects. However, this can occur. The most well-documented occurrences have been in China, where poorly stored sugarcane became mildewed, and when consumed led to severe illness and death, especially in children (Spencer, Ludolph, & Kisby, 1993). Between 1972 and 1989 there were more than 900 cases, with around 10% mortality. Following consumption of the mildewed sugarcane, nausea, impaired vision, convulsions and coma develop. In those who survived the coma many remained mute and incontinent, while others had varying degrees of dystonia. These effects were permanent. Magnetic resonance imaging (MRI) indicated substantial bilateral damage to the putamen and globus pallidus, with more variable damage to other brain areas (e.g., caudate nucleus). Animal neurotoxicology suggests that 3-NPA disrupts mitochondrial metabolism by inhibiting succinate dehydrogenase. It is unclear why this effect seems most potent in particular brain areas (notably the basal ganglia in rat models).

5.2.3.3   Soapberries

Two members of the genus *Sapindus* (soapberry) – the ackee fruit and lychee – are known to contain high levels of hypoglycin-A and methylenecyclopropylglycine (MCPG) when unripe (this applies especially to the ackee fruit). If unripe fruits are consumed (ackee) or consumed in excess (lychee), this can disrupt gluconeogenesis and β-oxidation of fatty acids, resulting in a significant fall in blood glucose. In a child, especially a malnourished one who has not recently eaten, this fall in blood glucose may be sufficient to induce convulsions, coma and death (Shrivastava, Kumar, & Thomas, 2017). Those who recover appear to have ongoing cognitive dysfunction, the origins of which are not fully understood (Spencer & Palmer, 2017).

5.2.4   Flavourants

5.2.4.1   Wormwood and Absinthe

Absinthe is a pale green-coloured spirit (around 60–80% ethanol by volume), which is manufactured by macerating several herbs, but primarily wormwood leaves, in ethanol. It is traditionally drunk with a small quantity of sugar to mask the bitterness of the wormwood extract and diluted with water. This acts to bring the volatiles out of suspension in the ethanol, liberating a pleasant floral/herbal smell and flavour (Lachenmeier et al., 2006). Absinthe was the most popular drink in France and much of Europe in the nineteenth century. It was cheap to produce (using industrially sourced ethanol as a base) at a time when wine prices were high, and was made popular by returned serviceman who had drunk it as a universal prophylactic in the French Algerian wars of the 1840s. By the mid-1850s a syndrome termed absinthism was becoming increasingly recognised. This was described as having both an acute and more chronic presentation. Acutely, heavy consumption of absinthe led to excitation and euphoria, hallucinations, followed later by vomiting, dizziness, depression and occasionally seizures (Lachenmeier et al., 2006). Chronically, users experienced seizures, blindness, hallucinations, nightmares, psychosis and progressive mental deterioration. Faced with a growing recognition of the ills associated with absinthe consumption, pressure built to ban this drink, and setting aside Spain and the Czech Republic, absinthe was prohibited across Europe by the start of World War I.

It has been argued that the primary psychoactive and neurotoxic constituents of wormwood are α- and β-thujone. (There is often little data on each of these isomers individually and where they are distinguished, this is noted in the text below.) Thujone is a monoterpene with structural similarities to tetrahydrocannabinol (THC), although research suggests that it does not exert any effect on cannabinoid receptors (Patočka & Plucar, 2003). The key question was whether thujone was actually responsible for absinthism – and there are good grounds to think it was not. Many of the effects originally attributed to thujone can arise from consumption of alcohol (e.g., euphoria, convulsions on withdrawal, dependence, mental deterioration). Methanol contamination of the industrial ethanol used to manufacture cheap absinthe was known to occur at that time, and as we detail further here, methanol is neurotoxic and can cause blindness. In addition, cheap absinthe used herbs other than wormwood that were toxic (e.g., sweet calamus), including the poisons copper sulphate, to give the fake absinthe its characteristic green colour and, antimony chloride to mimic the milky clouding after the addition of water. Further evidence that thujone is not particularly toxic can be seen in the re-legalisation of absinthe in 1991 by the European Union, albeit with strict upper limits on the amount of thujone (set at 35 mg/L).

However, there is some evidence to suggest that thujone can be both neurotoxic and neuroactive. In mice, a dose of 45 mg/kg bodyweight is the LD50, with death ensuing from seizures, and sub-lethal doses are also seizure inducing (Patočka & Plucar, 2003). In humans, we could find only one study that examined the acute effects of thujone. Dettling, Grass, and Schuff (2004), using a repeated measures design, administered ethanol, ethanol plus 10 mg of thujone, and ethanol plus 100 mg of thujone, with measures of mood and attention being administered before, and at two time intervals following intoxication. The higher dose of thujone exhibited two effects that were independent of ethanol: it decreased attentional capacity and increased arousal/anxiety. Thujone exerts its effects on the brain in several different ways. It is a reversible modulator of the GABA-A receptor, and a competitive inhibitor of the GABA-gated chloride channel (Patočka & Plucar, 2003). In addition, it affects other ligand-gated ion channels, including the serotonin 5HT3 receptor and the nicotinic acetyl-choline receptor (Sultan, Yang, & Isaev, 2017). While it seems unlikely that drinking absinthe would generate thujone levels sufficient to produce neurotoxic effects, it is possible that chronic exposure *might* lead to neurological damage, with seizures as the principal consequence (Millet, Jouglard, & Steinmetz, 1981).

5.2.4.2 *Myristicin*

Myristicin (or methoxysafrole) is the main volatile in nutmeg and mace, as well as being found in far lower concentrations in dill, celery, parsley and black pepper (Hallström & Thuvander, 1997). The neurotoxic effects of myristicin emerge when significant quantities of nutmeg or mace are consumed (5–15 g), with nutmeg containing around 3% myristicin per gram – equivalent to a dose of between 150 and 450 mg of myristicin (Stein, Greyer, & Hentschel, 2001). Most consumption in this range is deliberate and an attempt to obtain a psychoactive effect for which nutmeg has been renowned since the middle ages. In one study using a 400 mg dose of myristicin in 10 participants, only 6 reported any effects (Truitt et al., 1961). Four reported positive effects, mild euphoria and feelings of irresponsibility, freedom and alertness, with two feeling nauseous and anxious with tachycardia. The latter description matches hospital reports of acute nutmeg intoxication, but also including hallucinations, dry mouth and excitability – with these symptoms lasting several hours (Hallström & Thuvander, 1997). The effects of myristicin seem to be exerted by one of its metabolites, 3-methoxy-4,5-methylene-dioxyamphetamine (MDA), which is also a primary metabolite of MDMA.

5.2.4.3 Anisatin

Anisatin, neoanisatin and pseudoanisatin are three neurotoxins found in high concentration in Japanese star anise (*illicium anisatum*). The star-shaped fruits of this plant closely resemble those of Chinese star anise (*illicium verum*) – which also contains neurotoxins but at far lower concentrations (namely veranisatin A, B, and C; Ize-Ludlow et al., 2004). There have been several reports of poisoning, which appear to have resulted from Chinese star anise being adulterated with Japanese star anise. As a tea, Chinese star anise is used for its alleged calmative effects on the digestive system by adults, children and infants. As this generally exposes the individual to higher single and cumulative doses, it is with this form of preparation that most anisatin poisonings are known. Shortly following ingestion, jitteriness and hyperexcitability are observed, followed by vomiting, nystagmus and seizures – with most making a full recovery (Ize-Ludlow et al., 2004). These effects are generated by the picrotoxin-like effect that anisatin has, with it being a non-competitive GABA antagonist (Matsumoto & Fukuda, 1982).

5.2.5 Contaminants of Milk and Honey

5.2.5.1 Trematol (Milk Sickness)

Many plants that livestock eat are toxic and many of these toxins find expression in milk (Panter & James, 1990). In the eighteenth and early nineteenth century as settlers spread out across the US Midwest, thousands died – including Abraham Lincoln's mother – from what became known as Milk sickness (Niederhofer, 1985). This disease also afflicted cattle, sheep and goats, with the first signs being anorexia and inactivity, followed by characteristic tremors of the nose, flanks and limbs that were worsened after physical activity – hence its name the 'trembles' (Panter & James, 1990). As the illness worsened, it resulted in a characteristic stiff gait and abnormal posture, followed by coma and death. If the animal was nursing, their offspring would also develop this same illness. Outbreaks were sporadic, but notably worse after periods of drought when pasture lands were depleted of grass. Observations from native Americans, simple experiments on farms and the collection of reports from local doctors suggested that the source of milk sickness was two plants – White snakeroot (*Ageratina altissima*) and Rayless goldenrod (*Isocoma pluriflora*), both of which tended to be eaten by stock when other fodder was unavailable.

Trematol, the poisonous extract from these plants, is composed of several benzofurans, including tremetone, dihydrotremetone and

6-hydroxytremetone. Which of these chemicals alone or in combination is neurotoxic remains to be ascertained, as at least tremetone alone (the original suspect agent) does not appear to have the same toxic profile as that resulting from the whole plant extract (Davis, Lee, & Collett, 2015). In humans, consumption of milk from animals that have fed on these plants, or the consumption of their meat, produces the potentially fatal milk sickness. This resembles the animal form, with loss of appetite, weakness and vomiting, severe constipation, muscle spasms and the characteristic trembling, worsened by exercise, ending in coma and death (Dolan, Matulka, & Burdock, 2010). Trematol seems to produce some of its toxic effects on the body by blocking lactic acid metabolism (hence the link with physical activity). However, as the specific agent remains to be identified, there is uncertainty surrounding its mode of action, especially on the central nervous system.

5.2.5.2 Grayanotoxins

Grayanotoxins are ingested by humans when they consume honey from bees who have harvested pollen and nectar from certain plants. Historically, honey poisonings occurred in the United States when bees fed on Rhododendron species and other members of the *Ericaceae* family. Currently, most grayanotoxin poisonings occur in the Black Sea region of Turkey, from bees feeding on two particular Rhododendron species. The grayanotoxins constitute a group of around 60 diterpene toxins. Poisoning usually happens after consumption of honey bought from one producer, as toxins are generally highly diluted in commercial honeys that pool supplies. The honey may have a bitter aftertaste and burn the throat, with symptoms developing rapidly after ingestion. These include a burning and tingling mouth, nausea, vomiting, dizziness, weakness and confusion, visual disturbances, heavy sweating and salivation, and potentially life-threatening drops in blood pressure and heart rate (Gunduz et al., 2008). These effects result from grayanotoxins' effects on voltage-gated sodium channels, leaving them open and the neuron hyperexcitable. Fatalities from grayanotoxin poisoning are now uncommon due to effective medical management of the vascular-related complications.

5.2.6 Other Contaminants and Miscellaneous Sources

5.2.6.1 Methanol

Methanol ingestion can occur when people consume incorrectly distilled spirits, and while there are many instances of this occurring in developed countries, outbreaks of methanol poisoning from home distillation are more common in the developing world (Barceloux et al., 2002). Methanol itself is not neurotoxic. It is initially metabolised in the liver with the enzyme alcohol dehydrogenase into formaldehyde and then by aldehyde dehydrogenase into formic acid – the principal neurotoxic agent. As ethanol has more than 10 times the affinity for alcohol dehydrogenase than methanol, drinking contaminated spirits means that the signs of methanol poisoning are delayed, relative to someone consuming methanol on its own for suicide or intoxication.

Formic acid has two main effects. Peripherally, it selectively damages the neurons in the eye, leading to the characteristic consequence of methanol poisoning – permanent visual impairment. Its second effect is to inhibit cytochrome oxidase. It is not as efficient in this process as carbon monoxide or cyanide, but is sufficiently good to cause oedema and cell death of brain tissue (Salzman, 2006). This brain damage is selective, and occurs in the putamen, extending into the white matter of the frontal and occipital regions as well (Hantson, Duprez, & Mahieu, 1997; Salzman, 2006). Why this process targets the putamen initially is understood, but it has been suggested that this brain region may have unusually poor venous drainage allowing a higher build-up of formic acid. The consequences of this damage, especially if the person goes untreated, are extrapyramidal symptoms, with akinesia and rigidity being the principal ones. Methanol poisoning can be effectively treated if it is detected rapidly, thereby minimising visual loss and putamen damage, but as its initial presentation resembles ethanol intoxication, differential diagnosis can be challenging (Holt & Nickson, 2018).

5.2.6.2 *Polychlorobiphenyls (PCBs)*

PCBs refer to a range of organic chlorinated compounds that were used up until the late 1970s as coolants in electrical transformers. PCBs are highly oil soluble. This is important because transformers were also sometimes filled with mineral or vegetable oils as coolants, and crucially the *same filling equipment* was used for both PCBs and these oils. Thus, nearly all transformers filled with oil were contaminated with PCBs.

PCBs as a class can be divided into coplanar and non-coplanar varieties. Coplanar PCBs are highly toxic, but have little direct effect on the brain. Non-coplanar PCBs are less toxic, but have multiple adverse effects on the brain, both acutely and chronically. While these effects can be readily separated in animal models, the many instances of human poisoning generally involve exposure to PCB mixtures (Aoki, 2001), and there have been many instances where PCB-contaminated oil has entered the human food chain (e.g., Belgium – through animal feed (Covaci, Voorspoels, & Schepens, 2008); Japan – Yusho disease from contaminated rice bran oil (Aoki, 2001)). The classic signs of coplanar toxicity are chloracne, endocrine disruption, with less-dominant neurological signs such as fatigue, headache and peripheral neuropathy – these probably resulting from the non-coplanar PCBs. Animal data indicates multiple indirect and direct effects on the brain of non-coplanar PCBs (Aoki, 2001), including alterations in thyroid function (and then effects on brain function), alterations in protein kinase C activity in the cerebellum and various effects on neurotransmission (acetylcholine and dopamine). Non-coplanar PCBs may also alter brain development in children, causing cognitive impairments and life-long alterations in structure and function that are still poorly understood (Aoki, 2001).

5.2.6.3   Thiaminases

A number of plant and insect species can lead to very rapid onset thiamine (vitamin B1) deficiency, with life-threatening neurological consequences. These events tend to occur in people who are already marginally thiamine deficient, who subsist on refined carbohydrates (and especially with cassava, which contains thiamine-binding cyanogenic glycosides) and hence have low intake of thiamine (Adamolekun, 1993). Thiaminases are present in several food stuffs in low quantities, such as certain fish, coffee, fermented fish sauce, tea leaves and betel nut, and excess consumption of these foods in individuals with marginal deficiency could induce a deficiency state. The two documented examples relate to the consumption of the *Nardoo* fern by Australian Aborigines and silkworm larvae by West Africans. For the *Nardoo* fern, traditional methods of preparation (grinding and washing) eliminate the thiaminase prior to consumption, but there have been reports of consumption without adequate preparation, leading to coma and death. Consumption of silkworm larvae has been studied in some detail as it provides a useful source of protein. Unfortunately, consuming these larvae results in nausea, vomiting and dizziness, followed in the subsequent hours by visual disturbances (nystagmus), ataxia, confusion, coma and death if untreated (Adamolekun, 1993; Nishimune et al., 2004). These symptoms can be readily reversed by the administration of thiamine. Both the *Nardoo* fern and silkworm larvae contain unusually high levels of thiaminases, which are not deactivated by cooking, and which rapidly deplete bodily supplies of thiamine, inducing an acute deficiency syndrome.

5.2.7 Conclusion

Most acute dietary neurotoxins come from plants, fungi, protists (dinoflagellates, diatoms) and bacteria – organisms where chemical defence against ingestion would be useful. While this argument has seen much support for plants (alkaloids) and fungi (alkaloids), it is less obvious why protists or bacterial species would produce toxins that affect humans but not their more immediate consumers such as fish or shellfish. In these cases, it may be that protists utilise these agents for completely different purposes. One suggestion is that they serve to alter the behaviour of other protists of the same species (Cusick & Sayler, 2013), and so as they need to exert an effect on other protists, they do so via cell signalling systems (i.e., gated ion channels) and their neurotoxicity arises out of this function. As consumers become increasingly taken with the idea of artisanal local produce, many acute neurotoxic syndromes that had all but vanished as a consequence of industrialised agriculture may reappear – notably via milk, fungal and plant contaminants (Panter & James, 1990). However, as we will see in the next section, industrialised agriculture has generated its own unique share of neurotoxic poisonings.

5.3 Chronic Dietary Neurotoxins

The same selection criteria as for the acute dietary neurotoxins apply to the selection of topics in this section, with one key exception, here the neurotoxic effects emerge after a period of exposure. This section covers infectious proteins, poisonous cycads, lathyrism, konzo, tropical ataxic neuropathy, and β-carbolines. These are followed by the chronic dietary contaminants, lead, mercury, arsenic, aluminium and pesticides. The causes and consequences of these chronic dietary neurotoxins are summarised in Table 5.2.

5.3.1 Infectious Neurotoxic Proteins

Proteins are normally folded into specific forms that are integral to their effective biochemical function. However, certain proteins seem vulnerable to conversion from their normal folded form into a misfolded form. These mis-folded forms then act to convert other normally folded forms of the same protein into the misfolded form. This can result in a vicious cycle of autocatalytic conversion, causing the misfolding of every single protein of that type, with catastrophic effects on the brain and body (Aguzzi,

Table 5.2. *Chronic dietary neurotoxins*

Agent	Food	Name	Neurotoxicity	Link to primary mechanism	Primary effectPD/AD[1]
Prion protein	Flesh/beef	Kuru/BSE[2]	Autocatalytic protein misfolding	Dementia	AD
a-Synuclein	Meat	PD	Autocatalytic protein misfolding	PD?	PD?
b-Methylamino-L-alanine	Cycad/flying fox	Guam ALS[3]	Protein misfolding, oxidative stress	ALS	PD
b-N-oxalylamine-L-alanine	Grass pea	Lathyrism	Glutamate agonist, oxidative stress	Spastic paraparesis	–
Linamarin (cyanate)	Cassava	Konzo	Uncertain	Spastic paraparesis	–
Uncertain	Cassava	TAN[4]	Uncertain	Late-life onset paraparesis	–
b-Carbolines	Cooked meats	ET?[5]	Uncertain	Tremorgenic	PD/AD?
Lead	Organ meat/seafood	–	Multiple pathways	Uncertain effects of diet	–
Mercury (methyl mercury)	Seafood	–	Protein misfolding + other effects	Vision, movement, coma	–
Arsenic (inorganic forms)	Rice	–	Protein misfolding + other effects	Mood, learning, memory	–
Aluminium	Tea/coffee	–	Inflammation, protein misfolding	Cognitive impairment	AD?
Pesticide (organophosphates)	Fruit/grain products	–	Acetylcholinesterase inhibitors	Cognitive impairment	PD/AD?

[1] Parkinson's disease/Alzheimer's disease.
[2] Bovine spongiform encephalitis.
[3] Amyotrophic lateral sclerosis.
[4] Tropical ataxic neuropathy.
[5] Essential tremor.

Baumann, & Bremer, 2008). It is also now apparent that more than one misfolded form of a particular protein can exist, and that each specific misfolded form can result in a different symptom profile, as well as being useful in identifying the source of infection.

In this section we examine the only well-established example, the prion protein, and also an emerging candidate, the α-synuclein protein. For both of these cases, we document the evidence that favours a dietary route of infection. Before turning to the prion protein, two caveats are necessary. First, the term prion is used in the literature to refer both to a specific type of protein *and* to the general phenomenon of infectious misfolding proteins. Second, as far as we know, these infectious proteins are just that – proteins – and so as 'lifeless' chemicals they would seem appropriate to include here among other chemical neurotoxins. While this assumes that these infectious proteins are as 'lifeless' as paraquat or mercury, there are some anomalies in the evidence that are yet to be resolved. The most intriguing is that misfolded proteins made in the laboratory (which appear to be 'nature' identical) seem far less infectious (if at all) than those obtained from an infected human or animal. This would suggest that some additional component (of an unspecified nature) is needed to enable the prion to function as an infectious agent (Sigurdson, Bartz, & Glatzel, 2019).

5.3.2   The Prion Protein

The prion protein is most concentrated in neuronal tissue, so while it is expressed throughout the body, it is especially abundant in the brain and spinal cord. The prion protein is highly conserved amongst mammals, suggesting its biological importance. However, it does not have one clear role, rather a variety of different functions, some of which involve the whole prion protein and others that rely on specific fragments of it (i.e., sheered of by proteolytic enzymes). In the foetus the prion protein is important to neural development, while post-development it serves a variety of roles in the cell membrane relating to cellular adhesion, synapse formation, axon guidance, protection against oxidative stress, myelin sheath integrity, ion homeostasis and cellular signalling (Sigurdson et al., 2019).

The importance of this protein for neuronal function becomes evident when it is disrupted. In around one person in a million, each year, the gene that codes for it undergoes a spontaneous mutation that results in an aberrant version, which is misfolded. The misfolded version then starts to convert the normal folded prion into the misfolded form resulting in rapid cognitive decline and dementia, with most people dying within 1 year of clinical onset. This disease was first documented 100 years ago by two different German neurologists and so has the double-barrelled name of Creutzfeldt–Jakob disease (CJD). As this form of CJD is the commonest, and arises via spontaneous mutation, it is termed sporadic CJD. There are also familial forms of abnormal prion folding, which are inherited, and these manifest in a variety of different disease forms, including fatal familial insomnia and Gerstmann–Straussler–Scheinker syndrome. Both of these diseases affect the central nervous system and are rapidly fatal once the disease manifests. The final category is the one of most interest here, namely the acquired variant CJD. Three routes of acquisition have been documented. The first is iatrogenic, from corneal grafts, blood and surgical instruments that have been in contact with or come from a person with CJD (of whatever form – variant, sporadic, familial). One of the reasons that prion infections are so troubling is that the misfolded versions of this protein are highly stable, so even autoclaving or exposure to proteolytic enzymes has little effect. The second and third routes of acquisition involve ingestion of the misfolded prion protein – and we examine this issue in the next two sections.

5.3.2.1 Kuru

In the early 1950s, Western medical and field officers started to make the first patrols into the Eastern highlands of New Guinea, which was then an Australian protectorate. It soon became apparent that an unusual neurological disease was present, particularly amongst members of the Fore linguistic group, and those from different language groups that were contiguous with it. This comprised a total population of around 30,000 people spread over many small villages dotted in dense jungle covering several hundred square miles, with no formal roads or airstrips and little means of communication with the outside world (Beasley, 2012). Formal medical investigation started in 1957, and it was noted that around 70% of cases were adult females, with most of the remainder being male and female children. Adult males formed only around 2% of cases. From conversations with villagers, it emerged that the disease had first appeared in the 1920s and gradually spread to encompass all of the Fore region. The epidemic started to decline as contact with Westerners increased, and no new cases were identified in people *born* after 1959. The total estimated death toll was around 2,700, with the last person dying in 2009 (Whitfield et al., 2017).

The disease was initially described by two Australian doctors, Zigas and Hornabrook and was called by villagers the shaking illness – kuru – in the Fore language. The incubation period for the disease varied between 4 and 30 years, for genetic reasons that are now well understood (more later). Once symptoms started to occur, it took between 6 and 24 months for the patient to die, with the disease being uniformly fatal. Initial physical symptoms started with ataxia, with the only unusual cognitive feature being emotional lability, characterised by inappropriate laughter or tears. As the disease progressed, the ataxia worsened to the point that walking unassisted was no longer possible, and dysarthria and convergent strabismus occurred. The sufferer then became bed ridden, being unable to stand, sit or raise their head or move. This progressive loss of voluntary control then affected swallowing, bladder and bowel movements, with death resulting from aspiration pneumonia, starvation or infected bed sores. It was noted that there was no dementia and that kuru sufferers were cognitively intact throughout the disease (Collinge, Whitfield, & McKintosh, 2006).

A combination of deft detective work by the Australian doctors, along with experimental work using neural tissue samples obtained from dead patients, led the US researcher Gajdusek to conclude that it was some form of infectious agent (he believed it was a virus), as injection of the tissue into chimpanzee brains resulted in the same disease. Field work revealed that the likely route of infection was from the Fore's funeral rites, which involved the cooking and eating of the dead. In this process, women and children were mainly fed the brains and spinal cord, placing them at most risk of infection. Examination of the misfolded prion protein revealed that it was of the same type as observed in sporadic CJD. Based on the observation of the epidemics time course, it is presumed that a Fore person died of sporadic CJD, and their body was eaten by family and friends. The consumers of the more infectious nervous tissue then developed CJD themselves, and died either fairly soon after consuming the tissue or after a delay of some years – only then to be eaten themselves, further spreading the infection.

Another interesting finding was that those who developed the disease after a short incubation period possessed a particular type of the prion protein that disposed them to a more rapid transition to the misfolded form. Heterozygosity at codon 129 of the prion protein confers resistance to the disease. The vast majority of people who consumed infected tissue but did not develop kuru until they were in their 50s or 60s were heterozygotes. In contrast, those that died more rapidly from consuming the neural tissue were homozygotes at codon 129. A fascinating corollary to this story is that the heterozygote form of the prion protein is over-represented in all human populations, suggesting that collectively we have all been exposed to bouts of infectious prion disease.

Even before the Western medical and field officers realised that the funeral rites were transmitting kuru, they and the local missionaries let it be known that this practice had to stop, and disease transmission was soon extinguished well before the full mechanics of the infection process were understood. It would, however, take another epidemic to unravel more specific details about the true nature of the infectious agent.

5.3.2.2   Mad Cow Disease

The UK epidemic of mad cow disease was first officially detected on a Sussex farm in the winter of 1984, with cow 133 exhibiting an unusual posture (see Figure 5.2), weight loss, poor coordination and tremors. Within a few months the cow was dead, and other cases had started to

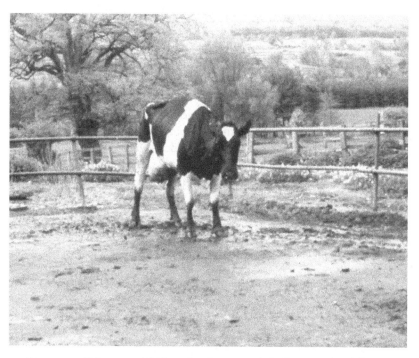

Figure 5.2   Dairy cow exhibiting splayed stance typical of an animal with bovine spongiform encephalitis (BSE)

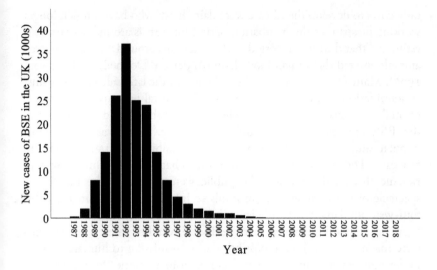

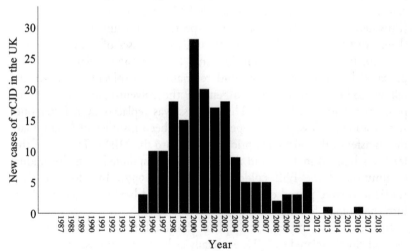

Figure 5.3   Upper panel – New cases of BSE in the UK over the last 30 years; lower
panel – New cases of variant Creutzfeldt–Jakob disease (vCJD)

emerge across the whole of the UK (see Figure 5.3, upper panel). Mad cow
disease (bovine spongiform encephalitis; BSE) is now estimated to have
infected 1.1 million head of UK cattle, with 4.4 million slaughtered in an
attempt to cull affected livestock, and around 160,000 animals dying from
the disease itself. As the average age at slaughter of a cow is 2.5 years, the

only cows to develop the disease were dairy herds who have a much longer working lifespan, as the incubation period for BSE is around 5 years. It is estimated that during the period of the epidemic, around 750,000 infected animals entered the human food chain (Anderson, Donnelly, & Ferguson, 1996). Many of these were slaughtered without the later safe guards against contamination of meat with tissue from the central nervous system or use of offal – the latter being an ingredient of 'beef' baby food. As the size of the BSE epidemic became public knowledge, there was considerable popular and media concern about the possibility of transmission to humans. The initial response from the Thatcher government was to ridicule this possibility, and the public were treated to the unedifying spectacle of the then agriculture minister John Selwyn Gummer and his four-year-old daughter, Cordelia, eating British beef burgers.

As the realisation dawned that the disease could be infectious, attempts were made to minimise the possibility of transmission to humans, and to understand where the disease had come from in cattle. Suspicion soon centred on meat-and-bone meal (MBM), which was fed to calves (Prusiner, 1997). MBM was a high-protein supplement derived from sheep, cattle, pig and chicken offal, and the carcases of animals deemed unfit for human consumption. Up until the late 1970s, MBM had been prepared by dissolving the ground remnants in a solvent to extract the tallow, followed by heating to remove the solvent-tallow, leaving the protein-rich greaves behind. This process was replaced by a faster one-step heating process, which appears to have been insufficient to eliminate the transfer of the misfolded prion protein into the MBM. The use of this feed was banned in 1988 and this directly corresponded with the gradual diminution of the BSE epidemic (Prusiner, 1997). In addition, tight restrictions were placed on the entry of beef and bovine-related products into the human food chain.

In May 1995, 19-year-old Stephen Churchill died from a disease that seemed closely related to CJD, especially as his brain on post-mortem had the highly characteristic spongy appearance. Stephen, who had a particular liking for sausages and beef burgers, was nearly 50 years younger than the average age of onset for sporadic CJD, in addition to having a slightly different pattern of symptom onset. Soon, other cases in young people started appearing (mainly) in the UK, with 178 confirmed cases since Stephen's death (National CJD Research and Surveillance Unit, 2017) – see Figure 5.3, lower panel. This variant form of CJD, has a median age of onset of 27, and a median duration of illness to death of 14 months (Heath, Cooper, & Murray, 2010). Unlike sporadic CJD, variant CJD has an initial psychiatric manifestation, with depression, social withdrawal, anxiety and psychosis, alongside painful sensory symptoms. As the disease progresses it comes to more closely resemble sporadic CJD, with involuntary movements, ataxia and dementia.

It took several years to provide convincing evidence that the specific misfolded form of the prion protein responsible for BSE was the causal agent for variant CJD in humans. Several key pieces of evidence accumulated. First, the direct injection of neural material from BSE-affected animals into the brains of mice induced a similar disease to BSE, as did neural material from variant CJD sufferers (Gill et al., 2013). Second, the neuropathological changes seen in cows with BSE and people with variant CJD are extremely similar, with the characteristic spongy appearance of the brain on post-mortem (Prusiner, 1997) – see Figure 5.4. Third, a few cases were detected where the abnormal prion protein was detected in the body prior to illness – in the lymph system, appendix, and coeliac ganglions in some victims – indicative of an infectious gut-to-brain pathway (Collee & Bradley, 1997). Fourth, and perhaps most tellingly, misfolded prion proteins come in particular forms, which characterise different infection sources. All of the tested BSE and variant CJD cases have the same strain of abnormal prion protein (Hill, Desbruslais, & Joiner, 1997).

It is now suspected that the abnormal prion protein is ingested in contaminated beef products, and that the protein is sampled by microfold

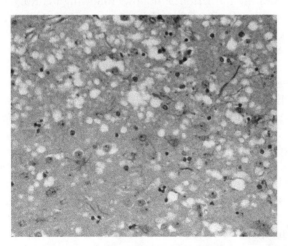

Figure 5.4   Characteristic spongy appearance of the brain on post-mortem of a cow with BSE

cells, which form part of each Peyer's patch – gut lymphatic tissue. This sampling is undertaken to monitor potential pathogens in the gut, but in the case of the abnormal prion protein, no immune response occurs and the protein is then in close proximity to branches of the autonomic nervous system (Sigurdson et al., 2019). This is one possible route, but there are others, including direct movement through the gut wall if it is inflamed (i.e., leaky), and through pinocytosis into subepithelial tissue, which in both cases would bring the prion protein into proximity of nervous tissue. It has then been suggested that it moves via retrograde axonal transport to the brain. Once in the brain, and having entered a neuron, the abnormally folded prion protein starts the autocatalytic conversion of all normal prion proteins into the abnormal misfolded form.

The autocatalytic conversion of proteins to the abnormal folded form disrupts neuronal proteostasis in several ways. Proteolytic enzymes can no longer break down the misfolded prion protein, and this seems to have a knock on effect, slowing the degradation of other proteins. This disrupts the functioning of the endoplasmic reticulum – a major cellular locus of protein production – and initiates one pathway to cell death (apoptosis). Another seemingly independent route of neurotoxicity is via the abnormal prion protein's effect on the neuronal membrane. Here, it alters membrane permeability, generating abnormal ion channel currents and triggering signalling cascades that also induce apoptosis. The combined result of this assault is loss of neurons, gliosis (hypertrophy of astrocytes), and the formation of hollows following neuronal loss, giving the tissue at the microscopic level its characteristic spongy appearance (Aguzzi et al., 2008).

While there is considerable relief that the scale of the human epidemic is limited to the loss of 178 lives, there is a concern that there may be a second wave to the epidemic, in much the same way as happened before with kuru. Indeed, there is evidence to suggest that a number of genotypes favoured early onset of variant CJD, but especially being homozygous on codon 129 of the prion protein (Prusiner, 1997). As many thousands of people must have been exposed to the BSE abnormal prion, this offers one explanation as to why more did not initially succumb. Another reason is that it may be more difficult to contract due to difficulties associated with cross-species transmission. Nonetheless, there have now been several attempts to determine the prevalence of infection by examining tonsil and appendix tissue harvested and stored from UK hospital patients across the 1990s and 2000s. Examination of multiple tissues series suggests that around 500 people per million are infected (Gill et al., 2013). Whether these individuals will go on to develop variant CJD or infect other people via blood transfusions or tissue donations remains to be seen.

5.3.2.3 α-Synuclein

Parkinson's disease is a progressive neurodegenerative condition, characterised by its effect on the motor system, impaired sense of smell, and gut-related symptoms (e.g., constipation). There are a cluster of diseases that share some core symptoms with Parkinson's, including dementia with Lewy bodies, multiple systems atrophy, and corticobasal degeneration. One common neuropathological feature of all of these illnesses is that on post mortem, the patient has abnormal clusters of the α-synuclein protein either as fibrils, Lewy neurites or Lewy bodies – these differing in size and shape – which sometimes occur in combination with other proteins. It is strongly suspected that the development of these α-synuclein clusters is a causal step in cell death, as Lewy bodies are a typical feature of dopaminergic neurons in the substantia nigra when affected by Parkinson's disease.

Like CJD, Parkinson's disease has both familial and sporadic forms, with the sporadic form being by far the most common (Goedert, Clavaguera, & Tolnay, 2010). There are now a number of neuroscientists who suspect that Parkinson's *may* be a prion-type disease, with some abnormal change to the structure of α-synuclein protein occurring via spontaneous mutation or some form of environmental trigger, with this then altering the conformation of other α-synuclein proteins. Consistent with this hypothesis is the key observation that the abnormally folded α-synuclein is especially prone to aggregation (Killinger & Labrie, 2017). At least three pieces of evidence support a prion account. First, as with other infectious disease of the brain (e.g., Rabies), there is a systematic propagation through the brain. Second, α-synuclein from patients with multiple systems atrophy can infect mice, with *some* susceptible animals developing a similar disease (Tamgüney & Korczyn, 2018). Third, Parkinson's disease patients who have had foetal tissue grafts show evidence on post mortem of Lewy bodies in this tissue, consistent with an infectious agent (Olanow & Brundin, 2013). Fourth, prior to any of the classic presenting motor signs, Parkinson's disease seems to affect both the olfactory bulb and enteric nervous system, and both of these have been identified as potential entry points for some form of disease-initiating event (Borghammer, 2018).

Evidence for a gut-based point of disease onset is intriguing. Some evidence points to the detection of abnormal α-synuclein pathology in enteric nervous system tissue before disease onset, although these findings are controversial (Borghammer, 2018). Better established are the effects of vagotomy, as the vagus nerve has been suggested as a primary route of entry of abnormally folded α-synuclein into the brainstem. Various forms of vagotomy used to be deployed to treat stomach ulcers, including partial and full truncal sections. Partial sections should have little effect on misfolded α-synuclein spread, but one would expect that complete truncal vagotomies would serve to prevent any misfolded α-synuclein reaching the brain. Consistent with this notion, data suggests a lower incidence of Parkinson's disease in patients with truncal vagotomies, but not partial vagotomies (or no vagotomy at all; Borghammer, 2018). A further piece of evidence is that diseases which serve to make the gut leaky and inflamed, such as appendicitis and *Helicobacter pylori* infection (the causal agent for stomach ulcers), seem to increase Parkinson's disease risk, arguably by making it easier for the misfolded α-synuclein to enter the body. In addition to this, there is also evidence that the gut microbiome of Parkinson's disease patients may play some role in generating the misfolded α-synuclein, as faecal transplants from Parkinson's disease patients to transgenic mice prone to Parkinson's disease enhances α-synuclein pathology (Killinger & Labrie, 2017). Finally, it should be stressed that the nasal epithelium is an equally plausible site of entry for an environmental trigger and the gut hypothesis is just one amongst a number of possible scenarios – all of which may be valid – to explain the origins of sporadic Parkinson's disease.

If the gut does provide a point of entry for an infectious misfolded α-synuclein protein, what is the source? All of the animals we eat have α-synuclein in their muscles and to a far lesser extent in milk. As with the prion protein, misfolded α-synuclein seems particularly stable and so should resist any change generated by cooking. Animal α-synuclein differs from human α-synuclein at codon 53, with threonine in animals and alanine in humans. The threonine α-synuclein seems more susceptible to misfolding and aggregation, in that familial early onset Parkinson's disease is characterised by a mutation at codon 53, with a threonine substituted for an alanine (Killinger & Labrie, 2017). Some environmental event relating to food or food preparation, our gut, etc., may cause the more readily misfoldable animal α-synuclein to misfold, and this in turn may be one trigger for the progressive autocatalytic conversion of human α-synuclein to the misfolded variety. If this were possible, then there should be evidence linking diet to Parkinson's disease.

There have now been several investigations into the links between Parkinson's disease and diet (Honolulu Heart Study, Nurse Health

Study, Health Professionals Follow-Up Study), but there is still much uncertainty surrounding protective and risk-related factors, with the probable exception of coffee (protective). The food most likely to be a risk factor if the protein misfolding hypothesis has a dietary basis is meat. As described earlier, meat contains significant quantities of α-synuclein, with other animal products such as milk and cheese containing far less. An additional consideration is the way that meat is cooked. Browned or blackened meat contains an array of carcinogenic heterocyclic amines (HCA). At least some of these HCAs are neurotoxic to dopaminergic cells in animals (Trp-P-1 and 2; PhIP; Agim & Cannon, 2015) and others, especially harmane, are elevated in the blood of people with Parkinson's disease (and essential tremor). HCAs may then be directly neurotoxic to the dopamine system, but they may also facilitate the misfolding of α-synuclein in the gut (or other points of first contact between HCAs and α-synuclein in the body).

Dietary data has not consistently identified any link between meat consumption, however operationalised (red, white, etc.), and Parkinson's disease (e.g., Agim & Cannon, 2015; Anderson, Checkoway, & Franklin, 1999; Killinger & Labrie, 2017). However, if high HCA levels are required in addition to meat exposure, this particular combination does not appear to have been explored. In contrast to meat, there has been consistent evidence (including a recent meta-analysis) linking milk and cheese consumption to heightened Parkinson's disease risk, with this analysis also revealing a linear dose-response relationship (Jiang et al., 2014). There is also a link to dietary saturated fat intake and heightened risk for Parkinson's disease, but here the evidence is more inconsistent, at least in part because it suggests that some fats may be protective (notably PUFAs; Agim & Cannon, 2015). Whether a dietary-driven α-synuclein misfolding hypothesis is correct now depends upon whether exposure to HCAs and meat is predictive of Parkinson's disease, or whether some dietary component of dairy products or form of saturated fat enables misfolding.

5.3.3 β-Methylamino-L-Alanine (BMAA)

In the years after World War II, American epidemiologists identified rates of amyotrophic lateral sclerosis (ALS) and Parkinson's dementia complex (PDC) in Guam, as being substantially higher (100–200×) than in mainland United States (Kurland, 1988). Both the Guam-ALS and PDC diseases were very similar, but not identical, to sporadic ALS and PDC observed outside of Guam. For ALS the similarities were a progressive and painless weakening of skeletal muscle, with upper motor neuron signs (i.e., arising in the brain/spinal cord), but its unusual features were neurofibrillary tangles in the hippocampus and subcortical areas, and an age of onset (M = 45 years) some 20 years younger than the sporadic or familial forms. For PDC, the symptoms included cognitive decline, classic parkinsonian features (e.g., rigidity, bradykinesia), with similar pathology in the substantia nigra and subcortically, including neurofibrillary tangles – but again with an earlier age of onset (M = 55 years). Post mortems on healthy indigenous Guamanians (Chamorro people) also revealed neurofibrillary tangles, and the suspicion that many people had sub-clinical features of ALS and PDC.

As part of the search for environmental factors that might account for the anomalous number of cases in Guam, other ALS hotspots were progressively identified, including two villages in the Kii peninsula of Japan, the Auyu people of West Irian, clusters around certain North American lakes with large cyanobacterial blooms, and among returning veterans of the Gulf War; however, the Guam hotspot was by far the standout in size. A series of conferences was organised in the early 1960s to discuss cause, and initial interest focussed on the carcinogen and neurotoxin methylazoxymethanol – but animal experiments did not support this suggestion (Karamyan & Speth, 2008). While this particular agent may have been incorrect, its dietary source proved more instructive – the cycad – a large plant looking similar to a palm tree. The seeds from these plants were used to make flour using a ritualised method of preparation. The seeds were soaked in water multiple times over several days – the final rinse water was then given to chickens, and if they lived, the seeds were dried, ground, baked and eaten as tortillas or dumplings – a rather pointed indication of their potential toxicity (Brenner, Stevenson, & Twigg, 2003).

Chemical examination of the cycad seeds by Bell and colleagues revealed the presence of β-methylamino-L-alanine (BMAA; Karamyan & Speth, 2008), which they suspected might be a neurotoxin. Preliminary investigations using intraperitoneal injection in chicks confirmed this, with the immediate presence of motor symptoms, which intensified with higher dose and dissipated after a day or so. However, investigations into BMAA largely ceased as it was viewed as an acute neurotoxin, unlike the chronic effects observed in people. This changed in the 1980s with work by Spencer (Kurland, 1988). Using oral dosing of BMAA in monkeys over several weeks, he observed the subtle onset of ALS-like motor symptoms, but with notable intra-individual variation (i.e., some monkeys seem far more susceptible than others). Higher doses and longer exposure worsened symptoms, and post mortem inspection revealed significant pathology in the spinal cord and motor cortex, but only occasionally in the substantia nigra. This pathology was characterised by neurofilaments, the presumed precursor of neurofibrillary tangles.

Spencer's work aroused significant interest and a flurry of extension and replications in various animal species – with mixed results. The critics noted that the dose of BMAA used was equivalent to a human consuming almost their own weight in cycad flour each day; that the time course was decades, not weeks; and that the monkeys were well nourished – unlike many of the Chamorro people who had had to endure near starvation under the Japanese occupation during the war. These critiques and some of the failures to replicate in other species reignited the search for other neurotoxic agents, leading a number of researchers to focus on certain cycad sterols. However, as Karamyan and Speth (2008) outline, this turned out to be an unpromising line of enquiry, mainly because many of the potential sterol agents are routinely consumed by many people, and at high concentrations, and from multiple plant sources. In addition, there were some fairly good reasons to rebut criticisms of Spencer's work particularly those on dosing (and see below), as dosing does not scale linearly with body size. Smaller animals often need several times the dose that would be suggested by scaling down from humans or monkeys (Karamyan & Speth, 2008).

Several new findings have directed attention back to BMAA. The first, was that cycad-based flour was not the only source of BMAA in the Chamorro diet. Flying foxes feed on cycads, accumulating considerable quantities of BMAA. Flying foxes are considered a delicacy in Guam and were consumed in large numbers by the Chamorro, providing a further rich dietary source of BMAA (Murch, Cox, & Banack, 2004). The second was that understanding of BMAA bioavailability had focussed on free BMAA, when in fact dietary sources provided considerable amounts (especially flour) of protein-bound BMAA (Murch et al., 2004). The intriguing notion was that the protein-bound form could serve as a reservoir in the body of BMAA, with its gradual release and incorporation into proteins, causing cumulative damage over many years. Indeed, it had been something of a mystery that Chamorro people who had left Guam when young to live elsewhere, still had a significantly elevated risk of ALS. If they possessed a reservoir of BMAA, a heightened risk of illness would be expected.

A further piece of evidence was a large study conducted in vervet monkeys (Cox et al., 2016). The focus here was on pathology (no behavioural data was reported), and the monkeys were either given the same dose as in the Spencer study or one more equivalent to that experienced by the Chamorro. Over 140 days (noting that vervet's normal lifespan is 30 years), the animals were dosed with BMAA, and then postmortemed at the end of the experiment. The high dosage condition showed extensive neuropathology, characterised by neurofibrillary tangles. More interestingly still, was evidence of similar neuropathology in the human equivalence dose condition (all relative to undosed controls), but with damage concentrated particularly in the entorhinal cortex, as well as the amygdala and frontal cortex. Tau pathology (i.e., neurofibrillary tangles) in the entorhinal cortex is particularly noteworthy, as this is the same structure initially affected by another neurodegenerative condition, Alzheimer's disease.

There have now been quite extensive investigations into the neurotoxicity of BMAA and it is apparent that it exerts multiple adverse effects on the brain (see Cox et al., 2016; Delcourt et al., 2018; Van Onselen & Downing, 2018). First, it appears to alter protein folding in two independent ways. One involves the incorporation of BMAA directly into proteins substituting for alanine and serine, while the other suggests damage to extant proteins. The former has been suggested to cause amyloid protein to clump and the latter has been argued to result in hyperphosphorylation of the tau protein, leading to the destruction of cellular microtubule networks and the formation of tau clusters (Cox et al., 2016). BMAA can also effect proteins in another way, by interfering with their capacity to function as enzymes, with amylase, catalase and glutathione-S-transferase all affected (Van Onselen & Downing, 2018). Third, BMAA may bind with metal ions, which can both generate free radicals, damaging cellular function and serving to catalyse reactions that are deleterious to cellular function, including disturbing protein synthesis in the endoplasmic reticulum (Murch et al., 2004). Fourth, BMAA can adversely affect NMDA and AMPA receptor function, and can serve as an agonist to both receptor types, causing cell death via excitotoxicity (Murch et al., 2004). Fifth, it has been suggested that neuromelanin (such as in the substantia nigra) serves to sequester neurotoxins, including BMAA. With chronic exposure, neuromelanin becomes saturated, dysfunctional and allows these neurotoxins to escape, initiating both local cell death and more distant adverse consequences from these agents. With BMAA's extensive capacity to disrupt neural function, its presence in the Chamorro diet, and more recent links between BMAA exposure and ALS (e.g., living near lakes with 'algal' blooms generated by cyanobacteria that synthesise BMAA), it seems likely that BMAA is responsible for Guam ALS and PDC.

5.3.4 Lathyrism

The grass pea (*Lathers sativus*) is resistant to pests, drought and flood, and it will grow in saline and nutrient-poor soils. This makes seeds from the grass pea an ideal food source when crops fail (Xu et al., 2017). Unfortunately, while incidental consumption of grass pea seeds does not appear harmful, subsisting on them is. It has been known for several thousand years that consuming grass pea seeds results in a particular set of symptoms termed lathyrism (Manna et al., 1999). Hippocrates in *Of the Epidemics* wrote, 'At Ainos [in Thrace] all men and women who ate peas continuously became impotent in the legs and that state persisted' (Barrow, Simpson, & Miller, 1974). Over the last 200 years many outbreaks of lathyrism have occurred in Europe and Asia, with more recent ones in India, Bangladesh and Ethiopia. The Ethiopian outbreaks were associated with famine – as with the others – and left tens of thousands of people with varying degrees of disability (Ludolph et al., 1987). All outbreaks of lathyrism are strongly correlated with periods of food insecurity and famine, and, crucially, with consumption of the grass pea.

Lathyrism is a form of permanent bilateral spastic paraparesis (partial paralysis of the lower limbs; Manna et al., 1999). It has three modes of presentation: (1) sudden onset, with weakened legs or falling; (2) subacute onset, with walking difficulties; and (3) insidious onset, with very gradual impairment in mobility (Ludolph et al., 1987). Symptoms may include very frequent urination, pain and numbness in the limbs (or hind legs in animals, who are also affected), developing into varying degrees of disability: (1) mild, characterised by a particular type of gait in which the person walks on the ball of their feet while tilting forward at the pelvis; (2) moderate, with a staggering gait, where a crutch is needed for walking; and (3) severe, with tonic paraplegia, such that the person has to crawl or use a wheelchair to get about. The disease affects pyramidal tract neurons in the spinal cord and neurons in cortical areas that control leg movements (Manna et al., 1999).

The agent believed responsible for lathyrism is β-N-oxalyl-L-α,β-diaminoproprionic acid (β-ODAP; also known as β-N-oxalylamine-L-alanine (BOAA)), which is a non-protein amino acid (Xu et al., 2017). The evidence for this claim is based upon the correlation between high levels of consumption of grass pea seeds, the presence of β-ODAP in the seeds, the capacity of β-ODAP to induce a similar syndrome in monkeys and, as we describe later, the well-established neurotoxicity of β-ODAP in experimental animals and neuronal tissue (Spencer, Roy, & Ludolph, 1986). There are however, two things to note. First, while heavy dietary reliance seems necessary for lathyrism to emerge, it still affects some people much more than others. Considerable investigation has led to the idea that ingestion of sulphur-containing amino acids methionine and cysteine is protective against the neurotoxic effects of β-ODAP. Indeed, the amino acid profile of grass pea seeds is notably deficient in these two amino acids, and so whole reliance on this food stuff would also generate a dietary deficiency, one that could be ameliorated if other food stuffs were being consumed. The second thing of note is that there is little explanation as to the neuro-selectivity of β-ODAP. This has led some to suggest that perhaps other compounds in the grass pea seed might be responsible. One line of investigation has looked at nitrile compounds, many of which are also neurotoxic or become so after bacterial or chemical degradation (Llorens, Soler-Martín, & Saldaña-Ruíz, 2011). One attraction of these types of compounds is their neuro-selectivity, but there is no overwhelming evidence as yet that they are responsible for lathyrism.

β-ODAP is neurotoxic via three main routes (Van Moorhem, Lambein, & Leybaert, 2011), but as noted earlier, it is still unclear why it appears to target the spinal and cortical circuitry controlling the movement of the legs (or hind limbs in animals). First, β-ODAP is an AMPA glutamate receptor agonist. This has been demonstrated in several studies, most notably by the observation that the AMPA receptor blocker 1-naphthyl acetyl-spermine prevents the excitotoxic build-up of calcium ions that β-ODAP induces (Van Moorhem et al., 2011). Relatedly, β-ODAP inhibits the sodium-ion-dependent high-affinity glutamate transport system, resulting in an accumulation of extracellular glutamate. Second, dietary deficiency of sulphur-containing amino acids reduces the amount of glutathione, which is involved in clearing excess free radicals. β-ODAP increases free radical production in mitochondria – further enhanced by high calcium ion levels – and the reduced availability of glutathione leaves this toxic effect unchecked. Finally, the build-up of calcium ions also starts to affect the endoplasmic reticulum, increasing the incidence of misfolded proteins. The impact of all of these effects is to induce neuronal apoptosis. While these mechanisms are largely understood, it is the selectivity of the effects that remains a significant unknown.

5.3.5 Konzo

The Yaka people of the Democratic Republic of the Congo (DRC) have a magical device to aid hunting called a Konzo, which results in an animal running as if its two hind limbs were tied together (Kashala-Abotnes, Okitundu, & Mumba, 2019). This illustrates a key symptom of this eponymous disorder, which shares some interesting similarities with lathyrism and has some differences too. The key differences include initial presentation being mainly in children and child-bearing-age women (in contrast to young men for lathyrism), sudden symptom onset (varies in lathyrism) and differences in symptom profile (more later). Konzo is also associated with consumption of another food stuff – bitter cassava (*Manihot esculenta*). Like the grass pea, cassava grows on poor soil, is less labour intensive than other crops (important in HIV-affected villages), is highly drought tolerant and the edible root will even survive burning of the aboveground parts of the plant (Kassa, Kasensa, & Monterroso, 2011). Unfortunately, cassava contains cyanogenic glycosides, notably linamarin, which are toxic. These are usually dealt with by a series of processing steps involving pulverisation, washing, fermentation and sun drying. In conditions of drought and famine, processing steps are constrained by environmental (minimal water) or societal (war) conditions. The consequence of inadequate processing is Konzo, as seen in several sub-Saharan countries (DRC, Central African Republic, Tanzania, Mozambique) over the last 100 years (Cliff et al., 2011).

Konzo is typified by a sudden onset of muscular weakness in the legs after significant physical activity (e.g., a long walk). This occurs with some acute sensory symptoms in the legs (numbness, tingling), visual disturbances and swallowing difficulties (Kashala-Abotnes et al., 2019). As with lathyrism, this can leave a person with varying degrees of disability from impairments that are only visible when the person is asked to run to total immobility. Konzo is sometimes associated with optic neuropathy, and more frequently with anorexia, with some degree of weight loss (and stunting in children). The extent of motor deficits is not restricted just to the legs, but there is some impairment of fine motor control in the hands and arms, which is as persistent as the spastic paraparesis (Boivin, Okitundu, & Makila-Mabe Bumoko, 2017). Cognitive deficits have also been observed, notably in visuospatial skills and problem solving (more prominently in boys), but whether these occur as a consequence of the neurotoxins in poorly processed cassava or are a result of the greater social disadvantage experienced by Konzo sufferers remains to be addressed (Boivin, Okitundu, & Makila-Mabe Bumoko, 2013).

The precise neurotoxic agent in poorly processed cassava that is responsible for Konzo is beginning to emerge and it is plausible that it involves more than one agent. The cyanogenic glycoside linamarin is metabolised in the body to acetone cyanohydrin and then to cyanide, which is broken down via three pathways: (1) the principal one is through the enzyme rhodanese to thiocyanate, which is then expelled in urine; (2) a further pathway is to cyanate, with this being a more prominent route if the person's diet does not supply adequate sulphur-containing amino acids; and (3) the smallest route ends with 2-aminothiozole-4-carboxylic acid (Kassa et al., 2011). There are multiple toxic agents here. Acetone cyanohydrin selectively damages thalamic brain areas in rat models, but has no specific effects on motor areas (Nzwalo & Cliff, 2011) – so could be responsible for cognitive deficits. Cyanide, while being a potent metabolic toxin, is not known to have specific effects on the motor system. Linamarin causes reversible hind limb tremors in rat models, but not a Konzo-like presentation. The most likely agent seems to be cyanate. It is neurotoxic in animal models and produces a Konzo-like syndrome in monkeys (Kassa et al., 2011). As we noted above, it is produced in greater quantities when the person has a dietary deficiency in sulphur-containing amino acids. Indeed, like the grass pea in lathyrism, cassava is deficient in these types of amino acids and in addition (again like the grass pea), toxins become more concentrated in the food under drought conditions.

That cassava is the causal agent is well established. Konzo sufferers report relying on cassava prior to symptom onset, and all studies that have looked have found higher concentrations of thiocyanate and linamarin, and lower concentrations of sulphur-containing amino acids, in the urine of Konzo sufferers, relative to controls (Cliff & Nicala, 1997; Nzwalo & Cliff, 2011). The impact of the neurotoxin/s in cassava seem to be focussed on the upper motor neurons, which run from cortical areas controlling movement, terminating either in the brain stem (corticobulbar tracts) or the spinal cord (corticospinal tracts). As with lathyrism, it is unclear why there is such specificity for motor neurons, especially as the toxic agent seems to be different.

5.3.6   Tropical Ataxic Neuropathy

Tropical ataxic neuropathy (TAN) is characterised by similar gait abnormalities as Konzo and lathyrism, but with much more pronounced sensory deficits, including deafness, blindness and impairments in proprioception, balance and touch (Netto et al., 2016). Unlike these other conditions, TAN occurs more in older people with its prevalence peaking in the fifth and sixth decade, and there is also some improvement of symptoms with time. There is some evidence that TAN has a dietary cause, in that cassava consumption has been consistently linked to this illness (Adamolekun, 2011). Dietary intake of sulphur-containing amino acids may be protective, as it assists with the metabolism of cyanide via the less harmful thiocyanate pathway (see Konzo earlier). Deficiency in other sulphur-containing compounds that donate sulphur to enable the cyanide–thiocyanate pathway has also been proposed as a contributing factor (notably thiamine deficiency (vitamin B1)). Indeed, some have gone as far to suggest that TAN is fundamentally a vitamin B group deficiency syndrome (see Chapter 9); however, there are several reports of TAN sufferers with adequate blood levels of thiamine and other B-group vitamins (e.g., Madhusudanan et al., 2008). It seems possible that TAN reflects an interaction between some type of as-yet-unspecified dietary deficiency combined with chronic sub-acute exposure to the toxic metabolites of cassava consumption (see Spencer & Palmer, 2012, for a broader perspective on the interaction between nutritional deficiency and susceptibility to dietary neurotoxins).

5.3.7   β-Carbolines

β-Carboline alkaloids (notably harmane, but also harmaline, norharmane, harmine and around 200 other congeners) are formed endogenously in low concentrations, but the majority are ingested, particularly from cooked meats (Maillard reaction products), coffee and alcoholic drinks (Louis, 2008). β-Carbolines alkaloids, and especially harmane, are neurotoxic, inducing tremors in animal models and humans. Several studies have now identified higher blood harmane levels in people with the neurological condition termed essential tremor (e.g., Louis et al., 2005). Essential tremor is characterised by a 4–12 Hz kinetic tremor of the arms and hands, visible when reaching or manipulating objects. In addition to being a risk factor for the development of Parkinson's and Alzheimer's disease, it has a variety of other related (poor balance, rest tremor) and seemingly unrelated cognitive and psychiatric symptoms (anxiety, depression, social phobia, executive dysfunction; Louis, 2008).

While essential tremor has a significant genetic component, it is largely a sporadic disease and so there has been interest in the environmental factors that might predispose to its development. Because a major source of β-carbolines come from diet, two studies have examined whether cooked meat consumption is linked to this disorder (i.e., high β-carboline content). One study found no link between meat consumption and the presence or absence of essential tremor, while a second study found an association, but only in males (Louis et al., 2005; Louis & Zheng, 2010). A significant confound is that eating meat may simply be easier if a high degree of tremor is present (Lavita et al., 2016). However, in healthy controls, blood harmane levels are significantly correlated with meat consumption, but not in people with essential tremor, which may suggest that higher levels of blood harmane in this disorder have an endogenous source (i.e., non-environmental). More generally, whether dietary sources of β-carbolines modify the risk of developing essential tremor or other motor-related disorders is not currently known.

5.3.8 Lead

Although oral poisoning with lead (referring here to the metal, its salts, etc.) is rare, dietary exposure constitutes a significant component (40–80%; Tahvonen, 1996) of total lead intake. The key question then is whether normal dietary intake, which in Europe is somewhere around 0.024 mg/day (Millour, Noël, & Kadar, 2011; Ysart, Miller, & Croasdale, 2000), can cause brain damage. Three caveats need to be borne in mind when considering this question. First, nutritional deficiency in calcium and iron increases the risk of neurotoxic damage from lead. Second, children are far more vulnerable to the effects of lead than adults, and especially those from disadvantaged backgrounds. Third, the effects of lead are cumulative.

Exposure to lead in food has fallen significantly over the last three decades, with at least some of this resulting from reductions in environmental lead levels such as the move away from leaded petrol (Ysart et al., 2000). However, what was considered a safe level of exposure has also changed quite dramatically, moving in the 1960s from 60 μg/dL to the current recommendation of 10 μg/dL. But even with this lower threshold, there does not appear to be any level of lead that is 'safe', and adverse effects on brain systems in animal models can be demonstrated at nano and picomolar concentrations – well within the current 'safe' threshold (Lidsky & Schneider, 2003).

Across various studies, there are some consistencies in those foods that are found to have the highest lead concentrations, these being organ meats;

seafood, especially shellfish; and wines and beverages (Millour et al., 2011; Ysart et al., 2000). It is unclear if dietary lead exposure produces any of the characteristic neurotoxic effects seen in adults or children who have been exposed to lead via other means – notably inhalation of lead-contaminated dust (e.g., IQ lowering, delinquency, poor scholastic achievement, multiple neurocognitive deficits; see Finkelstein, Markowitz, & Rosen, 1998; Mason, Harp, & Han, 2014).

5.3.9   Mercury

5.3.9.1   Mercury in Food

Mercury comes in three main forms: elemental, inorganic and organic (Clarkson & Magos, 2006). While exposure to elemental mercury vapour has some neurotoxicity (mad hatters, etc.), in the main, mercury vapour and inorganic mercury primarily affect bodily systems, especially the kidney, gastrointestinal tract, cardiovascular and immune systems, and the lungs. Typically, poisoning with these forms of mercury does not involve ingestion via food, rather it is the organic forms of mercury that are of special interest in respect to diet. Two main groups of organic mercury compounds exist, those involving methyl mercury and those involving ethyl mercury. Ethyl mercury tends to be less neurotoxic than methyl mercury, as it degrades to an inorganic mercurial form, resulting in more bodily symptoms. In contrast, methyl mercury is highly neurotoxic, with relatively little effect on other bodily systems (Clarkson & Magos, 2006; Holmes, James, & Levy, 2009).

Humans disperse somewhere around 2–3,000 tonnes of elemental and inorganic mercury into the atmosphere each year, from the burning of coal, smelting, chlorine production, paper mills and waste incinerations being the main sources. This is in addition to a more variable but equally large contribution from natural sources, such as forest fires, volcanoes and crust degassing. This atmospheric mercury is very widely dispersed around the earth, and dissolves into the oceans, where it is metabolised by phytoplankton into its organic methyl mercury form. This rapidly bioaccumulates through the food chain, concentrating in large predatory fish and marine mammals – with almost a millionfold biomagnification from the bottom to the top of the food chain (Ceccatelli et al., 2013). Not surprisingly then, predatory fish and marine mammals are the principal dietary sources of methyl mercury, with negligible contributions from other sources (Holmes et al., 2009).

5.3.9.2   Methyl Mercury Poisoning

Although there have been documented reports of methyl mercury poison-ings going back to the 1940s, these were single incidents and it was not until the disasters of Minamata in the 1950s that the neurotoxic conse-quences of exposure became apparent. Minamata is situated on the west-ern side of Kyushi island, Japan, and is the location for the large Chisso chemical plant, which at the time manufactured important chemical pre-cursors for the plastics industry, fertilisers and a myriad other chemical products (see Figure 5.5). The factory had two major waste discharge pipes, one of which exited more locally into Minamata bay and the other dispersed more widely into the Shiranui sea. The owners were aware that the plant's waste products might cause harm, but it was a major employer with good political connections and its attitude to the environment was probably in line with most others in the chemical industry at that time: 'The chemical industry is essential to Japan today and some damage to marine life should be tolerated' (Harada, 1995). If the damage had been confined to dead fish, that might have been acceptable, but the factory had been manufacturing the key plastic ingredient acetaldehyde since the 1930s, using inorganic mercury and manganese dioxide as catalysts. In August 1951 they changed catalysts, now using ferric sulphide and methyl mercury, and discharged waste from this process directly into Minamata bay – and from 1958 onwards – into the Shiranui sea. It is estimated that an equivalent of 82 tonnes of elemental mercury was deposited into the marine environment, with 14 tonnes in the form of methyl mercury. The latter was rapidly bioaccumulated by the marine life of the Shiranui sea, and then consumed in varying quantities by the 200,000 people who lived around the contaminated area (Harada, 1995). Discharge did not stop until 1968, when the plant finally fitted a closed-cycle waste disposal system.

Although estimates vary, from an 'official' figure of 2,230 cases to a more realistic 10–20,000 cases and 900+ deaths (Ceccatelli et al., 2013), the effects of consuming methyl-mercury-contaminated seafood soon became apparent. Before human cases emerged, local people observed large numbers of fish, belly-up, and swimming in circles, shellfish open and rotting, seagull deaths, and a strange epidemic amongst the large feral cat population, with bizarre rotational movements of their bodies. This ended with the almost complete disappearance of feral cats. Human cases were exemplified by constriction of the visual field, with intact central vision but peripheral blindness, difficulty with voluntary muscle

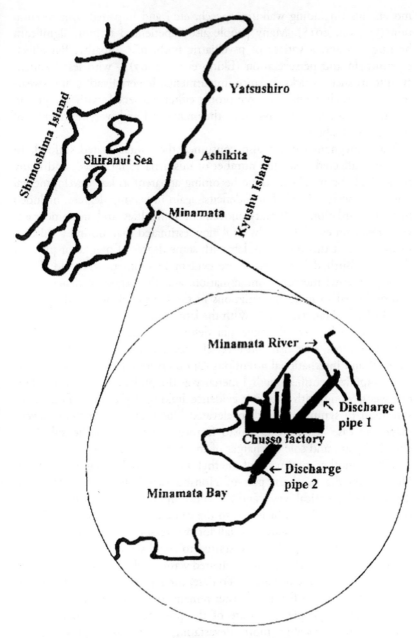

Figure 5.5   Location of the Chisso factory and its discharge pipes

movements (including walking, speech, etc.) and impaired somatosensation (Jackson, 2018). Many people also experienced tremor, significant hearing loss and a variety of psychiatric problems – apathy, flat affect, egocentrism and perseveration (Ekino et al., 2007) – with less frequent symptoms such as ticks, balance impairments, hypersalivation and sweating, and muscle pains. The symptoms either worsened, with the person lapsing into a coma and dying, or they remained with varying degrees of permanent disability.

Many pregnant women also consumed the contaminated seafood. In the worst affected areas, the number of miscarriages increased, and many babies had abnormalities, these becoming apparent as key developmental milestones were missed. These deficits, again in varying degrees, included mental retardation, voluntary movement difficulties and in some cases gross deformities of the limbs. It is now estimated that around a third of infants born at this time were left with some degree of mental or physical disability. Birth defects were more evident in mothers who had higher levels of methyl mercury contamination, and the degree of deficit could also be linked to monthly variations in the Chisso plant's production of acetaldehyde (Harada, 1995). With the large and growing number of adult cases, the emergence of congenital deformities, and the environmental impact on birds, cats, fish and invertebrates, the disaster started to attract national and international attention. All observers – local and from overseas – rapidly identified methyl mercury as the probable toxic agent. This discovery, along with growing evidence linking degree of seafood consumption to symptoms, and to elevated blood and hair mercury levels, made the case against the Chisso factory unassailable – the sole large chemical plant and sole discharger of mercury in the region.

When another outbreak of methyl mercury poisoning occurred in Niigata (on the northern part of Honshu island, Japan) – again from discharge of chemical waste and the consumption of contaminated fish – there could be little doubt left as to the cause of 'Minamata disease'. The number of acute cases started to fall for two reasons – and not because of any official action. Local people started to avoid seafood, and the Chisso factory started to discharge contaminated waste solely into the Shiranui sea where it more readily dispersed. To date, the saga of adequate compensation and recognition for this disaster remains on-going in Japan.

While many people are aware of the poisoning of Minamata, fewer know of the arguably more devastating Iraqi wheat poisoning of 1971–1972 (Bakir, Damluji, & Amin-Zaki, 1973). Iraq received several large shipments of wheat seed, which was destined for sowing, not for eating. The seed had been sprayed with a methyl-mercury-based fungicide, which included a bright red dye, and each sack was marked with skull and crossbones. Large quantities of this wheat got into circulation as food, after the wheat was washed to remove the dye. As the dose of methyl mercury was so much higher than from seafood in Minamata, symptoms appeared quite rapidly – the same as those documented in Minamata. Official figures suggest around 6,000 people were hospitalised and 500 died, but contemporary analyses suggest that more like 40–50,000 people were affected in varying degrees, with many being left with permanent disability (Sanfeliu et al., 2003).

5.3.9.3 Methyl Mercury Pathogenesis

Both neuroimaging data and neuropathology were undertaken on the Minamata victims. The changes to the brain were fairly consistent across adults. There was a characteristic atrophy of the cerebellum, and at the microscopic level there was selective destruction of granule cells, with purkinje cells left intact (Clarkson & Magos, 2006; Korogi et al., 1998). There was also selective damage to the calcarine region of the occipital lobe, with the degree of damage typically reflecting loss of peripheral vision. The motor and somatosensory cortex also demonstrated atrophy, and where hearing loss occurred, there was usually damage to the transverse gyrus of the temporal lobe (Korogi et al., 1998). Examination of foetal brain tissue suggests a far more extensive degree of damage, with incomplete growth of the cortical layer and neurons not reaching their designated destination. Animal and human studies both suggest that foetal and infant brains are highly sensitive to the effects of methyl mercury – more so than adults – and at lower doses (Castoldi, Johansson, & Onishchenko, 2008; Clarkson & Magos, 2006).

Methyl mercury forms a complex with the amino acid cysteine, which then resembles the amino acid methionine. This allows methyl mercury to be readily moved across the blood brain barrier on the large neutral amino acid carrier. Methyl mercury then disrupts cell membranes – both that of the blood-brain barrier (making it leaky, which may facilitate further entry of methyl mercury) and also of neurons, disrupting cellular calcium levels and adversely affecting neuronal signalling. There is also disruption of mitochondrial function through increased oxidative stress. The production of proteins by the endoplasmic reticulum is also affected, resulting in inclusions of methyl mercury, with misfolding. Microtubule assembly is also disrupted by inclusion of methyl mercury into its protein scaffolding. While the cell attempts to limit these effects using glutathione, selenoprotein p and metallothionenes, when these become overwhelmed the cellular damage results in apoptosis (Sanfeliu et al., 2003). The mystery here is why methyl mercury is initially selective to the cerebellum and calcarine cortex, and why in these regions only particular cell types succumb to its effects. This picture is further complicated by the fact that metabolism of methyl mercury can generate elemental mercury in the brain, and how this contributes to the pattern of deficit is not understood either.

5.3.9.4   Fish: Is It Safe?

Apex fish predators and marine mammals contain higher levels of mercury than any other form of food, and so an important question is whether consumption of such seafood is safe. In an attempt to address this question, there have been several cross-sectional studies and three larger longitudinal ones on groups who consume a lot of seafood (Castoldi et al., 2008; Grandjean, Weihe, & Jørgensen, 1992). It is the three well-powered longitudinal studies that are of special interest here, as these include large numbers of infants (due to their acknowledged sensitivity to methyl mercury) followed through to their teenage years. All three studies tracked cognitive and physical development as well as assessing foetal and current levels of mercury exposure. The Faroes study, following more than 900 infants from birth up to 14 years, initially found few effects linked to foetal methyl mercury exposure, but effects became evident at around 6–7 years old and when retested at 14. Exposure was linked to lower IQ, poorer coordination and impaired motor performance at 6–7, and at 14 years. The New Zealand study used a smaller cohort of around 200 infants. It found some evidence of developmental impairment early on, and lower IQ and poorer coordination at age 6. The Seychelles study followed more than 700 infants and found no evidence of impairment at any wave of testing.

These results have provoked some controversy because of their disagreement. The New Zealand study is arguably dependent on one outlying observation that had a particularly high level of methyl mercury exposure – removal of this case weakens these data. While the Faroes study was well controlled for confounding variables, the effects of PCBs on development and their interactive effects with methyl mercury may be problematic. The diet in the Faroes is also unique in having a Whale meat/blubber component, which contains more methyl mercury than fish and PCBs too (Grandjean et al., 1992). PCB exposure also tended to be lower in the

Seychelles population and higher in New Zealand, so the combination of these two chemicals *may* be particularly deleterious. The Seychelles group also tended to have lower methyl mercury doses than the two positive studies, and there is also recognition that genetic differences might account for some of the divergence in findings between study populations (Castoldi et al., 2008). While these observations suggest that low dose methyl mercury may adversely affect the developing foetus, this has to be balanced against the well-acknowledged benefits of dietary fish consumption and by the practicalities of available protein sources in peoples whose staple has traditionally been seafood.

5.3.10   Arsenic

Arsenic is highly toxic, it is a potent carcinogen, is linked to cardiovascular disease and is a known neurotoxin (Tyler & Allan, 2014). Exposure to arsenic occurs via anthropogenic sources (e.g., pesticides, mining, chemical industry) and from the contamination of ground water by mineral arsenic. While there have been occasional food-based poisonings from anthropogenic arsenic, such as that involving the use of arsenic contaminated beer (Vahidnia, van der Voet, & de Wolff, 2007), the vast majority of poisonings arise from mineral sources of arsenic. It is estimated that somewhere around 100 million people are chronically exposed to toxic levels (i.e., >10 ppb) of arsenic in drinking water. Not only is arsenic ingested via drinking, but it contaminates food preparation, and plants and animals exposed to water from the same source. Rice is particularly effective at taking up arsenic, and as in many regions with the highest water-arsenic levels, the local people are also heavy consumers of rice (i.e., Bangladesh, West Bengal). Rice is now recognised as a significant independent source of arsenic exposure (Majumder & Banik, 2019).

Arsenic is present in the environment in several different forms, elemental, organic and inorganic, and it is the inorganic forms which contribute the most to its toxic effects. The inorganic types arsenite (valence state III), normally present in freshwater/food, and arsenate (valence state V), normally present in anaerobic groundwater, are of particular importance. When ingested, they enter the body via the intestines, with arsenite being transported across the blood-brain barrier by acquaglycoprotein 9, where it then accumulates in the brain. Arsenate is initially metabolised by the liver, generating several more toxic arsenic compounds, which can then transit the blood-brain barrier (Escudero-Lourdes, 2016). While the body actively excretes arsenic in urine and bile, it would seem that chronic exposure even just above the notional safe threshold can lead to bioaccumulation in the brain and other tissues.

Most of the neurotoxic effects that have been studied in humans and animals result from low-level chronic exposure (i.e., in ppb and ppm doses). The human studies usually use either urinary arsenic levels or those of the persons drinking water supply as indices of exposure. In children, there is convincing evidence that consistent exposure, even in the ppb range, results in broad intellectual impairment and a reduction in IQ, with notably specific effects on learning and memory, and with a link to the presence of attention-deficit hyperactivity disorder (Tyler & Allan, 2014). In adults, there is a similar neurocognitive profile linked to arsenic exposure, but in addition it is also associated with a greater likelihood of mental health problems, especially anxiety, depression and low mood. The foetal exposure literature is equivocal, with some studies reporting later developmental delay and others not.

The neurotoxic effects and mechanisms of inorganic arsenic have been studied (Escudero-Lourdes, 2016). At a systems level, animal data finds that arsenic impairs multiple aspects of hippocampal function, including its capacity for long-term potentiation and for the generation of excitatory post-synaptic potentials. Arsenic also impairs the function of the glucocorticoid receptor, and reduces hippocampal neurogenesis. All of these effects likely impact learning and memory, and the latter two may impact mood, with the hippocampus being less able to inhibit the hypothalamic–pituitary–adrenal axis's stress response, and with impaired neurogenesis linked to depression (Tyler & Allan, 2014). At a cellular level, arsenic affects multiple pathways because it can substitute for phosphorous, disrupting metabolic processes, and also because it binds to certain amino acids, namely those with thiol groups, especially cysteine. There are multiple consequences from this. Binding to cysteine causes enzyme dysfunction, prompts protein aggregation and damages microtubules; substituting for phosphorous causes mitochondrial stress and apoptosis signals; and its metabolic disruption causes oxidative stress and a proinflammatory response (Escudero-Lourdes, 2016). This in turn inhibits cellular autophagy of misfolded proteins, allowing this arsenic-driven process to accelerate, as well as switching the kynurenine pathway to shift away from metabolising tyrosine into serotonin – again with potentially adverse effects on mood. The shift in the kynurenine pathway, also results in an increase in neurotoxic metabolites, such as quinolinic acid, which are selectively neurotoxic to the hippocampus.

5.3.11 Aluminium

Aluminium compounds are abundant in the environment and humans are exposed to them in several ways. The principal means of exposure is in food. Sodium aluminium phosphate is a widely used emulsifying agent (food additive E541), and in its acid form it is employed as a leavening agent in commercial bakeries. Aluminium sulphate is also used as a food additive (firming agent E520). In addition, many plants concentrate aluminium salts, notable examples being tea and coffee, with tea being able to provide as much as 945 mg of aluminium per kg dry weight (Stahl et al., 2018). In addition to food, aluminium sulphate is used as an adjuvant in vaccines, is widely consumed as an antacid (e.g., Gaviscon), and almost universally drunk, being used in water purification as a flocculant (either as aluminium sulphate or hydroxide). Finally, aluminium cookware, containers, etc. can also leach aluminium, especially if in contact with warm food acids (e.g., cooking marmalade).

In the United States, the average total daily exposure is around 7–8 mg (i.e., all sources including inhalation, skin absorption from cosmetic products, etc.) with much of this coming from food. While bioavailability of aluminium in the gut is higher in water (around 0.3%) than in food (around 0.1–0.3%), the amount of aluminium in water (around 0.2 μg/L) is far smaller than in food (mg quantities; Yokel, Hicks, & Florence, 2008). How aluminium is transferred across the gut wall into the bloodstream is not understood, but once in the blood, typical plasma levels of aluminium in the United States are around 0.002 mg/L. Aluminium can reach the brain and it appears to do so by using the same mechanism as iron. The glycoprotein transferrin is known to weakly bind to aluminium, and transferrin can move across the blood-brain barrier in a receptor-mediated manner (Fishman et al., 1987). While most aluminium is not absorbed by the gut and hence leaves the body as part of faeces, the plasma fraction is mainly excreted via urine and bile.

The effects of aluminium on the human brain are controversial. This is not so much about its neurotoxicity, but rather about the specific claim that it can cause or contribute to Alzheimer's disease (e.g., see www.alz.org/alzheimers-dementia/what-is-alzheimers/myths, where the US Alzheimer's society lists 'aluminium causes Alzheimer's' as a myth). Turning first to the uncontroversial claim that aluminium is neurotoxic, two sources of evidence indicate this. Animal data demonstrate both in vivo and in vitro that exposure to aluminium directly (i.e., by immersion of tissue or injection into the brain) or indirectly via oral ingestion at high or human-like doses results in demonstrable neuropathology and adverse changes in cognitive performance (Mizoroki, Meshitsuka, & Maeda, 2007). A key target region is the hippocampus, with related effects on learning and memory. In terms of neuropathology, in mice, chronic low-level oral exposure in drinking water can generate an inflammatory response in the brain, with microglial and astrocyte activation (Bondy, 2010). Indeed, aluminium seems to produce a wide variety of adverse effects on neurons. At a general level it alters ion balance, leading to a build-up of intracellular calcium. It also impacts protein folding, notably of key enzymes in mitochondria, as well as disrupting the function of the endoplasmic reticulum. It also disrupts DNA repair. Aluminium promotes oxidative stress, at the same time as disabling some of the mechanisms for reducing reactive oxygen species. The upshot of all of these adverse effects is apoptosis, and loss of neuronal tissue (Frisardi et al., 2010).

The second line of evidence for neurotoxicity comes from human studies, drawing on three sets of data outside the dietary domain. One is the haemodialysis literature, where aluminium salts were employed in the dialysate (i.e., the fluid in a dialysis machine which is on the other side of the permeable membrane to the blood flowing through the machine). Patients on prolonged dialysis and who were exposed to this form of dialysate were prone to develop dialysis encephalophy (impaired voluntary movement, psychosis, leading to convulsions and coma). This condition was largely eradicated by eliminating the use of aluminium salts in the dialysate, suggesting their responsibility for this condition (Jack, Rabin, & McKinney, 1983).

A further source of evidence comes from industrial exposure in welders and smelter workers. Several studies indicate exposure-related impairments in working memory, attention and visual memory, but noting that cognitive impairments have not been found in all studies (Inan-Eroglu & Ayaz, 2018; Kandimalla et al., 2016). A final source of evidence comes from acute exposures. The most notable example was the Camelford incident, where 20 tonnes of aluminium sulphate was accidentally discharged into the drinking water of 20,000 local people. A large number subsequently reported becoming unwell before there was any official acknowledgement of the incident, with gastrointestinal symptoms, muscle pain and concentration and memory problems forming the bulk of reports (Altmann, Cunningham, & Dhanesha, 1999). These reports persisted, and so a group of 55 residents were tested to determine cognitive impairment, 3 years post-exposure. Testing revealed impairments on the symbol digit coding test and a reaction time test, but not on other cognitive domains (e.g., memory) – a pattern the authors had also reported in patients exposed to aluminium in dialysis, but who had not developed dialysis encephalophy. These test results suggest a general cognitive impairment, as the tests (symbol digit coding, reaction time) are not specific to any particular brain region/function. Taken together with the animal findings, these data would suggest that aluminium is neurotoxic in humans.

What is controversial, however, is whether exposure to aluminium is a cause or contributor to Alzheimer's disease. There are four main bodies of evidence to consider, each of which has been questioned for different reasons. First, was the finding of aluminium in amyloid plaques and neurofibrillary tangles in the brains of people who had died of Alzheimer's disease. This finding is controversial because at that time it was technically difficult to identify aluminium accurately in bodily tissues. Most, later, more accurate attempts have failed to find any evidence of aluminium at all – although two more recent studies did (Morris, Puri, & Frye, 2017). The second line of evidence concerns exposure to aluminium in drinking water and Alzheimer's disease risk. Killin et al.'s (2016) systematic review of this literature was strongly supportive of a link; however, this conclusion is controversial because variability in aluminium exposure from other sources, especially diet, should completely overwhelm any signal from variability in water levels – particularly as dietary sources of aluminium are not typically controlled for. This concern motivated a number of studies that form the third line of evidence, namely whether dietary exposure to aluminium increases Alzheimer's disease risk. Studies have examined tea drinking (rich in aluminium), general dietary estimates of aluminium intake and antacid use (this generates very high levels of exposure). This body of literature has uniformly found no link between these sources of dietary aluminium and Alzheimer's disease (Kandimalla et al., 2016). These findings remain controversial because so many unmeasured variables may affect aluminium intake and absorption (e.g., individual genetic differences, difficulties in estimating aluminium dietary exposure, etc.; Exley, 2017). Finally, there is the animal literature, with the idea being to search for neuropathology reminiscent of human Alzheimer's disease following aluminium exposure. Setting aside the suitability of any animal model to capture all of the complex neuropathology of Alzheimer's disease, this literature is inconclusive. While key studies find evidence in transgenic mice of increases in amyloid β following aluminium exposure, other studies do not (Bondy, 2016).

Overall, proponents of the view that aluminium is a causative agent of Alzheimer's disease cite the socio-scientific history of lead neurotoxicity.

As Bondy (2016) notes, humans have a 3000-year history of lead usage, with neurotoxicity being recognised since 700 BC, but only since the 1980s has there been a gradual and grudging acknowledgement (and action) on the consequences of low-level lead exposure. In contrast, human use of aluminium only dates back 200 years, and restrictions on exposure would be financially costly for this large industry. Only more research will determine if this analogy is correct.

5.3.12   Pesticides

Pesticides refer to chemicals used to control a variety of plant and animal species that reduce agricultural productivity. Herbicides are the most prominent in terms of quantity used, but it is the insecticides – also used in high volumes – that are of special interest because they are aimed at killing animals from the class *Insecta*, with whom we share many neuro-chemical similarities. The first wave of insecticides in the 1940s was dominated by the organochlorines such as DDT (dichlorodiphenyltrichloroethane), but these were phased out in the 1970s due to their persistence in the environment and potential adverse effects on human health (endocrine disruptor, carcinogen). DDT is a neurotoxin and kills insects by altering the flow of ions through nerve membranes, leading to a generalised hyperexcitability of the nervous system and death. The organochlorines were replaced by the organophosphates, which are less immediately toxic to humans, degrade rapidly in the environment and so do not bioaccumulate (e.g., Lazartigues, Thomas, & Banas, 2013). This group is now being displaced by carbamates, which have a less toxic profile than the organophosphates, principally because they cannot pass the blood-brain barrier. Both carbamates and organophosphates exert their effects mainly by inhibiting acetylcholinesterase activity (irreversibly for organophosphates and reversibly for carbamates – linking to their toxicity), resulting in a build-up of acetylcholine in the synaptic cleft, with greater neural activity followed by suppression (Sidhu, Singh, & Kumar, 2019).

Chronic exposure to organochlorines and organophosphates has been studied quite extensively in agricultural workers, exterminators and in those who manufacture these chemicals. This body of work has highlighted that low-level exposure is associated with various adverse effects to health, including neurotoxic consequences, the most deleterious being an increased risk of developing Parkinson's disease (Wirdefeldt et al., 2011). Dietary exposure alone involves a chemical burden at least a few orders of magnitude less than that experienced by those who work directly with these chemicals. Perhaps not surprisingly then, the literature is inconclusive as to whether exposure at the concentrations encountered in food are harmful (Rosas & Eskenazi, 2008).

Most attention has been on foetal and infant exposure to organochlorines and organophosphates, via the mother (e.g., blood levels and in milk). There are studies that find adverse effects of exposure and ones that do not. Adverse effects are typically mild developmental delays for organochlorines, but for organophosphates the potential adverse consequences may be more severe, with links to ADHD and pervasive developmental disorder. For children and adults, most exposure (to organophosphates) occurs through grain products and fruit (Szenczi-Cseh & Ambrus, 2017). However, there is no obvious link between consuming these particular food types and higher rates of Parkinson's disease (Wirdefeldt et al., 2011). Although many consumers remain concerned about ingesting pesticides, diet-induced neurotoxic effects do not seem to pose a significant risk.

5.3.13 Conclusion

A number of interesting themes emerge from this literature. One concerns the connections between exposure to dietary neurotoxins and the degenerative diseases of old age, suggesting at the broadest theoretical level that these diseases reflect cumulative environmental insults, of which diet is one contributor. Another is the way in which poor nutrition (especially sulphur-containing amino acids) can heighten vulnerability to dietary neurotoxins, with lathyrism, konzo and TAN being more obvious examples. Less obvious examples may be lead, arsenic and methyl mercury exposure, where it has been suggested that dietary iron, calcium and selenium may be protective, and that their deficiency may enhance vulnerability. A further theme is the putative interactive effects of chronic dietary neurotoxins with other toxins and neurotoxins. These are understudied and difficult to disentangle, but clearly occur (e.g., lead and cadmium, mercury and PCBs, arsenic and manganese).

In addition to these emerging themes, it is also important to mention two examples that we left out. One is the goitrogens, of which Cassava is an important example, and there are several others (e.g., *brassicae* species). The goitrogens are not directly neurotoxic, but lead to an iodine-deficiency syndrome (see Chapter 2 and 9) that affects brain development and function. The other concerns exposure to the environmental breakdown of plastics in the sea and their accumulation in seafood – so-called micro- and nanoplastics. We did not include these because at the moment it is unclear if they exert neurotoxic effects in humans and other mammals. However, an emerging body of work in fish and marine invertebrates suggests they are neurotoxic, and there is a growing suspicion that they may also harm us (Prust, Meijer, & Westerink, 2020).

5.4   General Conclusion

Apart from the considerable human disease burden that results from dietary neurotoxins, it is their capacity to shed light on other significant scientific questions that makes them so interesting. Among the chronic dietary neurotoxins, protein misfolding often emerges as a cause of neuronal dysfunction. Not only may this offer one way to understand specific brain region and cell type effects (i.e., via impact on a specific protein/s expressed solely in that region/cell type), but it also merges into the prion literature, as a pathway to neurodegenerative disease. Among the acute dietary neurotoxins, the most interesting question is a different one, namely what functional goal do these poisons serve. Although this can be clearly addressed for plant alkaloids, it is far less clear what function many of the potent marine neurotoxins have. As these contribute significantly to the human poison burden, understanding their function may be important in predicting outbreaks and managing risk.

CHAPTER 6

Neuroprotective Effects of Diet

6.1 Introduction

As covered in Chapter 4, a nutritionally poor-quality diet – particularly a Western-style diet (WS-diet) – is increasingly understood to exert adverse effects on neurological function. Consumption of a WS-diet impairs learning and memory, and is associated with increased risk or severity of psychological, neurological and neurodegenerative disease. The physiological mechanisms underlying these effects include inflammation, oxidative stress, blood-brain barrier permeability, reduced brain derived neurotrophic factor (BDNF) and gut dysbiosis (covered in Chapter 4). Conversely, healthy dietary patterns (e.g., Mediterranean diet) and certain dietary components (e.g., polyphenols) have antioxidant and anti-inflammatory properties (Estruch, 2010; Yoon & Baek, 2005), and beneficially impact the gut microbiota (De Filippis et al., 2016; Telle-Hansen, Holven, & Ulven, 2018). Considering there are a multitude of neurological conditions which are associated with increased oxidative stress, neuroinflammation and gut dysbiosis, this raises the question of whether using diet (see Table 6.1 for a summary of the key diets that have been studied) to reduce this pathology can improve the course and outcomes of these neurological conditions. This is the focus of this chapter.

6.2 Mediterranean Diet

The Mediterranean Diet (MedDiet) incorporates high intakes of fish, fruits, vegetables, legumes, wholegrains, olive oil and nuts, and minimal intake of processed foods, including hydrogenated or trans-fats, refined grains and added sugar. The MedDiet became of interest based on observations that, relative to Western countries, people living in Greece, Italy and Yugoslavia tend to have greater longevity and lower rates of cardiovascular disease, cancer and other chronic health conditions (Keys et al., 1986;

Table 6.1. *Summary of recommendations for Mediterranean, DASH, MIND and Ketogenic diets*

Food	Diet			
	Mediterranean	DASH	MIND	Ketogenic
Fruit	Yes	Yes	Yes	Yes**
Vegetables	Yes	Yes	Yes	Yes**
Berries	–	–	Yes	–
Leafy greens	–	–	Yes	–
Wholegrains	Yes	Yes	Yes	No
Beans	–	Yes	Yes	Yes**
Poultry	Yes	Yes	Yes	Yes
Fish	Yes	Yes	Yes	Yes
Red meat	Reduce	No	No	Yes
Oils	Olive oil	–	Olive oil	Any oil
Nuts	Yes	Yes	Yes	Yes
Seeds	Yes	Yes	–	Yes
Dairy	Limited	Low fat	Reduce	Yes
Alcohol	Limited	–	Limited	Limited
Processed foods	Reduce	–	–	Reduce
Sweets	Reduce	Reduce	Reduce	Limited
Sodium	–	Reduce	–	–
Saturated fat	–	Reduce	–	–

* DASH = Dietary Approach to Stop Hypertension, MIND = Mediterranean-DASH Intervention for Neurodegenerative Delay.
**Allowed if within carbohydrate range.

Willett, 1994). Although the initial interest in the Mediterranean diet was sparked by the Seven Countries study (Keys et al., 1986), which has been widely criticized for failing to include several countries that did not fit the pattern of results, there is now a vast literature investigating the beneficial effects of this traditional dietary pattern. Many more recent studies have linked MedDiet to reduced risk of chronic diseases, including cardiovascular disease, diabetes and cancer (Serra-Majem, Roman, & Estruch, 2006). Here, we address the evidence for the benefit of MedDiet for conditions that affect the brain.

There are several possible mechanisms through which MedDiet may exert beneficial effects on brain health. There is evidence that MedDiet can modify cardiovascular risk factors such as body weight, blood pressure, fasting blood glucose and atherosclerotic dyslipidaemia (Estruch et al., 2018). These in turn are likely to improve blood flow to the brain.

Indeed, adherence to MedDiet is associated with reduced cerebrovascular disease on MRI (Scarmeas et al., 2011). MedDiet has also been shown to reduce oxidative stress and neuroinflammation (Vetrani et al., 2013), and has also been linked to beneficial modification of gut microbiota (Lopez-Legarrea et al., 2014).

6.2.1 Cognitive Performance

For the MedDiet, a systematic review reported that in three cross-sectional studies, higher MedDiet intake was associated with a higher cognitive score combining memory, language, processing speed and visuospatial function (Petersson & Philippou, 2016). Of 18 longitudinal studies, MedDiet intake was associated with better working memory and verbal fluency, processing speed, verbal memory and immediate and delayed recall. Five RCTs were also identified, with four showing improved cognition. Notably, the single RCT that did not demonstrate cognitive improvement in the MedDiet group was a small ($n = 25$), within-subjects, 10-day intervention conducted in young adults (McMillan et al., 2011). One study with a sample of 176 (mean age = 53) from the UK, demonstrated reduced confusion in the MedDiet group (Wardle et al., 2000). The remaining three studies were subpopulations of the Prevencion con Dieta Mediterrania (PREDIMED) trial. Older adults at risk of cardiovascular disease were randomized to one of two MedDiet intervention arms (one supplemented with nuts, the other with olive oil), compared to a low-fat diet control group. Though the primary outcome was cardiovascular prevention, subsets of the trial were examined in relation to changes in cognition. In 522 participants, both MedDiet groups performed better on the mini mental state exam (MMSE) and clock drawing than the low-fat diet control after 6.5 years on the diet (Martinez-Lapiscina et al., 2013). In 285 participants who were addition-ally evaluated by a neurologist, the MedDiet with olive oil group per-formed better on verbal fluency and memory tasks and had a lower risk of mild cognitive impairment (MCI; Martinez-Lapiscina et al., 2014). However, neither of the above studies included cognitive information at baseline. In 334 participants who completed repeated cognitive assess-ments, both of the MedDiet groups showed improved cognitive function over 4 years on a battery of memory, attention and executive function tests, whereas the low-fat control group demonstrated cognitive decline (Valls-Pedret et al., 2015).

6.2.2 Depression and Anxiety

Diet has been of increasing interest as a modifiable risk factor for the common mental health disorders of depression and anxiety. Overall, systematic reviews consistently show that healthy eating patterns are associated with reduced risk of depression in adults (Lai et al., 2014), young adults (Collins et al., 2020) and children (O'neil et al., 2014). MedDiet has emerged as the healthy diet pattern having the most evidence of an association with depression. A meta-analysis of nine cross-sectional studies showed that greater MedDiet adherence was linked to a 28% lower odds ratio for depression; however, there was no association between MedDiet and depression across four cohort studies (Shafiei et al., 2019). In contrast, a separate meta-analysis reported that MedDiet adherence was associated with lower risk of depressive symptoms across time (Molendijk et al., 2018). Two RCTs have shown that a MedDiet pattern can improve depression symptoms in adults with a diagnosis of depression (Jacka et al., 2017; Parletta et al., 2019).

Though anxiety has received less attention, a similar relationship appears to exist. In cross-sectional studies, MedDiet adherence has also been linked to lower risk of anxiety (Sadeghiet al., 2021; Sanchez-Villegas et al., 2009). And, although anxiety was a secondary outcome in one of the RCTs described before, improvements in anxiety symptoms were also observed following 12 weeks of a MedDiet pattern (Jacka et al., 2017).

The likely mechanisms are consistent with those described in Section 6.2.1, and in Chapter 4. Both chronic inflammation and oxidative stress have been implicated as a causal pathway in depression and other mental health disorders (Anderson et al., 2014). Animal models have shown that alterations in gut microbiota can increase depressive and anxiety-like behaviours (Dinan et al., 2019). The HPA axis is strongly implicated in the pathophysiology of psychiatric disorders. For example, greater than 60% of people with depression exhibit alterations to HPA-axis activity, including elevated levels of cortisol production and ACTH levels (Naughton, Dinan, & Scott, 2014). Higher adherence to MedDiet has been linked to lower cortisol levels and lower levels of inflammatory biomarkers (Carvalho et al., 2018). Furthermore, cortisol has been associated with higher levels of tumour necrosis factor (TNF; i.e., greater inflammation) and higher adherence to MedDiet appears to counteract this association. Relatedly, BDNF has been implicated in the pathogenesis of depression and anxiety, with decreased hippocampal BDNF levels associated with depressive behaviours, and observations that antidepressants enhance the expression of BDNF

(Martinowich, Manji, & Lu, 2007). In a subpopulation of participants in the PREDIMED study who had depression at baseline, those in the MedDiet plus nuts group had higher levels of plasma BDNF after 3 years compared to the low-fat diet control group (Sánchez-Villegas et al., 2011). The underlying mechanisms of action by which diet may influence mental health (i.e., neuroinflammation, oxidative stress, epigenetics, mitochondrial dysfunction, gut–brain links, tryptophan metabolism, HPA axis, BDNF) have been reviewed comprehensively by Marx et al. (2021). While much of these data are based upon animal studies, they offer a convincing and plausible picture of how diet can impact mental health via multiple interacting pathways.

6.2.3 *Neurodegenerative Conditions*

The results of several meta-analyses show MedDiet is protective against the development of MCI (mild cognitive impairment)/AD (Alzheimer's Disease), when measured by brief cognitive screening or *Diagnostic and Statistical Manual of the American Psychiatric Association* (DSM) criteria (Singh et al., 2014; Sofi, Macchi, & Casini, 2013; Wu & Sun, 2017). There are several possible mechanisms that may explain the neuroprotective effects of MedDiet in AD. Atrophy in AD has been associated with neuroinflammation, oxidative stress, reduced blood flow and gut micro-biome changes (Frisardi et al., 2010a; Petersson & Philippou, 2016), which are factors modified by MedDiet as described in Section 6.1.2. MedDiet has also been associated with reductions in AD pathology, beta-amyloid and tau, using PET imaging markers (Matthews et al., 2014; Merrill et al., 2016). And on MRI, greater MedDiet adherence is associated with larger overall brain volume and greater grey matter volume in brain regions typically affected in AD, such as the temporal lobes and hippocampus (Gu et al., 2015; Mosconi et al., 2014; Staubo et al., 2017).

A limited body of research has investigated links between MedDiet and other neurodegenerative conditions. Closer adherence to the MedDiet has been linked to reduced odds of Parkinson's disease (PD) and later age of onset of this disorder (Gao et al., 2007; Okubo et al., 2012). In 600 individuals with PD in Italy, while overall MedDiet consumption was not significantly different to matched controls, people with PD consumed less fruit, vegetables, fish, milk and cereals compared to controls, these being important components of the MedDiet (Alcalay et al., 2012). In Huntington's disease, while MedDiet adherence was not associated with disease onset (Marder et al., 2013) – as might be expected given the genetic basis for this condition – it was associated with better-quality of life (Cubo et al., 2015; Rivadeneyra et al., 2016).

6.2.4   Other Neurological Conditions

The ability of a MedDiet to reduce neuroinflammation and oxidative stress, and benefit the gut microbiome, should in theory also confer benefit in the treatment of other neurological diseases where these mechanisms are likely to be important. Indeed, studies suggest that MedDiet consumption lowers risk of multiple sclerosis (MS) (Jahromi et al., 2012; Sedaghat et al., 2016). People with MS with high fish, fruit, vegetable, and legume intake (i.e., components of MedDiet) report better mental and cognitive quality of life (Hadgkiss et al., 2015). A randomised controlled trial (RCT) in 20 individuals with MS revealed that a combination of 10 days caloric restriction followed by a 6-month MedDiet improved subjective attention, concentration and memory; however, the design meant it was not possible to tease out the beneficial effects of diet versus caloric restriction (Choi et al., 2016).

6.3   Dietary Approaches to Stop Hypertension (DASH) Diet

The DASH diet recommends higher intake of fruit, vegetables, low-fat dairy products, whole grains, poultry, fish and nuts, and recommends reducing intake of red meat, sweets and sugar-containing beverages. The primary difference with the MedDiet is that the DASH diet places no emphasis on consuming oily fish, plus the DASH diet is heavily focused on reducing sodium intake. This is not surprising, given that the DASH diet was developed specifically to help lower blood pressure. Considering the beneficial effects of the DASH diet on cardiovascular risk factors, some studies have also investigated its potential to improve cognitive function and reduce risk of neurodegenerative and neurological conditions.

6.3.1   Cognitive Performance

Prospective studies in older adults have shown the DASH diet is linked to less cognitive decline after 4.1 years (Tangney et al., 2014), and with better cognitive function after 11 years (Wengreen et al., 2013). In women aged more than 70 years, adherence to the DASH diet over an 11-year period (1984–1995) was associated with better average cognitive function in the next 6 years (1995–2001), and specifically better verbal memory and performance on a brief telephone screening tool (Berendsen et al., 2017).

However, in this study, adherence to the DASH diet 1984–1995, was not related to *change* in cognitive function over 1995–2001, which may suggest that people need to remain on the DASH diet to maintain cognitive benefits. One RCT investigating the effect of DASH diet on cognition over a 4-month period showed psychomotor speed improved in those assigned to the DASH diet, compared to the usual diet control group (Smith et al., 2010a). The group receiving the DASH diet with exercise and caloric restriction improved on measures of executive function, memory and learning, whereas improvements in those domains were not observed with the DASH diet alone.

6.3.2   Neurodegenerative Conditions

Higher adherence to a DASH diet has been shown to be related to a lower risk of MCI and AD (Morris et al., 2015b). There has only been limited research examining links between DASH diet and other neurodegenerative conditions, perhaps because a revised version of this diet, focused on neurodegenerative conditions, quickly emerged (see Section 6.3.4).

6.3.3   Depression

There is increasing evidence that depression is linked to hypertension (Meng et al., 2012). Moreover, both depression and hypertension are associated with elevated inflammation, oxidative stress and hyperactivation of the HPA axis (Dinh et al., 2014; Hamer & Steptoe, 2012; Perez-Cornago et al., 2014). Due to the potential benefit of the DASH diet on hypertension and other depression risk factors, it has been of interest to investigate the relationship between DASH diet and depression. Cross-sectionally, DASH diet adherence was associated with lower depression symptoms in Iranian adults (Valipour et al., 2017) and adolescent girls (Khayyatzadeh et al., 2018). In 14,051 individuals without depression symptoms at baseline, DASH diet was associated with lower depression risk after a follow-up period of approximately 8 years (Perez-Cornago et al., 2017). In older adults (mean age 80.4), those with higher adherence to the DASH diet had lower rates of depressive symptoms over a 6.5-year follow-up (Cherian et al., 2020). An RCT of 102 women with migraine showed that, as well as reduced migraine severity, the DASH group had lower depression symptoms compared to controls (Arab et al., 2021). However, this finding cannot be generalized to the broader population as the improvement in depression symptoms may have been secondary to reduced migraine severity. To our knowledge, there are no clinical trials evaluating depression symptoms as a primary outcome following DASH diet.

6.3.4   Other Neurological Conditions

Little research has focused on DASH diet and other neurological conditions. As described earlier, DASH diet was shown to reduce migraine severity compared to a control diet in an RCT. Retrospective analysis of two large cohort studies, the Nurses Health Study and the Health Professionals Study, found no association between DASH diet pattern at baseline and risk of developing MS over a 4-year follow-up (Rotstein et al., 2019).

6.4   Mediterranean-DASH Diet Intervention for Neurodegenerative Delay (MIND)

The MIND diet is a new dietary pattern designed specifically to reduce risk of dementia. As the name suggests, it is based off the principles of the MedDiet and DASH diets. It is very similar to these diets, encouraging high intake of vegetables, whole grains, fish, nuts and olive oil. However, the MIND diet additionally recommends increased intake of leafy green vegetables and berries, and reduced intake of red meat, cheese, butter/margarine, fast fried foods, pastries and sweets. In prospective studies, the MIND diet was associated with reduced risk of cognitive impairment observed over a 12-year period in older adults who were aged 60–64 years at baseline (Hosking et al., 2019). In older adults (average age 81.4 years), the MIND diet was associated with slower rate of cognitive decline over 4.7 years, and when participants with MCI at baseline were analysed separately, the MIND diet was shown to be even more protective (Morris et al., 2015a). The MIND diet was associated with reduced risk of AD over 4.5 years in participants aged 58–98 years, and appeared to confer a greater reduction in dementia risk compared to the DASH diet and MedDiet (Morris et al., 2015b). Finally, the MIND diet has also been associated with lower depressive symptoms over a 6.5-year period in older adults (Cherian et al., 2020).

6.5   Ketogenic Diet

The ketogenic diet (KD) is high in fat and low in carbohydrate, typically at a ratio of 4:1. It was designed to mimic a fasting state, without depriving the body of adequate protein for growth and development. Under normal conditions, the brain utilises glucose as its primary sources of energy by breaking down carbohydrates through a process called glycolysis. When the predominant caloric source switches to fat, the body resorts to mobilizing fatty acids from fat stores, which are then metabolised by the liver to produce ketone bodies. The brain is able to use ketones in order to generate cellular energy. This shift in energy metabolism appears to reset cellular metabolic dysfunction and neuronal activity by: (1) reducing glutamate-mediated apoptosis and increasing GABA-mediated inhibition (Gano, Patel, & Rho, 2014; Gasior, Rogawski, & Hartman, 2006); (2) reducing oxidative stress by decreasing reactive oxygen species (Sullivan et al., 2004); (3) increasing levels of antioxidant agents (Milder, Liang, & Patel, 2010); (4) increasing mitochondrial biogenesis (Bough et al., 2006); and (5) reducing inflammation (Kim do et al., 2012).

A challenge of this diet is that it is considered unpalatable, and frequently reported side effects include gastrointestinal upset, weight loss and increases in serum lipids (McDonald & Cervenka, 2018). As such, less strict KD variants have emerged, including lower ratio KD (e.g. 3:1 or 2:1), the Modified Atkins Diet (MAD; typically a 10–20 g/day carbohydrate limit), or medium-chain triglyceride oil (MCT) supplementation (e.g. coconut or palm kernel oil).

6.5.1 Epilepsy

The original ketogenic diet was described by Wilder in 1921 and proposed to treat epilepsy (Wilder, 1921). It has primarily been used to treat paediatric epilepsy, with 30–60% of children achieving a 50% reduction in seizures, which is defined as therapeutic success. In adults, a meta-analysis revealed a combined efficacy rate of the KD of 52% for the classic KD and 34% for the MAD (Ye et al., 2015). Improvements in cognition are reported in both children and adults with epilepsy who consume a KD, and may be due to both reduction in seizures as well as ability to withdraw from medications (Nikanorova et al., 2009). In a randomized controlled trial, 26 children and adolescents between the ages of 1–18 years on KD for 4 months showed reduced seizure frequency and severity, as well as greater improvement in receptive vocabulary and simple reaction time, compared to the 22 patients in the care-as-usual group (Lambrechts et al., 2016). There were no improvements in tasks assessing motor activation or integration of visual and motor abilities. In adults with refractory epilepsy, there are subjective reports of improvements in alertness and concentration following KD (Mosek et al., 2009; Sirven et al., 1999). However, other studies, which have utilised objective neuropsychological testing, have not shown any consistent change in cognition despite reductions in seizure frequency (Lambrechts et al., 2012; Veggiotti et al., 2010). It may be that early intervention with the KD is necessary to prevent developmental delay occurring. This interpretation is supported by studies suggesting improvements appear to be largest in the youngest children (Ramm-Pettersen et al., 2014).

6.5.2   Malignant Gliomas

Malignant gliomas are the most common type of brain tumour, with glioblastoma multiforme (GBM) being the most aggressive type. Despite surgical resection, radiotherapy and temozolomide, response to treatment is poor and less than 10% survive 5 years (Anton, Baehring, & Mayer, 2012). KD has been explored as a therapeutic option as, unlike brain cells, cancer cells cannot utilize ketone bodies effectively. To meet the demands of rapid proliferation, tumour cells have high rates of glycolysis, thus rely on glucose as the main energy source for sustaining growth (Warburg, Wind, & Negelein, 1927). Hyperglycaemia is negatively associated with survival in GBM patients (Derr et al., 2009).

In studies using a mouse glioma model, KD as an adjunct to radiation therapy reduced blood glucose, increased blood ketones and extended life (Abdelwahab et al., 2012), reduced tumour vasculature (Woolf & Scheck, 2015) and reduced reactive oxygen species (Abdelwahab et al., 2010) compared to a control diet group. Studies examining the use of KD for the treatment of brain tumours are typically case studies. In 2010, a 65-year-old woman with GBM was treated with a kilojoule-restricted (<2,510 kJ/day) KD combined with radiation and chemotherapy after partial tumour resection. After 2 months on the diet, there was no observable brain tumour, whereas 10 weeks after the diet was stoppe, tumour recurrence was detected (Zuccoli et al., 2010). In a pilot study of 20 adults, patients who achieved stable ketosis on a KD had a trend toward increased progression-free survival (Rieger et al., 2014). However, in other studies, adults treated with KD showed evidence of tumour progression by 12 months in a case series of 6 adults (Champ et al., 2014), and by 12 weeks in another case series of 2 adults (Schwartz et al., 2015). Overall, though KD appears to be safe and tolerable in the treatment of GBM, in the absence of control groups it is not possible to draw conclusions about its efficacy.

6.5.3 Traumatic Brain Injury

Rodents maintained on a KD have been shown to have improved cognitive outcomes following traumatic brain injury (TBI), including improved recovery of memory function (Appelberg, Hovda, & Prins, 2009). The physiological mechanisms underlying these improvements include reduced cerebral oedema, apoptosis and improved cerebral metabolism (Deng-Bryant et al., 2011; Hu et al., 2009; Prins, Fujima, & Hovda, 2005). These effects appear to be age dependent, with KD conferring neuroprotection in young but not adult rodents (Deng-Bryant et al., 2011). To our knowledge, there are no human studies that investigate KD in TBI.

6.5.4 Multiple Sclerosis

In an animal model of multiple sclerosis, ketogenic diet has been shown to reduce neuroinflammation, with corresponding dampened motor disability and attenuation of memory dysfunction (Kim do et al., 2012). One randomized controlled trial has been undertaken, assessing the impact of KD for 6 months, compared to diet as usual in 20 patients with relapsing-remitting MS. The KD group self-reported improved health-related quality of life, including mental and cognitive health, compared to the diet-as-usual group (Choi et al., 2016). However, it is difficult to establish a blinded control condition in such trials due to the nature of the intervention, therefore, future studies would benefit from objective neuropsychological testing rather than subjective report of cognitive improvement.

6.5.5 Aging and Neurodegenerative Conditions

In aged rats, KD administered for three weeks significantly improved learning and memory (Xu et al., 2010). This was associated with increased angiogenesis and capillary density, suggesting KD may support cognition via improved vascular function in aging. In 20 older adults with AD or MCI, an MCT diet was linked to improved performance on a brief screening tool covering several cognitive domains, including attention, memory, language and praxis (Reger et al., 2004). However, this effect was observed only for those individuals without the Apolipoprotein-E e4 allele suggesting these subjects are better able to utilize ketones than APOE e4 carriers. In 23 older adults with MCI, ketosis was induced using a very low carbohydrate diet (5–10%) and was shown to improve verbal memory performance compared to a high-carbohydrate diet (50%), with improved memory positively correlated with ketone levels (Krikorian et al., 2012b). In one further RCT in 152 individuals with AD, MCT consumption improved performance on a cognitive screening test (ADAS-Cog) compared to placebo (Henderson et al., 2009).

6.5.6   Autism Spectrum Disorder

Autism spectrum disorder (ASD) is a neurodevelopmental disorder that is characterized by problems with social interaction and communication, and restricted or repetitive behaviours. KD has been hypothesized to improve symptoms in ASD through its anti-inflammatory properties, improved mitochondrial function (Lee, 2012) and changes in gut microbiota (Rawat et al., 2021). In animal models, KD attenuated some autistic features, for example showing increased sociability and decreased repetitive behaviour (Castro et al., 2017). We are aware of only one randomized controlled trial in humans, which found improvement on the Childhood Autism Rating Scale (CARS) in those consuming a MAD diet for 6 months, compared to a gluten-free, casein-free diet (El-Rashidy et al., 2017). A prospective follow-up study of 30 children over 6 months (Evangeliou et al., 2003), and a single case observed over 16 months (Żarnowska et al., 2018), similarly showed improvement on the CARS. In addition, clinical improvements on both the CARS and the autism diagnostic observation schedule-2 (ADOS-2) were observed after 3 months on a KD/gluten-free/MAT diet (Lee et al., 2018). Notably, there was a great deal of variability in the diet protocols used across all of these studies, including MAD, MCT and KD. However, considering individuals with ASD often have extreme food selectivity, flexibility in the dietary regime may be necessary to engage this population.

6.6   Nutritional Components That May Contribute to Neuroprotection

6.6.1   Polyphenols

Polyphenols are natural compounds found in plant-based foods. They are classed into two subgroups; flavonoids and non-flavonoids. The subgroups of polyphenols and their dietary sources can be seen in Table 6.2. Polyphenols are proposed to exert beneficial effects on the brain due to their antioxidant, and anti-inflammatory properties (Yoon & Baek, 2005). In addition, they can modulate intracellular processing cascades and gene

Table 6.2. *Polyphenols and their dietary sources*

Class	Subclass	Example compound	Natural source
Flavonoids	Anthocyanins	Cyanidin, malvidin, delphinidin	Berries, grapes, red wine, cherry
	Flavonols	Quercetin, myricetin	Rhubarb
	Flavones	Apigenin, luteolin	Red onion, leek
	Flavanones	Hesperitin, naringenin	Broccoli
	Flavanols	Epicatechins, epigallocatechins,	Celery, parsley
	Epigallocatechin gallate	Capsicum	
	Isoflavones grapes, wine, cocoa, apricots, beans, green tea, soybeans, miso	Genistein, daidzein	Citrus fruits
Phenolic acids	Caffeic acid, ferulic acid	Coffee, cereals	
Phenolic alcohols	Hydroxytyrosol	Olives	
Curcuminoids	Curcumin	Turmeric	
Stilbenes	Resveratrol Pomegranate	Grapes	
Lignans	Secoisolariciresinol Garlic	Lentils, linseed	
Tanins	Condensed	Procyanidins	Cocoa, chocolate
	Hydrolyzable	Gallotannins, ellagitannins	Mango, pomegranate

expression, thus can increase synaptic plasticity to have a direct effect on memory formation and storage (Vauzour, 2017). Furthermore, their anti-diabetic, anti-thrombotic and anti-hypertensive actions exert a positive effect on the vascular system, which may also improve cerebral blood flow (Khurana et al., 2013). As such, the potential for polyphenols in the prevention and treatment of cognitive decline in aging and neurological disorders has attracted a lot of interest.

6.6.1.1   *Age-Related Cognitive Decline*

Epidemiological studies have shown that increased consumption of poly-phenols is associated with better cognition in middle-aged and older adults without dementia. A review of 28 papers concluded that overall higher dietary polyphenol intake does have beneficial effects on cognition for healthy or mildly cognitively impaired older adults, with the most beneficial polyphenol sources being berry fruit juices and isoflavone sources such as soy protein or soy isoflavone supplements (Lamport et al., 2012). Since that review was published, additional studies have shown increased consumption of polyphenols assessed using urinary bio-markers are associated with better immediate memory in individuals aged 55–80 years (Valls-Pedret et al., 2012) and with lower risk of cognitive decline over 3 years in adults more than 65 years old (Rabassa et al., 2015). In middle-aged adults, higher total polyphenol intake assessed using die-tary records was associated with better language and verbal memory, assessed after a follow-up of 13 years (Kesse-Guyot et al., 2012).

Grape juice is rich in polyphenols, including flavonoids, resveratrol and anthocyanins, and a relatively easy way to increase polyphenol intake in intervention studies as it can be matched for taste (Stalmach et al., 2011). Healthy women aged 40–50 who consumed grape juice for 12 weeks showed benefits across several measures of cognition, including verbal recall, executive function and lateral tracking, compared to placebo (Lamport et al., 2016). Similarly, older adults with MCI showed improved memory, together with greater activation in the anterior and posterior right hemisphere on functional neuroimaging, following grape juice supplemen-tation for 16 weeks (Krikorian et al., 2012a). A review of RCTs examining the effects of flavonoids on cognition reported that 9 out of the 15 included studies reported significant improvements in cognition following flavonoid supplementation compared to a control group (Macready et al., 2009).

With regard to specific polyphenols, higher intake of blueberries and strawberries, rich in anthocyanin, was associated with reduced cognitive decline in adults more than 70 years old (Devore et al., 2012). Blueberries consistently improve hippocampal plasticity and memory function in animal studies (Casadesus et al., 2004; Ramirez et al., 2005).

Cocoa is high in epicatechin, catechin and oligomeric procyanidins (Lazarus, Hammerstone, & Schmitz, 1999). In middle-aged adults, con-sumption of a cocoa-containing drink resulted in significantly enhanced positive mood compared to placebo after 1 month, but no effects were observed for cognition (Pase et al., 2013). Healthy older adults who consumed a high cocoa diet for 3 months had better memory performance compared to placebo on a pattern separation task, and this was accompa-nied by enhanced activity in the dentate gyrus, the area of the hippocam-pus responsible for neurogenesis (Brickman et al., 2014). Curcumin is a polyphenol found in the yellow spice turmeric. In adults aged 60–85, 1 month of curcumin supplementation improved working memory and mood compared to placebo (Rainey-Smith et al., 2016). Resveratrol is found in grapes, red and white wine, dark berries and cocoa. In overweight but otherwise healthy individuals aged 50–80 years, 26 weeks of resveratrol supplementation resulted in better verbal memory performance and increased functional connectivity in the hippocampus (Witte et al., 2014).

6.6.1.2 Alzheimer's Disease

In rat models of AD, improvements in learning and memory have been observed following grape seed (Lian et al., 2016), curcumin (Hoppe et al., 2013), lychee (Sakurai et al., 2013), dark chocolate (Madhavadas et al., 2016), green tea (Haque et al., 2008), red wine (Wang et al., 2006) and cinnamon (Frydman-Marom et al., 2011) supplementation. Apart from their antioxidant and anti-inflammatory properties, additional underlying mechanisms for reducing AD pathology may be the ability for polyphenols to lower levels of amyloid-beta plaques (Hirohata et al., 2007; Ono et al., 2008). In addition, grape skin anthocyanin (GSA) extract, can inhibit acetylcholinesterase (Pervin et al., 2014). There are few studies conducted in humans. In older adults with dementia, daily consumption of cherry juice, rich in anthocyanin, improved verbal fluency and short- and long-term memory after 12 weeks compared to a control juice (Kent et al., 2017). The cherry juice group also showed reductions in systolic blood pressure, but not markers of inflammation (CRP and IL-6).

6.6.1.3 Depression and Anxiety

Polyphenols are proposed as a promising candidate for reducing symptoms of depression and anxiety through the same mechanisms of reducing neuroinflammation and oxidative stress, and positive effects on adult hippocampal neurogenesis (Dias et al., 2012). The literature supporting effects of polyphenols is summarized very well in a recently published systematic review of observational and interventional studies that assessed depression symptoms in relation to polyphenol intake (Bayes, Schloss, & Sibbritt, 2020). In 17 of the 20 observational studies, higher polyphenol intake was significantly associated with decreased symptoms of depression. Of 17 interventional studies, which assessed the effect of polyphenol supplementation for individuals with elevated depressive symptoms or with a diagnosis of depression, 12 found a statistically significant positive effect, 4 found a positive effect that was not statistically significant, and only two observed no difference between groups. The polyphenols identified as being effective in the review included soy isoflavones, tea flavanols, cocoa flavanols, coffee hydroxycinnamic acid, walnut flavonols, citrus flavones and resveratrol.

The literature regarding anxiety is not as extensive as the depression literature. Animal studies have shown reduced anxiety behaviours in rodents supplemented with blackberry juice (Guzmán-Gerónimo et al., 2019), bilberry leaves (Sidorova et al., 2019), chlorogenic acid (Bouayed et al., 2007), green tea polyphenol-epigallocatechin gallate (EGCG; Vignes et al., 2006), and a polyphenolic combination of quercetin, xanthohumol and phlorotannin-rich extract (Donoso et al., 2020). A meta-analysis revealed that cocoa-products significantly reduced anxiety symptoms in seven studies with 429 human participants, with a medium effect size (Fusar-Poli et al., 2021).

6.6.1.4 Neurodevelopmental Disorders

The green tea flavonoid, ECGC, has been explored as a therapeutic tool for Down syndrome due to its ability to inhibit dual specificity tyrosine-(Y)-phosphorylation-regulated kinase 1A (Dyrk1A), in mouse models of Down syndrome (Souchet et al., 2019). Elevated levels of Dyrk1A are caused by trisomy 21 in Down syndrome, and are thought to be related to altered ratio of neuronal excitation and inhibition (Dowjat et al., 2007). Inhibition of Dyrk1A by ECGC administered prenatally, resulted in improvement in novel object recognition memory in mice (Souchet et al., 2019). In an RCT of 84 patients with Down syndrome, the group given ECGC together with cognitive training, demonstrated better visual recognition memory, inhibitory control and adaptive behaviour, compared to the group that received cognitive training with placebo (de la Torre et al., 2016). These findings provide support for larger-scale Phase 3 trials.

Animal models of ASD have similarly been used to examine the therapeutic potential of polyphenols. Oral palmitoylethanolamide and luteolin was shown to reduce non-social behaviours in mice (Bertolino et al., 2017). Learning and memory deficits in young mice with experimentally induced autism were attenuated by green tea consumption (Banji et al., 2011). Prenatal resveratrol administered subcutaneously was shown to prevent social deficits in offspring (Bambini-Junior et al., 2014). Resveratrol administered orally for 4 weeks restored the sensory and behavioural alterations in a rat model of ASD, and this was proposed to be due to suppression of oxidative stress, mitochondrial dysfunction and neuroinflammation (Bhandari & Kuhad, 2017). In an open label, phase 2 clinical trial, including 40 children aged 4–10 years with ASD, an oral polyphenolic formulation of luteolin, quercetin and quercetin glycoside rutin was shown to improve autistic behaviour and reduced serum levels of inflammatory markers compared to baseline (Tsilioni et al., 2015).

6.6.1.5 Other Neurological Conditions

Animal studies have investigated the potential for various polyphenols to improve cognition across a range of neurological conditions. Resveratrol has been shown to prevent impaired memory induced by chronic stress (Liu et al., 2014a), diabetes (Schmatz et al., 2009), traumatic brain injury (Sonmez et al., 2007) and ischaemic stroke (Li et al., 2016) in rats. Curcumin at doses of 50–300 mg/kg has been demonstrated to significantly improve learning and memory in experimental animal models of epilepsy (Ahmad, 2013; Choudhary et al., 2013; Jiang et al., 2015; Kaur, Bal, & Sandhir, 2014; Kaur et al., 2015; Mehla et al., 2010; Reeta et al., 2011), traumatic brain injury (Sharma, Ying, & Gomez-Pinilla, 2010; Sharma et al., 2009; Wu, Ying, & Gomez-Pinilla, 2006), diabetes (Kuhad & Chopra, 2007), human immunodeficiency virus (Tang et al., 2009), stress (Xu et al., 2009b) and cigarette-smoke (Jaques et al., 2012, 2013). These effects of curcumin were associated with normalization of hippocampal levels of BDNF, synaptic plasticity and markers of inflammation and oxidative stress. In an animal model of MS, curcumin also reduced the severity and duration of symptoms, the number of inflammatory cells, and T cell proliferation, though no investigation of cognition was reported (Natarajan & Bright, 2002; Xie et al., 2009).

Despite the promise of these animal studies, there are few human studies other than those examining age-related cognitive decline discussed earlier. Pomegranate extract, high in punicalagins, anthocyanins and ellagic acid, administered twice per day 1 week prior to surgery, attenuated postoperative memory deficits compared to placebo (Ropacki, Patel, & Hartman, 2013).

6.6.1.6 Summary: Polyphenols

While many of the supplement studies are at concentrations that would be difficult to obtain solely through diet (Rainey-Smith et al., 2016; Witte et al., 2014), the epidemiological studies presented do suggest that dietary consumption of polyphenols is associated with improved cognition, at levels that could be achieved through diet (e.g. >600 mg/day polyphenols or >495 mg/day flavonoids have been used as cut-offs (Lamport et al., 2015; Rabassa et al., 2015). As 200–300 mg polyphenols are available per 100 g of various fruits (e.g., grapes, apples, dark berries) and 100 mg per cup of tea or a large coffee (Llorach et al., 2012), such a level is clearly reachable from diet. Moreover, the supplement literature can guide which diet sources should be sought out. Overall, while there are numerous preclinical studies demonstrating the therapeutic potential of polyphenols across a range of conditions that affect the brain, clinical trials are now required to provide an evidence base supporting recommendations for their use in humans.

6.6.2   Omega-3 Fatty Acids

Omega-3 fatty acids (O3FA) are a group of polyunsaturated fatty acids (PUFAs) that play a critical role in brain development and function. The primary O3FAs are eicosapentaenoic acid (EPA) and docosahexaenoic acid (DHA). DHA is particularly concentrated in neural tissue, and is an important component of the phospholipid bilayer that surrounds all neurons (Kaplan & Greenwood, 1998). O3FAs have reported anti-inflammatory and antioxidant properties (Simopoulos, 1999), and they are vital for maintaining cell membranes, synaptic transmission and energy storage (Heinrichs, 2010). Humans are unable to synthesize O3FAs, and therefore they must be obtained through dietary sources (Simopoulos, 1991). Both EPA and DHA can be obtained by eating oily fish, and the use of fish oil as a dietary supplement has been the focus of much research in this field (Jenkins & Josse, 2008). Other dietary sources rich in O3FAs include krill oil, walnuts and oils such as flaxseed, canola and wheatgerm (Tou, Jaczynski, & Chen, 2007).

6.6.2.1   Neurodegenerative Conditions
The literature in this field is established enough that there have been several systematic reviews conducted. Overall, the benefit of O3FA supplementation appears to be dependent on severity of the disease. Patients with MCI generally show positive results in intervention studies of EPA and DHA supplementation, whereas no benefits are gained for patients with AD (Cederholm, Salem, & Palmblad, 2013). Consistent with this, a randomized, double-blind trial of 219 patients with MCI reported significantly better full-scale intelligence quotient following 12 months of 2 g/day DHA supplementation compared to placebo (Zhang et al., 2017). In addition, there were significant differences in hippocampal volumes bilaterally. Other reviews have reported positive effects of O3FA supplementation for those with mild AD, but not in severe AD (Ajith, 2018; Canhada et al., 2018). These findings suggest O3FA supplementation must occur early in the disease course to have observable effects.

Lowered levels of O3FA in the brain can alter dopamine systems in a manner that may increase the risk of developing PD (Healy-Stoffel & Levant, 2018). In a rat model, O3FA supplementation for 4 weeks prevented the behavioural and neurochemical disturbances associated with drug-induced PD (Barros et al., 2017). In various observational studies of patients with PD, higher O3FA intake was associated with a lower risk of PD (Abbott et al., 2003; De Lau et al., 2005; Gao et al., 2007), and reduced PD progression (Mischley, Lau, & Bennett, 2017). There are very few RCTs investigating O3FA supplementation in PD. One RCT found that 6 months of supplementation with fish oil (DHA 800 mg/day and EPA 290 mg/day) resulted in lower depression symptoms compared to placebo, but no difference in disease severity (Pomponi et al., 2014). Similarly, 3 months supplementation with fish oil (EPA 720 g/day and DHA 480 mg/day) reduced depression symptoms but not parkinsonian symptoms (da Silva et al., 2008). Finally, an RCT in 60 patients with PD found reduced disease severity in a group provided 1,000 mg O3FA from flaxseed oil, plus 400 IU vitamin E supplements for 12 weeks, compared to a placebo group (Taghizadeh et al., 2017). However, the effects of O3FA cannot be teased apart from Vitamin E in this study.

6.6.2.2   Depression and Anxiety

There are several systematic reviews and meta-analyses investigating the effect of O3FA supplementation in depression. We are aware of three meta-analyses that have reported an overall beneficial effect of O3FA supplementation on depression symptoms, and that EPA is more effective than DHA in major depressive disorder (Grosso et al., 2014; Liao et al., 2019; Mocking et al., 2016). The typical dose of EPA administered in these RCTs was mostly 1 or 2 g/day. In one of the meta-analyses, meta-regression showed that beneficial effects of O3FA supplementation were greater in participants taking antidepressants (Mocking et al., 2016). Furthermore, O3FA supplementation has been shown to decrease severity of depression symptoms among patients treated with, but resistant to, antidepressants (Jazayeri et al., 2008; Nemets, Stahl, & Belmaker, 2002; Peet & Horrobin, 2002). These findings suggest O3FAs may improve antidepressant response.

A systematic review and meta-analysis of 19 intervention studies including 2,240 participants showed that O3FA supplementation resulted in improvement in anxiety symptoms compared with control arms (Su et al., 2018). Analysis of subgroups showed that the association of O3FA treatment with anxiety was stronger in those with a clinical diagnosis as opposed to reported symptoms, and that a higher dose (>2 g/day) was more effective than lower doses (<2 g/day). In terms of mechanisms, RCTs conducted in student populations have shown that compared to placebo: (1) O3FA supplementation for 3 weeks can reduce anxiety induced by university exams, together with decreasing salivary cortisol levels (Yehuda, Rabinovitz, & Mostofsky, 2005), and (2) 12 weeks supplementation can reduce anxiety symptoms and concurrently lower inflammatory markers (Kiecolt-Glaser et al., 2011).

6.6.2.3   Other Neurological Conditions

Various animal studies have shown that O3FAs administered either prior to or following traumatic brain injury (TBI) can attenuate learning and memory deficits. (Mills, Hadley, & Bailes, 2011b; Pu et al., 2013; Wu, Ying, & Gomez-Pinilla, 2004). There are multiple mechanisms through which O3FAs may be beneficial to TBI recovery, including reducing axonal injury, inhibition of apoptosis, preventing hippocampal volume loss, increasing BDNF levels, inhibition of pro-inflammatory cytokines and reducing oxidative stress following the injury (Bailes & Mills, 2010; Mills et al., 2011a, 2011b; Wu, Ying, & Gomez-Pinilla, 2007). Human research has been restricted to a small number of case studies for whom O3FA supplementation was provided in hospital following TBI. However, improvements cannot be teased apart from the natural trajectory of recovery following TBI. Therefore, RCTs are required to demonstrate the efficacy of O3FAs for improving recovery in this population.

For people with multiple sclerosis, a meta-analysis which included seven studies showed O3FA supplementation was associated with reduced relapse rate, and beneficial effects on inflammatory markers and glutathione reductase (AlAmmar et al., 2021). A meta-analysis of four RCTs conducted in people with multiple sclerosis showed that O3FA supplementation had no significant effect on level of disability, or serum levels of pro-inflammatory cytokines IL-1B and IL-6 (Sedighiyan et al., 2019). However, there was a significant relationship with TNF-α, suggesting an anti-inflammatory effect.

6.6.2.4   Neurodevelopmental Disorders

Numerous trials have examined the effects of O3FA supplementation on symptoms of neurodevelopmental conditions such as ADHD and ASD. A meta-analysis of double-blind RCTs for ADHD showed the effect sizes for O3FA supplementation were small for parent ratings (ES = 0.17) and teacher ratings (−0.05) of symptoms (Pelsser et al., 2017). More recently, an RCT investigating O3FA supplementation for 3 months in children and adolescents with ADHD found greater reduction in ADHD ratings in the placebo group (Cornu et al., 2018). Several meta-analyses have found no evidence to support the use of O3FAs in reducing the core and associated symptoms of ASD (Bent, Bertoglio, & Hendren, 2009; Horvath, Lukasik, & Szajewska, 2017; James, Montgomery, & Williams, 2011). As such, there is little evidence to support the efficacy of O3FA supplementation for reducing the core symptoms for either of these disorders.

6.6.3   Summary: Nutritional Components

We have elected in this chapter only to cover the nutritional components with the greatest evidence base – polyphenols and O3FA. However, we acknowledge there are a range of other possible therapeutic components that we have not addressed and for which there is an emerging evidence base. Particular vitamins and minerals may be therapeutic, for example vitamin B12, or folate, may improve memory function in adult women (Bryan, Calvaresi, & Hughes, 2002). Vitamin E may attenuate cognitive impairment following TBI in animals and reduces cognitive decline in older adults (Perkins et al., 1999; Wu, Ying, & Gomez-Pinilla, 2004). Choline may ameliorate memory impairments secondary to seizures in rats (Holmes et al., 2002). The number of studies examining individual nutritional components in isolation is extensive. However, in the search for individual components that can be isolated and provided in supplement form, are we losing sight of the bigger picture? Taking the contents of Chapter 4 and this chapter together, it seems sensible to conclude that one cannot, for example, consume a WS-diet for decades and expect a polyphenol or omega-3 supplement to remediate the chronic adverse effects of such a diet. Ethical considerations probably prevent this question from ever being answered empirically (at least in humans), but it seems a tough possibility to consider nevertheless. What is perhaps a more reasonable issue is that there are numerous nutritional components of healthy diets that are beneficial for brain function and that may interact synergistically, and the ideal would be to consume a broad range of them through a varied, non-processed diet. A more detailed discussion of the merits and demerits of research on individual dietary components, and some of the broader issues surrounding this, can be found in Chapter 10 (see Sections 10.3.2 and 10.3.3).

6.7   Conclusions

This chapter provides a summary of the research examining the potential for diet to be used as an intervention to improve brain function in a range of neurological conditions. There are commonalities in the mechanisms underlying these diets, including their ability to reduce oxidative stress and inflammation and improve mitochondrial function. There is also some overlap in these diets as, for example, MedDiet, DASH and MIND all tend to be high in polyphenols, and all of the diets described result in reduced intake of processed foods, which as described in Chapter 4, have numerous adverse effects on the brain.

It should be noted that most studies do not propose that diet interventions should replace pharmacological and other medical treatments, but rather to be used as an adjunct to existing treatments. One advantage of diet interventions is that they are non-invasive and relatively low risk, with no side effects and are largely consistent with dietary recommendations aimed at improving other aspects of physical health. However, more extreme diets such as the ketogenic diet can cause ketoacidosis (unrestrained, abnormally excessive levels of ketone bodies) and may require close monitoring of ketone levels.

There are other disadvantages to diet interventions. When compared to pharmaceutical intervention, adherence to a prescribed diet can be difficult to achieve. There are potential cognitive, motivational, time and financial constraints that can prevent individual participants from engaging in a diet intervention. Furthermore, evaluating the effects of diet interventions can be more difficult than drug trials as it is difficult to obtain a true 'placebo' group with zero intake of the diet or nutrients in question, blinding participants to the diet they are consuming is impractical, and there is great variability in the level of adherence to the diet. Nevertheless, it is encouraging that despite these barriers, there is an increasing amount of literature to support the use of diet and diet components to improve brain function across a range of neurological conditions.

CHAPTER 7

Food-Related Drugs and Food as a Drug

7.1 Introduction

This chapter focuses on drugs that are commonly consumed as part of our diet, and on aspects of our diet that have been construed as having drug-like effects. The numbers are impressive. Approximately 2 billion people regularly drink alcohol, 6 billion regularly consume caffeine, and the whole of the world's 7.8 billion people consume food, with many now exposed to the types of food that *may* cause dependence. Consequently, the effects of these drugs – and perhaps of certain foods as well – is potentially profound, especially in their effects on the user and their capacity for dependence and harm. These form the main focus for each section on alcohol, caffeine (and theobromine) and food.

7.2 Alcohol

The archaeological record suggest that humans have deliberately consumed alcohol since Neolithic times. It serves several roles. It is a food, supplying energy at 7 kcal/g and contributing 16% of the energy intake of an adult American 'social' drinker (Traversy & Chaput, 2015). It is also made from food, with grain, for example, making bread, porridge, beer and spirits (Dietler, 2006). It serves an important ritualistic role in several religions, and as an intoxicant in many traditional celebrations and gatherings. In more recent times it has been commodified and marketed, with widespread availability, but at significant personal and societal cost (Moodie et al., 2013).

Approximately one-third of the world's adults are alcohol consumers, drinking an average of 6.4 L of pure alcohol per year (Peacock et al., 2018). More men consume alcohol than women (40% of male adults vs 25% of female adults), and while 18% of the world's adults report heavy episodic drinking (>60 g alcohol on one occasion in the last month), men are again over-represented here, relative to women (Global Burden of Disease 2016 Alcohol Collaborators, 2018). While men's use of alcohol involves more public drinking and drunkenness, risk-taking and aggression, women's use is less public, and is more associated with managing negative emotion (Erol & Karpyak, 2015). This distinction is becoming less apparent in Westernised nations, reflecting its likely sociocultural basis.

There is some controversy over claims that regular low alcohol usage may reduce all-cause mortality (Stockwell et al., 2016), even when setting aside arguments over whether this putative effect is caused by alcohol per se or by the polyphenols in beer and wine (Arranz et al., 2012). There is, however, no doubt that alcohol causes significant personal and social harms. Alcohol addiction is the most prevalent substance use disorder, with some 64 million adults estimated to have a problem in managing their consumption of this drug (Peacock et al., 2018). Alcohol represents a significant health burden on society. It is linked to 60 acute and chronic diseases, it was responsible for 2.8 million deaths in 2016, and was the seventh leading cause of premature death in 2016 (Global Burden of Disease 2016 Alcohol Collaborators, 2018). Again, men are over-represented in alcohol-related morbidity and mortality, and these problems are more common in alcohol-tolerant societies, with Europe having one of the highest age-standardised mortality (33/100,000) and drug-dependence rates (108/10,000).

An enormous amount has been written about alcohol, and there is also a very large body of associated research – enough to fill several books. The aim here is provide a general overview as alcohol usage pertains to brain and behaviour, because as the statistics above suggests, alcohol is a very consequential part of human diet.

7.2.1   Metabolism

It might seem odd that humans are able to metabolise alcohol. However, this capacity is present in all eukaryotes, and in humans a small quantity of alcohol is generated routinely by microbial fermentation in the gut – a condition that can become quite problematic in the rare instances of auto-brewery syndrome. Primary absorption of alcohol occurs in the small intestine, with stomach-associated absorption becoming more significant if it is also filled with food (Eckardt et al., 1998). Some metabolism of alcohol to acetaldehyde by the enzyme alcohol-dehydrogenase (ADH) can occur in the stomach, but the liver is the primary site for alcohol clearance from the body. The liver also uses ADH to break alcohol down to acetaldehyde, which is this then broken down to acetate and fed into the Krebb's cycle for energy. The liver has two additional enzymes, cytochrome P450 and catalase, which can break down alcohol, but in an acute drinking episode most metabolism involves ADH. The brain can undertake some very limited metabolism of alcohol, using cytochrome P450 and catalase (Zakhari, 2006). This is important because while acetaldehyde does not seem to pass through the blood-brain barrier, its in situ production means it can potentially affect brain function, as with acetate. Indeed, animal data suggests that some of ethanol's psychoactive effects, especially relating to its addiction potential, may be mediated by acetaldehyde, with acetate contributing to impaired motor control (Deitrich, Zimatkin, & Pronko, 2006).

Alcohol preferentially dissolves in water. So for a given body weight, the more water that it contains, the lower the blood alcohol concentration. As women tend to have less water than men, for the same body weight, for a given quantity of alcohol they will tend to have a higher blood alcohol content (Erol & Karpyak, 2015). Apart from bodily composition, many factors influence the speed with which blood alcohol rises on drinking (e.g., rate of drinking, food, carbonation, genetics) and how rapidly the body can remove alcohol (e.g., age, diet, sex, smoking status, time of day, genetics). An important factor is a person's drinking history. Regular drinkers develop tolerance for the physiological effects of alcohol, such that a progressively higher dose is required to obtain the same effect. There is some evidence of acute tolerance within a single drinking bout, but it is chronic tolerance that is responsible for most of the reduced physiological effects of this drug (Feldman, Meyer, & Quenzer, 1997). This occurs through increased efficiency of metabolism (e.g., cytochrome p450 starts to play a bigger role in breaking down alcohol; the liver increases in size) and from alterations in receptor sensitivity. These alterations allow an alcoholic to tolerate levels of blood alcohol that would kill an unseasoned drinker (i.e., exposures in the range of 50–200 mM).

7.2.2 *Acute Effects on Behaviour*

This and the next section (on brain impacts) examine the effect of acute alcohol exposure in the 2–20 mM (blood alcohol concentration, BAC) range – and under more exceptional circumstances, up to 50 mM (BAC), drawing on relevant animal and human data. This captures the full acute exposure range of most human 'social' drinking (Harrison et al., 2017), with its broad array of behavioural changes. These include its: (1) subjective effects (affect, change in consciousness, stimulation and sedation); (2) anxiolytic effects; (3) reinforcing effects; (4) impacts on cognition and performance; (5) impact on appetite; and (6) impact on aggression – all of which are covered in turn. It is important to be aware of the many situational variables that moderate these effects, the most notable being expectations about what alcohol will do, the environment in which it is consumed, the gender and drinking history of the consumer, who it is consumed with, the psychological and neuropsychological profile of the drinker and their genetic disposition (Eckardt et al., 1998; Heinz et al., 2011). In some cases – aggression, for example – these factors are essential for understanding alcohol's effects, while for others they serve to varying degrees as moderating factors.

A person who drinks a few times a week, and then in moderation, is able to detect that they have ingested an intoxicant, when present in the range of 2–7 mM BAC, even when controlling for expectancy bias. At these concentrations, alcohol is reported to exert a stimulatory effect, but as BAC increases participants report more sedation, ending in unconsciousness. A broadly parallel inverted U shape occurs for affective reactions to alcohol, with lower doses judged as pleasant and higher doses as unpleasant, culminating in nausea and vomiting. There is some evidence that animals also show this biphasic response.

Alcohol also has some anxiolytic effects. Self-report findings tend to be more consistent than those using physiological measures, and there is also variability dependent on the type of stress task employed. There are two robust findings. First, participants who are anxious report a reduction in anxiety on consuming alcohol, even in expectancy-free designs. Second, animal data also indicate anxiolytic effects, although higher concentrations are required in mice, than in rats, with alcohol-dosed animals more likely, for example, to walk on the unprotected arms (i.e., risk of falling) of the elevated plus maze – with similar behaviour on other forms of anxiety tests.

The capacity of alcohol to reduce anxiety, at least in some people, and for alcohol consumption to result in feelings of pleasure and stimulation, offer three plausible routes by which this drug can reinforce further consumption. Animal data provide some support for these ideas. Mice seem especially sensitive to the stimulant effects of alcohol, something not found in most rat strains. Both rats and mice form aversions for places associated with alcohol consumption, suggesting that they do not enjoy their initial experience with alcohol. Indeed, human novice drinkers often start by consuming alcohol products that are high in sugar (and sometimes fat) to mask the aversive irritant taste (Copeland et al., 2007). Similarly, if rats are introduced to alcohol in this way, they too come to bar-press for alcohol, after a period of fading the alcohol–sugar mixture to alcohol alone. Presumably, animals come to learn that the consequences of drinking alcohol – but not to excess – is rewarding.

Alcohol starts to impair psychomotor performance in the range of 9–11 mM BAC on relatively simple tasks such as reaction time, tracking, vigilance and attention. More complex tasks reveal deteriorated performance at lower doses of alcohol, and for particularly complicated tasks like driving, impairment is linear with BAC, even when below most countries' legal limits (Esgate, Groome, & Baker, 2005). A characteristic feature of more extensive drinking bouts is either lost periods of time or amnesia for the latter part of the drinking bout. Animal data indicates that even low concentrations of alcohol are sufficient to impair hippocampal-dependent learning and memory, and it is this memory system (i.e., episodic/auto-biographical memory) which also seems to be affected by more significant drinking bouts. A further cognitive effect of alcohol is on executive function, namely the capacity to use, plan and prioritise information from a variety of cognitive systems for the execution of complex tasks. Such tasks are diverse and common parts of day-to-day life, and range from driving to social interaction. Simpler aspects of executive function are also affected, resulting in reduced self-control, and greater disinhibition and impulsivity (Oscar-Berman & Marinkovic, 2007).

As alcohol is a contributor to overall energy intake in most drinkers, and as alcohol is often consumed before a meal (to varying degrees from an aperitif to several beers), with a meal and after a meal (liqueurs, port, brandy, etc., or perhaps just more beer), there has been a lot of interest in its effect on appetite (Traversy & Chaput, 2015). The majority of experimental studies indicate that acute consumption of alcohol before a meal stimulates additional food intake, and independent of expectancy effects. It is unclear if it can also drive eating when a person is sated.

One of the most disturbing features of alcohol consumption is its capacity to make certain people in certain situations behave in an aggressive manner (Heinz et al., 2011). The caveat here is that this is not a universal effect, as the animal data illustrates. Low doses of alcohol increase aggression in many species, but only when the animal has some individual-level dysfunction (e.g., raised in a deprived environment, raised without a mother, etc.). The same appears to apply to humans, and three sets of factors are important. The first are situational variables, such that many drinking contexts may provide multiple occasions for the expression of aggression, due to some individuals being more likely to aggress and others more likely to say or do things that provoke. The second are individual factors, particularly a person's expectations about the aggression-inducing properties of alcohol, cultural sex roles and aggressive disposition. The third concerns alcohol's ability to impair aspects of executive functioning, especially self-control, self-reflection and evaluation of short- versus long-term costs. Where this system is already dysfunctional (e.g., in attention-deficit disorder, recovered traumatic brain injury), then alcohol further erodes the capacity to regulate aggressive behaviour. So while alcohol does not directly fuel aggression, it increases the probability of an aggressive outburst, and especially so in the 'optimal' context.

7.2.3   Acute Effects on the Brain

Alcohol has been described as a promiscuous drug, because it affects so many different brain systems. Its full range of effects is still not understood, nor indeed are its impacts on specific receptors that it affects, nor is there any more than a broad understanding of the linkage between its behavioural consequences and their neural basis. A further complication is that as the concentration of alcohol in the brain increases, the number of transmitter and secondary messenger systems that are affected by its presence also increases, as do the interactions within and between these elements (e.g., the dose-dependent transitions from stimulation to sedation, pleasure to displeasure reflect dose-dependent changes in alcohol's impact on the brain). This goes someway to explain the variability in findings about alcohol's effect on the brain in the animal literature (Eckardt et al., 1998). As with the preceding section on behaviour, the focus here is on lower-range alcohol concentrations, typically in the 2–20 mM range, but including up to 50 mM, but here we draw far more heavily on the animal literature.

There is agreement that a major target of alcohol is the gamma-aminobutyric acid (GABA) type A receptor (Doweiko, 2009; Eckardt et al., 1998; Feldman et al., 1997; Förstera et al., 2016). GABA is the brain's major inhibitory neurotransmitter. When a neuron with GABA type A receptor is activated, this opens a channel, which allows chloride anions to flow, making it more difficult to depolarise the neuron. GABA type A receptors can be made up of many different subunits. Alcohol does not affect the part of the receptor that binds GABA, rather it affects one or more of the non-GABA-sensitive subunits (probably 20+ combinations).

One it definitely attaches to is a site on the delta subunit, allowing it to modulate receptor function, making the neuron harder to depolarise and thus reducing its capacity to inhibit other neurons (Förstera et al., 2016). GABA type A receptors with the delta subunit are found in several brain areas that relate to alcohol's impact on behaviour. This includes the cerebellum, where it inhibits firing of granule cells, which in turn affects activity of Purkinje cells that project to cortical and subcortical sites, probably accounting for alcohol's impact on co-ordination/fine motor skill. It inhibits firing of GABAergic neurons in the ventral tegmental area (brain reward substrate), amygdala (anxiolytic effects – which seem to be mediated in part by the subunit that benzodiazapines attach to), hippo-campus (amnesia), thalamus (arousal/sedation) and in the neocortex (Harrison et al., 2017). The general reduction in inhibition in the neo-cortex is one reason why alcohol so broadly disrupts cognition (e.g., executive functions), and especially those processes that require response inhibition (i.e., the exercise of self-control).

Alcohol also inhibits the glutamate neurotransmitter system – the brain's main excitatory transmitter – by serving as a weak receptor antag-onist for the NMDA-type glutamate receptor possessing the NR2B sub-unit. This, and the other inhibitory effects that alcohol exerts on glutamate transmission (via the non-NMDA ionotropic receptor) impact function in the hippocampus (amnesia), amygdala (anxiolytic effect) and parts of the cortex. Indeed, in the hippocampus, alcohol inhibits long-term potentia-tion, providing one basis for its capacity to impair memory when intoxi-cated. An additional inhibitory effect is also exerted via alcohol's effect on the glycine receptor, which like the GABA type A receptor is also a chloride channel, and acts to reduce the likelihood of depolarisation. Glycine receptors affected by alcohol are known to occur in the hippo-campus (amnesia), brain stem (respiration) and in the cortex (Förstera et al., 2016)

There are also acute effects of alcohol on the serotonergic and dopami-nergic system. In addition to affecting one class of serotonin receptor (5HT3), alcohol stimulates firing of serotonergic neurons, contributing to the drug's anxiolytic effects. Alcohol also stimulates dopamine produc-tion in the mesolimbic reward pathway, of which the ventral tegmental area is part (see earlier). This change in dopamine levels underpins the stimulatory aspect of low doses of alcohol in mice. Dopaminergic activity is further enhanced by the up-regulation of the serotonergic system, and by loss of GABAergic inhibition. All of these effects, including the stimulation of endogenous opioids by dopamine and serotonin activity, and directly by alcohol itself, contribute to its rewarding properties (Eckardt et al., 1998). Alcohol also enhances the sensitivity of the nicotinic receptor to acetylcholine (which also impacts dopamine release), and it indirectly (via many of the receptor changes described earlier) and directly up-regulates production of the cellular messenger cyclic AMP.

Many of the systems affected by alcohol also affect ingestive behaviour. In the peripheral nervous system, alcohol inhibits leptin and glucagon-like peptide 1, both of which contribute to increased food intake in animal models. The central effects on serotonin, GABA and opioids are all – at low to moderate alcohol doses – known to produce changes that favour increased food intake (Traverey & Chaput, 2015).

Finally, alcohol's capacity to increase aggression in some individuals reflects a multiplicity of changes that are favourable to reduced self-control, enhanced threat perception and an aggressive response. It has been noted that the pattern of dopamine release when under stress, shares parallels with the pattern of dopamine release when consuming moderate doses of alcohol (Heinz et al., 2011). Elevated dopamine levels in several brain structures are also associated with increased aggression in animal models (e.g., in meso-limbic structures), as are changes in serotonergic function that occur with alcohol. Increased amygdala activity driven by changes in serotonergic, dopaminergic and GABAergic systems enhances perception of threat, and reduced self-control due to alcohol's effect on executive function results in a heightened chance of an aggressive response.

7.2.4 Chronic Usage and Dependence

Chronic usage of alcohol occurs on a spectrum from the innocuous to the harmful, depending on the amount of alcohol consumed, years of usage and the age, health status and gender of the drinker. Greater alcohol use over a longer period of time, continuing throughout the lifespan, in the presence of other chronic health conditions, and in men, is associated with a greater probability of an alcohol use disorder. Unhealthy drinking likely to impair health can be regarded as consuming more than 3–4 standard drinks per day (at 8–10 g of alcohol per standard drink), on most days of the week, for more than 5 years (Oscar-Berman & Marinkovic, 2007; Schuckit, 2009). This type of drinking pattern will ultimately affect physical health, increasing risk for cancer, stroke, heart disease, seizures, brain injury and malnutrition. Indeed, 20% of general practitioner visits in the United States involve an alcohol-related problem, and chronic usage and dependence results in a shortening of the lifespan by around a decade

(Schuckit, 2009). In addition to physical health, chronic use of alcohol has been identified, both acutely and chronically, as a probable cause of depression and suicide, and depression and other mental health conditions may themselves result in unhealthy drinking. Around 25% of alcohol-dependent men and 50% of alcohol-dependent women are clinically depressed (Conner et al., 2009).

The basis for diagnosing a person as having some type of substance-abuse disorder involving alcohol typically relies on either the criteria of the American Psychiatric Association's Diagnostic and Statistical Manual (DSM; version 5) or those of the World Health Organisation in the form of the International Classification of Diseases (ICD; version 11; see Table 7.1). Both DSM and ICD describe a very similar alcohol dependence disorder, which is termed 'alcohol use disorder' (AUD) in DSM and 'alcohol dependence' in ICD (Saunders et al., 2019). ICD has additional

Table 7.1. *Diagnostic criteria for alcohol dependence*

Diagnostic system
    Criteria and notes

Diagnostic and Statistical Manual of the American Psychiatric Association, Version 5
    In the past year:

1. Drinking more or longer than intended
2. More than once wanted to cut down or stop but could not
3. Spending a lot of time drinking or getting over its after-effects
4. Wanting a drink very badly
5. Drinking interferes with home, family or job
6. Continued drinking even when causing trouble with friends and family
7. Stopped normally pleasurable activities to drink
8. More than once got into situations from drinking that could lead to harm
9. Memory blackouts or drinking even though it may lower mood/increase anxiety
10. Need to drink more to get the same effect
11. Withdrawal symptoms occur when drinking stops

Two or more criteria met indicates an alcohol use disorder, with severity defined as: Mild 2–3 criteria met, Moderate 4–5, Severe, 6+.

World Health Organisation's International Classification of Disease, Version 11
    In the past year (or with 1 month or more of continuous alcohol use):

1. Impaired control over alcohol use – starting, amount drunk, stopping, craving
2. Alcohol use becomes a priority – takes precedence over interests, responsibilities, health, personal care, even if problems occur
3. Biological adaptations to alcohol use – tolerance, withdrawal symptoms, usage to manage withdrawal

Two or more criteria met indicates alcohol dependence disorder.

classifications, capturing patterns of use that are harmful, but less severe than dependence, and hazardous use, which is less severe than harmful, but that is likely to result in harm, and place a person at risk of later dependence. This gradation is also reflected in DSM's AUD, with clinician rating of mild, moderate or severe.

Lifetime risk for alcohol use disorder is around 10% of drinkers in the United States (i.e., approximately 7% of all US adults with an alcohol dependence problem). Looking at harmful use, 30–50% of regular US adult drinkers in the last year experienced some alcohol-related harm, from the mild (missing work/school) to the more serious (drink driving) – with similar rates in teenage drinkers (Schuckit, 2009). Hazardous use of alcohol is particularly pronounced in young drinkers, with 60% having experienced an episode of drunkenness by age 18. Overall, alcohol is responsible for 2–4% of all adult deaths and this drug constitutes the major source of referral to drug-dependence services.

7.2.5 Brain and Behavioural Impacts of Chronic Usage

Around half of the people with AUD who do not evidence any overt cognitive impairment will have detectable changes in their brain and neuropsychological profile (Oscar-Berman & Marinkovic, 2007). There are many plausible causes. Damage to the liver (e.g., increasing neurotoxic agents like ammonia) and circulatory system (e.g., resulting in mini-strokes), falls when drunk (e.g., causing brain haematomas), seizures from alcohol withdrawal, and malnutrition from poor diet, can all injure the brain. In addition to these routes, alcohol exposure has several more direct impacts: (1) Acetaldehyde, the first breakdown product of alcohol, can bind to proteins, nucleic acids and phospholipids in the brain, compromising their function (Deitrich et al., 2006). (2) Alcohol increases the quantity of reactive oxygen species in the brain. (3) It also decreases production of brain-derived neurotrophic factor. (4) It contributes to increased excitotoxicity through its effect on the excitatory neurotransmitter glutamate. As well as these routes, alcohol impairs the function of multiple organ systems in the body, which in turn causes systemic inflammation, which also affects the brain. The most general impact from all of these avenues of attack is neuroinflammation, which is evident in post mortem examination of the brains of people with alcohol use disorder (Zahr, Kaufman, & Harer, 2011).

The most frequently noted imaging abnormality in alcoholic individuals without any obvious cognitive impairment is ventricular enlargement (Zahr & Pfefferbaum, 2017). This is accompanied by a number of other degenerative changes, which seem to be more likely in the right hemisphere of the brain. The frontal lobes are reduced in volume, and there is also reduced blood flow and glucose metabolism, and reduced number of neurons on post mortem. This is associated with executive impairments, and hence impairment in complex tasks such as emotional regulation, social interaction, work, driving, etc., which are characteristically impaired in both acute and chronic alcohol use (Oscar-Berman & Marinkovic, 2007).

The limbic system is another brain area that seems particularly susceptible to alcohol's effects. The mamillary bodies are reduced in volume, as is the hippocampus, and the latter has reduced neurogenesis in the dentate gyrus, reduced white matter volume and decreased axonal diameter on post mortem. The amygdala is also smaller, and functional imaging in people with alcohol use disorder suggests both blunted response to emotionally arousing stimuli and corresponding reductions in amygdala activation, relative to controls. There are also alterations in the hypothalamus, some of which relate to the hyporeactivity of the hypothalamic–pituitary–adrenal axis, induced by alcohol. The cerebellum is also reduced in volume, particularly with white matter loss, and volume reduction here is also linked to reduced frontal volume and impaired executive functioning. There are also more general white matter volume reductions, evident in the corpus callosum and in other cortical and subcortical tracts (Zahr & Pfefferbaum, 2017).

A scientifically and medically important question is the degree to which these effects are reversible following a period of abstinence. This is scientifically important because some of the volume reductions attributed to chronic alcohol use could in fact turn out to reflect predispositions to alcoholism. This case has been made for the amygdala, but the finding that volume reductions here are at least partially reversible following abstinence argues against it. Imaging after recovery indicates ventricular shrinkage, with increases in brain volume reported in most of the brain areas that are affected by chronic alcohol use (Zahr & Pfefferbaum, 2017). The extent of recovery is varied amongst individuals, and this variability is not understood. Recovery also seems to be partial, and principally driven by re-myelination. Both the effects of chronic usage and recovery have been modelled in animals with similar conclusions to the findings in humans.

While the type of changes documented here are commonly encountered in people with AUD, there are a smaller subset who develop more profound brain-related diseases that are triggered either directly by alcohol or by the alcoholic lifestyle (Zahr & Pfefferbaum, 2017). The most important example of the latter is Wernicke's encephalopathy, and

Table 7.2. *Alcohol-related neurological syndromes*

Condition	Occurrence, cause and key features
Wernicke's encephalopathy	12–18% of AUD*, thiamine deficiency, classic symptom triad (ataxia, confusion, ophthalmoplegia)
Korsakoff's syndrome	Rare follow-on from Wernicke's encephalopathy, severe and permanent amnesia
Hepatic encephalopathy	50% of liver cirrhosis patients, confusion/delirium
Central pontine myelinolysis	Rare, resulting from hyponatremia, movement problems (loss of voluntary control of face, limbs)
Marchiafava–Bignami disease	Very rare, corpus callosum lesion, confusion and movement problems (speech and walking difficulties)
Alcoholic cerebellar degeneration	Rare, cerebellar lesion, movement problems (nystagmus, walking and speech difficulties)
Alcohol-related dementia	Unclear, frontal damage, frontal-type dementia

*Alcohol use disorder.

Korsakoff's syndrome, which are largely a consequence of a thiamine-deficient diet, with these disorders being examined in Chapter 9. Table 7.2 details the specific neurological syndromes linked to alcohol use and the alcoholic lifestyle, including an indication of their rarity. Hepatic encephalopathy occurs concurrently with liver failure. The liver's incapacity to function results in high levels of ammonia that are neurotoxic to the brain. Its effects are rapid, producing confusion, delirium and impaired coordination. Imaging indicates white matter abnormalities (corpus callosum, frontal lobes, corticospinal tracts), and damage to basal ganglia.

Central pontine myelinolysis also results from white matter damage, and on imaging reveals itself with a characteristic 'bat-wing' lesion in the pons. This syndrome is triggered by an electrolyte disturbance, which animal models suggest then damages the blood-brain barrier, allowing metabolites into the brain that would not normally be present. This condition manifests as an inability to control movement. A further condition, characterised by specific demyelination, is Marchiafava–Bignami disease, which damages the corpus-callosum, resulting in confusion and speech and movement problems. Alcohol can also specifically affect the cerebellum, and in particular the vermis, by damaging its Purkinje cells. This results in the alcoholic cerebellar degeneration, with abnormal eye movements, difficulty walking and speaking. A more contentious condition is alcohol-related dementia, as it arguably overlaps with hepatic encephalopathy, Wernicke's encephalopathy and Korsakoff's syndrome. That it exists as a unique condition is suggested by its occurrence in younger men, with intact liver function and without overt thiamine deficiency, who present with significant and degenerating executive function impairments. Imaging and post mortem examination suggest specific frontal degeneration. What is notable for most of these syndromes is that they share many overlapping abnormalities with functioning alcoholics. This would suggest that individual vulnerabilities may allow specific alcohol-related brain abnormalities to worsen.

7.2.6   Dependence

7.2.6.1   Transition into Problem Drinking

The transition to alcohol dependence involves an interplay between a person's genetic predispositions to addiction and their environmental circumstances. Several environmental factors have been identified that predispose to an AUD (Schuckit, 2009; Sher, Grekin, & Williams, 2005). Less supervision and less supportive and warm parent–teenager relationships are a risk factor, as well as a peer group that is permissive of over-consumption, encouraging risky behaviour and delinquency. More general societal attitudes are also relevant, such as the tolerance for public drunkenness, the availability and price of alcohol, drinking's perceived function in society and the legal framework that governs consumption (e.g., drinking age, opening hours, enforcement).

Even when there is an overwhelmingly conducive environment, not everyone who drinks develops an alcohol use disorder. Multiple human and animal studies have confirmed that there is a highly robust genetic component to alcohol dependence, accounting for between 40% and 60% of the variance in who is or is not dependent (Schuckit, 2009). It is now well established that people carry multiple genes that contribute risk towards dependence, often for drugs in general, sometimes specifically for alcohol and in certain cases for indirect dispositions like anxiety. One set of genetic dispositions relate to alcohol metabolism (Dick & Bierut, 2006). There are many variants of the ADH enzyme that breaks alcohol down into acetaldehyde, with some being much faster at this than others. A slower breakdown of alcohol – its effects linger longer – by ADH is associated with a greater risk of AUD. As the build-up of acetaldehyde is aversive, a slower capacity to convert it into acetate is linked to a lower risk of an AUD.

There is also significant genetic variance in psychological variables, notably impulsivity (Dick et al., 2010). Prospective longitudinal studies indicate that greater levels of trait impulsivity, which has a significant genetic basis, is linked to a greater risk of developing an AUD. Animal data also supports this contention. Other psychological factors with a genetic component linked to risk of an AUD are neuroticism (i.e., propensity for negative emotionality), presence of psychiatric illness (anxiety, depression, mania), anti-social personality disorder and other forms of drug dependence.

In addition to metabolic dispositions and psychological traits, there are several gene variants that affect brain neurochemistry that confer risk of an AUD (Vengeliene et al., 2008). Initial sensitivity to alcohols effects is subject to variability via the form of NMDA and GABA A receptors. The capacity of alcohol to reinforce further consumption is linked to several factors – variation in dopamine, serotonin and cannabinoid receptors; opioid reward system; and the anxiety-related corticotrophin releasing factor/neuropeptide Y system. Certain polymorphisms in all of these systems confer additional risk of an AUD.

7.2.6.2   Problem Drinking

Many different models have been proposed to explain how problem drinking is maintained (Sher et al., 2005). That is, what drives continued use in the face of the multiple costs of drinking – financial, social and health. Even with the high level of interest in addiction and alcohol dependence in particular, and with use of animal models and human research, there is no clear 'winning' model. In all likelihood, components of several models may be explanatory of an individual's drinking, with different component mixes for different people, dependent on their genetic make-up and environmental circumstances. There are four basic types of models. First, reward models, where consumption of alcohol induces pleasure, and it is this pleasure that motivates consumption. Second, tension-reduction models, which are particularly pertinent to anxiety-prone people, whereby drinking removes anxiety. Third, pharmacological models, whereby drugs of addiction, including alcohol, sensitise motivational pathways, so that the drug becomes a bodily need in a broadly analogous manner to food and water. Fourth, deviance proneness, where excessive drinking is viewed as indulgence in one delinquent behaviour amongst many others (e.g., smoking, violence, theft, vandalism).

In parallel to theoretical models of dependence, there is a lot of data on the changes that occur in the alcohol-dependent brain, typically using animal models (Vengeliene et al., 2008). The acute effects of alcohol reduce inhibition in the neocortex via its effect on the GABA

A receptor. Dependence is associated with varying changes (often a reduction) in the density of GABA A receptors in different parts of the brain, including in the reward-related mesolimbic dopamine system. The endocannabinoid system increases in activity with dependence, and changes have also been documented in the acetylcholine, opioid and corticotrophin-releasing factor/neuropeptide Y systems.

Ceasing to use alcohol when dependent produces withdrawal symptoms in the majority of dependent users (Schuckit, 2009). These start within several hours of the last drink, peaking 48 hours later and are much reduced after 96–120 h. Depending on length of dependence, and the length of the last drinking bout, withdrawal can range from mild to life-threatening. Symptoms includes anxiety, insomnia, pounding heart, sweating, increased blood pressure, hallucinations and, in the most severe cases, seizures, confusion and delirium. Once this has been endured, the dependent user has to avoid drinking. This is made difficult by the presence of cues associated with consumption – internal states (stress, low mood, excitement); other drugs (smoking); the sight, smell or sounds linked to drinks and drinking; and the taste of alcohol and its effects. All of these can induce craving, a phenomenon that is now acknowledged as a defining part of alcohol dependence (see Table 7.1).

Craving has been studied in animal models and with neuroimaging in people with and without alcohol use disorder. Animal craving models rely on measuring the degree to which an animal will work to obtain alcohol, with effort *presumed* to equate to desire. Animal data suggests a high degree of fractionation of craving (Vengeliene et al., 2008). First, by type of craving. This can manifest as desire for the rewarding aspects of alcohol, involving changes in mesolimbic dopamine pathways, and relief from withdrawal, which is argued to involve alterations in the GABA and glutamate systems. The second concerns the type of cue that induces craving. Stress-related craving seems dependent on the serotonergic and corticotrophin-releasing factor/neuropeptide Y systems. Smoking-triggered alcohol craving involves acetylcholine, and drinking-associated cues draw upon multiple systems (dopamine, serotonin, cannabinoid, opioid, glutamate). One unifying feature across all cue types seems to be GABAergic involvement.

Human neuroimaging data reveal an equally complex picture, but for a different reason. Schacht, Anton, and Myrick (2012) undertook a meta-analysis of the large number of functional imaging studies examining people with alcohol use disorder's response to alcohol-related versus non-alcohol-related cues. A proportion of the studies also included non-dependent drinkers, an important feature as will become clear. The first finding was that exposure to alcohol-related cues (relative to non-alcohol-related ones (whether these were motivationally salient – sex, food, etc. – or not does not make much difference)) produces activations across a broad range of brain structures, but notably in the mesolimbic dopamine system, anterior cingulate cortex and prefrontal cortex. All of these brain areas have been implicated in reward processing. The surprising finding here was that the degree of activation of these reward-related brain sites *was not greater* in alcohol-dependent drinkers. Rather, when people with alcohol dependence were contrasted against non-problem drinkers, to examine differences in their response to alcohol-related and non-alcohol-related cues, the outcomes indicated differential activations of superior temporal cortex, posterior cingulate cortex and the precuneus. The authors suggest that these differences reflect the greater associated memories, salience and value of drinking cues to people with dependence, or, alternatively, these structures are somehow involved in suppressing reward-related activations in dependent users. The simple idea that a craving cue elicits a greater reward-related response in a dependent person is not supported by these findings. Indeed, as the animal data also indicate, craving is a complex multifaceted phenomenon that is not well understood. It is, however, an important aspect of dependence.

7.2.7   Developmental Impact

7.2.7.1   Foetal Exposure

Foetal exposure to alcohol can result in a range of adverse health outcomes. Unlike alcohol dependence, where there are formalised diagnostic criteria, for foetal exposure to alcohol these are still being developed. The Institute of Medicine in the United States developed the first set of diagnostic guidelines. While these have been criticised on many grounds, they are important because they identify the general framework of adverse health outcomes that flow from foetal alcohol exposure, and in particular they specify the general characteristics of the neurodevelopmental disorder caused by alcohol consumption during pregnancy (Brown et al., 2019). Under the umbrella label of foetal alcohol spectrum disorder (FASD), they outline four manifestations: (1) FAS – foetal alcohol syndrome; (2) pFAS – partial foetal alcohol syndrome; (3) ARND – alcohol-related neurodevelopmental disorder; and (4) ARBD – alcohol-related birth defects (i.e., abnormalities of heart, bone, kidney, brain, etc.). The distinction between FAS and pFAS is the reduced severity of the latter, ARND shares just the behavioural and brain features of FAS and pFAS, and ARBD covers all of the physical abnormalities (including to the brain) that result from foetal alcohol exposure. We will use the term FASD to refer to this broad spectrum of effects, with a focus on brain and behaviour.

FASD ultimately reflects a spectrum of disability. Regular heavy foetal exposure to alcohol, especially with periods of binging and withdrawal, produces a characteristic syndrome. This is composed of a particular facial structure with a smooth philtrum, a flattened bridge of the nose, reduced eye openings, low positioned ears, a thin upper lip, brain damage – both physical and behavioural manifestations – and growth deficiency. That alcohol should affect the foetus is not surprising. It can pass through the placenta into the foetus, and alcohol is a known teratogen (Schneider, Moore, & Adkins, 2011). Alcohol's effect on foetal development is profound. It increases rates of stillbirths, spontaneous abortions, prematurity and low-birth-weight babies (Popova et al., 2017), and does so in a dose-dependent manner, with risk starting to increase linearly from a maternal intake of around 10 g of alcohol per day (Patra et al., 2011). Setting aside the vulnerability to toxic-insult that occurs during foetal development, with its cell proliferation, migration and differentiation, the foetus does not have the capacity to break down alcohol (i.e., no ADH).

Studying FASD in humans comes with some problems. Apart from the definitional issues, which make epidemiological study difficult (i.e., is everyone using the same definitions. etc.), there are also important measurement concerns. One relates to the difficulty in getting accurate recall of alcohol usage during pregnancy, both in terms of the limitations of human memory and because of social desirability effects (Lebel, Roussotte, & Sowell, 2011). Another is the timing of alcohol usage, which may be particularly important as it is highly likely there are periods of time when the foetus is uniquely vulnerable, most especially during the early stages of pregnancy (Schneider et al., 2011). This may be why an infant can have severe brain- and behaviour-related problems but no facial abnormalities, because at least in mice the facial abnormalities only develop with alcohol exposure during a particular period of gestation (Lebel et al., 2011). Alcohol is often just one of several drugs that may be used during pregnancy, with tobacco being particularly problematic as it is also a teratogen. If the mother is a heavy drinker or dependent, she may pass genetic traits to her offspring that share features with some of the adverse effects of foetal alcohol exposure, making it difficult to discern causation. Causation is also problematic in this context because any form of drug dependence produces disruption in a persons' life – unstable relationships, unsafe accommodation, stress, insecure food supply and poor nutrition. All of these can directly and indirectly affect foetal and child development.

Approximately 630,000 infants every year are born with FASD. Statistics around drinking during pregnancy indicate that Russia, the UK, Denmark, Belarus and Ireland have the highest intakes, and the Gulf states some of the lowest. Prevalence rates for FASD per 1,000 live births per year (Popova et al., 2017) are highest for South Africa at 58.5, followed by Croatia (11.5), Ireland (9), Italy (8) and Belarus (7), with the Gulf states and other countries that consume little alcohol having the lowest. South Africa's very high aggregate rate reaches more than 130/1,000 live births in Eastern Cape, its poorest province. Here, a combination of socially acceptable drinking and drunkenness, unemployment, home-brewed alcohol, poor nutrition, high rates of unplanned pregnancies and lack of awareness about the adverse effects of alcohol on the foetus all contribute to the observed rate of FASD.

FASD has many comorbidities, including physical deformities, chromosomal damage, ADHD, oppositional-defiant disorder and conduct disorder. It has a lifelong course, associated with academic failure, drug abuse, heightened risk for depression, contact with the criminal justice system and the need for supported living (Popova et al., 2017). Effects on development are apparent very early, with FASD infants showing habituation deficits and poorer suckling, reflexes and motor maturity than healthy infants (Schneider et al., 2011). Longitudinal studies suggest that there is no safe level of alcohol exposure during pregnancy, but effects become harder to detect where exposure is lower. This is because individual differences (e.g., maternal age, parity, genes) and variability in when the same quantity of alcohol may have been consumed start to produce effects in some infants/children, but not in others (Eckardt et al., 1998). What is clear is that the more the alcohol drunk during pregnancy, the greater the negative effects.

There has been a lot of research on children exploring the impacts of foetal alcohol exposure. The findings from neuropsychology, post mortem brain studies and imaging all indicate (again) a spectrum of presentations sharing the same essential features, but differing in magnitude, reflecting the degree of alcohol exposure during pregnancy. A consistent finding is that IQ is reduced, along with academic capacity for maths and language. Where alcohol exposure has been significant, IQ's between 70 and 80 are observed, falling in the latter case two standard deviations below the mean (i.e., lowest 2.5% of the population). Executive function and its subcomponents are also consistently impaired, along with a reduced capacity to learn and retain verbal and visual material (Mattson, Crocker, & Nguyen, 2011). Motor function, such as hand-eye coordination, postural stability and gross/fine motor skills are all poorer. At least in the most severe cases of FASD, most neuropsychological domains are impaired, with effects on IQ and executive and motor functions most evident in less severe cases.

The brains of children with FASD have also been studied. On autopsy, a general finding is smaller head and brain (microencephaly), an abnormal corpus callosum, enlargement of the ventricles and a smaller-than-expected cerebellum (Donald et al., 2015). MRI points to the same general conclusions, with a smaller brain with reductions in white and grey matter, corpus callosum almost absent in more severe cases, a smaller hippocampus and cerebellum even after correcting for brain volume, and abnormalities in the basal ganglia – with these types of effects evident in preschoolers, teenagers and adults exposed to alcohol as a foetus (Donald et al., 2015; Lebel et al., 2011). Diffusion tensor imaging has been used to explore damage to white matter tracts, which seem particularly susceptible to alcohol exposure, with the corpus callosum, anterior and posterior fibre bundles and cerebellar tracts notably affected.

Neurometabolism is also abnormal, with reduced levels of choline, indicating myelination abnormalities, and with disruption of most metabolites being evident (Donald et al., 2015). There have also been many attempts to link the neuropsychological abnormalities to brain structure and function. Links have been observed between executive function and cerebral blood flow in frontal areas, and what is interesting here is that even when task performance is similar, imaging abnormalities remain. Executive deficits have also been linked to the integrity of the corpus callosum, and verbal learning and memory deficits with impaired hippocampal function. The most consistent linkage can be made between brain volume and IQ, as a number of studies have observed moderate-sized correlations between total brain volume and IQ (an r of around 0.4).

These data are correlational. As noted earlier, people exposed to alcohol in utero may also have been exposed to a number of other adverse events/agents, which might explain the observed pattern of deficits. However, there are two bodies of data that suggest very strongly that alcohol is responsible. Both come from animal studies – noting caveats about differing brain development, etc. – where alcohol exposure can be carefully controlled and other explanations excluded. The first concerns animal models of foetal alcohol exposure, where the studies focus on the impacts on brain and behaviour. Imaging of young rodents exposed to alcohol in utero show reductions in brain volume, ventricular enlargement and selective volume reduction in the basal ganglia, hippocampus and cerebellum (Donald et al., 2015). Corpus callosum abnormalities do not appear to have been observed, which is surprising not only because alcohol causes the death of oligodendrocytes that generate the myelin sheath for neurons in animal models, but also because of its prominence in studies of human FASD (Sherbaf et al., 2019). Aside from this difference, there is a general similarity in alcohol's gross impact on animal and human foetal brain development.

There are also parallels for alcohol's behavioural impacts, although these are less clear-cut than the anatomical findings. In rodent and primate models, habituation is slowed in neonates following foetal exposure, and as the animals develop, coordination and muscle tone are impaired. In humans, executive dysfunction is prominent, but evidence for this in animal models is mixed, and in rodents it may be more sensitive to the timing of the insult than in humans (Schneider et al., 2011). Hyperactivity and inattention are also observed in some studies but not all, but higher levels of exposure do seem to produce a more consistent picture (i.e., in primates – hyperactivity, impaired motor development and cognition).

A second line of evidence suggesting that alcohol is responsible for the deficits seen in FASD in humans comes from the finding in animal studies that alcohol can damage the developing brain via multiple causal pathways (Eckardt et al., 1998; Goodlett & Horn, 2001). Animal data have provided strong evidence that during development, the brain is most susceptible to the effects of alcohol. Table 7.3 details eight routes that have been identified by which it can harm the foetal brain. Both animals and humans seem to have peak points of vulnerability during foetal brain development, notably around gastrulation and during neuronal proliferation, migration and differentiation. The general finding from the animal literature that alcohol impairs foetal brain development, the clear causal pathways to damage and the large human pool of data all indicate that alcohol causes damage to the foetal brain.

7.2.7.2   Exposure during Adolescence and in Old Age

In countries where alcohol is readily available, drinking usually starts during the teenage years, with binge drinking and drunkenness common in this age group. There are two questions of interest here. First, as the teenage brain is still maturing, with reductions in grey matter volume and increasing myelination and white matter volume, alcohol might permanently damage this maturation process. Second, and relatedly, is whether

Table 7.3. *Routes of alcohol's toxic effects on foetal brain development*

Type	Key effects
Altered gene expression	Alcohol interferes with normal gene expression
Oxidative stress	Alcohol generates reactive oxygen species and inhibits cellular antioxidants, leading to mitochondrial dysfunction
Excitotoxicity	Periods of alcohol withdrawal result in alterations to the NMDA receptor, increasing calcium flow into neurons
Glucose transport	Alcohol alters expression of cellular glucose transporters and reduces uptake of glucose
Neuronal proliferation	Alcohol impairs operation of the IGF-1 receptor, interfering with the regulation of neuronal proliferation
Glial cells	Radial glia cells coordinate neuronal migration but alcohol causes them to prematurely mature into astrocytes, disrupting migration
Neurotransmitters	Alcohol adversely affects the development of the serotonin system and alters the function of the glutamate system
Cell adhesion	Alcohol disrupts cell adhesion

exposure sensitises the brain in some way, making addiction in general more likely. This is an issue not only because brain maturation also involves changes to the mesolimbic dopamine reward system, but because alcohol in teenagers may produce a different drug experience to alcohol in the fully mature brain (Spear, 2018). Namely, teenagers may experience more of alcohol's positive rewarding and socialising properties, while being less aware of its capacity to impair judgement, motor skills, etc. The problem here is cause and effect. The things that tend to predict drinking in teenagers are risk factors for alcohol abuse in adults (both genetic and environmental), and, in turn, these same risk factors are linked to the type of adverse scholastic and drug-dependence outcomes, which alcohol use might be predicted to generate. Two basic approaches have been used to unravel this (Spear, 2018): First, using longitudinal studies, where participants are matched at baseline in, say, scholastic performance, to determine what differences emerge when drinking starts in some but not in others. The outcome from such studies is unclear, with some evidence of impaired learning and memory, but with these effects reversible following cessation of drinking. Where imaging has been used, there is some indication that drinking during the teenage years slows maturational processes, especially myelination. The second source of data comes from animal models. Here, evidence for neurocognitive effects is also ambivalent, but there is some indication that teenage exposure may increase motivation to drink. In sum, there are no clear answers as yet, but there is enough evidence for suspicion, particularly given the effects on the foetal brain.

Low to moderate alcohol consumption during middle age seems to be linked to a reduced risk for cognitive decline and dementia, an effect that now seems quite well established (Rehm et al., 2019). However, heavy drinking during middle age or old age is associated with an elevated risk for dementia, notably of the alcohol-related forms discussed earlier (see Table 7.2), but also for vascular dementias and age-related cognitive decline. It has been noted before that the degenerative changes observed in the aging brain – ventricular enlargement, frontal atrophy, sulcal widening – share features in common with alcohol-related brain effects. More importantly, the aging brain is more vulnerable to alcohol's toxic effects, especially those to the corpus callosum, hippocampus and cerebellum (Oscar-Berman & Marinkovic, 2007). It may be for these reasons that even light to moderate drinking in old age is associated with adverse brain outcomes and cognitive decline (Rehm et al., 2019).

7.2.8   Conclusion

Alcohol imposes major costs on society, the full extent of which is still being uncovered, particularly concerning foetal and adolescent exposure effects. It is useful to keep these extensive harms in mind when reading the final section in this chapter on food addiction. Alcohol use disorder is a paradigmatic example of addiction, and thus a useful 'yardstick' to evaluate other claims of addiction.

7.3   Caffeine

Caffeine (1,3,7-trimethylxanthine) is a purine class alkaloid found in more than 100 species of plants. Its presence in plant leaves seems to deter herbivores, while in fallen seeds it leaches into the surrounding soil and suppresses germination of other seeds. Most caffeine-containing foods and drinks derive from a small number of plant species, as outlined in Table 7.4. Tea, coffee and cocoa products are the most widely consumed, and while caffeine is the main psychoactive compound (and its metabolites), other agents are also present that can potentially affect brain function. The most frequently identified is theobromine, which is also a metabolite of caffeine, and which is briefly discussed in Section 7.4. L-theanine and chlorogenic acid also co-occur in tea and coffee, respectively (Schuster & Mitchell, 2019). While these compounds may be

Table 7.4. *Principal sources of dietary caffeine*

Plant species	Product (note)
Camelia sinensis	Tea (East Asia, drunk after dried leaves steeped in hot water)
Ilex paraguariensis	Yerba-maté (South America, prepared as a tea-like drink)
Coffea arabica	Coffee (Yemen, now 60–80% of world coffee production)
Coffea canephora	Coffee (W. Africa, now 20–40% of world coffee production)
Theobroma cacao	Cocoa (tropical South America, prepared as drink and food)
Paullinia sp.	Guaraná (Amazon basin, prepared as a tea-like drink)
Cola sp.	Kola nuts (W. Africa, chewed, and basis for cola flavouring)

psychoactive alone or act synergistically with caffeine, caffeine is almost certainly the most important agent by virtue of its far higher concentration and its capacity to induce effects in isolation.

In the United States and Canada, per capita average consumption of coffee is around 350 L per year, and around 200 L per year in Europe. The European figure is brought down in part because Ireland and the UK are primarily tea-drinking nations, while Nordic countries consistently come out as the highest caffeine consumers per capita. Caffeine content in tea and coffee can differ markedly, with coffee varying from 250 mg/100 mL (espresso) to 40 mg/100 mL (coffee bags), and tea from 6 to 35 mg/100 mL dependent on brewing time. Much lower caffeine contents are found in soft drinks and cocoa beverages (1–15 mg/100 mL), with baking and milk chocolate sometimes higher (up to 120 mg/100 g), and with energy drinks usually in the 'coffee range' (de Paula & Farah, 2019; McLellan, Caldwell, & Lieberman, 2016). In terms of caffeine consumption, in wealthy countries the elderly are the biggest consumers (150–170 mg/day), followed by adults (140–150 mg/day), adolescents (80 mg/day) and children (30 mg/day). With total annual world coffee production of 9.7 million tonnes, tea production of 5.8 million tonnes and cocoa production of 5.2 million tonnes, it is not surprising that more than 80% of the world's population consumes a caffeine-containing product each day (de Paula & Farah, 2019).

Caffeine is absorbed mainly in the small intestine. Peak salivary caffeine is reached around 45 min after ingestion, and peak plasma caffeine in 30–120 min post ingestion, with a half-life of 3–7 hours (de Paula & Farah, 2019; Temple et al., 2017). Caffeine readily crosses the blood-brain barrier, it easily traverses the placenta and can also pass into a lactating woman's milk. The metabolism of caffeine is principally undertaken by the liver, with it being broken down to paraxanthine (80%), theobromine

(15%) and theophylline (5%). These metabolites are broken down further and excreted through the kidneys. Metabolism is reduced during pregnancy, and is slower in the foetus and infant than in children and adults, resulting in longer periods of foetal and infant exposure to caffeine following consumption during pregnancy and lactation (Temple et al., 2017). Smoking acts to increase caffeine metabolism, reducing its half-life, and driving increased consumption in smokers.

The European Food Safety Authority sets an upper limit of 400 mg per day of caffeine as safe in adults. This value is lower for pregnant women, at 200 mg per day. The rationale for this is based on a variety of data (increased risk of low-birth-weight babies, higher rate of spontaneous abortion), including studies in mice, which indicate foetal exposure can disrupt neuronal migration, resulting in mild cognitive deficits and a heightened propensity for seizures (Temple et al., 2017). There is no human data indicating that caffeine adversely affects foetal development or that it impairs development. In children and adolescents, there are links between caffeine usage and delinquency, and while the caffeine content of products consumed by this group are much lower, due to lower body weight the mg/kg dosage may end up being much higher than for adults consuming coffee. There may be unforeseen consequences of this for potentiating reward (e.g., drugs of abuse, and perhaps also sucrose/fructose in caffeine-containing beverages), which are discussed later in this section.

7.3.1 Effects of Caffeine

Unlike alcohol, where a fairly ready distinction can be made between the effects of acute and chronic usage, this dichotomy is far less useful for caffeine. Nearly all caffeine users consume it every day, unlike alcohol, so most caffeine users are chronic users. While it is useful to look at the long-term impacts of caffeine consumption, which is considered later, most of the literature on caffeine's effects has to take into account chronic usage. This is because chronic usage can reveal a different picture of caffeine's effects than acute usage in non-users, and, more importantly, as chronic usage is the norm it is important to understand what its effects look like in what is the majority of the population. Even more importantly, there are now grounds to suspect that many of the cognitive benefits of caffeine only manifest under conditions where the drug is administered during withdrawal (i.e., every morning in most people) or under conditions of fatigue and sleep deprivation (Ferré, 2016; James, 2014; Temple et al., 2017).

Caffeine exerts a number of effects on bodily systems. It is ergogenic, meaning that many types of physical performance are enhanced by its consumption (McLellan, Caldwell, & Lieberman, 2016). It is a mild diuretic; it has dose-dependent effects on blood pressure, heart rate and vasodilation; and it also alleviates pain (Temple et al., 2017). Caffeine interferes with sleep, and does so in adolescents, adults and the elderly (Clark & Landolt, 2017). While the ergogenic and pain-relieving effects of caffeine seem to be unaffected by chronic usage, this does weaken caffeine's capacity to impair sleep, serve as a diuretic and affect cardiovascular function. In other words, tolerance develops to certain aspects of caffeine's physiological effects.

When a caffeine-deprived user is provided caffeine at a dose equivalent to a cup of coffee, relative to a placebo condition controlling for expectancy bias, participants describe significant increases in subjective well-being, alertness and energy. This positive state can serve as a reinforcer in humans and animals (although it is difficult to get animals to intercranially self-administer caffeine; Ferré, 2016). Caffeine administration can increase preference for and liking of co-occurring flavours and places, and especially so when they are encountered during caffeine withdrawal (Meredith et al., 2013). While overnight is sufficient to initiate caffeine withdrawal, which peaks 20–48 hours after the last dose, some people experience more pronounced symptoms than others (and this seems to have a substantial genetic component, shared with alcohol and nicotine). Common features of caffeine withdrawal are headache, poor concentration, flu-like symptoms, fatigue and low mood, with parallel states found in animal models, in newborn babies whose mothers were heavy caffeine users, and in soft drink-consuming children who cease consumption. These symptoms, which are typically mild and last just a few days, are easily reversed by the administration of caffeine (de Paula & Farah, 2019; Meredith et al., 2013).

Determining whether caffeine has beneficial cognitive effects in a person who is not caffeine- or sleep-deprived is still contentious. There is no doubt that in sleep-deprived people, caffeine significantly improves information processing speed, reaction time, attention and aspects of executive function, in addition to real-world tasks like driving (Irwin et al., 2020). Similarly, the claim that caffeine improves reaction time, vigilance and attention in people who are caffeine-deprived and in withdrawal, is also uncontentious (James, 2014). Some research designs, using caffeine naïve participants and those that control for withdrawal effects, do indicate a residual benefit, enough for the authors of leading reviews in this area to conclude that there is an independent effect of caffeine above and beyond that of withdrawal/fatigue-reversal (McLellan et al., 2016). Others contend that these effects arise solely from withdrawal amelioration and performance improvement under conditions of sleep deprivation/fatigue (Ferré, 2016; James, 2014; Temple et al., 2017). There is also some uncertainty around the extent of caffeine's effects on learning and memory, with no clear effects on short-term memory and a possible benefit to long-term memory.

7.3.2   Caffeine and the Brain

Caffeine exerts its main effects on adenosine receptors. Adenosine is produced in all cells of the body mainly as a consequence of metabolism of its phosphorylated forms (ADP, ATP). Adenosine levels rise dramatically following significant bodily stress (e.g., hypoxia, ischaemia) where it serves a protective role. Both adenosine and its phosphorylated forms can act as neurotransmitters binding to the Purine 2 class of receptor, while adenosine alone activates the Purine 1 class of receptor (DeNinno, 1998). The Purine 1 class has four subtypes, A1, A2a, A2b and A3, and caffeine is a high-affinity antagonist for all four (Jacobson et al., 2020), its structure similar to adenosine (see Figure 7.1). The A1 and A2a forms are high-affinity adenosine receptors, while the A2b and A3 are low-affinity forms. The latter are probably involved in mediating its high concentration protective role, while the former are involved in generating an inhibitory tonus over ascending arousal and dopaminergic systems (Borea et al., 2018; Ferré, 2016). Both the A1 and A2a receptors are expressed at multiple locations in the body, where they mediate many of caffeine's physiological effects (e.g., cardiovascular, diuresis). In the brain, the A1

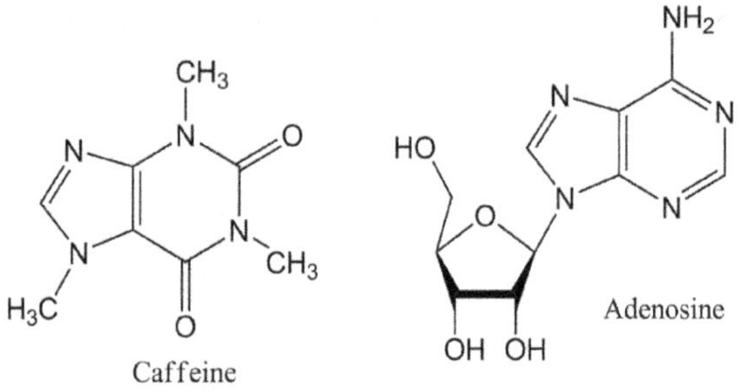

Figure 7.1   Structural similarity of caffeine and adenosine

receptor is widely distributed, while the A2a receptor is more restricted, occurring at high density in the striatum, olfactory tubercle and hippocampus (Grosso et al., 2017), and at a lower density in the cortex.

During daytime, adenosine starts to accumulate in the extracellular space of the basal forebrain, hypothalamus and cortex. Primarily via the A2a receptor (as suggested by knockout mice studies), this increases inhibition of: (1) ascending cholinergic neurons in the basal forebrain, (2) corticofugal neurons from the prefrontal cortex, (3) the pontine ascending arousal system and (4) hypothalamic histaminergic and orexinergic neurons. This normally serves to induce fatigue and sleepiness, and is effectively blunted by consumption of caffeine, which blocks these effects increasing alertness and reducing tiredness (Ferré, 2016; Ribeiro & Sebastião, 2010). Regular caffeine exposure seems to up-regulate the adenosine system, and it may be this that results in withdrawal symptoms, when caffeine consumption ceases.

Caffeine also generates a positive affective state (e.g., sense of well-being), which is related to its capacity to act as a reinforcer – in addition to removing the state of dysphoria induced by withdrawal. These effects are probably mediated by caffeine's effect on the A1 and A2a receptors located in the striatum, and in particular on the mesolimbic dopamine system (Borea et al., 2018; Ferré, 2016). First, caffeine blocks presynaptic A1 receptors increasing dopamine release. Second, the A1 receptor forms a complex with the D1 dopamine receptor (A1D1 heterodimer) on GABAergic striatal neurons, and caffeine inhibits adenosine's effect here, increasing dopamine transmission. Third, two A2a adenosine receptors form a receptor complex with two dopamine D2 receptors (A2aD2 heterotetramer), which potentiates the effects of dopamine. The first and second dopamine-related mechanisms are prone to rapid tolerance, while the third is not. Indeed, there is evidence that caffeine use leads to an increase in the number of A2aD2 heterotetramer receptors.

There is conflicting evidence as to whether caffeine results in dopamine release in the shell of the nucleus accumbens, which seems to be a specific characteristic of drugs of abuse (Nehlig, 2016). Nonetheless, the D2 receptor is the target of many such drugs, with them acting as agonists at this site. As described earlier, caffeine indirectly effects the D2 receptor by its binding to the A2aD2 heterotetramer. This has led Ferré (2016) to suggest that caffeine exposure might potentiate the effects of drugs of abuse. An additional concern is the presence of caffeine as an additive in sugar-sweetened carbonated drinks, which are widely consumed by children. The interesting question here is whether the presence of caffeine might also potentiate the rewarding properties of sugar, which would further reinforce their consumption.

Caffeine exerts a number of other effects. Some of these occur only at concentrations beyond those encountered in routine use (Monteiro et al., 2019). These are the inhibitory impacts on phosphodiesterases, which produce anti-inflammatory effects, the blockade of calcium reuptake via ryanodine receptors, and effects on the GABA A receptor. Caffeine is also a weak inhibitor of monoamine oxidase, and while this would be expected to increase dopamine, norepinephrine and serotonin levels, it does not seem to be relevant to caffeine's mood-enhancing properties (Jacobson et al., 2020). Caffeine also inhibits acetylcholinesterase, resulting in an increase in acetylcholine in the synaptic cleft, but whether this has any effect on behaviour is also unclear. A further effect is on glutamate, as there are A1A2a heterodimers where adenosine binding leads to glutamate release, which is blocked by caffeine (Borea et al., 2018; Kolahdouzan & Hamadeh, 2017).

7.3.3   Caffeine Abuse

The diagnostic and statistical manual of the American Psychiatric Association (DSM-V) includes two caffeine-related diagnoses – caffeine intoxication (caffeinism) and caffeine withdrawal – and identifies one condition requiring further study – caffeine use disorder (Wesensten, 2014). Caffeine withdrawal was discussed in Section 7.3.1, and there is general agreement that this occurs, and that in a minority of people it may be sufficiently unpleasant to warrant clinical attention. Caffeine intoxication occurs after acute exposure to a large dose/s (figures vary as to what dose this corresponds to, but it is well in excess of normal consumption, and in the order of grams of caffeine ingested). It generates anxiety, agitation, gastrointestinal disturbance and supraventricular and ventricular arrhythmias, which, if the dose is high enough, can kill (the LD50 for caffeine in humans is about 200 mg/kg). Caffeine-related deaths are rare and result from either suicide with caffeine tablets or accidental overdose of diet 'preparations' containing caffeine (Cappelletti et al., 2018).

Caffeine use disorder has three core elements: (1) persistent desire to cut down/control use but an inability to do so, (2) continued use even when it is known to be causing harm and (3) withdrawal symptoms on cessation of use or use to avoid withdrawal. Studies of prevalence in the general population are small and limited, and suggest (probably with big error bars) that somewhere between 6% and 9% of the population might satisfy the core elements of a caffeine use disorder (Meredith et al., 2013). As Budney, Lee, and Juliano (2015) discuss, there are significant risks associated with the introduction of this diagnosis in DSM-V. One is over-diagnosis and the other is trivialisation of the notion of substance use in the public's mind, and bringing psychiatry/psychology into disrepute (not unreasonable, when you consider the jokes/memes that would likely arise from the inclusion of this as a psychiatric disorder). However, there is also a good reason for considering it. There are certainly people who need to cut down use for medical reasons, notably pregnant women and people with certain cardiac conditions, and at least some of these people report significant difficulty in reducing or stopping caffeine (Meredith et al., 2013). The clincher is likely to be public perception of caffeine, and as long as this remains positive it is hard to see caffeine abuse being taken with the seriousness that it *may* deserve.

7.3.4   Long-Term Caffeine Effects

Lifetime caffeine usage may confer benefits by reducing the risk of age-related cognitive decline and Alzheimer's and Parkinson's disease. A 2015 meta-analysis found that coffee drinking was linked to a small reduction in risk for all forms of cognitive decline, but the effects for caffeine overall were equivocal (Kim, Kwak & Myung, 2015). Animal data certainly suggests that caffeine may be protective or even ameliorative, with multiple potential causal pathways for these effects mediated in particular via adenosine receptors (Kolahdouzan & Hamadeh, 2017; Monteiro et al., 2019). For Parkinson's disease, meta-analytic results are more definitive, with a relative risk reduction of 0.72 on three or four cups of coffee per day (Nehlig, 2016). In this case there is a clear benefit for men, but far less so for women, which has been attributed to the effects of oestrogen. Animal data are also supportive. Caffeine not only acts to reduce the likelihood of development of a chemically induced animal model of Parkinson's disease, it also may improve symptoms following damage (Kolahdouzan & Hamadeh, 2017; Monteiro et al., 2019). Whether caffeine may have utility in the treatment of Parkinson's disease is unclear, but the evidence is quite supportive for it providing a protective effect.

Finally, caffeine also seems to reduce the risk of stroke and depression (Nehlig, 2016). Two large prospective studies, suggest that two to three cups of coffee a day are linked to a 15% reduction in likelihood of depression, and four or more, with a 20% reduction. This has been confirmed in other studies, using caffeine intake from all sources, and, relatedly, caffeine use is also linked to a reduced risk of suicide. For stroke, two meta-analyses have found a reduction in risk of all stroke types for coffee consumption in the range of two to eight cups per day. These effects on depression and stroke seem to be well supported with consistent findings in the literature.

7.3.5   Conclusion

Caffeine consumption is ubiquitous, and its harms seem minimal. It is an interesting drug because its effects on reward pathways are indirect, and so more subtle than other drugs that can induce dependence. Questions remain over whether it confers cognitive benefits above and beyond countering the effects of its withdrawal (i.e., caffeine deprivation), and whether when caffeine is combined with sugar-sweetened beverages it might potentiate use (dependence?) of these products via its effect on brain reward pathways.

7.4   Theobromine

Theobromine (3,7-dimethylxanthine) is produced in the body as part of the breakdown of caffeine. The main food source of theobromine is cocoa products, especially chocolate. Dark chocolate contains the most at around 1 g/100 g, with much lower concentrations in milk chocolate at 0.1–0.5 g/ 100 g (Cova et al., 2019). Caffeine is also present in chocolate (at a ratio of 1 part caffeine to 5 of theobromine), which is important to mention as this dose is sufficient to induce psychoactive effects. Theobromine is an adenosine receptor antagonist like caffeine, but it is a less potent one. It has a longer half-life than caffeine, but with lower toxicity (Stavric, 1988; about 180 30-g milk chocolate bars are needed for lethality). Theobromine is at best only a weak stimulant, with limited effects on human cognition and alertness (e.g., Baggott et al., 2013; Judelson et al., 2013). Its effects on the body's physiological systems are qualitatively similar to caffeine, but perhaps with greater potency. It is unlikely that theobromine plays any significant role in chocolate's popularity.

7.5   Food

This section focusses on whether food can be a primary cause of an addiction – a food addiction. Unlike alcohol, cocaine or opium, where it is possible to live your whole life without consuming these substances, it is not possible to live without eating food. This singular fact makes the idea of food addiction particularly challenging. Before discussing this issue, it is important to deal with another. This book is focussed on the effects of food and drink on brain and behaviour. However, a reasonable proportion of food addiction research relates to obesity, which is often envisaged as an endpoint for food addiction. Such research is engaged in finding parallels between the obese brain and the addicted brain. To some degree it is a reasonable presumption that at least *some* obese people become obese because they have a food addiction (Gilbert & Burger, 2016). In some of these cases there may be an overlap with a recognised clinical condition – binge-eating disorder – which has 'addiction-like' features (Davis, 2017). Nonetheless, many obese people probably do not have a food addiction as their weight gain is slow and gradual over several decades (Rogers, 2017; Ziauddeen, Farooqi, & Fletcher, 2012). In addition, there are multiple causes of obesity that have little to do with addiction – neurodevelopmental (e.g., Prader-Willi syndrome; von Deneen, Gold, & Liu, 2009), hormonal (e.g., congenital leptin deficiency) and medical (e.g., hypothalamic tumours; Carter et al., 2016). In this section we focus where possible on studies of people of normal weight, and on longitudinal animal models (i.e., lean animals fed particular types of food or macronutrient) to avoid the confounds (i.e., heterogeneity of cause) that come from conceptualising (and focussing on) the obese as endpoints of addiction.

7.5.1 Defining Addiction as It Applies to Food

Approaches to defining what food addiction might be have been heavily influenced by the *Diagnostic and Statistical Manual of the American Psychiatric Association* (DSM5). This offers two types of addictions. The first is substance use disorder, which covers a range of drugs like alcohol, tobacco, stimulants and opiates, and has been the focus of the earlier part of this chapter. The second is behavioural addiction, which at present includes just one form, gambling (with sex-addiction as a possible future inclusion). Part of the problem for food is that it remains unsettled where it sits (if at all) within this structure.

As we noted earlier, a key definitional problem for the notion of food addiction is the fact that food is necessary for survival. Clearly this is not the case for drugs of abuse or gambling (and sex too – although the evolutionary ramifications would be severe). So how can you have an addiction to something that is necessary for survival and, thus, everyone engages in? There are at least three responses to this question. The first is not particularly controversial, and simply says that addictions come in degrees. For example, many people gamble and use alcohol without abusing them, but ordinary use shades into abuse, and the degree of abuse varies from mild to severe. This is reflected in the DSMV diagnostic criteria for both forms of addiction (i.e., severity is categorised). It also represents a major area of research to uncover risk factors for addiction to food (e.g., Davis et al., 2007).

The second response, and one that seems less frequently encountered in the literature, is that eating per se could be the problem, not what is being eaten (Fernandez-Aranda, Karwautz, & Treasure, 2018). In this case there is not a food addiction, but rather an eating addiction. There is not a lot to say about this conception here. This is not because it is unimportant, but rather because there is not a lot of research on it, and it also seems to fall outside of the domain of this book (i.e., focus on food and drink as a cause).

The third response is that only certain foods cause problems, especially modern, highly (or ultra-) processed foods, which it is argued are completely different from those encountered in traditional diets (e.g., Moubarac et al., 2014). We examine the notion of ultra-processed foods in more detail later in this section, but suffice it to say here that such foods are designed to be highly palatable, and it may be this characteristic which is problematic. High palatability may lead to alterations in brain motivational systems (encompassing the processes of food reward, learning and desire) in a manner that resembles the action of drugs of abuse. Importantly, this needs to be conceptualised as a behavioural addiction because these foods are not acting *directly* on the brain like drugs of abuse do, but *indirectly* via the perceptual system (encompassing here both exteroceptive and interoceptive signals). That aside, it is *conceivable* that certain chemical constituents and/or derivatives of modern highly processed foods could directly affect the brain (e.g., rapid changes in blood glucose may be one candidate). This then would be more akin, but certainly not identical to, a substance use disorder.

The main focus in this section will be on behavioural addiction to highly palatable ultra-processed foods. There is not sufficient evidence to suggest (at the moment) that any common constituent and/or derivative of our diet exerts a *direct* effect on the brain analogous to the way that alcohol and nicotine do, for example, and so while plausible it is not pursued further. There is though substantial evidence that certain types of diet, particularly those containing a lot of modern highly processed foods, are neurotoxic. The relevance of this to addiction is not currently clear, and its behavioural consequences are not usually thought of as being 'addiction-like'. However, the term 'vicious circle' has been used to describe its effects on appetite regulation, in the way that these diets undermine self-control and promote further intake of such foods (e.g., Hargrave, Jones, & Davidson, 2016). As this type of model is discussed in Chapter 4, it is not mentioned further here.

7.5.2 Food Addiction as a Behavioural Use Disorder

The essence of this model of food addiction is that modern, highly processed foods are engineered to be very palatable. High palatability may both encourage frequent use and cause changes to the brain's motivation/reward systems. These changes may mirror, to varying degrees, changes that occur when using drugs of abuse. While this general type of model has been popular in the literature (e.g., Hauck, Cook, & Ellrott, 2020; Rogers, 2017; Ziauddeen et al., 2012), it is typically aligned with a substance use disorder framework rather than a behavioural addiction one. To reiterate, our conceptualisation as a behavioural addiction seems difficult to dismiss, because all drugs of abuse affect the brain directly (e.g., opiates bind to opioid receptors), while foods – and gambling and sex – exert their effects on the brain indirectly via neurosensory pathways. This seems a key conceptual difference. It may also be functionally important too, as it likely limits the rapidity and extent to which highly palatable foods can alter brain systems, and the nature of the changes that are possible. While we have not seen a detailed systematic examination of this issue, it seems noteworthy that you cannot overdose on food in the same way you can on drugs of abuse. Put more bluntly, ER does not see people who overdosed *that night* on crisps, pizza, chocolate or sugar-sweetened beverages.

The notion of food addiction is very popular amongst the general public and has a long medico-social history (Davis, 2017). Chocolate addiction was first described in the 1890s, obesity was discussed as a form of food addiction in the 1950s (e.g., Randolph, 1956) and several food-addiction-related self-help groups have come into being over the last 50 years (e.g., Overeaters Anonymous, Food Addicts Anonymous). There is also a widespread fascination with the idea that certain foods can act like drugs of abuse. However, this is probably to think of things the wrong way round. Perhaps what is truly remarkable is how drugs of abuse hijack elements of the brain's motivation/reward systems (e.g., Carter et al., 2016; Kenny, 2011). The evidence for this is broad (and discussed further later) and

Table 7.5. *Diagnostic criteria for gambling disorder*

Diagnostic and Statistical Manual of the American Psychiatric Association, Version 5
  Criteria and notes
In the past year:
  1. Needs to gamble with greater amounts of money to achieve desired excitement
  2. Is restless/irritable when attempts to cut down or stop
  3. Has repeated unsuccessful attempts to control or stop gambling
  4. Preoccupied with gambling
  5. Often gambles when distressed
  6. Chases losses
  7. Lies to conceal involvement in gambling
  8. Jeopardises/loses relationships, jobs, educational opportunities, etc. due to gambling
  9. Relies on others for money
Two or more criteria met indicates an alcohol use disorder, with severity defined as:
Mild 4–5 criteria met, Moderate 6–7, Severe, 8–9.

extends even into what appears to be a key difference between drugs of abuse and food. Namely, eating leads to satiety and cessation of intake via multiple neuro-hormonal signals. In contrast, drug use ceases either when supplies run out or the person becomes too intoxicated to ingest more. However, it turns out that self-administration for a range of drugs of abuse is enhanced by hunger and suppressed by satiety (Carr, 1996) and that, in turn, highly palatable processed foods can impair capacity to experience hunger and satiety (Stevenson & Francis, 2017).

The characteristics of a substance use disorder are detailed in Table 7.1 for alcohol, and for a behavioural addiction – gambling disorder – in Table 7.5. There are some important differences between the two, most notably in the greater emphasis on the pharmacological features of tolerance and withdrawal for substance use (criteria 10a, 10b, 11a and 11b), and its de-emphasis for gambling (criteria 1 and 2). Food addiction does not seem particularly well accommodated by either set of criteria, although the underlying notion of compulsive use is central to both behavioural addictions and substance use disorders. If neither of these diagnostic schemes are ideal, how does one go about diagnosing a food addiction for purposes of research or therapy?

7.5.3   *Diagnosing Food Addiction*

The Yale Food Addiction Scale (YFAS) in its various guises has been the main published instrument to assess food addiction (Gearhardt, Corbin, & Brownell, 2009; Meule & Gearhardt, 2014; Schulte & Gearhardt, 2017).

There are other approaches, such as Ruddock et al. (2017), and although these have taken a rather different direction, emphasising appetitive drive and dietary control (which sound interestingly similar to other constructs in the field of appetitive behaviour – as measured by the Three Factor Eating Questionnaire – dietary restraint and hunger), this approach like the YFAS owes its origins to DSM-IV and DSM-V conceptions of addiction.

The original version of the YFAS was based on seven criteria from the substance dependence diagnosis from DSM-IV (Gearhardt et al., 2009). The YFAS has subsequently been revised to encompass DSM-V changes (Meule & Gearhardt, 2014), alongside shorter formats based on factor analysis of scale items (Schulte & Gearhardt, 2017). The YFAS has a self-report symptom checklist format (a summary form is presented in Table 7.6), reflecting themes of compulsivity and impairment of everyday activities outside of eating. While the YFAS owes its genesis to substance use disorder, it shares with the DSM-V gambling disorder criteria a de-emphasis on the pharmacological notions of tolerance (symptom 9 in Table 7.6) and withdrawal.

The YFAS has been widely administered, and so it is possible to make some remarks about how extensive food addiction may be, at least according to this scale (noting there are various ways to define whether someone does or does not have a food addiction – absolute or graded; it is the

Table 7.6. *Symptom checklist from the modified YFAS, version 2*

Summary symptoms and notes
Eating habits in the past year, especially relating to highly palatable processed foods:
1. Eating to the point of feeling physically unwell
2. A lot of time spent feeling fatigued due to overeating
3. Avoiding activities because they might lead to overeating
4. Would or do eat certain foods in response to distress
5. Eating behaviour causes distress
6. Significant problems in life due to eating
7. Overeating gets in the way of everyday duties
8. Continued overeating even though it causes emotional difficulties
9. Eating the same amount of food no longer gives the satisfaction it used to
10. Strong urges to eat certain foods
11. Failed attempts to cut down or stop eating certain foods
12. So distracted by eating that it could/did result in being hurt
13. Friends/family worried by the person's overeating
Symptoms need to be clinically significant for them to fall into these ranges:
Mild food addiction (FA) 2–3 symptoms, Moderate FA 4–5 symptoms, Severe FA, 6+ symptoms.

absolute mild+ that is generally counted here, but noting that counts in the reports here can combine earlier and later versions of the YFAS). Pursey et al.'s (2014) metanalysis of prevalence data suggest that around 11% of adults with a normal BMI meet minimum criteria for YFAS food addiction, with higher rates in women and older people. A subsequent systematic review by Long, Blundell, and Finlayson (2015) estimated that around 7% of the normal weight adult population had a YFAS-defined food addiction. A representative national sample from Denmark (Horsager et al., 2020) observed a prevalence of 8.5%, but this includes obese individuals. Obese people have higher rates of YFAS-measured food addiction, suggesting that in normal-weight individuals prevalence would be less than 8.5%. In sum, according to the YFAS, around 1/10 to 1/15 normal-weight adults have a food addiction.

The YFAS has attracted a certain amount of criticism (e.g., Long et al., 2015; Rogers, 2017). The scale asks participants to think about *foods they have problems with*, which brings us back to the issue of what constitutes a problem food, and what commonalities, if any, such foods have (Long et al., 2015; Westwater, Fletcher, & Ziauddeen, 2016). We turn to this topic in the next section. Another criticism concerns the validity of the YFAS 'diagnosis' of food addiction. This has attracted a lot of concern (Long et al., 2015; Rogers, 2017; Westwater et al., 2016). There is no doubt that YFAS scores are higher among obese people and in people with binge-eating disorder, but whether this provides validation is unclear. Many obese people, and people with binge-eating disorder, have considerable difficulty in controlling their food intake – but does this mean they are food addicts?

7.5.4 Which Foods May Be Addictive?

One starting point has been to ask people when completing the YFAS what sort of foods they have problems with (i.e., what foods are they thinking of when answering questions like those in Table 7.6). The top 10 are (in order): chocolate, ice cream, chips, pizza, cookies, crisps, cake, popcorn, cheeseburgers and muffins. The least frequently mentioned foods are apples, corn, salmon, banana, carrot, brown rice, cucumber, broccoli and beans (Schulte, Avena, & Gearhardt, 2015). One characteristic that links all of the top 10 problem foods is that they are highly processed, a conclusion that the authors also focussed on. Another obvious characteristic of these top 10 problem foods is that they are regarded by many people as highly palatable.

A further study also utilised participants completing the YFAS to examine the macronutrient/tastant profile of their problem foods. Markus et al. (2017) reported that it was the combination of high fat with either high sugar or high salt/umami, which constituted the largest group of problem foods. Not surprisingly, fat and sweet, and fat and savoury, encompass almost entirely the items identified by Schulte et al. (2015) reflecting again food processing and, relatedly, high engineered palatability.

The focus on processing as a key characteristic of problem foods has emerged from another quarter, namely identifying diets associated with weight gain and obesity. In a systematic examination of different food classification schemes, the best (in terms of specificity, coherence, concision, practicality and generalisability) was the NOVA system (Moubarac et al., 2014). This characterises foods and drinks as falling into three main categories: (1) unprocessed and minimally processed foods (e.g., frozen or fresh peas, dried or fresh fruit, eggs); (2) processed culinary ingredients (e.g., plant oils, flour); and (3) ready-to-consume products. This last-mentioned category divides into two, processed food products (e.g., bacon, tinned fish in oil, fruit in syrup) and ultra-processed products (e.g., chips, cookies, ready-to-eat meals, etc.). Not only do nearly all of the problem foods identified by Schulte et al. (2015) fall within the ultra-processed category, these foods are not surprisingly designed to appeal to the palate. That is they contain fats, salts and sugars to maximise palatability, and they are extensively tested on sensory evaluation panels to ensure that this goal is achieved. Ultra-processed foods constitute 58% of the energy intake of US adults, and people in the highest quintile for consumption for these food types are more likely to be obese (Juul et al., 2018).

In the extensive animal literature exploring food addiction, the focus has generally been on macronutrients, with an acknowledgement that their palatability is likely to be an important consideration. Sugar (sucrose, sometimes glucose) has been widely used, originally by Hoebel and his associates, Avena, Rada, and Hoebel (2009) and Wiss, Avena, and Rada (2018). In humans, sugar alone is consumed mostly in the form of drinks (Mountain Dew, Coke, Pepsi, orange juice, cordials, etc.), even though it occurs in many processed foods with fat (fruit yoghurt, chocolate mousse, etc.). Consumption of sugar in recent decades is confronting. It increased from 5 kg/per capita in the 1800s to 70 kg/per capita in 2006 (Tappy, 2012). High intake of sucrose is detrimental to health because it causes an unduly rapid rise in blood glucose, it drives dental caries and impairs certain aspects of brain function (see Chapter 4).

Most people consume sweetened products because they like the taste (and not forgetting its post-ingestive effects, which are independently reinforcing), something we have in common with rats and mice – although the strength of this preference reliably varies both in people and animals. In the laboratory, an animal model of sugar addiction has been developed, which has several interesting behavioural (impaired control, craving) and biological (tolerance, biochemical similarities) parallels with drugs of abuse (Avena et al., 2009; Wiss et al., 2018). However, to obtain this addictive behaviour, selected animals have to have carefully restricted (1–3 h) daily access to sucrose or glucose (dissolved in water – at a concentration roughly equivalent to 1–2 teaspoons of sugar in a cup of tea) over a protracted period of time (3 weeks). Free access does not produce this dependence model, and as other observers have remarked, the rather specific circumstances necessary to generate this sugar addiction means it has limited generalisability to humans as a model of addiction (although it may arguably serve as a model of binging). Perhaps more importantly, and as described in the previous section, sugar-only foods do not seem to be those that are reported as a 'problem', rather it is foods containing fat, either in savoury form or mixed with sugar.

Neither restricted access to fat alone or to fat–sugar/savoury mixtures seems to produce the same type of addiction model in animals as restricted access to sugar does. While there are some parallels of the sugar addiction model in biology (striatal dopamine changes) and behaviour (place preference) to substance use disorder, the withdrawal component (i.e., tremors, anxiety), either spontaneously from target-food withdrawal or naloxone precipitated, has not been consistently observed (Avena et al., 2009; Pandit et al., 2012). Unrestricted exposure to fat, fat/sugar and cafeteria diets (i.e., chips, cookies, etc.) typically leads to weight gain, suggesting a dysregulation of intake control, something that is not seen with the sugar addiction model (Hone-Blanchet & Fecteau, 2014). Apart from the sugar addiction model (and noting its problem of ecological validity), it is hard to characterise the consequences of exposing animals to palatable foods – which is what most of these diets involve – as *causing* an addictive behaviour.

In sum, what the data seems to tell us is that people report that highly palatable foods can be 'problematic' and that such foods are typically ultra-processed. Rats and mice also like to eat these same foods, and if they are given unrestricted access to them, on average they start to gain weight, as with people. Perhaps the problem here is that it is only certain people who are at risk of becoming 'food addicts'. Indeed, for many of the original studies on sugar addiction in rodents using the restricted access paradigm, animals were selected based on their preference for sucrose (Westwater et al., 2016). Similarly, the YFAS finds most people do not report food addiction even though nearly everyone is exposed to ultra-processed foods. It seems, then, a reasonable proposition that risk factors could be a key moderating variable.

7.5.5 Risk Factors and Addiction

There are a range of risk factors for addiction, which overlap with risk factors for obesity, supporting the idea discussed earlier that obesity can be conceptualised (*in part* – see Introduction to this section for limitations of this view) as an endpoint of food addiction. These overlaps include genetic dispositions for particular receptor subtypes (Taq 1A allele for the D2 dopamine receptor; A118G allele for the mu opioid receptor) involved in motivational processing, impulsivity, cue reactivity and sensitivity to reward (Davis et al., 2007; He et al., 2014; Stice et al., 2011; Ziauddeen et al., 2012).

If food addiction is conceptualised independently from obesity, then the approach would be to examine for relationships between risk factors known for addiction and YFAS score/diagnosis – *ideally* only where body weight is not a confounding factor. There is some data pertinent to this but most is not clear-cut. The behavioural activation system (BAS) is a biologically based personality characteristic reflecting sensitivity to reward, and higher BAS scores are linked to a greater propensity for addiction. However, there is no relationship between the BAS and the YFAS (Gearhardt et al., 2009), although the other facet of Gray's model the behavioural inhibition system (BIS) is related, but the BIS has not generally been considered a risk factor for drug abuse. A caveat: this study also included people who were overweight and obese, but as no BAS-YFAS link was observed, BMI is unlikely to be a confound.

Impulsivity is reportedly higher in people scoring higher on the YFAS, when this is assessed both by self-report and behavioural measures. However, these studies used only female samples and did not exclude overweight or obese participants, which makes interpretation problematic (see Pursey et al., 2014). Consistent with greater impulsivity in higher YFAS scorers is the observation in a large Norwegian study that ADHD is more common in people scoring higher on the YFAS (Horsager et al., 2020). This sample also contained overweight/obese participants and there was a significant relationship between weight status and ADHD, which again could have mediated the relationship observed between the YFAS and ADHD. This same study also revealed that rates of alcoholism were higher among higher YFAS scorers, an effect not obviously attributable to body weight, as there was no correlation between BMI and alcoholism in this study (but noting these have been found by others). There have also been some preliminary examinations of whether receptor subtypes linked to drug abuse are more prevalent in higher YFAS scorers. So far only one has been detected, relating to certain protein kinases involved in drug addiction (Gordon et al., 2018).

In sum, there is *some* evidence linking people who score higher on the YFAS to the same sort of biological risk factors as for addiction, but in almost all cases the concern is that these links may reflect overlaps between obesity and addiction. Clearly this risk literature is not developed well enough at the moment to provide a clear answer.

7.5.6   Compulsion to Eat

The core idea of food addiction is that certain people feel compelled to eat palatable food. The main evidence for this is simply that people report it. This is reflected in two key constructs of the YFAS (see Table 7.6). The first are constructs around compulsive use – craving, preoccupation and impaired control. The second concerns the consequences of the first, namely its impacts on a person's life. Starting with craving, this occurs for particular foods, especially palatable ones like chocolate, and is predictive of overeating and weight gain (Boswell & Kober, 2016). The occurrence of food cravings in people with no sign of eating psychopathology is common and well documented (Hill & Heaton-Brown, 1994; Lafay et al., 2001; Martin et al., 2011). Craving does seem to be more common in people with a higher YFAS score (Pursey et al., 2014), and this is probably not a consequence of confounding by inclusion of people with higher BMI, as BMI is unrelated to food craving (Boswell & Kober, 2016). Craving is also a common phenomenon in substance use disorder, especially during withdrawal (Sayette, 2016), but rather obviously this is restricted to those who have become dependent on a particular drug. So while craving drug X is specific *to people* with drug dependence for X, food craving does not share the same specificity – it's common. Of course, this could simply be that nearly everyone is exposed to highly palatable processed foods.

Excessive preoccupation with food and impaired capacity to regulate intake are reported to occur for food, and especially palatable foods like chocolate (Gordon et al., 2018). Indeed, the two questions most commonly answered in the affirmative on the YFAS both concern impaired regulatory capacity, with an inability to control intake ('can't cut down') and an inability to stop ('ate more than planned'; Horsager et al., 2020; Meule & Gearhardt, 2014). Beyond these self-reports there is as yet no behavioural evidence of heightened preoccupation and impaired regulatory capacity in higher YFAS scorers.

A notable difference between both the substance use and behavioural addictions in DSM-V, and food addiction, concerns the consequences of dependence. Clearly this is a very significant feature of drug use and gambling, with financial loss, relationship breakdown, interaction with the criminal justice system and work/study impairments being common. These types of severe consequences are not reported in the food addiction literature (Gordon et al, 2018) nor are they routinely identified on related questions on the YFAS, as the least frequently answered items concern the impacts on relationships and routine obligations (Horsager et al., 2020; Meule & Gearhardt, 2014). One contributing factor here is that highly palatable foods are cheap, easy to obtain and socially sanctioned. Indeed, when an opioid-dependent person is prescribed methadone they can lead a more normal life, as it frees them from the economic imperative of supporting an expensive opiate habit and its associated criminal and social consequences. So, this difference between traditional dependencies and food *may* be less important than it first appears. There are also the mental health consequences. People with higher YFAS scores do report being more depressed (Pursey et al., 2014), but whether this is uniquely linked to the adverse consequences of food addiction, obesity or other eating psychopathology is not clear.

A final source of evidence for compulsive eating comes from animal models. However, as we described earlier there are major concerns over the ecological validity of some of these models. This is because the ones that most parallel substance use disorder are the restricted access paradigms (Avena et al., 2009; Hone-Blanchet & Fecteau, 2014). Certainly, this type of model generates evidence of compulsive use, with rats, for example, prepared to risk electric shock to obtain access to target foods (Avena et al., 2009). More generally, restricted access models do not parallel the environmental circumstances that are presumed to occur for humans – effortless access to cheap palatable food at any time. When animals are provided with these same circumstances, they gain weight and at least some become obese (Pandit et al., 2012). This certainly does parallel what happens in humans, but it is probably not addiction.

7.5.7 Biological Aspects of Compulsive Use

In humans, food reward and motivation can be partitioned into three temporal aspects. The first is when food is anticipated. The second is when food is consumed, with the somatosensory system and the chemical senses as the dominant mediums. The third is in the hours following eating, when food is digested and signals concerning the food's nutritional qualities pass to the brain (Small & DiFeliceantonio, 2019). In humans, anticipation, consumption and gut signals are all capable of stimulating a central component of the brain's motivation/reward system – the striatum (He et al., 2014; Pelchat et al., 2004; Small, Jones-Gotman, & Dagher, 2003; Tellez et al., 2013). A further key aspect of food reward occurs when endogenous opioids are released on anticipation and consumption of food (Mercer & Holder, 1997). It has been suggested that learning about, anticipation of, and habitual aspects of food consumption are supported primarily by dopamine release in the striatum, while pleasure mainly arises from stimulation of the brain opioid system (Barbano & Cador, 2007; Carter et al., 2016). Importantly, many other structures (notably lateral hypothalamus, orbitofrontal cortex, insula, amygdala, hippocampus, prefrontal cortex) and neurochemicals (endocannabinoids, serotonin, grehlin, leptin) have significant roles in reward processing (i.e., learning, modulation, regulation), but the striatum, dopamine and endogenous opioids are core components.

Perhaps not surprisingly, drugs of abuse uniformly affect these three core components, especially in the transition to dependence. Initially, drugs of abuse stimulate dopamine release in the striatum when they are consumed, and this is suspected to shift with exposure to anticipation, such that drug-associated cues come to result in larger dopamine release than during consumption (Carter et al., 2016; Ely, Winter, & Lowe, 2013). Drugs of abuse also induce characteristic changes in gene regulation in the striatum (indexed generally by increases in delta Go/Gi switch regulatory protein 3 (FOSB) and decreases in cyclic amp-response element binding protein (CREB)) as well as altering various aspects of the endogenous opioid system (Kenny, 2011). If food, and especially highly palatable food, is capable of inducing compulsive use, then it would be expected to affect the same three core elements of reward processing in a similar manner.

Animal data demonstrate that consistent exposure to a highly palatable diet (weeks to months) causes increases in delta FOSB and decreases in CREB in the striatum (Alsiö et al., 2012; Gordon et al., 2018). There are two points to make about this finding – apart from its similarity to the effects of drugs of abuse. First, hunger also up-regulates delta FOSB, and hunger is associated with food seeking, making the potential link here to a 'strong motivated state' (*possibly* compulsive) aimed at obtaining palatable food (Kenny, 2011). Second, there is also the suggestion that delta FOSB levels may be permanently elevated in animals exposed to palatable food when they are young, such that exposure to palatable diets later in life produces increased consumption relative to naïve animals (Kenny, 2011). What does not seem clear at this stage is the *degree* of change in delta FOSB/CREB relative to drugs of abuse, and hence behaviourally, its impact on compulsive seeking of palatable foods. While abused drugs are known to fuel property crime to support their use, as can starvation (see Chapter 8), it is hard to believe that someone who is not starving but is deprived of Mars bars, chips and Coke would steal or harm others to obtain these snack foods. It *may be then* that the urge to consume is elevated for highly palatable foods, but not to the same degree as for drugs of abuse or with starvation.

Consistent with up-regulation of delta FOSB and the down-regulation of CREB, there are also alterations in striatal dopamine function associated with palatable food consumption. In animals, exposure to palatable diets reduces D2 receptor density in the striatum and produces a blunting of dopamine release on consumption (Alsiö et al., 2012; Gordon et al., 2018). It is not clear though if there is a similar transition pattern to drugs of abuse with a switch to more dopamine release during anticipation than during consumption. One suggestive parallel is the finding that exposure to palatable diets speeds the transition from action to habit, which is also dependent on changes to striatal dopamine function (Corbit, 2016; Gilbert & Burger, 2016). For opioidergic pathways, there is good evidence in animals that exposure to palatable diets leads to alterations in function at multiple points, and that a return to normal chow after prolonged exposure to palatable food is also linked to dysregulation of this system (Alsiö et al., 2012). It seems then that the animal literature offers a suggestive picture (and noting that restricted access models also implicate these same systems; Wiss et al., 2018), in which palatable foods do engender changes in the core components of the motivational/reward system, with the caveat that these changes are almost certainly not as dramatic as for drugs of abuse.

The human literature addressing whether palatable food use results in a similar pattern of brain changes to addiction is limited to functional neuroimaging, with the key focus being striatal activation. The presumption here is that 'users' (of palatable food) will have a more vigorous anticipatory striatal response to palatable food cues than 'non-users', with this relationship reversed on consumption. Three papers have explored this (and see also Tey et al. (2012) for some interesting behavioural data on blunted sensory-specific satiety for frequently eaten high palatability foods). Gearhardt et al.'s (2011) study was the first, comparing two BMI matched groups that differed in their YFAS score, so crudely food addicts ('users') and non-food addicts ('non-users'). Participants were scanned under two conditions: with cues to a palatable milkshake (i.e., anticipation) and on its consumption. Analyses were reported both by grouping and also using YFAS score as a continuous variable. The correlational approach revealed no relationship between YFAS score and striatal activity on either anticipation or consumption trials. The grouping approach revealed greater striatal activity in the YFAS food addicts during anticipation (as predicted), but no difference on consumption (not as predicted). There were also differences in ancillary reward structures (prefrontal and orbitofrontal cortex), but the core focus was the striatum, and the core hypothesis was only partially supported, and then only in the grouping approach.

Two further studies using adolescent participants have examined differences between regular consumers and non-consumers of a particular palatable food (Coke and ice cream), while scanning during cue presentation (anticipation) and on consumption. Burger and Stice (2012), using an ice-cream-flavoured milkshake, found that there was no difference in striatal response to cues for the milkshake (not predicted), but on consumption, striatal response was blunted in participants who habitually ate ice cream (predicted). This is partial support again, but this time just for the consumption part of the hypothesis. Burger and Stice (2014) conducted another study, this time using Coke. Again there was no anticipatory difference in striatal activation by whether a participant was a habitual Coke drinker or not (not predicted) nor this time was there any difference in striatal response on consumption (not predicted).

The human data are not very supportive of the idea that food addicts or those who routinely eat highly palatable foods have an 'addiction-like' pattern of striatal activation. These same questions have been explored far more extensively in obese participants and here too it remains unclear what impact palatable foods have on the striatum (Gilbert & Burger, 2016; Ziauddeen et al., 2012). So while the animal literature offers some support for parallels between changes to the function of core reward systems following palatable food exposure and drugs of abuse (and with the important qualification that it is just somewhat similar), the human biological evidence is inconclusive.

7.5.8 Conclusion

Medicine currently conceptualises two forms of addiction: to substances and to behaviours. Food addiction seems to fit better into the behavioural addictions because food does not directly affect the brain in the way that drugs like heroin or methamphetamine do. The indirect nature of food's impact (i.e., via sensory neurons) on the brain probably imposes limits on the severity of any resulting dependence. Food is unusual amongst the behavioural addictions (i.e., gambling, possibly sex) in that it is necessary for individual survival. This raises the problem of whether you can be 'addicted' to something that you physically require on a regular basis. One way out of this impasse is to emphasise that only certain foods have addictive potential, namely ultra-processed foods, which are engineered to be highly palatable. It is arguably their high palatability that results in the adverse changes to reward systems observed in animals exposed to these foods – changes which resemble those seen in animals exposed to addictive drugs. In humans, the evidence for a behavioural food addiction to ultra-processed palatable food in lean and otherwise healthy people relies almost exclusively on self-report. Currently, there is no strong evidence that such people have individual characteristics that are known to predispose towards addiction and there is no strong evidence that their brains' reward processes show changes of the sort that are expected in addiction.

An important consideration is whether the whole concept of food addiction is a useful one. It does seem to be an interesting question as to whether certain foods are overwhelmingly identified as a 'problem' by many people, and the food addiction literature has stimulated interest in identifying such foods (Schulte et al., 2015). But having identified them it seems that palatability is the key issue, and this and people's ability to regulate consumption of these foods has been a focus of appetitive psychology for decades. It is unclear if adding the concept of 'addiction' provides any novel insights (Rogers, 2017). On the other hand, there may be a group of people, of normal weight, who really struggle to regulate their intake of these problem foods. To the extent that the YFAS or similar instruments helps identify these people, it may be beneficial in directing them to some form of clinical intervention or support. However, perhaps the most compelling reason for studying food addiction is to shift the narrative of blame away from consumers and towards food manufacturers. It is well understood that food manufacturers have contributed to a narrative in which overeating is perceived as a personal failure of self-control (Herrick, 2009). This places blame directly on the consumer. Clearly, finding scientific evidence that highly palatable processed foods may have an 'addiction-like' effect on consumers upends this narrative, and puts the cause of overeating back on manufacturers (Cassin et al., 2019). This is unpopular with the food industry, because the likely consequence is regulation that may hurt profits. From a public health perspective, regulation has been highly successful in reducing tobacco use through limiting affordability, availability and acceptability (Capewell & Lloyd-Williams, 2018). Of course, this is premised on their being evidence for food addiction, and this is not currently established.

There is a flip side to the claim that food addiction may drive overeating. The concept of addiction is highly stigmatising (Cassin et al., 2019) and certainly if this is added in the context of obesity, there would be a double stigma – towards the obese body and towards the person as being an addict. Moreover, instilling the idea that overeating of palatable foods is outside of self-control and the product of addiction may make it harder for people to change (or want to change) their behaviour (Rogers, 2017). How powerful a disincentive this may be is not yet known (but see Hardman et al., 2015). As the opening section on alcohol should have made clear, addiction to this chemical is a significant medical and social problem. Some researchers have been concerned that applying the label addiction to overeating chips, chocolate and Coke can be seen to trivialise the harms from the likes of alcohol or gambling (Long et al., 2015). Clearly there is some merit in this argument, especially as the functional impairments of YFAS-defined food addict do not resemble those of people with chemical or gambling dependencies.

7.6   General Conclusion

The extent of alcohol's harms are large – worldwide, perhaps as many as 64 million people have difficulty controlling how much they drink. It is also well documented, but there are still areas where its adverse impacts are actively being examined, notably with foetal and adolescent exposure. For caffeine, usage far exceeds that of any other drug, in the order of 80% of the world's population consume it daily, but its harms seem minimal. Perhaps the only areas of concern are its possible foetal impacts and the effect it has when combined with sugar in soft drinks. For food addiction, as characterised here as a behavioural dependence for ultra-processed foods engineered to be highly palatable, the very concept of addiction remains contentious. Its harms do not begin to approach those of alcohol, other drugs or gambling, and a case can be made that applying the very concept of addiction to food may be counterproductive (i.e., trivialisation of addiction, additional stigmatisation of the obese, an excuse to avoid action on controlling food intake). Nonetheless, an addiction approach has forced us to reflect on whether there is something unique about the effects of ultra-processed foods engineered to be highly palatable and this may be its scientific legacy.

CHAPTER 8

Starvation and Caloric Restriction in Adults

8.1 Introduction

This chapter concerns starvation in fully grown animals and humans. Experimental studies in adult animals are unusual because it was originally thought that dietary effects on the brain were limited to the foetus, infant and child (see Chapter 2). The two main experimental themes in the developmental literature have been the neuroanatomical and behavioural impacts of protein-deficient (malnourishment) and energy-restricted diets (undernutrition). In the adult literature this nutritional distinction is not generally made. Instead, the terms starvation, or in less extreme circumstances fasting (self-imposed starvation); semi-starvation; food/energy/dietary restriction; and dieting are used. Only starvation and fasting involve the cessation of food intake (i.e., macro- and micronutrient deficiency), while the other terms usually refer to nutritionally adequate diets, but typically with just less energy than the body needs.

The human literature can be divided into short-term (a week or less) and longer-term studies (weeks to years), varying in form from laboratory-based experiments (e.g., Minnesota starvation study; Keys et al., 1950) to naturalistic observations (e.g., hunger strikes, concentration camps). All of these are examined here. Central to this chapter, and cutting across each topic, are the impacts of starvation on the brain and cognition; its effects on mood (particularly depression), appetite and behaviour (e.g., amorality); the traumatic context in which starvation often occurs; and the impact of initial body weight on its effects. The chapter also considers involuntary weight loss during aging and disease (e.g., cancer anorexia and cachexia), the psychological sequelae of recovery from starvation (e.g., episodes of binge eating) and calorie restriction for longevity in animals and people.

8.2   Animal Studies

It was thought that protein malnourishment and undernutrition in adult animals, raised on an adequate diet, had little impact on brain and behaviour. This perspective probably arose as developmental impacts were presumed to occur because of the energy and protein needs particular to growth (e.g., Morgane, Austin-LaFrance, & Bronzino 1993; Morgane, Miller, & Kemper, 1978). A small number of studies have now examined the impact in healthy adults of protein malnourishment and undernutrition regimens. Contrary to expectation, they do find adverse effects on the brain.

8.2.1   Adult Animal Studies of Protein Malnourishment

The major focus of research has been on the hippocampus, because of its importance to learning and memory and its well understood synaptic organisation. This uses rats given ad libitum access to a low-protein chow (resulting in a 50% reduction in protein), contrasted with an energy-matched control group on standard chow. Three studies have quantified the effects of this diet on hippocampal cell density. Paula-Barbosa, Andrade, and Castedo (1989) examined granule cell numbers in the dentate gyrus and pyramidal cell numbers in the CA3 region. Irrespective of whether the low-protein diet had run for 6, 12 or 18 months, both cell types were significantly reduced relative to controls. Andrade, Maderia, and Paula-Barbosa (1995b) used the same three exposure durations, but also included a recovery group (6 months low-protein diet and 6 months control diet). Duration again had no effect, with the same abnormalities evident at 6 months. The recovery group had identical abnormalities, suggesting that 6 months of dietary rehabilitation did not remediate cell loss. The third study (Lukoyanov and Andrade, 2000) included additional behavioural tests of spatial memory, inhibitory avoidance and emotional responsiveness. Here 6 months of a low-protein diet was used, including a recovery group (6 months low-protein followed by 2 months of control diet). Behaviourally, the low-protein diet impaired retention on the spatial learning task, but not initial learning or short-term memory; had no effect on avoidance learning; and blunted emotional reactivity on the open field test all of these effects were absent in the diet recovery animals. Anatomically, the results were identical to the previous studies, with these effects also present in diet recovery animals.

Low-protein diets also affect the neuronal spine density and synaptic connectivity of neurons in the hippocampal system. Spine density in the entorhinal cortex is reduced after 1 month of a low-protein diet (Brock & Prasad, 1992). Twelve months reduces synaptic connectivity between the axonal projections (mossy fibres) of granule cells in the dentate gyrus onto pyramidal cells in CA3 (Andrade, Madeira, & Paula-Barbosa, 1995a), as does 6 months for projections onto pyramidal cells in CA2 (Lukoyanov & Andrade, 2000). Diet recovery had no effect on the latter, but remediated the former.

While low-protein diets reduce the density of hippocampal granule and pyramidal cells, they have a different effect on certain interneurons in the dentate gyrus. Six months of a low-protein diet increased the number of parvalbumin-type interneurons (Cardoso et al., 2013; Hipólito-Reis et al., 2013). This may be neuroprotective, as these interneurons mop up excess extracellular calcium ions generated during protein deprivation, which can contribute to cell death. In addition, the parvalbumin interneurons exert an inhibitory effect, which probably counters the excitatory consequence from the loss of a further cell type, namely calretinin immunoreactive interneurons (Hipólito-Reis et al., 2013). Diet recovery had no effect on parvalbumin interneuron numbers, which remained increased (Cardoso et al., 2013).

There is only limited study of the impacts of adult starvation on other brain areas. Anatomically, a 6-month low-protein diet had no effect on cell density in the rat prefrontal cortex (Paula-Barbosa et al., 1988), but effects have been found elsewhere. Paula-Barbosa et al. (1989) reported that 12 and 18 months exposure to a low-protein diet resulted in a reduction in granule cell density in the cerebellum. These effects were not evident at 6 months, unlike those they observed for the hippocampus. Brock and Prasad (1992) also explored dendritic spine densities in other regions beyond the hippocampus, following a 4-week low-protein diet. Spine density was significantly lower in the striatum, and while no effects were reported for frontal and parietal cortices, the trend was lower here as well. Finally, adult mice fed for 1 month on a 5% protein diet (Sato, Nakagawasai, & Tan-No, 2011) had significantly reduced brain weight.

Behaviourally, three studies have examined for deficits beyond the hippocampus. Alaverdashvili, Li, and Paterson (2015) and Alaverdashvili et al. (2017), using an ultra-low-protein diet, tested for motor-related abnormalities driven by the observation that malnutrition in elderly people predicts impaired motor behaviour. As expected, there was impaired usage of the forelimb and hindlimb, as well as postural changes, these being correlated with alterations in motor cortex biochemistry. This suggests a central deficit, in addition to the effects of the low-protein diet on peripheral muscle and nerve tissue. Sato et al. (2011) observed several behavioural alterations in mice fed a low-protein diet. These animals were less anxious than controls on the elevated plus maze, as well as being generally more active.

In conclusion, there is consistent evidence for adverse changes in hippocampal anatomy and synaptic connectivity, resulting from death of granule and pyramidal cells, following a low-protein diet. Re-feeding does not generally repair these changes. Beyond the hippocampus there is some evidence of neuronal (cerebellum, striatum) and behavioural abnormalities after a low-protein diet, including in motor behaviour, anxiety and activity.

8.2.2 Adult Animal Models of Undernutrition

The literature on energy restriction for longevity and age-related disease reduction (see later in the chapter) is quite extensive, and overlaps with work on adult undernutrition. To separate these literatures we selected a criterion based on Mattson (2005) defining an undernutrition study as one using a diet in which intervention animals are fed 50% or less of the control group's diet and/or where the intervention animals weigh less at the end of the study than at the start. In addition, the period of undernutrition had to be at least a week, so that it is more relevant to chronic undernutrition than to an acute fast. The resultant undernutrition literature has two distinct focuses – behavioural/anatomical studies (predominantly hippocampal again) and stress.

8.2.2.1 Behavioural and Anatomical Studies

Three reports, each using different animal species and undernutrition protocols, have observed impaired hippocampal function and/or structure. Villain et al. (2016) fed a group of lemurs 40% of the diet provided to a control group for a 2-week period and examined the effects on their motor, learning and memory abilities. Degree of weight loss in the diet group was significantly correlated with greater impairment on a hippocampal-dependent learning and memory task. In a second study, this time using mice, Hao et al. (2000) reported that animals fed 40% of the control's diet for 1 week were significantly impaired on the eight-arm radial maze over all days of testing, a procedure sensitive to hippocampal function. In addition, dopamine and noradrenalin levels were reduced in the hippocampus and hypothalamus – the only two regions tested (i.e., implying that it is hard to know how selective this effect really is). The third study, using rats (Yanai, Okaichi, & Sugioka, 2008), reduced available food such that animals at the end of the 13-week restriction period weighed slightly less than they did at the start. While no group effect was evident on the Morris water maze, they did find differences on another hippocampal-sensitive task, the 30 min delay condition of a delayed matching to place task – with poorer performance in the diet-restricted group. They then examined if neurogenesis in the dentate gyrus was impaired in the diet-restricted group. It was, and the degree of impairment was correlated with poorer performance on both the delayed matching to place task, and the Morris water maze.

Beyond the hippocampus, only two other areas have been examined. Yucel, Warren, and Gumusburun (1994) exposed a group of rats to 50% of the diet provided to controls, for a 4-week period. The cerebellum was examined to determine granule cell density and synapse numbers – but no differences were evident. Finally, Warren, Freestone, and Thomas (1989), using the same dietary regimen, examined layers II–IV of the visual cortex, and found dietary restriction increased neuronal connectivity here.

8.2.2.2   *Stress Response to Undernutrition in Animals*

One or two days without food results in the activation of the hypothalamic–pituitary–adrenal axis, and the release of corticosterone, in both rats and mice (Jahng, Lee, & Yoo, 2005; Kim et al., 2004; Makimura, Mizuno, & Isoda, 2003). Food restriction over more protracted periods exerts the same effect (Armario, Montero, & Jolin, 1987; Hao et al., 2000; Holmes, French, & Secki, 1997; Yanai et al., 2008). Three studies have further examined this stress response. Carr et al. (1998) gave an intervention group of rats 50% of the food provided to an ad libitum control group. At the end of a two-week restriction period, the animals were killed and Fos-like immunoreactivity was determined in multiple brain regions. Greater Fos-like immunoreactivity was observed in most brain regions tested, indicative of a generalised cellular stress response. A second study by Heiderstadt et al. (2000) adjusted the treatment group's diet so that they lost weight, stabilising at 80% of their initial body weight, with controls maintained on an ad libitum diet. Corticosterone levels were significantly elevated at the end of the 5-week restriction period, suggesting the rats were stressed and had not adapted to the dietary regimen (and see for similar findings: Hao et al., 2000; Yanai et al., 2008). Heiderstadt et al. (2000) also observed rats' behaviour on an open field test, and found heightened activity – the opposite of what is observed from animals stressed by immobilisation, shock or injury. A third study, Jahng, Kim, and Kim (2007), exposed a treatment group of rats to 50% of the food eaten by ad libitum controls, over a 5-week period. Diet-restricted animals had heightened corticosterone levels at the end of the experiment. Animals were also tested on the Porsolt swim test (a measure of helplessness/depression) and on the elevated plus maze (an anxiety measure). Diet-restricted animals had greater periods of immobility on the Porsolt swim test, indicative of helplessness/depression, and spent more time in the closed arms of the elevated plus maze, indicative of anxiety. These animals also had significantly reduced serotonin turnover in the hippocampus and hypothalamus – consistent with a depressive reaction to stress.

It is plausible that increases in corticosterone reflect changes in feeding schedules (e.g., Armario et al., 1987). However, the ubiquity of the finding of corticosterone increases across so many designs, including those with ad libitum access to food, suggests that it is the stress of undernutrition that causes the corticosterone increase. The consequences of continued corticosterone release, which also occurs with ad libitum protein-deficient diets (Alaverdashvili et al., 2015), is damage to the hippocampus (McEwen, 2007). Corticosterone down-regulates neurogenesis in the dentate gyrus and causes the loss of granule cells (Gould & Tanapat, 1999). These corticosterone-induced hippocampal effects also impact behaviour, both in terms of impaired learning and memory (e.g., Vyas et al., 2002), but also in an increased propensity for depression, which may result from the reduction in neurogenesis (Pittenger & Duman, 2008). In sum, the stress induced by undernutrition and protein malnourishment in adult rodents seems to be a contributory cause, via elevated corticosterone, to hippocampal dysfunction.

8.2.3 Animal Studies: Conclusion

Protein malnourishment and undernutrition for greater than a week exert adverse effects on brain and behaviour, and especially to the hippocampus, learning and memory, and mood. This may in part be due to the stress of food deprivation and malnourishment. In addition, some studies report heightened activity levels in response to protein malnourishment or undernutrition. Food deprivation and excessive activity are particularly well studied in the context of activity-based anorexia, where food-deprived rats with access to a running wheel will run themselves to death (Lamanna, Sulpizio, & Ferro, 2019). This propensity for increased activity with food deprivation is driven by the hypothalamic–pituitary–adrenal axis, and so increased activity can also be seen as another part of the animal's stress response to malnourishment and undernutrition (e.g., Duclos et al., 2005). More generally, it is surprising how few studies have examined starvation effects in adult animals, especially in the context of anorexia nervosa (i.e., determining if brain abnormalities precede (predispose to) or follow starvation in this disorder) and recovery from starvation.

8.3   Human Studies

This next section forms the main part of the chapter, and is divided into the short-term and longer-term effects of restricted access to food. This division is a natural one in the literature, with the 'intervention' in most experimental or naturalistic studies lasting less than a week, in contrast to the starvation, hunger strike, anorexia and malnourishment literatures, where periods can range from months to years.

8.3.1   Short-Term Studies

There have been three types of investigations into the short-term effects of stopping eating: (1) deliberate experimenter-instructed fasts; (2) naturalistic religious fasts, notably Ramadan, with its repeated daily fasts over a 1-month period; and (3) self-initiated energy-restriction diets. While the latter may persist longer than a week, they do not readily fit with longer-term studies because adherence to the restriction process is typically intermittent or cyclic.

8.3.1.1   Experimenter-Instructed Short-Term Fasts
One finding that is undisputed is that after a period of several hours or days without eating, food becomes progressively more salient. In particular: (1) attention to food-related cues increases (Maran et al., 2017; Piech, Pastorino, & Zald, 2010), (2) an attentional bias to food-related words occurs (Mogg et al., 1998, (3) there is an improvement in memory for food-related stimuli (Morris & Dolan, 2001) and (4) there is an increased willingness to work to obtain food (e.g., Raynor & Epstein, 2003). There has also been interest in determining if a short period without food impacts more general aspects of cognition. With this in mind, fairly extensive cognitive batteries have been run on participants who have fasted, often under laboratory conditions, for 24–48 hours. Comparisons are typically made within subjects, to a non-fasting period, with this occurring in a counterbalanced order before or after fasting.

Examining the seven studies detailed in Table 8.1, the conclusion is that short-term fasting has little effect on general measures of cognition, in either obese (Solianik & Sujeta, 2018; Solianik, Sujeta, & Čekanauskaite, 2018) or normal-weight participants (Green & Rogers, 1995; Lieberman, Bukhari, & Caldwell, 2017; Lieberman, Caruso, & Niro, 2008; Solianik et al., 2016; Ståhle, Ståhle, & Granström, 2011). The only detectable effects were on reaction time (but see Gutiérrez et al., 2001), with evidence in two studies for slowing and reduced speed of finger tapping, but with faster reaction times in one. This last effect was in a study that tested weightlifting athletes at the start and end of the fasting period (Solianik et al., 2016), rather than comparing performance across two different sessions much further apart in time as with the other designs – so it could be a practice effect.

It has been claimed that short-term fasting is linked to increases in anger and hostility (MacCormack & Lindquist, 2019), and that this forms part of a more general reaction characterised by an increasing focus on self and the conservation of resources (Petersen et al., 2014). As detailed later, these types of changes do characterise more significant episodes of hunger (i.e., famine), but in experimental settings where deprivation is short lived, well powered experiments only find small effects and then on only certain measures of greed (Hausser et al., 2019). In particular, tasks that involve no interaction with others, such as mock charity donations pick up increases in greed (i.e., smaller donations when hungry), whilst resource allocation games involving reciprocity and cooperation generally do not. The notion that hunger may more broadly contribute to anti-social behaviour has been the source of a number of interesting but largely untested hypotheses (Benton, 2007; Nettle, 2017).

There has also been interest in whether acute hunger affects mood. Of the six studies examining mood, two found that a 48-hour fast had no impact, with three others reporting, respectively, greater tiredness, anger and jitteriness. Only one study (Lieberman et al., 2017) found more extensive effects, with the fast period resulting in increases in tension, anxiety, fatigue and confusion – but noting that this study also included a significant aerobic exercise component, which might be responsible for this. The general conclusion, and one echoed in a broader systematic review (Benau et al., 2014), is that short-term fasting does not exert any consistent effect on mood or on general cognition. (Also note the parallels here to the studies described in Chapter 2 on the impacts of missing/ having breakfast; this had little impact on cognition too.)

Table 8.1. *Studies examining the effects of short-term fasts on general measures of cognition and mood*

Study	Fast in hours	Sample	Mood effect of fast	Effects of fasting	General cognitive tests (summary)	
					Null effects of fasting	
Green et al., '95	24	21 students	More jittery	Finger tapping slowed	Vigilance, attention, memory	
Lieberman et al., '08	48	27 soldiers	Minimal effects	None	RT[1], vigilance, memory, reasoning	
Lieberman et al., '17	48	23 soldiers	Extensive effects	None	RT, vigilance, memory, reasoning	
Solianik et al., '16	48	9 athletes	Angrier	Faster RT	RT, memory, perception	
Solianik et al., '18	48	9 obese	None	Varied RT effects	Memory, psychomotor, self-control	
Solianik and Sujeta, '18	48	11 obese	Tired	None	Memory, psychomotor, self-control	
Ståhle et al., '11	48	12 CD[2]	Not assessed	Slowed simple RT	Memory, self-control	

[1]Reaction time.
[2]Community dwelling.

Five reports have focussed on a more hypothesis-driven examination of the cognitive effects of fasting. People with anorexia nervosa demonstrate both a tendency to 'stay' on set shifting tasks (i.e., deciding to 'stay' with a familiar way of undertaking a task vs shifting to a new approach when needed) and show weak global coherence (i.e., focussing on minutiae rather than on the bigger picture; Smith et al., 2018). One way of trying to determine if a difference in cognition between people with anorexia nervosa and healthy controls is a consequence of starvation versus a pre-existing disposition (more later) is to see if the difference emerges in healthy controls when food-deprived, fasted or starved. Five reports examined the impact of varying fast periods on set shifting (five reports) and global coherence (one report), with the outcomes summarised in Table 8.2.

For set shifting, there are two ways to assess an effect. First, determine if reaction times are slowed when a shift is required following a period without food. The two well-powered studies (Bolton et al., 2014; Pender, Gilbert, & Serpell, 2014) found a shift cost with fasting, but no effect was observed in the two studies that had smaller sample sizes (Giles, Mahoney, & Caruso, 2019; Piech et al., 2009). One study (Solianik et al., 2016) found a shift benefit after fasting, but this study (as described earlier) involved contrasting performance at the start and end of the fasting period (i.e., practice effects are a concern here). The second way to assess if set shifting is affected by fasting is to look at the number of errors made on shift trials. In this case, there was no favourable evidence. Error rates were either observed to increase when fasted, for both shift and stay trials (Bolton et al., 2014; Giles et al., 2019; Piech et al., 2009), or were not affected by fasting (Pender et al., 2014; Solianik et al., 2016). Turning to central coherence, one study finds that fasting shifts processing to the local (over global) relative to sated testing (Pender et al., 2014). So while this supports the idea that short-term fasting produces a focus on minutiae at the expense of the larger picture, for set shifting the effects are inconsistent.

Neuroimaging has also been used to study differences between the fasted and sated state – with fasting periods comparable to those used in behavioural studies (i.e., 24–48 h). The majority find increased brain activation to food-related pictures in the fasted state, when contrasted to the sated state. This increased activity is observed in the amygdala, hippocampus and orbitofrontal cortex (meta-analysis of five studies; van der Laan et al., 2011), and more broadly in some individual studies extending to the hypothalamus, insula and basal ganglia (Del Parigi, Gautier, & Chen, 2002; Morris & Dolan, 2001). These effects are larger when the

Table 8.2. *Studies examining the effects of short-term fasts on set shifting and central coherence*

Study	Fast in hours	Sample	Testing set shifting effects on reaction time	Effects on error rates	Testing coherence
Bolton et al., '14	16	56 students	Shift cost (slower) when fasted	More errors on all trials when fasted	Not tested
Giles et al., '19	48	23 soldiers	No effect	More errors on all trials when fasted	Not tested
Pender et al., '14	18	60 students	Shift cost (slower) when fasted	No effect	Lower global coherence
Piech et al., '09	5	16 students	No effect	No effect[1]	Not tested
Solianik et al., '16	48	9 athletes	Shift benefit (faster) when fasted	No effect	Not tested

[1] Another manipulation; cueing with food did impact error rates and there was some evidence of an interaction with fasting state, but the results were not decisive.

food pictures are of high-energy, palatable foods (Goldstone, Prechtl de Hermandez, & Beaver, 2009). Evoked response potential (ERP) studies point to a similar conclusion with greater neural activity toward food than non-food pictures when fasted, relative to sated, and with activity mainly in the temporo-parietal regions (e.g., Stockburger et al., 2009). While not all studies have found differences in response to food pictures between the fasted and sated states (Uher et al., 2006), the general consensus is that greater attention towards food stimuli follows short-term food deprivation, with this reflected in greater neural activity in brain areas involved in the control of appetite.

8.3.1.2 Religious Fasts

In Medieval Europe, nearly one-third every day was designated for religious fasting, although many were not observed (Vandereycken & van Deth, 1994). In the modern era, the most well-known religious fast is Ramadan, which occurs over the ninth month of the Islamic calendar. During this period Muslims refrain from food, drink, tobacco and other bodily pleasures, and focus on their spiritual life, charitable deeds and community. Practically, this means eating a morning meal called *sahur* (also *suhur, shour*) before sunrise, abstaining from all food and drink in the day, and then eating a main meal after sunset called *iftar* (*ftour*). This pattern is then repeated for the whole of the Ramadan period, culminating in the religious festival of Eid al-Fitr and the lifting of the fast.

Several researchers have tried to use Ramadan as a natural experiment, to examine the impacts of fasting on cognition. This is made difficult by a number of confounds. Apart from fasting, Ramadan also involves stopping caffeine, nicotine and fluid intake of any kind during daylight hours. So in addition to being fasted, participants may be experiencing nicotine withdrawal, missing their tea or coffee, and be thirsty. People also need to rise early in order to partake in *sahur*, and so many end up sleeping far less than they normally would or sleeping in and not having food or drink at all (perhaps especially undergraduate research participants). Needless to say, what is eaten and drunk is also likely to vary considerably from one person to another. Not only do these confounds interfere with observing any clear effect of food restriction they also make people irritable (i.e., smoking cessation, sleep deprivation; Kadri, Tilane, & El Batal, 2000), which is not conducive to good performance on tests of cognition. Finally, because Ramadan is based on a lunar calendar, with the period of fast each day dictated by sunrise and sunset, the demands of the fast vary from year to year (e.g., summer vs winter) and from location to location (short day length vs long day length). While the studies here are broadly similar in this last regard, being conducted in the Middle East or South East Asia, concerns about sleep, nicotine, caffeine, fluid and mood all need to be kept in mind.

Four studies have examined the cognitive impacts of Ramadan, with two finding some evidence of impacts and two not. Tian et al. (2011) tested cognitive function in 18 athletes during and after Ramadan, with a pre-Ramadan familiarisation test to reduce the likelihood of practice effects. They found some improvement in processing speed and visual attention during morning testing during Ramadan relative to the control testing, with a decline in verbal learning and memory during afternoon testing. Mood was not assessed, and sleep was reportedly reduced during Ramadan – which might account for poorer afternoon performance. The study went to some lengths to standardise cognitive testing sessions by asking subjects to refrain from caffeine and nicotine on the Ramadan *and* control tests, and by the provision of meals for participants on test days.

Yasin et al. (2013) tested 30 students during and after Ramadan on maths and memory problems. They found no effect on performance, and noted no change in reported sleep time, as this was compensated for by daytime napping or by skipping *sahur*. This parallels the outcome of the two final studies. Najafabadi et al. (2015) tested 15 athletes pre- and post-Ramadan, finding little effect on the two tested measures, digit span and Stroop. Chamari, Briki, and Farooq (2016) examined sustained attention and reaction time, before, during and after Ramadan, in 11 athletes. Sustained attention improved across the course of the study (a probable practice effect) with no effect on reaction time. Participants also reported greater sleep disturbance. In sum, Ramadan fasting seems to have little effect on cognition.

A final religious fast study focussed on the impact of a single day of abstinence – the Jewish fast of the 10th of Tevet (Doniger, Simon, & Zivotofsky, 2006). Here, 46 students were tested, with almost all participants completing the cognitive test battery first on the fast day and then again at a later time point (interval between sessions varying from 1 to 90 days). Two points need to be noted. First, testing order (93% getting tested fast first) predisposes to finding impairments on the fast day due to practice effects. Second, while smoking was not included in this fast, drinking was, and so caffeine consumption is likely to be markedly reduced on the fast day, which is not likely to benefit cognitive performance. Multiple impairments were observed on fast day performance when contrasted to the control day, with poorer non-verbal memory, verbal IQ, information processing speed, verbal and visuo-spatial function. No effects were evident for response inhibition, verbal memory, Stroop or finger tapping. As the general finding of the short-term fasting studies in the previous section seems to be 'little effect on cognition', the suspicion must be that confounds like caffeine or nicotine deprivation or practice effects are more likely causes of the impairments reported in this study.

8.3.1.3   Dieters and Dieting

Scientists studying dieting have examined if having to deal with hunger and preoccupation with food (especially in an environment where it is constantly available), may produce cognitive deficits (Jones & Rogers, 2003; Polivy, 1996). People who consciously restrict their food intake (i.e., dieting) have a range of common features (e.g., avoiding fatty foods) termed 'dietary restraint' (King, Polivy, & Herman, 1991). This has been measured using several different questionnaires and people reliably vary on this dimension (Hawks, Madanat, & Christley, 2008). Several studies have looked at whether preoccupation with food that occurs during dieting, and/or in individuals who score high on dietary restraint, is related to impaired cognition.

One approach to studying this problem contrasts three groups of subjects: (1) current dieters who score high on dietary restraint ('diet and restraint group'), with this group actively restricting food intake and preoccupied with what they eat and their body weight; (2) people not currently dieting but who still score high on dietary restraint ('restraint group'), and so who are preoccupied with what they eat and their body weight; and (3) people not currently dieting who score much lower on dietary restraint ('neither group'). Preoccupation with food should be graded across these three groups, being highest in the 'diet and restraint group', intermediate in 'restraint group', and lowest in the 'neither group'. If preoccupation with food causes cognitive deficits, then these should follow this gradient.

Four studies have adopted this approach. Green et al. (1994) employed tests of sustained attention, reaction time, working memory and finger tapping. Excepting finger tapping, poorest performance was observed in the 'diet and restraint group', then the 'restraint group', with the 'neither group' evidencing the best performance. This suggests that greater preoccupation with food translates into greater impairment on sustained attention, reaction time and working memory. Green, Elliman, and Rogers (1997) tested working memory, focussed attention and finger tapping. For working memory, the *best* performance was observed in the 'restraint group', and for focussed attention performance was *poorest* in the 'restraint group', with no differences on the tapping test. This set of outcomes does not favour the same interpretation nor is it apparent why both the best *and* the worst performance should be localised to the 'restraint group'.

In a third study, Green and Rogers (1998) focussed on components of the working memory system, testing the visuospatial scratchpad (mental rotation), the articulatory loop (phonological similarity) and the central executive (Tower of London task). The 'diet and restraint group' performed best on the mental rotation task and worst on both the phonological similarity task and on planning the most complex moves on the Tower of London task. The 'restraint group' and the 'neither group' had very similar outcomes on all tests. It is not clear why mental rotation performance should be best in the 'diet and restraint group' as preoccupation with food might be expected to impact all aspects of working memory performance.

Finally, Green, Rogers, and Elliman (2000) asked participants to imagine their favourite holiday on some trials and their favourite food on others, while undertaking a reaction time task. Performance between groups was identical in the favourite holiday image condition, but for food images, reaction time was slowed to the same degree in both the 'diet and restraint group' and the 'restraint group', relative to the 'neither group'. This suggests that holding food images in mind impairs response performance in individuals who exhibit high levels of dietary restraint. In sum, these four studies are inconsistent, but they do suggest that in *some circumstances* (although it is not clear what these are) preoccupation with food is linked to poorer information processing on executive-type tasks.

Another approach has also been used. Participants varying in dieting status are provided different sorts of food (e.g., chocolate or carrot) to see if these yield different cognitive impacts. The idea here is to try and trigger some of the same food-related thoughts that occur during dieting, and see what effect this has. In one study, current female dieters undertook a battery of three cognitive tests – working memory, focussed attention and finger tapping – in the presence or absence of chocolate (Green et al., 2000). This had no impact on test performance. In a further study, dieters and non-dieters were tested on the same cognitive battery, before and after eating a chocolate bar (Jones & Rogers, 2003). An impairment in short-term memory (i.e., poorer immediate recall) was observed in dieters who consumed the chocolate.

The working memory system has been a particular focus of study because preoccupying thoughts about food should exert their deleterious effects primarily on this system. Kemp, Tiggemann, and Marshall (2005) and Kemp and Tiggemann (2005) both examined several aspects of the working memory system in female dieters and non-dieters. Both studies identified deficits in working memory, especially in the operation of the central executive, which was poorer in dieters. Impairment on tests of the phonological loop were evident in one study, but not in the other, and neither found any effects for the visuospatial sketchpad. Dieters were also found to have more preoccupying cognitions and these were in some cases related to the central executive deficits. Meule (2016) also contrasted female dieters and non-dieters, in addition to collecting information about how successful they had been at weight loss dieting. On a test of working memory using food and non-food stimuli, dieters were poorer on the food-related task, and especially so if they had been unsuccessful at dieting. Dieters also reported being more depressed, but the effect of this variable on cognition was not examined.

These studies do suggest that intrusive thoughts about food may impair cognition. The working memory system seems most susceptible to such intrusions, but effects on sustained attention and reaction time were also reported. What is perhaps of more interest is what *causes* these intrusive food-related thoughts. Dieters and hungry participants remember more material about food from stories relative to controls, and pay more attention to food-related words – all suggestive of preoccupation (Polivy, 1996) – as with the literature reviewed at the start of this section. One possibility is that thoughts about food are usually under some degree of inhibition, which intensifies when sated and relaxes when hungry (e.g., Attuquayefio et al., 2016; Kanoski et al., 2007). By extension, more extreme states of deprivation, seen after protracted periods of time without food, would see progressively greater lifting of inhibition to the point where it was no longer in effect. Consequently, *any* food-related cue, internal or external, however remote the association, would result in a flurry of food-related thoughts. Such intense preoccupation with food is routinely observed in reports of deep starvation – as detailed later.

8.3.1.4 Conclusion

The general finding from short-term experimental studies and religious fasts is that they have few impacts on general cognition, but do result in a greater preoccupation with food. There is a small but detectable increase in greed on certain tasks. Mood does not seem to be affected, although this is more difficult to assess in the religious fast studies, due to various confounds (sleep, smoking, thirst and caffeine). The study of dieters suggests that restricting food intake results in preoccupation with food, with these effects sometimes being detectable on working memory tests. There has been little exploration of how these food-related cognitions (i.e., preoccupation with food) occur.

8.3.2   Longer-Term Studies

This section examines longer-term (greater than 1 week) experimental and observational studies, including case reports, of the effects of varying degrees of starvation.

8.3.2.1   The Natural History of Famine

Famines are extended periods of food restriction experienced by certain groups of people in a particular region. Periodic famines have probably occurred since the advent of agriculture and the development of the first towns and cities (Prentice, 2005; Stubbs & Turicchi, 2020). There is a rich historical literature describing the effect of famine on people's mind and body, with additional sources of information coming from stories of survival (e.g., the Donner Party, Scott's ill-fated Antarctic expedition (McCurdy, 1994)) and the extensive medical and historical literature on World War II (Dutch hunger winter of 1944, Siege of Leningrad 1941–1944, Warsaw ghetto 1941–1943, Great Bengal famine 1943–1944, and the multiple concentration and death camps run notably by the German and Japanese governments (e.g., Burger, Sandstead, & Drummond, 1945; Keys et al., 1950; Leyton, 1946)). Apart from these war-time atrocities, humanity witnessed multiple large-scale famines in the twentieth century. Twenty-five million died in the Ukraine famine in 1921, somewhere between 15 and 43 million in the 'difficult three-year period' in China between 1959 and 1961, a million in Bangladesh in 1974, between 0.2 and 3.5 million in North Korea in 1996, and 70,000 in Sudan in 1998 – and there were many others (e.g., Collins, 1995; Prentice, 2005; Scrimshaw, 1987). It is hard to comprehend these numbers, a view echoed by Stalin, who said: 'one death is a tragedy, a million is a statistic'.

In trying to understand the effect on human behaviour of famine, it is important to consider the body's physiological adaptations to starvation and the physical symptoms that accompany this, as well as the frequently traumatic context in which starvation occurs. Both will contribute to the constellation of behavioural changes identified across the famine and survivalist literature – the focus of this section. Human and other home-otherms (i.e., warm-blooded animals) respond to starvation by lowering basal metabolic rate, ceasing reproductive activity (e.g., halting menstruation), and reducing upkeep of the digestive organs (Prentice, 2005). There are also shifts in the body's fuel usage. Under normal feeding conditions, energy needs are met by liberating glucose from both glycogen stores and from fatty acids derived from fat. If there is no food, a different pattern of fuel usage emerges over the days and weeks that follow and this occurs in three phases (Heymsfield et al., 2011). In phase one, the body utilises all of its remaining glycogen stores, it draws upon protein from the liver and gastrointestinal tract, and some visceral fat. In the second phase, consumption of visceral fat mass accelerates, with some usage of protein from muscle mass. In the third and final phase, other fat stores are simultaneously burnt alongside protein from muscle. Death then ensues.

Fat stores in humans are quite substantial, and especially so in obese individuals. Consequently, the body can subsist for a long period of time in the absence of food, this ranging from several weeks in a lean person (e.g., Devathasan & Koh, 1982; Kerndt et al., 1982), to several months in an obese person (e.g., Thomson, Runcie, & Miller, 1966). The physiological adaptations identified here coincide with a range of unpleasant physical symptoms that a starving person has to endure. In the early and mid-part of starvation the commonest encountered are: (1) lowered body temperature, feeling cold, and intolerance of this sensation; (2) diarrhoea and polyuria; (3) dizziness and postural hypotension; and (4) oedema (e.g., Collins, 1995; Keys et al., 1950; Leyton, 1946). In the later stages severe lethargy emerges to the point where even simple acts like raising one's hand may take several minutes to complete.

While the physical consequences of starvation are unpleasant, the context in which it occurs is likely to be as bad or worse (Scrimshaw, 1987). Keys et al. (1950) argued that it was not possible to tell what the true behavioural consequence of starvation per se were, because natural instances were generally so traumatic. As starvation can be held at bay by money to purchase food, starvation is likely to be accompanied by poverty, lack of warm clothes and fuel shortage for heating. There is likely to be no transport other than walking, there will be queuing and foraging for food – all a likely break with normal routine. Starvation brings with it diminished immunity to infection, so minor illnesses occur more frequently, and decent hygiene standards are likely to be hard to maintain if displaced from home, making this problem worse (e.g., gastrointestinal infections). More significantly, witnessing the suffering of children, family, friends and strangers is likely to be very disturbing. At its worst, concentration camp inmates witnessed daily beatings and deaths, and when Belsen camp was liberated by the British 11th Armoured Division there were more than 10,000 unburied corpses dispersed amongst the survivors (Mollison, 1946).

As the first British office to enter the camp, Major Leonard Berney later wrote, 'I remember being completely shattered. The dead bodies lying beside the road, the starving emaciated prisoners still mostly behind barbed wire, the open mass graves containing hundreds of corpses, the stench, the sheer horror of the place, were indescribable.' Clearly, trauma is a central feature of many people's experience of famine and starvation, and this needs to be borne in mind when considering effects on behaviour.

The natural history of starvation literature identifies three main areas of behavioural change: appetite, apathy/depression and amorality. Not surprisingly, the sensation of hunger figures prominently. Leyton (1946) served as a medical officer in several camps during World War II, whilst a prisoner of war (POW) of the Germans. He observed that '...on the POW diet it took about 3 weeks for a healthy man to become permanently and intensely hungry'. Similarly, in Keys et al.'s (1950) review of the natural starvation literature, reports of intense hunger are common. For example, Mikkeleson's forced Arctic overwintering in 1912 was accompanied by starvation, where he described how 'every fibre in one's body is clamouring for food' and that the sensation of hunger was so intense it amounted to pain. Indeed, several authors report that the intensity of this sensation may preclude focussing on any other mental activity, making attempts at deliberate distraction impossible (e.g., Leyton, 1946).

The intense desire to eat can be accompanied by changes in dietary behaviour. People report eating things that would not usually be considered food, but that in times of need *might* provide energy or stem hunger by filling the stomach. Boggiano et al. (2013) has made a study of this (termed concocting), and Table 8.3 provides some examples. Instances of concocting were also well documented by Keys et al. (1950). In apparent

Table 8.3. *Examples of concocting during periods of starvation*

Source	Concoctions
Boggiano et al. (2013)	Bulking out food with ground acorns or saw dust; pounding animal hides into a glue-like substance; soaked hard roots with mashed banana skins and mango pits; old shoes, deer skin and bones; watery stew from dirty potatoes and vegetables, with grit and stones
Burger et al. (1945)	Tulip bulbs, raw mangolds and wurzels
Keys et al. (1950)	Necrophagia, bark, twigs, dirt, rats, mice, dogs, cats, lizards, frogs
McCurdy (1994)	Necrophagia, active cannibalism, boiled animal hides
Morell-Hart (2012)	Dogs, mice, grass, carrion, harnesses, boiled animal skin

contrast, there are also reports of fastidiousness amongst starving people. One oft-cited example is the use of protein hydrolysate during re-feeding in World War II. This tastes very bitter and was widely refused (e.g., Lipscomb, 1945). Another were the complaints during the extensive Belsen re-feeding program, with people expressing a deep hatred of black bread and soup, and their expressed desire for white bread and solid food. These complaints were so frequently encountered that Mollison (1946) concluded that '. . .starving patients are fastidious about their food'. While desperation might drive concocting, these creations do not seem to be enjoyed. Rather normal food preferences may have to be voluntarily overridden. A final aspect of starvation is hoarding. Mollison (1946) reported that even dying Belsen inmates in the re-feeding hospitals would hide bread and meat under their pillow.

A second, widely reported aspect of behavioural change is the apathy and depression that engulfs the starving person. Looking through the mass of historical material reviewed by Keys et al. (1950), every description of starvation over the period of 700+ years examined included terms such as: gloom, apathy, depression, languor, exhaustion, debility, melancholy, irritability, negativity, lassitude, mental slowing, nervousness, hostility, introversion, loss of interest in personal hygiene and appearance, increased somnolence and loss of moral. This depressive state seems to lift fairly rapidly with re-feeding (Burger et al., 1945) – perhaps in equal part the result of relief from imminent death and the reversal of biological changes resulting from starvation.

Of all of the behavioural changes that accompany starvation, the most remarkable and widely commented upon is the loss of normal standards of moral behaviour. Table 8.4 documents examples taken from Keys et al.'s (1950) review and also from other sources. Together, they indicate a progressive shift from a normal (i.e., 'fed') altruistic stance to an intensely egocentric one during deep starvation. The consequences of this can be highly disturbing, with people lying and cheating to obtain food, stealing it even from loved ones, murdering for it, selling children, engaging in prostitution – indeed pretty much any act that will secure a meal. What is less clearly established is the extent of this moral collapse. It does not appear to be universal, nor does it seem to affect everyone to the same degree, so it may just amplify existing tendencies to delinquency. But this is a guess. While there has been a lot of scientific interest in understanding the consequences of starvation on hunger and mood (see below), its effect on moral behaviour has gotten less attention. Yet this seems one of the most deeply troubling and yet interesting aspects of human starvation.

Table 8.4. *Effects of starvation on morality*

Source	Actions/quotes
Keys et al. (1950)	'There was no charity left amongst us'; 'loss of appreciation of social ties'; people 'lied shamelessly for a chance to obtain food'; 'all social bonds strained, children abandoned, rioting and theft'; 'normal social relationships breakdown with an increase in theft and violent crime'
Leyton (1946)	The focus on food was such that '. . .the half-starved man would go to the greatest lengths of ingenuity and dishonesty to obtain small amounts of extra nourishment'; '. . .moral standards were completely in abeyance, for a man would steal his best friends rations or sell his overcoat for food. . .'; 'none of the hardships suffered by fighting men brought about such a rapid or complete degeneration of character as chronic starvation'
Lipscomb (1945)	'The most conspicuous psychological abnormality was a degradation of moral standards characterised by increased selfishness and it was more or less proportional to the degree of under-nutrition'
McCurdy (1994)	'. . .the two native American guides from Fort Sutter were consumed after probably being murdered by a member of the group'
Morell-Hart (2012)	A breakdown of even family ties with '. . .family members become competitors'
Prentice (2005)	'. . .each man has become a thief to his neighbour'

8.3.2.2 Hunger Strikes

Fessler (2003) defines hunger strike as a 'voluntary refusal of food in an attempt to achieve a political goal or other social manipulation'. Hunger strike is a powerful tactic because it sets authority a moral paradox – give in or bear the responsibility for the hunger striker's death. Many famous (e.g., Gandhi, Suffragettes), infamous (e.g., Irish nationalists in the Maze prison, Backpacker killer Ivan Milat) and lesser-known cases (e.g., a former President of South Korea, a US academic seeking to reverse a negative tenure request) have engaged in hunger strikes, and it is claimed that the numbers are increasing (Burkle, Chan, & Yeung, 2013; Fessler, 2003). The main interest in the hunger strike literature has been the issue of mental competence. For Western medicine, hunger strikers present a conflict between the autonomy of the person in choosing to starve versus the duty to keep a person alive. Both the British Medical Association's and the World Medical Association's statements on treating hunger strikers identify mental competence as crucial in the decision whether to agree to a person's wishes to starve or to provide treatment.

The consequences of hunger striking can be split into the earlier and later stages. Survival to death seems to vary quite markedly across different reports. For the Maze prisoners (Irish Republican Army detainees) in Northern Ireland, it was 45–61 days (Burkle et al., 2013), while Başoğlu, Yetimalar, and Gürgör (2006), in their detailed study of Turkish political prisoners, reported that some had *survived* fasts from 130–324 days. One difference may be the extent to which the person takes water and another may be secret feeding. Irrespective of this, the Turkish political prisoners had a mean BMI of 12.3 at the end of their fasts (more details later). The early stages of the hunger strike may be defined as the first 10 days or before 10% of initial body weight is lost (Burkle et al., 2013). The only systematic study of the early stages of hunger striking was of 33 South African male political prisoners (Kalk et al., 1993). They were examined for physical and mental symptoms after between 6 and 24 days of starvation. As in the studies of famine, these men reported significant weakness, dizziness, gastrointestinal symptoms (severe stomach pain, nausea, diarrhoea) but there was no mention of hunger or thirst. (It is not clear if this was not asked or was presumed so obvious that they did not need to be asked.) What did stand out was the high levels of depression reported (80%), nearly all of which were confirmed by psychiatrist interviews. So as with famine, depression is a key feature – not forgetting that these men had been detained without charge for months or years before commencing their hunger strikes. An important question then is whether the presence of depression can impair competence. Hindmarch, Hotopf, and Owen (2013), in a systematic review of the literature pertinent to this issue, found evidence that depressed people's capacity to appreciate the gravity of their situation is impaired, and that this impairment is proportional to the degree of depression. On this basis, competence *may* (i.e., the person may not be depressed) be impaired even in the early stages of a hunger strike.

In the later stages, as the person comes closer to death, the issue becomes less complicated. The only comprehensive study at this stage was conducted by Başoğlu et al. (2006). They followed 41 male and female political prisoners in Turkey who had fasted for a mean of 199 days. These political detainees had consistently refused all treatment, but when they became unresponsive, they were tube-fed and nutritionally rehabilitated. None of these treated individuals chose to restart their fast. During the period of initial recovery, symptoms of Wernicke–Korsakoff syndrome (see Chapter 9) were evident in all of the cases – both peripheral (e.g., nystagmus, neuropathy) and central (e.g., confusion, amnesia). Everyone also exhibited the amnestic symptoms even after months of rehabilitation. What is puzzling is that all of these people were provided thiamine supplementation to prevent Wernicke–Korsaksoff syndrome developing, in addition to re-hydrating solution (water, sucrose and salt) throughout most of their fasts. One possibility is that damage to the gut wrought by starvation impaired thiamine absorption, another is that an additional micronutrient deficiency stopped the utilisation of thiamine. Wernicke–Korsakoff syndrome has been observed in other cases of prolonged fasting (again where thiamine supplementation occurred; Devathasan & Koh, 1982), and so this may be a significant cause of mental impairment in the late stages of starvation.

8.3.2.3   Laboratory Studies

Most of the scientific studies considered in this section examine the impact of significant reductions in energy intake (10–25%) over a protracted period of time (weeks to months) rather than the effects of completely stopping eating – although there are a few such studies reported here. The earliest formal semi-starvation study is the post-World War I Carnegie Nutrition Laboratory Experiment (Butterly & Shepherd, 2010). Benedict (of the Harris–Benedict equation fame) had been studying metabolism and weight loss in the famous US 'Hunger artist' Agostino Levanzin (see Heymsfield et al., 2010 – Figure 1). Levanzin made his living by fasting in public, with people paying money to watch him (Vandereycken & van Deth, 1994). This spurred Benedict's interest and led him to conduct the first study of weight loss under formal experimental conditions. It lasted 4 months and the first tranche of healthy young male participants lost around 12% of their initial body weight. Some psychological examinations were also undertaken. They found few effects on cognition, but significant effects on motivation (extreme hunger, loss of interest in other activities, including sex) and emotion (irritability and low mood).

Similar types of psychological changes have also been observed in more contemporary studies. Five main study groupings emerge and so this section is structured accordingly. These are: (1) the Minnesota starvation study and (2) the Biosphere II period of semi-starvation, with both dealing with initially lean individuals; (3) medically supervised total fasting and (4) very low-energy diets – in overweight and obese people; and (5) laboratory restriction studies in lean people.

The Minnesota Starvation Study   This experiment was not motivated by a desire to study starvation, but rather to find the optimal way of re-feeding people who had experienced deep (i.e., severe) starvation in Europe during World War II. However, from a contemporary perspective, the study's enduring legacy remains its detailed examination of the biopsychological consequences of a 6-month period of semi-starvation. The outcome from this vast scientific enterprise, which included detailed physiological, psychological and sociological studies of the participants over a 1-year period, was published after the war in 1950 as a two-volume book (Keys et al., 1950). The first volume is primarily devoted to the physiological findings and the second to the psychological, and the details reported in this section come primarily from this source.

The participants were 32 male conscientious objectors who both volunteered to take part and who passed screening to ensure that they were physically and mentally healthy before commencing the study. The study had three main phases, with all of the participants housed at the University of Minnesota laboratory of physiological hygiene for the duration of the experiment. The first phase was a 3-month baseline period with the participants having an average weight of 70 kg and an energy intake of 14,644 kJ. The second phase was a 6-month period of semi-starvation. During this phase they had an energy intake of 7,332 kJ, were expected to undertake various jobs connected to the project, in addition to regular exercise that consisted of walking several kilometres per day. At the end of this phase participants had an average weight of 53 kg, their physical strength had declined by 30%, their basal metabolic rate had fallen 40%, their pulse rate had dropped from 56 to 38 beats per minute, and their body temperature had also fallen. All of the participants reported being persistently cold and even in the height of summer kept two or three blankets on their beds. A further notable physical symptom was the presence of oedema on their face, wrists and ankles (known as starvation oedema). Compliance with the dietary regimen was excellent, partly because the whole study was on-site with food provided and also because the participants, at least initially, were highly motivated. Nonetheless 4/32 participants were found to have obtained food outside of the experiment, with this being identified by slower-than-expected weight loss. Although the starvation period was fairly well tolerated by most of the participants – described in more detail later – four individuals developed major psychiatric problems during this phase of the study. Three appeared to have developed depression, which required temporary admittance to a psychiatric hospital. All three recovered and were able to complete the study. A fourth cut off a finger in an apparent attempt to end his participation. He also recovered and completed the experiment.

The key phase of the study – for the experimenters and participants alike – was the 3-month re-feeding phase, which utilised several different initial feeding programs (7,853–17,397 kJ), followed by a general phase of 21,832 kJ used for all participants. During this phase weight regain was mainly fat mass at the expense of the lost lean muscle mass. While the type of re-feeding program did not appear to make much difference (other than the conflict caused by some participants receiving more food during the initial re-feeding phase), by the end of the 3-month period when ad libitum access to food was permitted, participants gorged themselves and all table manners were abandoned in the complete focus on eating.

The studies' psychological findings can be divided into three parts, which are dealt with in this order: cognitive effects; personality, social and emotional impacts; and motivational effects. The cognitive effects are the simplest to present, as they found no evidence of any reduction in what they termed intellective functions. The battery included tests of spatial and verbal memory, word fluency, arithmetic, inductive reasoning, tests of perceptual speed, sentence completion and intelligence. Participants were examined at various intervals throughout the study and while the tests may not have had the psychometric properties of modern-day neuropsychological batteries, a repeated measures design and the broad range of functions examined should have enabled the detection of any obvious deficit. The absence of cognitive impairments is concordant with contemporary studies described later in this section.

In stark contrast were the effects on personality, social and emotional functioning and motivational systems. A flavour of these impacts can be gained by this quote from one of the participants (Samuel Legg), who was later interviewed about his experiences: 'The psychological effects of starvation are unbelievable. We went there because we were concerned about people abroad and wanted to do what we could to help those less fortunate than ourselves, and I think we lost that feeling after about 2 months (of starvation). At the end of 5 months of starvation our attitude was "to heck with the people abroad. I AM HUNGRY". That was all that was important. The only important thing left was whether I was ever going to get food. I was only interested in myself.' More detailed observations were made on the behaviour of all of the men by the experimental staff, and in addition the men completed personality inventories, rating scales and reports on all aspects of their social and psychological functioning during the study.

Formal psychological testing was undertaken using the Minnesota Multiphasic Personality Inventory (MMPI), which had just been developed at the University of Minnesota, and the Guilford/Guilford-Martin inventories. The former indicated that relative to the baseline period, participants became more anxious about their health, more depressed, more neurotic, more rigid in their thinking styles and had more schizotypal traits. There was no change in psychopathy, paranoia or mania, and only changes on the depressive inventory entered the clinical range. The Guilford inventories also documented a range of changes. These were an increase in introversion, depression and neuroticism, and a reduction in impulsiveness, general activity, leadership, and self-confidence.

Many of these changes were evident in observations of the men's behaviour. The nature of the interaction between participants changed over the starvation period. During baseline they had been engaged and lively participants, and had friendly warm interactions with each other and the staff on the project. As the study progressed into the starvation period, they became apathetic, depressed, tired and irritable. There was a loss of spontaneous activity, a marked reluctance to do their jobs, and a change in the nature of the group dynamics, from friendly to sombre, with stilted interactions, sarcastic humour and outbursts of temper over minor things. In common with reports of natural starvation, the men described a decline in libido across this period. This was tracked, alongside hunger and desire to engage in activity, on a monthly basis across the starvation period, with these data presented in Table 8.5. The change in libido coincided with a lack of interest in personal appearance. However, of all of the changes enacted by the semi-starvation diet, the one most frequently remarked on from staff observation and participant reports was egocentricity, which at its core reflected a preoccupation with meeting one's own need for food.

Table 8.5. *Changes in self-reported hunger, libido and desire for activity across the semi-starvation phase of the Minnesota starvation study, with the scale being from −5 (extreme decrease) via 0 (normal) to +5 (extreme increase)*

Variable	Baseline	Semi-starvation period (week)						Re-feeding period (week)	
		4	8	12	16	20	24	6	12
Hunger	0.0	1.2	1.6	2.0	2.0	2.1	2.5	1.8	0.9
Libido	0.0	−0.3	−0.8	−1.2	−1.3	−1.6	−1.7	−1.2	−0.8
Activity	0.0	−0.2	−0.4	−0.9	−0.6	−0.8	−1.2	−0.8	−0.2

Participant reports of hunger increased across the semi-starvation period (Table 8.5). Food cravings were common, with 72% of participants reporting an increase in craving frequency. Many participants – 60% – reported constant feelings of hunger, with this typically localised to the abdominal area. There was considerable individual variation both in the intensity of hunger, from mild discomfort to intense pain, and in its consistency across each day. In some participants the desire to placate hunger led them to filling their stomachs with acaloric fluids, such as water, weak tea or coffee. Others resorted to excessive gum chewing (40 packs per day for one man), nail biting and smoking.

Preoccupation with food was present in most cases, with only three claiming not to experience it and criticising the others for exhibiting what one of these men described as 'nutritional masturbation' and another as 'animal-like' behaviour. In the main, their thoughts (this word in free association would lead them to... *food for thought*, etc.), daydreams and conversation were dominated by food, although their night-time dreams were not. With the latter, participants were woken during REM sleep to spontaneously report their dreams, but these were rarely about food. The participants also discussed how the next meal would be eaten, and their eating rate slowed such that some of them would take 2–3 h to eat their meagre rations. Any food waste provoked intense negative responses from the group, as did any perceived attempt to obtain food from another participant. Just under half the participants started collecting recipes, and reading recipe and cookery books, and even those who did not engaged in related behaviours (e.g., one man compared the price of foods across advertisements in different print media). Around a third started to save up money (rather than spending their allowance on gum or tobacco) so that they would be able to buy extra food during the re-feeding phase. This preoccupation with food and incessant hunger gradually lifted during re-feeding, with the other adverse changes also diminishing as food became available. We consider the long-term consequences (decades) of partici-pating in this study – and of periods of starvation more generally – in a later section of the chapter.

Biosphere II Biosphere II (so named to prompt the question, 'what is Biosphere I?') was a 200,000 m³ closed biological ecosystem located near Tucson, Arizona. It was designed with planetary colonisation in mind, to test out whether such a facility could support a human crew with food, water and oxygen for an extended period of time. Since the facility was completed in 1987 it has hosted two studies of this sort, and the first of these is the focus here. The crew were composed of four men and four women, all of whom were lean and healthy, and who left Biosphere I to be 'sealed' inside Biosphere II in September 1991. The facility was 'unsealed' two years later and the crew released.

The interior consisted of several biomes, with a total land area of 12,700 m^2. Among these was an agricultural area, where some animals (chickens, pigs) were reared alongside a variety of food crops. The intention was to be fully self-supporting, but a series of unanticipated events – less sunlight than expected, insect pests, a mouse plague and reduced oxygen levels – conspired to reduce supply, requiring supplementation from emergency stores. This led to a rationing of supplies, with an energy intake of 7,400 kJ for the first 6 months, rising to 8,000 kJ for the remainder (Walford et al., 1999). This has to be set against the large energy expenditure of the crew, who were actively maintaining all of the biomes – that is they were working as farmers. While the diet was nutritionally complete, it did not provide sufficient energy, and male crew members lost 18% of their initial body weight and female members 10% (Walford et al., 1999).

Crew members were able to maintain their vigorous daily routine, including cognitively demanding scientific work, without any reported loss of intellectual capacity. There were also no reports of mental confusion, lethargy or weakness (Walford et al., 1999). However, crew members did report feeling constantly hungry. It has been suggested that this constant hunger, and the falling oxygen levels (equivalent later on to working at high altitude) probably contributed to the crew splitting into two factions. In this regard, the effects of the period of undernutrition sounds akin to the social effects observed in the participants of the Minnesota study. While crew members undertook a considerable daytime workload, voluntary physical activity declined over the 2-year study, which might seem logical (Weyer, Walford, & Harper, 2000). What is surprising is that this reduced voluntary activity persisted when crew members were re-evaluated 6 months after the end of the study, having both returned to their normal lives and a normal weight.

Medically Supervised Fasting During the 1960s, several papers appeared in the *Lancet* (Silverstone, Stark, & Buckle, 1966; Thomson, Runcie, & Miller, 1966) and the *Journal of the American Medical Association* (Drenick et al., 1964; Duncan et al., 1962) describing case series of obese people who had been put on supervised total fasts (i.e., no food) for documented periods ranging from a few days to a maximum of 249 days without food.

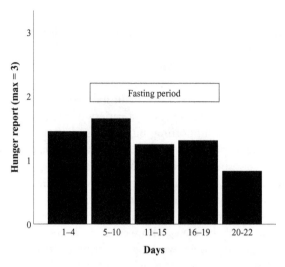

Figure 8.1   Little change in reported hunger during a period of total fast.
Source: Data adapted from Silverstone et al. (1966)

A surprising conclusion of these and some later studies was that the people undergoing these total fasts reported having diminished or even absent sensations of hunger as it progressed (see Figure 8.1). Whilst these long fasts did observe some of the same physical effects (e.g., cold intolerance, menstrual irregularities, postural hypotension, fatigue), mood was reported to be generally positive, even euphoric in some cases (Fisler & Drenick, 1987; Kerndt et al., 1982). The most notable findings then are the apparent absence of adverse effects on hunger and mood.

In the case of mood, this *may* be attributable to the length of the fast, which across all of these studies had a median value of 3 weeks. Indeed – and contrary to the general thrust so far – at least one laboratory study in lean participants using a 3-week total fast found no effects on standardised measures of mood, anxiety and depression, even though cortisol levels were elevated during the fast period reflecting physiological stress (Fichter, Pirke, & Holsboer, 1986). Perhaps then in healthy people in a safe laboratory context, a short-duration total fast *may* only have a minimal impact on mood.

In respect of absent hunger in these medically supervised fasts, several factors may be relevant. A notable one is that all of the participants were overweight or obese, in contrast to all of the other studies described so far that reported significant hunger in participants. It is known that food deprivation in the obese produces a different pattern of fuel usage to that in

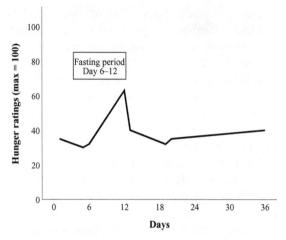

Figure 8.2 Hunger ratings increasing across a fast period.
Source: Data adapted from Johnstone (2007)

lean participants, and it has been suggested before that this may affect hunger (Stubbs & Turicchi, 2020). Another is the extent of hunger assessment during the total fast period. Silverstone et al. (1966) reports the only empirical examination of hunger, and this used just two reports per day, and these were made using a yes/no question format (with answers summed). A more recent and detailed study by Johnstone's group (Johnstone, 2007) suggests that measurement may be important. They had six obese individuals undertake a 6-day fast, with a 5.6% loss of initial body weight. Hunger was measured hourly during waking across baseline, fasting and follow-up periods. As can be seen in Figure 8.2 hunger ratings increased significantly above the baseline period and throughout the fast. This finding would seem to suggest that multiple measurement occasions using a response scale format are necessary to capture actual increases in hunger. Demand characteristics are a further relevant consideration. Obese participants in medical settings may be reluctant to reveal being hungry. This may reflect both their physician's belief that total fasting eliminates hunger (which they may have been told to entice them into this form of treatment) and that obese individuals are 'always hungry'. In sum, these reports do not allow any firm conclusion over the effects of fasting on hunger in the obese.

Dietary Restriction in Overweight and Obese People   In obese individuals, weight loss significantly improves cognition, a conclusion reached by both of the most recent systematic reviews (Siervo, Arnold, & Wells, 2011; Veronese, Facchini, & Stubbs, 2017). Veronese et al. (2017) examined cognitive outcomes from 13 longitudinal studies (total n = 551) and 7 randomised control trials (total treatment n = 328, control n = 140). For the longitudinal weight loss studies (median interval between tests = 24 weeks), irrespective of whether the weight loss (mean BMI went from 37.2 to 30.9) was from energy-restricting diets or bariatric surgery, improvements in attention, executive functioning and memory were observed, with no effects for motor speed or language. For the randomised control weight loss trials (typically of around 20 weeks duration) examining just energy reduction diets, the only consistent improvement was in memory. The mean age of participants in these studies was around 50 years. Whether similar patterns of cognitive improvement are seen in older participants is less clear, with at least one longitudinal study in 60–70-year-olds finding that *either* loss or gain in weight is associated with a higher risk of cognitive impairment at the end of the study period (Brubacher, Monsch, & Stähelin, 2004). Relatedly, dementia risk is significantly heightened (40% increased risk) in people less than 65 who are obese, but is somewhat reduced in those aged more than 65 (17% reduced risk; Pedditizi, Peters, & Beckett, 2016).

While cognition has been a focus of many studies examining the biopsychological effects of weight loss in the obese/overweight, the majority have focussed on mood, hunger and fatigue. This is because these may be important factors in undermining an overweight or obese person's willingness to persist with an energy-restricting diet. Two studies have reviewed the older literature focussing on state and trait mood, depression and anxiety. Wing et al. (1984) examined 10 prior studies, finding 4/10 reported no effect of the diet intervention on mood and 6/10 found that it led to an improvement. O'Neil and Jarrell (1992) reviewed five subsequent very-low-energy diets, with two reporting no effect on mood, two an improvement and one a worsening. The more recent literature is summarised in Table 8.6. Of the eight studies in Table 8.6 examining mood, five reported an improvement, two found some weak evidence of worsening mood and one reported no effect. This latter also measured cortisol, and there was some evidence of an increased stress response early during dieting, which had dissipated by the middle of the study. Summarising across all 23 studies – old and new – suggests 57% find weight loss improves mood, 13% it worsens it, and 30% it has no effect. Table 8.6 suggests a favourable effect on mood is most evident in studies with higher-BMI populations and larger sample sizes, which would suggest that

Table 8.6. *Energy-restricting diet studies with obese or overweight participants, where mood, hunger and fatigue, alone or in combination, were studied as outcomes*

Variable	Sample				Intervention		Outcomes		
	Size n =	Age M =	Sex m/f	BMI M =	Type	kJ/day (% weight loss)	Mood	Hunger	Fatigue
Foster et al. (1992)	76	41	f	38	26	1,758 (19) vs 2,763 (22) vs 3,394 (19)	Improved	Reduced	Stable
Burley et al. (1992)	8	–	f	34	2	1,700 (5)	Improved	Reduced	–
Buffenstein et al. (2000)	9	28	f	26	4	3,100 (8)	Worsened	–	More
Bryan et al. (2001)	63	50	f	35	12	6,960 (13)	Improved	–	–
Green et al. (2005)	75	32	f	28	8	6,270 (3)	No change	–	–
Johnstone (2007)	12	–	m	35	3 and 6	2,500 (5) vs 5,000 (9)	–	Increased	More
Williamson, Martin, and Anton (2008)	48	38	m and f	28	26	9,200 (10) vs 8,600 (10) vs 3,650 (14)	Improved	Reduced	–
Cheatham, Roberts, and Das (2009)	42	35	m and f	28	26	7,830 (9) vs 6,090 (9)	Worsened	Increased	More
Hussin et al. (2013)	31	60	m	27	13	5,850 (4)	Improved	–	Less

the effects of weight loss especially in the obese is likely to improve mood – in addition to cognition.

Many of the studies detailed in Table 8.6 also looked at the effects of their dietary interventions on hunger and fatigue. For hunger, the effects were mixed for the five studies that measured this variable, with three finding reductions and two finding some mixed evidence of increases. Of the latter two, Johnstone (2007) observed a small increase in hunger, but this was less marked than for fasting (see earlier) and tended to be most noticeable only in the first few days of energy reduction. Cheatham et al. (2009) suggested that the high glycaemic index condition (e.g., white bread, watermelon, rice bubbles) was associated with increases in hunger. However, eating this type of food is unusual in a typical low-energy diet (i.e., it is normally plant based with high fibre). So the tentative general conclusion would be that hunger across the energy-restriction period is reduced. Finally, for fatigue, three studies reported an increase in fatigue, one reported no change and another found weight loss invigorating. This last mentioned study was the only one conducted in an older sample.

Experimental Dietary Restriction in Lean People   While weight loss seems to bring cognitive and possibly mood benefits to obese and overweight participants, two studies have examined this using dietary restriction on lean and highly physically fit participants. Shukitt-Hale, Askew, and Lieberman (1997) randomised 34 male soldiers (M BMI = 19) to either a reduced energy intake condition (8,000 kJ) or a control condition (16,494 kJ), for the duration of a 25-day period of field exercises and then 5 days in garrison. Participants in the reduced-energy-intake group lost significantly more weight than controls (4 kg vs. 1.7 kg), but there were no effects on the cognitive variables measured (reaction time), nor in mood state, fatigue or other physical symptoms. In the second study, Karl, Thompson, and Niro (2015) varied both energy intake using a within-subject design (baseline period vs 30% reduction period) and the ratio of protein to carbohydrate using this as a between-group factor. As the latter factor did not interact with energy reduction, it is not further mentioned. The participants were normal or overweight (noting this is likely to be muscle rather than fat) young men and women, all physically fit army personnel, who undertook the intervention for 30 days, with a 10-day initial baseline period of normal energy intake followed by a 20-day 30% energy reduction period. Energy restriction was associated with improved reaction time, learning and memory tests, but as the tests were repeated it is likely that some of these changes were practice effects. Participants reported a worsening of mood during the energy-restriction period. These two studies suggest that periods of energy restriction in lean individuals are unlikely to cause any significant cognitive impairment – perhaps even the reverse – although they may worsen mood.

Laboratory Studies – Conclusion   Energy restriction in lean individuals does not seem to produce cognitive impairment beyond the interfering effects of dealing with hunger, low mood and irritability that occurs during food restriction or fasting. Egocentricity, in some cases leading to amoral behaviour, is another feature of semi-starvation. The effects of fasting and semi-starvation on overweight and obese people seems different. It improves cognition, especially memory; is associated with improved mood in many studies; and *may* not generate the same intense hunger as in lean individuals. It is unclear whether reduced hunger severity stems from physiological or psychological causes.

8.3.2.4   Anorexia Nervosa

Anorexia Nervosa (AN) is a relatively rare illness (prevalence ≈ 0.5%) characterised by: (1) restriction of energy intake leading to significant low body weight, (2) intense fear of weight gain and (3) disturbance of perception of body shape and weight (from APA DSM-V). AN classically manifests in adolescent girls around menarche, with loss of menses from significant weight loss. For researchers studying the causes of AN, an oft-cited difficulty is in disentangling the neurocognitive effects of starvation from pre-existing dispositions that cause AN (e.g., Hay & Sachdev, 2011). Kaye, Fudge, and Paulus (2009), in discussing this problem, distinguish between what they call trait and state effects. Trait effects are the ones that AN researchers are primarily interested in and are presumed to exist before disease onset (although this is difficult to establish due to the low prevalence of AN) and to persist into recovery (this forms the main type of trait test, noting the potential confound that any observed effect could be a 'scar' resulting from starvation). State effects are the direct effects of starvation, and what we are interested in here (note that the emerging literature on atypical AN, which has the same features as AN *but* without the low body weight, may represent another means at getting at state/trait distinction, but this *presumed* AN and atypical AN are essentially the same disease).

An additional reason to examine the AN literature in the context of starvation is because there is an extensive number of neuroimaging studies, providing potential insights into the starving brain. The important data

relevant to starvation effects is then to see what brain changes are ameliorated by re-feeding (and thus are a likely *consequence* of starvation). In this
regard there is some consensus. Positron emission tomography (PET)
scans have examined neurometabolism in AN. They find reductions in
metabolism in frontal, cingulate, temporal and parietal regions, which
return to normal after re-feeding (Cucarella, Tortajada, & Moreno,
2012; Frank et al., 2004; Kaye et al., 2009).

For magnetic resonance imaging (MRI), AN samples show reductions
in brain volume (cortical and subcortical), characterised by greater shrinkage of grey matter (5–6%) relative to white matter (3–4%), enlargement of
the sulci, dilation of the ventricles and an increase in cerebrospinal fluid –
again with all of these abnormalities diminishing in response to re-feeding
(Barona, Brown, & Clark, 2019; Cucarella, et al., 2012). The white matter
tracts of the corpus callosum, which connect the two hemispheres of the
brain, seem to be especially affected, with notably worse axonal coherence
during the starvation phase (Barona et al., 2019). There are also multiple
alterations in brain neurochemistry, especially for serotonin and dopamine
(using magnetic resonance spectroscopy), but disentangling these from
trait changes has proved challenging (Kaye et al., 2009).

There has been speculation as to why these brain-related changes occur
during starvation, but there is no consensus here. While starvation per se
seems the obvious answer (Fuglset et al., 2015), dehydration may also be
a contributory factor. Reduced fluid intake often accompanies AN, either
as a consequence of excessive exercise (i.e., fluid loss from sweating) or
from interoceptive abnormalities such that the person no longer feels
thirsty (Barona et al., 2019; noting that: (1) some authors report excess
fluid intake in AN (Calugi, Miniati, & Milanese, 2017) and (2) water
need when utilising fat as fuel is minimal (Cahill, 1970)). A further
possibility, and one that is an indirect consequence of starvation, is
hypercortisolaemia, with elevated cortisol driving brain shrinkage.
There is no consensus across studies as to whether elevated cortisol levels
sufficient to induce these type of changes occur in AN (Frank et al.,
2004). In addition, while the animal studies reviewed at the start of this
chapter do indicate that the neurobehavioural changes in memory function are probably stress driven (i.e., via cortisol), these effects are characterised by their specificity to the hippocampus. Hypercortisolaemia
looks to be a less likely explanatory candidate.

Cognitive impairments are a prominent feature of AN. The well-
established abnormalities are in cognitive flexibility (inflexible in AN), a
focus on specific detail rather than the bigger picture (termed central

coherence), attentional biases to food and body-related issues, and impairments in multiple aspects of working memory and in effective decision-making (Lang, Roberts, & Harrison, 2016; Ralph-Nearman et al., 2019; Smith et al., 2018). With the interest in disentangling the effects of starvation from the causes of AN, researchers have examined whether these cognitive deficits persist after re-feeding and weight regain. While not conclusive, there is general agreement that all of the impairments listed, with the exception of working memory, *persist* after recovery (Smith et al., 2018; and see Olivo et al., 2017). In respect of working memory deficits, it is interesting to parallel these to the dieting literature, where they too found some evidence of deficits in this domain during active dieting. There may be a common cause here, not from a deficit perspective, but instead from the intense preoccupation with food that occurs in AN (e.g., collecting cook books, worrying about food, etc.; Calugi et al., 2017) and in dieters. This may impair performance on working memory tasks due to the constant intrusion of food-related thoughts.

Two general features of starvation in initially lean people were low mood and apathy. In AN, negative emotionality (i.e., low mood) is considered to be a trait, both in terms of being a predisposing factor and also present following recovery (Bradley, Taylor, & Rovet, 1997; Kaye et al., 2009). There is general agreement, though, that starvation leads to a deterioration in mood and often clinical depression, which is significantly improved during re-feeding and weight gain (Accurso et al., 2014; Kaye et al., 2009). A more complicated picture unfolds with apathy and activity. At least some patients with AN engage in excessively high levels of exercise even when seriously malnourished – and this is a diagnostic feature of the restricting subtype of AN (e.g., Guisinger, 2003). Similarly, some have suggested that constant movements such as fidgeting also reflects a generally heightened activity state. However, survey studies find that excessive tiredness and lack of energy are some of the commonest symptoms of starvation reported in AN (Casper et al., 2020). It would seem that mental restlessness and drive for thinness are symptomatic of the disease – propelling fidgeting and excessive exercise – while tiredness and lack of energy are consequences of starvation (Casper et al., 2020).

People with AN exhibit many of the characteristics observed during studies of non-clinical populations who are starved. They are preoccupied with food, depressed, apathetic and lack energy. Unlike non-clinical starving groups, they have extensive neurocognitive impairments, pre-existing depression exacerbated by starvation, and sometimes a tendency for excessive exercise. Their unique contribution to understanding the neuropsychology of starvation are the effects on the brain, notably shrinkage and hypometabolism, although dehydration may be a contributing factor to these changes, something unique to AN. More intriguingly, the cognitive effects of starvation when AN-related effects are factored out seem to be very limited – restricted to working memory changes, and with these likely a consequence of preoccupation with food. We could find no anecdotal observations or studies of whether the egocentricity and presumably related amorality observed in other starving groups occurs in AN.

Anorexia and Cachexia Secondary to Cancer and Other Diseases Setting aside Hyperemesis Gravidarum, which in its most severe form can produce significant weight loss (15%+) during pregnancy (Fejzo et al., 2009), disease-related weight loss usually involves a combination of anorexia (loss of appetite) and cachexia. Cachexia is the loss of body mass, lean and fat, observed during chronic illness, and it can occur with or without anorexia. Either cachexia alone or more commonly anorexia-cachexia is found in between 60 and 80% of cancer patients (Advani et al., 2018; Sánchez-Lara, Arrieta, & Pasaye, 2013). It is especially common in the later stages of illness and in certain types of cancer (non-small cell lung cancer, head and neck cancers, pancreatic cancer), in chronic obstructive pulmonary disease, tuberculosis, with chronic heart failure and end-stage renal disease (Laviano et al., 2005; Laviano, Inui, & Marks, 2008). It is often a significant contributor to mortality from these diseases and a very major cause of reduced quality of life in people living with these illnesses.

There are some very notable physiological differences between cachexia-anorexia and starvation. In cachexia-anorexia, there is almost immediate loss of both muscle (sarcopenia) and fat mass. Both fat and protein reserves are lost at the same time, unlike in starvation, where fat loss occurs first, followed only in the later stages by loss of muscle mass (Laviano et al., 2005). A second difference is that there is no reduction in basal metabolic rate, and if anything it may be elevated, with additional loss of energy as heat. The causes are also different. Cachexia can drive weight down even in the presence of a normal appetite and energy intake. When combined with anorexia, weight loss effects become even more pronounced and rapid (Laviano et al., 2005).

The anorexic component is characterised by early satiety, alterations in taste and smell, meat aversion and nausea. This may arise from treatment side-effects including dysgeusia (unpleasant tastes) from radiation therapy, nausea and conditioned taste aversions from chemotherapy, and ulcers in the mouth and throat making eating painful. An additional cause comes from cytokines, released as a result of the body's immune system fighting the cancer or disease. Cytokines affect anorexigenic pathways in the hypothalamus, and especially the melanocortin system (Laviano et al., 2008). The motivational aspects of eating also seem to be altered, with abnormal neural responses to food images before and after a test meal, especially in the hypothalamus (Molfino, Iannace, & Colaiacomo, 2017; Sánchez-Lara et al., 2013). There is no data as yet to indicate whether anorexia-cachexia produces a neurocognitive-depression-fatigue profile, akin to that observed with starvation, as there is little data on its psychological sequelae.

8.3.2.5 Aging
Women typically reach their peak body weight between 55–65 and men between 34–54 (Omran & Morley, 2000). After this weight starts to fall, such that between the ages of 70–81, men will on average lose 6.6 kg in weight and women 5.7 kg, with this mainly being muscle loss (sarcopenia). Weight loss during aging is often assessed using a broad multidimensional measure of malnourishment that includes BMI, weight loss change, presence of gastrointestinal symptoms, and diet evaluations (e.g., Mini Nutritional Assessment, Elderly Nutrition Screening Tool; Omran & Morley, 2000; Tamura et al., 2013).

In Westernised countries, estimates of the reported community prevalence of malnourishment amongst the elderly vary enormously, from 1–15% (Fávaro-Moreira, Krausch-Hofmann, & Matthys, 2016) to 10–51% (Edington & Kon, 1997) and between 7 and 85% (Chen, Liu, & Hwang, 2016). This variability reflects the absence of any uniformly agreed definitions of what constitutes malnourishment during aging. Rates of malnutrition are higher in elderly samples admitted to hospital, being 39% in one report (Allen, Methven, & Gosney, 2013), 43% in a UK study (Edington & Kon, 1997) and between 35 and 65% in a systematic review (Fávaro-Moreira et al., 2016). In nursing homes, the figures are even higher. In one study, more than 70% of nursing home residents lost greater than 22 kg during their stay (Omran & Morley, 2000), with others estimating prevalence of malnutrition at between 20 and 60% (Fávaro-Moreira et al., 2016), 27 and 37% (Allen et al., 2013) and even up to 85% (Edington & Kon, 1997). In a representative cross-sectional study of US nursing homes, 12% were chronically malnourished and 4% had BMIs below 16 (Challa et al., 2007). The US Center for Disease Control figures estimate around 1.3 million people are in nursing homes in the United

Table 8.7. *Correlates of weight loss in the elderly grouped into categories*

Correlate	Comment
Medications	50+ linked to appetite loss, malabsorption and metabolic changes
Alcoholism	Common and linked to malnutrition
Oral factors	Perceptual decline, teeth, dentures, dysphagia
Gastrointestinal	Delayed gastric emptying, malabsorption
Poverty	Limited capacity to buy food
Social isolation	Limited capacity to obtain food
Dementia	Multiple impacts (e.g., refusing to eat, inability to prepare food)
Parkinson's	Increased energy expenditure
Depression	Most frequently identified in cross section but not longitudinal studies
Thyroid/adrenal	Dysfunctions affecting metabolism
Appetite hormones	Multiple changes that are anorexigenic to leptin, CCK, insulin, grehlin
Infections	Elevated cytokines (e.g., from TB, clostridium difficile)
Cardiovascular	Multiple impacts (e.g., pain on swallowing, metabolic effects)

States, which would translate to more than 50,000 elderly with BMIs <16 – a striking number of significantly underweight people.

While there is an extensive understanding of the correlates of weight loss in the elderly (see in Table 8.7), it is often difficult to know if these are causes or consequences. It is known that weight loss is predictive of all-cause mortality (Chen et al., 2016; Tamura et al., 2013), and of longer hospital stays and more complications (Edington & Kon, 1997; Omran & Morley, 2000). However, whether this results from the multiple factors linked to weight loss in the elderly that are also life-shortening (see Table 8.7) or from weight loss itself, its impact on immunity and healing capacity is not known. There are also strong associations between demen-tia and weight loss, but in this case it would appear that dementia probably drives reduction in body weight (Allen et al., 2013; Chen et al., 2016). There may be metabolic alterations in dementia as at least one study has reported high rates of malnutrition even though energy intake was intact (Omran & Morley, 2000). Certain behavioural changes especially in the later stages of dementia can actively interfere with feeding, such as refusal to eat, to open or close the mouth or swallow, head turning and spitting out food (Allen et al., 2013). There are also studies identifying a link between depression and weight loss (Chen et al., 2016; Tamura et al., 2013). Indeed, depression in the elderly seems to be more closely linked to reduced food intake and weight loss than it is in younger samples (Omron & Morley, 2000). Interestingly, the few longitudinal studies do not identify depression as a risk factor for weight loss (Tamura et al., 2013), while this is overwhelmingly the case in cross-sectional studies. This implies, as with other forms of starvation or semi-starvation, that depression may be a consequence of weight loss rather than a cause.

8.3.3   Recovery

Apart from re-feeding syndrome, an often fatal complication of providing nourishment too quickly to starving people (Friedli, Stanga, & Sobotka, 2017), those who recover from starvation experience mainly psychiatric and psychological consequences. In general terms, psychiatric complications arise from the traumatic experiences that may accompany starvation, so post-traumatic stress disorder (PTSD) figures prominently (e.g., Favaro, Rodella, & Santonastaso, 2000; Zohar, Giladi, & Givati, 2007). PTSD may contribute to abnormal patterns of eating, but there is some evidence that episodes of starvation, as well as intermittent periods of food availability and significant hunger, can generate eating-related pathologies. There are three literatures that deal with this. The first studies survivors of World War II, those who experienced starvation in concentration and prisoner-of-war camps, and those who participated in Key's Minnesota starvation study. This section also includes the few studies of the children and grandchildren of holocaust survivors, to see if they show any unusual patterns of ingestive behaviour. The second literature concerns the consequences for families, and especially children, from the lowest socio-economic groups of society, who experience intermittent food supply, with periods of no food and hunger. The final literature concerns the psychological and psychiatric impacts of long-term voluntary weight loss in individuals who can maintain a stable low – relative to prior to weight loss – body weight.

8.3.3.1   World War II

Around two-thirds of holocaust survivors experienced PTSD in the years immediately following the war and many also experienced severe starvation (Zohar et al., 2007). For example, in the Warsaw ghetto, rations were so inadequate even when supplemented with black market food (average energy intakes of 3,000–6,000 kJ per day) that 15–18% of the ghettos populace starved to death (Sindler, Wellman, & Stier, 2004). Several studies have examined holocaust survivors – mainly aged 70+ (i.e., 50+ years since the war) – to determine if they currently, or had in the past, experienced abnormalities in eating behaviour. One study found that survivors' relationship with food was unusual, in that they did not like to throw it away, even when spoiled, they stored excessive food, and some felt anxious when food was not immediately available (Sindler et al., 2004). However, these attitudinal impacts, which the interviewees directly attributed to their experiences of starvation, were only present in 50% of the interviewed survivors. Indeed, most remarked that the easy availability of food in the United States, their generally comfortable housing and lifestyle and the many years since their experiences had made the present more influential than the past (Sindler et al., 2004). Two other studies of holocaust survivors, which searched more specifically for formal eating pathology, including pre-clinical forms, found no evidence of abnormality (Bachar, Canetti, & Berry, 2005; Leon et al., 1981). As with Sindler et al. (2004), Leon et al. (1981) found only attitudinal effects – well-stocked pantries and an insistence on not wasting food.

Studies of holocaust survivor families have been inconclusive. Zohar et al. (2007) examined eating disorder pathology in children and grandchildren of holocaust survivors and age-matched controls. Degree of exposure to holocaust-related experience was measured on a continuous scale, using the number of relatives who were holocaust survivors, discussions at school and home about the holocaust, etc. The authors found a weak positive correlation between greater holocaust exposure and greater eating disorder pathology, and especially so in grandchildren. However, the most direct test, contrasting children and grandchildren of holocaust survivors with controls found no evidence of any increase in eating disorder pathology. A further study by Chesler (2005) contacted holocaust survivor's offspring and asked them to partake in a study concerning eating pathology. The resulting sample included several adult offspring (7/11) who either had clinical or subclinical eating disorder's (mainly binging). However, as the recruitment process directly stated the study aims, it is hard to know if people with eating psychopathology just self-selected or if it related to being a survivor's child. As Leon et al.'s (1981) study found no family psychopathology, the evidence for it affecting the eating behaviour of survivors' children is inconclusive at best.

The three studies of prisoners of war – from US, Canadian and Italian samples – come to a different conclusion. In the late 1980s there were still more than 75,000 ex-prisoners of war alive in the United States. These people had experienced imprisonment, torture and malnutrition (Speed et al., 1989). Speed et al. (1989) examined which particular aspect of their traumatic experience most closely related to the presence or absence of PTSD in 62 ex-prisoners of war. The sample on average lost nearly a third of their initial body weight during a mean captivity period of 1.5 years. The participants were questioned about all aspects of their experience and the investigators then examined which component was most predictive of PTSD, both on return from the war and at the time of test. In both cases the most significant predictor was body weight loss during incarceration, mirroring findings from another study of Dutch resistance fighters from World War II. Whether this finding is a consequence of the traumatic nature of starvation itself or whether starvation is a general marker for extreme ill-treatment is not knowable here, but it points to the difficulties of disentangling components of the natural starvation experience.

Two further prisoners of war studies find convergent evidence that experience of starvation is associated with a greater likelihood of binge eating (i.e., loss of control over food intake). Polivy et al. (1994) examined survivors of the ill-fated Dieppe raid of 1942, in which 5,000 Canadian troops participated, with 1,600 escaping back to the UK, 1,400 killed or wounded and 2,000 captured by Axis forces. They compared 67 men who had escaped with 198 who had spent the remaining years of the war in German prisoner-of-war camps. The escapees reportedly gained 4 kg of body weight over the 1942–1945 period, while the incarcerated group lost an average of 10 kg. Participants were interviewed about their current and past eating behaviour. Binge eating occurred with double the frequency (60%) in prisoners of war, relative to the escapees (30%), with this division being even starker for higher-frequency binging. Degree of binging was positively correlated with degree of weight loss, both in the whole sample and in just the prisoners of war.

A problem, of course, with the Dieppe study is that it does not examine the possible confounding effects of concurrent psychopathology. As the Speed et al. (1989) paper demonstrates, PTSD is likely to be higher in those experiencing larger weight loss and so perhaps this contributes or even drives any later-life binging effect. A report by Favaro et al. (2000) suggests this is not the case and that the binging results from starvation. They compared 51 Italian concentration camp survivors with 47 former partisans, on psychiatric and eating-related psychopathology measures. A third of concentration camp survivors reported episodes of binge eating (and 7/51 were currently bulimic) in contrast to 4% of the partisans group. Looking just at the prisoners of war, and comparing those with and without bulimic episodes, there were no differences in the degree of weight change during incarceration, length of incarceration or in rates of depression and PTSD. These findings suggest that the binge eating was a *probable* consequence of starvation, and this concurs with Polivy et al.'s (1994) data.

The 'probable' in the sentence was italicised because of data from the long-term follow-up of the Minnesota starvation study participants by Eckert et al. (2018). They obtained data on 20/36 participants, with 11 deceased (one of whom had left a detailed video interview and was included as a posthumous participant) and 6 who could not be found. Participants were aged 79 at the time of the study, and it was readily evident that all had led full and productive lives, pursuing careers in academia (6 professors), teaching, law, engineering and other professions. There was no evidence of any psychopathology, even amongst those who had exhibited psychiatric symptoms during the study, nor was there any evidence of binging or eating-related disorders. Participants were asked to recall their personal experiences of starvation. The motivational aspects of starvation were pre-eminent (i.e., apathy, lethargy, etc.), as with the preoccupation with food and hunger. During re-feeding, the participants also remarked on feeling a loss of control over eating, something that Key's had also observed. However, while Key's concluded that this was short-lived, the retrospective consensus was that it took nearly 2 years to fully normalise diet, attitudes to food, and body weight.

One aspect that they did recall, and for which we could not find any mention of in the two volumes about the Minnesota study (Keys et al., 1950), were changes in body self-perception. The participants reported three effects. First, and most interesting in relation to anorexia nervosa, was that some of the men were *unaware* of how thin they had become during the experiment. Second, some men thought that the study staff (i.e., Ancel Keys and colleagues) were fat and overweight (they were normal weight). Third, and more accurately given that most of the men gained fat mass rather than lean mass during re-feeding, several reported feeling fat after the study was over.

The most notable omission in their recollection of the effects of starvation, and as highlighted by Eckert et al. (2018), was the significant level of depression and irritability both observed by the study staff and also evident in psychiatric measures. Almost no mention was made of this, even though all other aspects of starvation were accurately recalled – and even including new material on body perception. In contrasting the findings of this follow-up with those of the prisoner-of-war studies, it is odd that heightened binging would be found in the latter but not the former. A few things stand out. Keys participants were highly intelligent (IQ 130+), they were in a supportive group and they were selected for participation based upon having a stable temperament. Of course some of these same factors would also hold true for the prisoners of war, and indeed these may be protective against developing later eating psychopathology, but the most notable difference is the level of concurrent trauma. Studying the Minnesota men suggests that you may need traumatic experience and certain person-specific characteristics for binging to occur following starvation. This conclusion, however, fails to explain why a propensity to binge was not detected in the holocaust survivors. Perhaps for these people, starvation was not the central traumatic theme of their captivity, and for this reason it was not a central theme of any subsequent psychopathology.

8.3.3.2 *Binging as a Consequence of Insecure Food Supply*

A further body of work suggests that binging may be induced without the need for starvation. Nettle (2017) has theorised that exposure to an intermittent and insecure food supply, with periods of no food or reduced intake, may contribute to the broader association observed between socio-economic status and its many adverse consequences (e.g., higher rates of obesity, drug use, crime). While the specifics of this theory are not relevant here, he does make the interesting claim that periods of binging, induced by intermittent hunger, may contribute to higher rates of obesity in poorer people (a similar theoretical claim is also made by others, in relation to the effects of intermittent dieting by researchers such as Herman and Polivy). This is a reasonable suggestion, because at least in the United States where most of this work has been undertaken, intermittent food supply among the poor is common.

Measures of 'food insufficiency', which focuses on various indices of child hunger (e.g., going to bed without having eaten), suggests an overall prevalence in the United States of 8% being described as 'hungry' – and with 21% deemed at risk of being 'hungry'. Amongst the poorest Americans, this is 21% described as 'hungry' and 50% at risk (Nettle, 2017). 'Food insecurity' is a further index, which focuses on the ability to have a safe, nutritious and continuous food supply. In the United States, 16% are defined as being food insecure and 6% as very food insecure, but among the poor this is 40% and 20%, respectively. These people – adults and children – experience repeated and erratic instances of hunger, with frequent uncertainty as to when or where the next meal will come from.

Food insufficiency and insecurity have measurable impacts. Rates of depression and suicidal thoughts and intentions are strongly related to food insecurity in adolescents, although food insecurity may just be a good marker of familial dysfunction (Alaimo, Olson, & Frongillo, 2002).

However, it is the relationship with eating psychopathology which is of special interest here. Three studies suggest a link between episodes of binge eating, food insufficiency/insecurity and obesity. Smith and Richards (2008) interviewed children drawn from families in homeless shelters in Minneapolis. They reported significant food insufficiency with 54% not getting enough food and 25% going to bed hungry. Only non-perishable foods (i.e., chips, chocolate, soft drink) could be kept in shelter rooms, and when this was available many participants reported over-eating. Olso, Bove, and Miller (2007) interviewed a sample of 30 adult women. Those who had grown up in low socio-economic status (SES) households were all obese, in contrast to 33% obese in those who grew up in higher-SES households. Many of the women growing up in low-SES households reported that as children they feared running out of food and that they ate more when food became available, especially highly palatable non-perishable foods.

The final study is particularly interesting as it more formally established eating-related psychopathology. Becker et al. (2017) assessed food insecurity, eating disorder pathology and dietary restraint in 503 people who were using a US food bank to supplement their food supply. They found that binging was positively associated with food insecurity. However, they also found that food insecurity was linked to greater compensatory behaviours, such as vomiting, laxative use and exercise. This implies that eating disorder pathology more broadly is higher amongst adults who are food insecure, but with the important caveat that variation in body weight was not included as a covariate (it was not measured), which may account for the higher rates.

8.3.3.3   Long-Term Voluntary Maintenance of Reduced Body Weight
While food insecurity and insufficiency are subjected to episodic food deprivation often by economic and political forces outside of their control, another group deliberately deprive themselves of food for the purposes of maintaining a reduced body weight after a period of dieting. Of course most people who try to diet are ultimately unsuccessful, but a small minority do appear to be able to lose weight and keep it off. These individuals have been studied as part of the US National Weight Control Registry. People self-enrol in this register if they have lost more than 14 kg and maintained this loss for at least one year.

Klem et al. (1998) examined these individuals to determine if they had any evidence of psychopathology, and especially in relation to eating. The sample consisted of 629 women (they had experienced a weight change from a BMI of 35 to one of 24) and 155 men (weight change from BMI of 37 to 26). There was no evidence of clinical or subclinical depression or other psychiatric symptoms, and longer time since initial weight loss ended was linked to lower scores on these measures. Dietary restraint was considerably higher than control samples, and similar to that encountered in actively dieting groups. The data on eating-related psychopathology was interesting. The authors noted that average binge rate for the sample was one per month. There was no US normative data to interpret this binge rate, but it appears higher than one might expect (i.e., we *presume* that binging, defined as a loss of feeling of control over food intake would be rare or absent in healthy normal weight controls). Moreover, there was a weak correlation between greater change in weight (i.e., pre to post diet) and binge-like behaviour. It seems that this population too showed *some* evidence of heightened binging behaviour following periods of self-imposed energy restriction.

8.3.3.4 Recovery: Conclusion

Most attention has been on binge eating as the only significant long-term consequence of starvation or extreme hunger. At least some evidence of binge eating was present in ex-prisoners of war, people who have experienced intermittent food supply and hunger (but noting the potential confound with obesity) and people who have voluntarily lost and maintained that lost weight. No evidence of binging was found in samples of holocaust survivors or participants of the Minnesota starvation study. One way of integrating these findings is to see binging as more likely to occur following a traumatic experience, where its central feature is significant hunger. This idea remains to be tested.

8.3.4 Energy Restriction and Longevity

While starvation is ultimately lethal, there may be circumstances where a degree of undernutrition, relative to ad libitum intake, is beneficial. Historically, research started in rats by studying the effects of adopting a moderate degree of energy restriction (20–30% less than ad libitum fed controls) during late adolescence and maintaining this for life. One consequence of this procedure – termed calorie restriction, or CR – is to significantly extend the average lifespan of common laboratory animals (e.g., worms, fruit flies, rats and mice). Another is that the CR animals show fewer signs of age-related degeneration of all bodily systems, including the brain (Shanley & Kirkwood, 2006).

In the last 20 years there has also been interest in whether all or some of the beneficial effects of CR can be obtained more easily by using intermittent periods of energy restriction (often referred to as intermittent feeding (IF) or restriction (IR)). Commercial weight loss programs have significantly shaped the nature of intermittent dietary regimens, with various subtypes emerging, including alternate-day fasting, periodic fasting (e.g., 2 days per week fasting) and daily time-restricted feeding. While there is emerging evidence about some of these types of fasting on body weight and metabolic parameters, less is known about their long-term consequences and their effects on brain and behaviour.

Most of the focus here will be on CR, but including intermittent forms when there is relevant evidence. There is no doubt that CR has primarily attracted attention because of its capacity to extend lifespan in laboratory animals. The evolutionary arguments about *why* this occurs (i.e., functional benefits) are worth considering, because they impact on what we might expect to happen to the brain. The basic idea is that for animals that cannot easily move to search for other food sources, they should shift into a mode where lifespan is extended, thereby increasing the possibility that they are still alive and able to reproduce when the environment becomes more favourable (Shanley & Kirkwood, 2006). This suggests lifespan extension should be more likely in organisms that cannot readily relocate, have limited food stores, and where the environment is unstable (i.e., intermittent food supply). For organisms in more stable environments, those who can draw on large fat/food stores, and for those capable of moving to new places to search for food, there should be less need for CR to extend lifespan. However, it has been argued that even if this account is correct, there may be an evolutionary conserved cellular response in all animals, which is activated by stressful circumstances, putting cells into a 'survival mode'. From a functional perspective, preservation of brain health should be important in lifespan extension (i.e., once the lean times are over, successful brain function is vital to coordinate feeding and reproduction), but whether putting a cell into survival mode would exert a long-term beneficial effect is less functionally obvious.

How the effects of CR arise to produce elongated lifespan is not fully understood. It is very likely that the brain, as the central metabolic controller (Mattson, 2005), is influential in coordinating organism-wide adaptations to CR (e.g., reductions in heart rate). At a cellular level, changes in mitochondrial function are important. When feeding is ad libitum, there is an over-abundance of free oxygen species from mitochondrial production of adenosine tri-phosphate. Free oxygen species cause damage to all cellular components, including DNA, and are one plausible mechanism for aging. Under conditions of CR, free oxygen species markedly diminish, and there is an alteration in the types of protein manufactured in the cell, with a shift to those with a protective function. This includes enzymes that reduce free oxygen species, assist protein and DNA repair, and in the case of the brain (Mattson, 2005), proteins that promote neural and glial cell survival, notably brain-derived neurotrophic factor (BDNF) and glial-derived neurotrophic factor (GDNF).

One thing that CR may not achieve, but which intermittent forms of energy restriction can, is metabolic switching (de Cabo & Mattson, 2019; Mattson et al., 2018). The brain normally utilises glucose as its fuel, but when bodily availability of glucose diminishes, with stores of glycogen expended, the body switches to burning fatty acids to generate ketones that the brain can use instead. The two main ketones, beta-hydroxybutyrate (BHB) and acetoacetate can enter the brain via the blood-brain barrier and can also be synthesised in astrocytes. This metabolic switching has two major impacts on cellular function in the brain. First, the brain detects the reduced availability of glucose, which down-regulates the production of the protein kinase mTOR, putting cells into a conserve, maintain, repair and reuse mode, in contrast to the more typical growth phase associated with enhanced mTOR activity. Second, the ketone BHB serves as a signal to up-regulate production of BDNF and to further inhibit mTOR. This is in addition to a more generalised response that mirrors the effects described in the preceding paragraph and, which in the brain, is triggered by heightened levels of the excitatory neurotransmitter glutamate (Mattson et al., 2018). It is unclear how the cellular effects induced by CR and intermittent energy restriction (via metabolic switching) relate – although it is clear they overlap.

The level of speculation about the beneficial and to a lesser extent harmful effects of CR and intermittent fasting in humans (e.g., Vitousek et al., 2004) has far exceeded what is known. Anecdotally, death rates have in certain circumstances been seen to fall when large segments of the population are effectively placed on CR (Most et al., 2017). The Danes in World War I and the Norwegians in World War II both saw mortality fall by a third during periods of enforced energy restriction. Okinawans have four to five times the rate of centenarians relative to comparable regions, and it has been suggested that an energy-restricted diet is one factor. Experimental evidence – the main focus of what follows – comes from two main sources. The first is the limited studies conducted on monkeys and great apes, the closest possible group upon which CR regimens can be ethically enacted. The second is the far briefer duration human studies, of which there are three. The CRON study follows members of the Calorie Restriction Society, who have voluntarily adopted a CR regimen. We could find no brain- or behaviour-related studies of this population, and in addition as they are self-selected it is not possible to know whether any beneficial consequences come from CR or the self-selection process (i.e., people likely to be interested in living a presumably very healthy lifestyle and with very high levels of self-control).

There have been two experimental studies of CR. The first is the CALERIE 1 trial, which had three arms, and recruited overweight middle-aged people for between 6M and 12M of CR or some variant thereof. The second is the CALERIE 2 study, which was a much larger multicentre clinical trial, with around 180 participants completing a 2-year intervention. It included normal-weight and overweight (M BMI = 25) middle-aged adults, contrasting 25% energy restriction with an ad libitum control condition. In addition to a couple of small-scale clinical trials, our knowledge of the behavioural, cognitive and brain effects of CR is limited to these studies. Most of the data has focussed on the effects of CR on hunger, psychopathology and cognition, and so the following sections are organised around these three themes.

8.3.4.1   Calorie Restriction and Hunger

If CR is to be considered as a practical means of extending well-span (and lifespan) the regimen needs to be tolerable. In reports of natural starvation and in the Minnesota study, hunger and persistent thoughts about food were evident, persistent, bothersome and sometimes painful. In CR and intermittent fasting studies, both human and animal, examination of hunger has *not* come to the fore. Some have claimed that this is deliberate, because these dietary regimens are so unpleasant that acknowledgement of this fact would dissuade most people from undertaking them (Vitousek et al., 2004). In animals, CR results in significant increases in activity before food is provided and there is also some evidence of stereotypy (Weed et al., 1997). However, the former is an extension of behaviour already observed in laboratory animals and the latter could equally result from housing/boredom rather than CR itself. So animal data offers little in regard to understanding hunger in CR.

As for humans, the literature suggests that people do not experience overwhelming hunger on CR or intermittent fasting regimens – but with some major caveats examined after the evidence is reviewed. In both the CALERIE 1 and 2 studies, subgroups completed the hunger scale of the three-factor eating questionnaire (TFEQ), which measures general experience of hunger and its behavioural consequences (Stunkard & Messick, 1985). Williamson et al. (2008) found that CALERIE 1 CR participants reported a small but significant reduction on the hunger scale at 6M. Marlatt et al. (2017) followed up a small number of the CALERIE 2 CR participants and ad libitum controls, but there was no difference in TFEQ hunger, even though CR participants still seemed to be adhering to the regimen. Another approach has been to ask participants to report both adverse and positive consequences of adhering to the CR or intermittent fasting regimen. Harvie, Pegington, and Mattson's (2011) CR participants (25% energy reduction) made no spontaneous complaints about hunger, while 15% of the intermittent fasting group did (very low calorie diet for 2 days per week). Adherence to the diet was also better in the CR group.

Three studies have used rating scales to evaluate hunger. Johnson, Summer, and Cutler (2007) conducted a small study (n = 9) to examine the effects of intermittent energy restriction (1 day CR, 1 day ad libitum) on asthma, with participants recording hunger every 2 h daily – reportedly for the whole study period, although only summary data is provided. Hunger was approximately 8% greater on fast days, and there was a general decline in hunger on both fast and ad libitum days across the 8 weeks of the study. Harvie, Wright, and Pegington (2013) compared two intermittent fasting groups with a CR group, and found initially that the intermittent groups were hungrier on fast days, but this effect had dissipated by the end of the 3M trial. Anton, Han, and York (2009) undertook the only study focussed solely on hunger, observing participants in the Pennington arm of the CALERIE 1 trial. Appetite ratings were obtained before breakfast on all of the days that participants were staying at the research facility – essentially during baseline and weeks 22–23. There were modest increases in all appetite ratings, including in the control group, which tended to mask what likely would have been significant increases in hunger and reductions in fullness (currently marginally significant alone) between baseline and the end of the study period (see Figure 8.3, left & right panels). In this report, with its detailed presentation, there do appear to be persistent increases in hunger and reductions in fullness – but absolutely nothing like the large and pervasive changes in the starvation/Minnesota studies.

As we noted earlier, these data come with caveats. First, with the exception of CALERIE 2 data, all of these studies were conducted on overweight and obese participants, who therefore had significant fat reserves in excess of those who undertook the Minnesota study – and

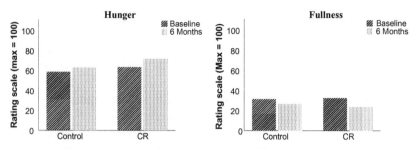

Figure 8.3   Ratings of hunger (left panel) and of fullness (right panel) taken at
baseline and at follow-up in the control and calorie restriction groups.
Source: Data adapted from Anton et al. (2009)

probably greater than those who experienced natural starvation. If normal-weight participants were placed on a CR or intermittent energy regimen, for purposes of extending well-span or lifespan, this difference could be important in whether hunger would be a major burden. The CALERIE 2 data are of particular interest in this regard, as these participants were in the normal to overweight range, and in fact this study had quite poor compliance, with less than 20% actually achieving the target level of CR. Whether poor compliance resulted from greater hunger is difficult to know, as apart from the follow-up TFEQ hunger scale data of Marlatt et al. (2017) we could find no reports of hunger-related measures for this study.

A second issue concerns support. Interventional studies represent the best possible circumstances for a particular dietary regimen to succeed. Being in a 'scientific study', as well as receiving support from numerous health professionals, are likely to motivate the participants in these trials. Indeed, in the CALERIE 1 study, this included sessions with both nutritionists and doctoral-level psychologists, and for the latter, this included discussion of managing the troublesome consequences of dietary restriction (i.e., presumably hunger and craving). As our main data source about hunger is from this study, it is hard to know the effects of these demand characteristics on participant responses. Finally, there is the issue of hunger measurement. This is a complex topic, because hunger is far from a simple response to changes in bodily state (Stevenson, Mahmut, & Rooney, 2015). Hunger is an individual difference, it has state and trait properties, it is not associated with one particular feeling (e.g., stomach rumbling), and is strongly affected by environmental variables (e.g., adverts, places and times linked to food, people eating, smell of food). An ideal approach would be some form of ecological momentary assessment over an extended period of time. However, if CR did produce extreme hunger, it is highly likely that the Anton et al. (2009) study would have detected it, but what effect CR might have on hunger in lean people still remains unknown.

8.3.4.2 Calorie Restriction and Psychopathology
The Minnesota study, observations of natural starvation and the psychological consequences of self-imposed weight loss in anorexia nervosa, suggest the possibility that CR or its variants might have adverse impacts on mood, vitality, libido and eating psychopathology (Vitousek et al., 2004). Rodent data also suggests that in some circumstances CR can induce anxiety and depression-like behaviours (Murphy, Dias, & Thuret, 2014). In humans, for mood, seven CR or intermittent energy restriction regimens have explored this. None found adverse changes, and 6/7 reported improvements. The positive outcomes were for the Pennington arm of CALERIE 1 (Williamson et al., 2008), the CALERIE 2 trial (Martin, Bhapkar, & Pittas, 2016), both arms of the Harvie et al. (2011) trial – based on symptom reports – all arms of the second Harvie et al. (2013) trial, the small intermittent energy restriction trial by Johnson et al. (2007) and a German CR trial (Prehn et al., 2017). The Marlatt et al. (2017) follow-up study of CALERIE 2 participants found no difference in mood between controls and CR participants. It is again important to note that these reports typically concern overweight and obese individuals, and positive mood changes with weight loss may reflect satisfaction with goal achievement and improved body image. Weight loss and maintenance of this loss in lean individuals may produce different outcomes.

Nearly all of the studies finding mood improvements also observed increases in self-reported vitality, but no study reported any change on quality of life measures (Martin et al., 2016; Marlatt et al., 2017). Two studies examined libido. The Martin et al. (2016) report on the main CALERIE 2 trial found some evidence of improvement in sexual function in men, but not in women, while the follow-up study observed just an increase in sexual fantasy in the CR group (Marlatt et al., 2017). Two further studies, both from the CALERIE trials, have examined for eating disordered psychopathology. It is important to bear in mind that both CALERIE 1 and 2 screened for psychopathology *before* recruitment – including eating disorders – so these studies address just whether CR per se invokes disordered eating. These studies cannot tell us whether CR would affect someone with a vulnerability to, or a history of, eating disorders. Both Williamson et al. (2008) and Marlatt et al. (2017) found little evidence of emergent eating-related psychopathology, but as with any group of food restrictors (i.e., dieters) there was an increase in dietary restraint and avoidance of forbidden foods. Neither of these studies found any evidence of increases in binge eating, and Williamson et al. (2008) reported a decrease in disinhibition (i.e., improved control over eating), relative to ad libitum controls. So at least in these psychologically healthy overweight and obese participants, calorie restriction did not have any immediately obvious adverse effects on disordered eating.

8.3.4.3   Calorie Restriction and Cognition

Several studies demonstrate that learning and memory of aging rats and mice is improved by CR and that the earlier in life this starts the greater the benefit (Mattson, 2005). However, it has been noted that animals in the wild often have body weights and dietary patterns that are more like CR animals than ad libitum fed controls in the laboratory, and so it could be that much of the beneficial effect on cognition results from the *absence* of overfeeding and excess weight in CR animals (Mattson, 2005). This also appears to be the case for studies of CR in monkeys (Bourg, 2018). In the two large-scale macaque studies (both involved CR vs ad libitum controls), one observed that CR resulted in significant extension of lifespan (Colman, Anderson, & Johnson, 2009; the Wisconsin study) and the other did not (Mattison, Roth, & Beasley, 2012; The National Institute of Aging (NIA) study).

The Wisconsin study, using 30% CR initiated in adulthood, not only observed that ad libitum controls had three times the rate of age-related mortality of CR animals, but that the CR animals also looked more youthful and had significantly fewer signs of age-related disease (Colman et al., 2009). The monkeys also underwent brain imaging. Some age-related changes in grey matter were independent of diet, notably to the frontal and temporal cortices. However, CR animals had preserved sub-cortical grey matter volume in the insula, putamen and caudate. CR also moderated age-related changes to the cingulate, temporal and dorsolateral prefrontal cortices, suggesting better preservation of executive and motor function. There is, though, a powerful alternative explanation, namely that these effects arose because of the diet that the ad libitum animals were fed, which was nearly 30% sucrose (getting close to a diet of Froot Loops or Coco Pops at 37% sucrose). In contrast, the NIH macaque CR study used a different diet, composed of only 4% sucrose. In this study (Mattison et al., 2012), there was no life extension effect, although the CR animals did show fewer signs of age-related disease. Unfortunately MRI measures were not obtained.

A final monkey study, this time using mouse lemurs (Pifferi & Aujard, 2019), compared 30% CR with ad libitum feeding. When all of the control animals were dead, just over a quarter of the CR animals were still alive, with median survival being 9.6 years, relative to 6.4 for controls. Before turning to the cognitive impacts of CR it is again important to note the effects of ad libitum feeding. Wild mouse lemurs normally weigh (at an equivalent time in the season) around 60 g – this is towards the *lower end* of the weight range of the CR animals (60–80 g). In contrast, the ad libitum controls weighed between 90–110 g. Both behavioural and imaging measures were obtained to assess brain function. Memory performance did not differ but there were some motor benefits in the CR group, although it was unclear if these resulted from reduced sarcopenia or better coordination (i.e., brain function). Imaging revealed a mixed picture. There was reduced grey matter volume in the CR animals relative to controls, but the CR animals had reduced white matter atrophy in contrast to controls. In sum, animal studies provide some evidence of benefit of CR on the aging brain, but it is unclear if these effects reflect the absence of damage induced by ad libitum consumption of food in controls.

Turning to humans, the evidence is also equivocal. On the CALERIE 1 trial, Martin et al. (2007) conducted an extensive neuropsychological battery at baseline, 3 and 6M, on the Pennington arm of the study. They found no evidence of beneficial or harmful effects of CR on tests of long- and short-term verbal learning and memory, visual memory or sustained attention. A cognitive battery (the CANTAB) appears to have been used on some or all of the CALERIE 2 trial participants, but as far we can tell only one sub-test from this data set has been published. They found evidence on one component of one sub-test of the CANTAB, measuring spatial working memory, finding a greater reduction in errors on this test over the trial (Leclerc, Trevizol, & Grigolon, 2020). They also found that this improvement was related to alterations in one cytokine measure (interleukin 6; Trevizol, Brietzke, & Grigolon, 2019). Cognitive improvements in overweight and obese participants are well documented (see earlier in this chapter) and so this change in working memory seems consistent, albeit a hard won benefit.

The two final human studies could equally be discussed under the banner of weight-loss-improved cognition in the obese, but were published as CR impacts on cognition in the elderly. Witte et al. (2009) randomised overweight healthy elderly to: (1) a 30% CR group, (2) a dietary enhancement group (with unsaturated fatty acids) or (3) an ad libitum control group for the 3M intervention. Participants completed a neuropsycholog-ical battery measuring verbal learning and memory, executive and short-term memory function. There was significant weight loss in the CR group, but not in the other two groups. Cognitive benefits were also restricted to just the CR group, finding improvement in delayed verbal memory – suggestive of hippocampal benefit. This was also found to correlate with increased insulin sensitivity and decreased C-reactive protein in the CR group. No other changes in neuropsychological function were observed.

In a second and more extensive study by the same group (Prehn et al., 2017), older obese (M BMI = 35) participants were randomised either to a control (diet as usual) or a CR condition. However, the CR condition was an 8-week period of 60% energy reduction, more reminiscent of a very-low-calorie diet than long-term CR, and this 8-week period was then followed by 4 weeks of a less rigorous but reduced energy intake regimen, and then 4 weeks of weight maintenance at 15% of their initial body weight. Both neuropsychological (as for the previous study) and MRI imaging were conducted at baseline, 8 weeks and at the end of the study (16 weeks). In the CR group at 8 weeks, relative to baseline and controls, delayed verbal recognition memory, delayed verbal recall, words learned and processing speed (trail making A) were improved. Structural changes on MRI were also seen (again relative to baseline and controls), with an increase in grey matter volume in the inferior frontal gyrus and right hippocampus, and reductions in grey matter volume in the right olfactory cortex, cerebellum and left post central gyrus. Resting state connectivity between the hippocampus, precuneus and angular gyrus increased in the CR group.

At 16 weeks, the delayed recognition memory effect was lost, suggesting that it was connected with the active weight loss phase, but all of the other neuropsychological gains were maintained, plus an improvement on verbal fluency (trail making B). MRI changes were less evident in contrasting to baseline (no comparisons of 8 weeks to 16 weeks were reported so it is not apparent whether the other changes may in part have been maintained). Reductions in right cerebellum grey matter volume were significant in the CR group (relative to baseline and control), but there were no alterations in functional connectivity. Some of the observed changes, notably delayed recognition memory and to a degree some of the MRI changes, may be attributable to the effects of energy restriction per se; however, most cognitive benefits were evident at 8 weeks and maintained to 16 weeks suggesting that whatever physiological changes had occurred (via the direct or indirect effects of CR), the benefits to cognition remained. In as much as these findings are interesting and important, they seem to better belong to the earlier section on weight loss in the obese/overweight and cognitive improvement. Indeed, as this section has repeatedly indicated, we do not know what effect CR will have on the brains of lean people.

8.3.4.4 Calorie Restriction: Conclusion

Many laboratory species, notably worms, fruit flies, rats and mice, live longer and healthier lives when on an energy-restricted diet. Attempts to translate this research to humans have been complicated by two factors. First, when testing CR in monkeys, many of the beneficial effects seem to come from *avoiding* the unhealthy diet and excess weight gain observed in ad libitum fed controls. Second, human research has mainly involved only short periods of CR in overweight and obese participants. In these people it is reasonably well tolerated, it improves mood, and in some cases yields cognitive gains in learning and memory – but all of these effects are similar to any weight loss program. What effects CR has on lean people, whether it is tolerable and desirable for them in the longer term, and if it delivers better health into old age, remains to be established.

8.3.4.5 General Conclusion

A person's initial body weight has a major effect on the sequelae of starvation. Overweight and obese people do not always react with extreme hunger or low mood to long periods of no food or restricted diet, but more typically show improved mood and cognition, especially learning and memory. This mirrors the findings of the calorie restriction literature, which has mainly focussed on overweight and obese people. In marked contrast are the findings from lean animals and people. Lean animals placed on protein and energy-deficient diets evidence adverse changes to hippocampal anatomy and function, which in part may be due to the physiological stress induced by these dietary regimens. Lean people show a constellation of starvation-related symptoms, notably acute hunger, low mood, irritability and egocentricity. The latter can morph in certain people into amoral behaviour in the search for food, and while this effect is well documented, it is little studied. At least in the early and mid-stages of starvation, cognitive changes are limited. They are generally restricted to the interfering effects of starvation symptoms (e.g., constant thoughts about food, hunger pain), although low mood can be a major issue in disrupting cognitive function, especially in relation to mental competence in hunger strikers. Cognition in advanced starvation has been little studied. It is seriously affected by micronutrient deficiencies, which can cause irreversible brain damage. On recovery, the nature of the starvation experience may be important in dictating the long-term mental health consequences. Binge eating often occurs during re-feeding, but persists in some individuals where starvation and acute hunger have been central traumatic features of their experience. Significant weight loss can also occur in other contexts. The adverse consequences of involuntary weight loss during anorexia, aging, cancer and other diseases are all major health problems, and in some cases (notably aging) have received little research attention.

CHAPTER 9

Essential Nutrient Deficiencies in Adults

9.1 Introduction

The global vitamin, mineral and supplements market is worth US $109 billion per year (*Financial Times*, August 17, 2020). Even with this massive nutritional input, many adults, including those who live in wealthy countries, do not obtain sufficient intakes of certain vitamins, minerals and essential macronutrients – with iodine, iron, zinc, selenium and vitamins B2, B6, C and D being notable examples. In this chapter the focus is on the neurocognitive impacts of essential nutrient deficiency states in adults, with the consequences for foetal and child neurocognitive development examined in Chapter 2.

A good starting point is to identify the nutrients that are covered in this chapter. The basic criteria are that the nutrient is a single chemical or related group of chemicals, it is vital for bodily functioning and it cannot be adequately synthesised in the body. Thus, all of the vitamins are examined, and all of the essential minerals – with the exception of hydrogen, oxygen, carbon and nitrogen – but with certain of their combinations included, namely the essential fatty acids and proteins. Hydrogen, oxygen, carbon and nitrogen were omitted because they are so abundant, constituting more than 95% of bodily mass. Applying the term deficiency to them seems wholly inappropriate and terms like starvation, dehydration or hypoxia are more fitting, and the first-mentioned was the focus of Chapter 9.

A common approach is taken for each vitamin, mineral or essential macronutrient. The biological agent or agents are first identified. This is important as there are often multiple dietary and bodily forms, and the foods within which they most commonly occur are described. How these chemicals are moved from the mouth to the central nervous system is also examined – noting that this is not always fully understood. The transport process is important as a number of deficiency states arise from a breakdown in one or more aspects of this process. Where available, data on who is deficient and why, is also provided. The normal functions of the chemical/s on the brain, both general (i.e., as with all cells in the body) and specific (i.e., to the brain) are presented, alongside the consequences of deficiency for neurocognitive function (drawing on animal and human data). The additional effects of marginal deficiency (in the case of vitamins termed hypovitaminosis) are also reported, and especially so in relation to aging, neurodegenerative diseases and mental health.

As described elsewhere in this book, an important consideration is the utility of focussing on a single chemical. Of course, this whole chapter is going to do just that, but a deficiency in one micronutrient rarely occurs in isolation and usually has knock-on consequences for other micronutrients. For example, supplementation with one micronutrient (e.g., zinc, folate) can cause or mask another deficiency (respectively for the last examples, copper and B12). Notwithstanding, the identification of specific micronutrients and their impact on bodily and brain function represent key developments for nutritional science, and so rightly deserve dedicated space.

9.2   Vitamins

9.2.1   Vitamin A (Retinoic Acid)

Vitamin A consists of three core compounds: retinol, retinal and retinoic acid. It can be obtained from animal sources in the form of retinyl palmitate, which is broken down in the small intestine into retinol. Retinol can also be obtained by the breakdown of a limited number of plant-based foods, with the primary sources being alpha, beta and gamma carotenoid. Retinol is the main form stored in the body, principally in the liver. This can be readily converted into retinal, which in the eye, when combined with opsin, forms light-sensitive chemicals (e.g., rhodopsin). Retinol can also be converted into retinoic acid, which is the main active form of Vitamin A for most cellular purposes (Shearer et al., 2012).

Retinoic acid exerts significant effects on the adult brain, with most research in animals. Vitamin A effects cells in the brain in at least three ways: it regulates DNA transcription (i.e., turning it on and off); it regulates protein kinase activity (i.e., turning proteins on and off); and it acts as a paracrine by diffusing from one cell into another. Certain brain areas appear to be especially sensitive to its effects, with three identified, namely the olfactory bulb, hypothalamus and hippocampus. Knockout mice that lack one of the three neuronal nuclear retinoid receptors have impaired hippocampal-dependent learning and memory. This same deficit, and others, can be obtained by placing an animal on a vitamin A-deficient diet (Cocco, Diaz, & Stancampiano, 2002). This impairs hippocampal, olfactory bulb and hypothalamic neurogenesis, synapse formation, and neuronal spine growth. In the hippocampus it stops long-term potentiation and depression (Misner, Jacobs, & Shimizu, 2001). In older rats, vitamin A bioavailability is significantly reduced in the brain, and dietary supplementation results in improvements in hippocampal-dependent learning and memory (Dumetz, Buré, & Alfos, 2020). This has led to the suggestion that reduced bioavailability of vitamin A may contribute to the neurodegenerative conditions of old age (Olson & Mello, 2010; Shearer et al., 2012).

There are currently no reports that vitamin A deficiency in adult humans results in readily observable neurocognitive impairment (noting that deficiency states are rare as liver stores are substantial). One reason for this is that people may not have looked, and another is that the first consequences of deficiency seem to be visual impairment. For several other essential nutrients, the brain defends its own supply even in the face of major bodily deficiency. Consequently, bodily deficiency signs (i.e., visual impairment here), may occur before any central deficiency symptoms emerge.

9.2.2   Vitamin B1 (Thiamine)

Vitamin B1 refers to a set of related water-soluble compounds, the four most important being free thiamine (the form found most commonly in food), thiamine-monophosphate, thiamine-diphosphate (the main active form) and thiamine-triphosphate. Most foods contain some thiamine, with somewhat richer sources being wholegrains, meat, fish, seeds, yeast, fruit and nuts.

Thiamine deficiency is not restricted to developing countries. Several groups are at risk in wealthier societies, most notably chronic alcoholics (estimates vary between 30 and 80% of this group; Kloss, Eskin, & Suh, 2018). Alcoholics are at risk of thiamine deficiency for multiple reasons (Arts, Walvoort, & Kessels, 2017): (1) alcohol needs to be metabolised and this utilises thiamine; (2) alcoholism is often accompanied by gastroenteritis which impairs thiamine absorption; (3) liver cirrhosis reduces the body's capacity to store thiamine (and liver stores are not substantial under normal conditions – around 1 month reserve); (4) alcohol may impair the bodies utilisation of thiamine; and (5) alcoholics often eat little and what they do eat is not particularly nutritious. Thiamine deficiency syndromes can also be observed in people who have undergone gastrointestinal tract surgery (for cancer; weight loss), pregnant mothers with hyperemesis gravidarum, people with eating disorders, those receiving intravenous feeding and in HIV/AIDS (Scalzo et al., 2015). Common factors here are poor absorption in the gut, inadequate thiamine intake, other micronutrient deficiencies (e.g., magnesium), high metabolic rate and drug interactions.

Thiamine is absorbed by the gut both passively and actively, and is carried in the blood in bound form. It crosses the blood-brain barrier by an active carrier process using the THTR1 and THTR2 transporters (Tiani, Stover, & Field, 2019). Thiamine performs both general and specific functions in the brain. It has a general function as a coenzyme for several steps in the metabolism of carbohydrates, fats and proteins in the Krebs cycle – a key catabolic pathway for energy generation. It also serves as a coenzyme for the generation of intermediaries in the Krebs cycle (alongside several other B vitamins) and in the metabolism of glucose. More broadly, it has anti-inflammatory functions and plays a role in gene regulation.

In the brain, thiamine is important in the production of myelin and the neurotransmitters acetylcholine, GABA and glutamate, and it has several roles in reducing oxidative stress and in maintaining the structural integrity of cell membranes (Hiffler et al., 2016; Manzetti, Zhang, & van der Spoel, 2014). Not surprisingly, given these multiple roles, deficiency has a significant impact on function, impairing energy production, allowing the build-up of excitotoxic levels of glutamate, increasing oxidative stress and causing loss of osmotic gradients across neuronal cell membranes (Kloss et al., 2018).

In Asian countries, adult thiamine deficiency usually manifests as the cardiac form called wet beriberi. In contrast, amongst Caucasians with thiamine deficiency, notably alcoholics and those derived from other causes (e.g., gastrointestinal surgery, extreme dieting; Karakonstantis, Galani, & Korela, 2020) it occurs almost universally as the neurological or dry beriberi form, known as Wernicke's encephalopathy (WE). This suggests a possible genetic basis for the difference in presentation between Caucasian and Asian populations (Chandrakumar, Bhardwaj, & Jong, 2019). There has in the past been some debate about the genesis of WE, especially whether it required a combination of alcoholism and thiamine deficiency to occur. A parallel debate has also taken place about the role of maternal alcoholism and thiamine deficiency in the pathogenesis of foetal alcohol spectrum disorder (FASD; Kloss et al., 2018). While FASD does seem to be caused by alcohol, WE occurs as a consequence of thiamine deficiency. Scalzo et al. (2015) compared the clinical presentation of WE in alcoholics with the pattern of neurological symptoms in non-alcoholic cases. WE is normally described as having a triad of symptoms: ophthalmoplegia (paralysis of the muscles surrounding the eye), ataxia and mental confusion – although this 'classic' triad is only seen in around 16% of cases (Chandrakumar et al., 2019). The pattern of symptom presentation in alcoholic and non-alcoholic cases was largely identical, suggesting a common aetiology in thiamine deficiency. This conclusion is further supported by animal models of thiamine deficiency. These do not involve administration of alcohol, yet produce a pattern of deficit that very closely resembles human WE (Zahr & Pfefferbaum, 2017).

Although the 'classic' symptom triad of WE purports to capture all key facets of the disease, the symptom profile of WE is varied. Initial presentation is typically non-specific (headache, abdominal pain, irritability, fatigue), and as WE develops, alongside ophthalmoplegia, ataxia and mental confusion, it can also include, anorexia, memory impairment, emotional dysregulation, hypothermia, hypotension, tachycardia, syncope, painful breathing, seizures and vocal aphonia – some of which overlap with wet beriberi (i.e., cardiac symptoms, vocal aphonia). The neural basis of these symptoms has been studied in some detail (Chandrakumar et al., 2019; Zahr & Pfefferbaum, 2017). There is bilateral loss of neurons and myelinated structures from the mammillary bodies, brain stem, cerebellum and hypothalamus. Damage to the brain stem contributes to visual impairments such as nystagmus, gaze palsy and abnormal reactions to light, in addition to vestibular abnormalities (balance), syncope, tachycardia, breathing difficulties and hypotension. Cerebellar changes contribute to ataxic gait, alongside a reduced capacity to utilise vestibular information. Hypothalamic changes can cause hypothermia, and excessive glutamate release can generate seizures. Hyperintensities on MRI are also seen in periventricular tissue, the hippocampus (which was not originally thought to be affected) and the orbitofrontal cortex – with the latter two probably implicated in memory and emotional dysregulation, respectively. Many of these same sites are also damaged when inspected post mortem. If WE is diagnosed (usually utilising the Caine criteria – see Table 9.1) and quickly treated with thiamine, most symptoms remit. However, if it is not rapidly treated, it turns into a chronic condition called Korsakoff's syndrome (KS) or, far more rarely, nutritional cerebellar degeneration (Arts et al., 2017). Korsakoff's syndrome is quite rare, with estimates varying from 0.005 to

Table 9.1. *Caine¹ criteria for the diagnosis of Wernicke's encephalopathy*

Clinical sign	Specific diagnostic features
Poor diet	Underweight, thiamine deficient, abnormal dietary pattern
Ocular abnormalities	Nystagmus, gaze palsy, ophthalmoplegia
Cerebellar abnormalities	Ataxia, dysmetria, abnormal coordination and alternation
Altered mental state	Disorientation, confusion, abnormal digit span, coma
Mild amnesia	Memory test failure on simple or complex tests

¹*Journal of Neurology, Neurosurgery & Psychiatry*, 62, 51–60, 1997.

0.05% prevalence. While there is no formal definition of KS, it has two key characteristics. First, it follows on from WE and second, it includes irreversible memory impairment. The primary mnemonic impairment is to episodic memory (i.e., recollection of specific personal events), with a far greater anterograde than retrograde deficit, and the sparing of childhood memories. Semantic memory (i.e., facts) is usually intact, as is procedural memory (e.g., riding a bike). Other cognitive deficits have also been documented in KS, the most frequent being to the executive system. In addition, people with KS tend to have flattened affect, they lack volition and especially in the early stages of KS they lack insight into their illness (Arts et al., 2017). This can result in confabulation ('honest lying'), where the person endeavours to explain gaps in their memory by generating often implausible stories. The cause of the severe memory impairment is believed to involve damage to the mammillary bodies and/or the anterior nuclei of the thalamus, disrupting the limbic-diencephalic memory circuit of which the hippocampus and amygdala form core parts.

There has been interest in whether thiamine hypovitaminosis might contribute to a number of conditions via an increase in oxidative stress, impairments to endoplasmic reticulum and protein misfolding, and immune disruption (abnormal autophagy). In Alzheimer's disease, a characteristic feature is reduced glucose metabolism. Low levels of thiamine may contribute to this, as plasma vitamin B1 concentration is known to be abnormally low in this disease (Liu, Ke, & Luo, 2017). In animal models, thiamine hypovitaminosis is linked to increased beta amyloid accumulation, plaque formation and the promotion of tau phosphorylation – all characteristics of Alzheimer's disease. However, thiamine supplementation does not have beneficial effects. In addition, thiamine hypovitaminosis has also been implicated in Parkinson's disease. This degenerative condition is linked to both lower cerebrospinal fluid levels of thiamine and to damage to one of the metabolic pathways in which thiamine serves as a coenzyme, in the substantia nigra. The latter is correlated with the severity of motor symptoms. There is some limited evidence that thiamine supplementation may assist in managing symptoms (Liu et al., 2017). Finally, thiamine hypovitaminosis correlates with depression in the elderly, while in young adults the reverse relationship has been observed, but with no evidence that supplementation in the former improves symptoms (Dhir et al., 2019).

9.2.3   Vitamin B2 (Riboflavin)

Vitamin B2 is found in three different forms in food, as free riboflavin in generally small amounts, and in two enzyme-bound forms, flavin adenine dinucleotide (FAD; most common form) and flavin mononucleotide (FMN; less common form). Rich sources of B2 are milk and dairy products, and meats, with other sources being fortified breakfast cereals, salmon and some dark green vegetables (Powers, 2003). FAD and FMN are broken down at the gut wall into riboflavin, which is then actively transported across the gut membrane and into the bloodstream. Deficiency states are not well investigated but are believed to be common even among well-nourished Westerners. This is because some 10% of the population have a genetic variant of the transporter protein that makes absorption less efficient (Kennedy, 2016). Other groups at risk include pregnant women and athletes, due to high metabolic demands; people who consume only small quantities of meat and dairy; and the elderly, who are less efficient at absorbing B2. Alcoholics are at special risk of deficiency and this often coincides with low levels of vitamin B1 (Langohr, Petruch, & Schrom, 1981). Indeed, vitamin B2 is directly and indirectly involved in the metabolism of B3, B6, B9 and B12, and so inadequacy of B2 has ramifications that extend beyond its specific effects (Powers, 2003).

FAD and, to a lesser extent, NAD serve as co-factors for a large family of enzymes termed flavoproteins, with most localised in mitochondria. The majority perform redox reactions (electron transfers) but their roles extend across a range of different functions critical to mitochondrial metabolism and cellular energy generation (Mosegaard, Dipace, & Bross, 2020). The deficiency disease associated with B2 spans from mild symptoms, such as a sore throat and skin ulceration (especially around the mouth and lips), to more severe manifestations, such as swollen tongue, anaemia and impaired nerve function. There is uncertainty about whether these symptoms overlap other B-group deficiency states. Somewhat more specific deficiency data comes from the study of children and adults who have abnormalities in the riboflavin transporter, and where a deficiency in B2 is definitely occurring. The main characteristics of this disease state, which was termed Brown–Vialetto–Van Laere syndrome until it became clear that it was a B2 transporter disease, are its neurological features – cranial nerve deficits, limb weakness, ataxia, feeding difficulties and dyspnoea (Jaeger & Bosch, 2016). Interestingly, individuals with this disorder, some of whom are only identified as adults (but noting that diagnosis usually occurs in infancy) are cognitively intact. This is also reflected in neuroimaging, with damage to cranial nerves, the brain stem and cerebellum, but with no evidence of damage to the cerebral cortex or hippocampus (Manole, Jaunmuktane, & Hargreaves , 2017).

Although the deficiency state does not seem to be associated with cognitive deterioration, it has been suggested that due to its prominent role in mitochondrial health that hypovitaminosis states like those of old age may impair cognition, and that supplementation in certain diseases may be beneficial. For the former, one Chinese prospective longitudinal study identified lower vitamin B2 levels to be associated with declines in general cognitive ability and more specifically with learning and memory (Tao, Liu, & Chen, 2019). For its effect on disease, vitamin B2 can serve as a prophylactic treatment for migraine, reducing headache frequency, although the precise mechanism is not understood. It has also been suggested that its neuroprotective effects (i.e., via mitochondrial health and reduction of oxidative stress), which may make it a potential adjunct treatment for neurodegenerative conditions (Marashly & Bohlega, 2017).

9.2.4 Vitamin B3 (Nicotinamide Adenine Dinucleotide)

The active form of vitamin B3 (NAD; Nicotinamide adenine dinucleotide) can be obtained by dietary consumption of nicotinamide or niacin, and from consumption of the amino acid tryptophan, which can then be converted into NAD (see Figure 9.1). Nicotinamide, niacin and tryptophan can all be obtained from animal protein sources and from nuts, mature wholegrains and fortified foods (Rennie et al., 2015). Some important plant-based sources of niacin are in the form of niacin glycoside (e.g., notably in corn) and these have low bioavailability unless the corn is processed by the addition of an alkaline solution (a process termed nixtamalisation) traditionally using either wood ash or slaked lime. Not only does this improve the flavour and texture of the corn, enabling it to be

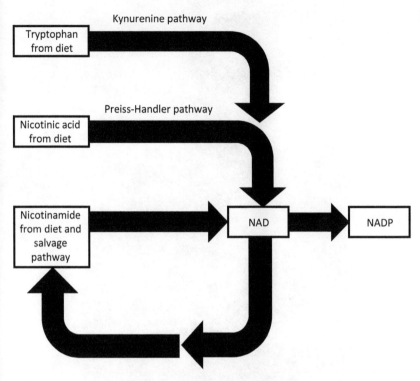

Figure 9.1   Generation of vitamin B3

formed into a dough, but more crucially it makes the niacin available for absorption by the gut (Gasperi et al., 2019).

Historically, a reliance on corn and access to minimal quantities of animal protein were the major contributory factors to the high prevalence of vitamin B3 deficiency – pellagra; see Figure 9.2 – between 1900 and 1940 in the southern parts of the United States. During this period more than 3 million people developed pellagra and more than 100,000 died (Rajakumar, 2000). As with many other nutritional deficiencies, it was at first believed to be an infectious disease. However, adept detective work by Dr Joseph Goldberger demonstrated that protein-rich foods ameliorated its effects, and that removing such foods from the diet, in a study done on prison inmates, resulted in the development of pellagra. The name pellagra comes from the Italian word for rough skin, and as the name implies this deficiency disease is characterised by its impact on skin exposed to sunlight (see Figure 9.2), as well as its effects on the gut and brain. This symptom

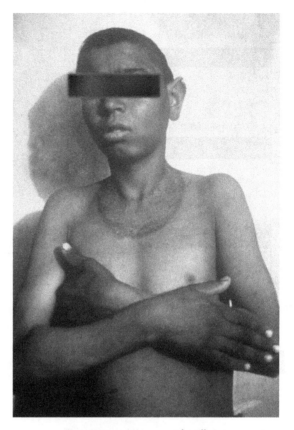

Figure 9.2   A person with pellagra

profile has traditionally been termed the three Ds: dermatitis, diarrhoea, and delirium, with some adding a fourth D – death (Brown, 2010).

Traditional cultures avoided pellagra by nixtamalisation, but contemporary cases now occur where diets have shifted to rely more upon refined carbohydrates with low animal protein intake. In industrialised countries, many of the same groups identified for the other B-group vitamins are vulnerable. People with digestive problems who cannot absorb nutrients efficiently (e.g., Crohn's disease), malnourishment from cancer or anorexia, certain drugs (e.g., isoniazid) and alcoholism can all impair absorption of niacin and nicotinamide (de Oliveira Alves, Bortalto, & Filho, 2017). Alcoholic pellagra is uncommon but can occur alone or in combination with the better recognised WE (B1 deficiency; Serdaru, Hausser-Hauw, & LaPlane, 1998). Differential diagnosis between

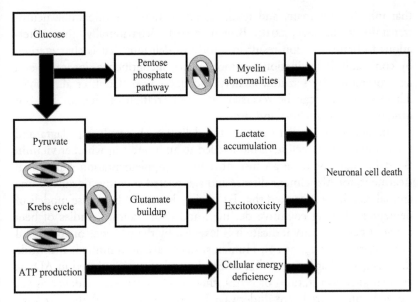

Figure 9.3   Points of impact (ovals with diagonal lines) of vitamin B3 deficiency on cellular metabolism and the routes to neuronal cell death

alcoholic pellagra and WE is difficult as both have neurological profiles that overlap, but the presence of the skin conditions associated with pellagra, and the absence of ocular signs, can distinguish the two (Cook, Hallwood, & Thomson, 1998; de Oliveira Alves et al., 2017).

One of the reasons that pellagra manifests as a skin, gut and brain disease is that it affects tissues with high energy requirements and cell turnover. This is because NAD plays a critical role in cellular metabolism, especially in the Krebs cycle and ATP production, and also in the synthesis of nucleotides used in DNA from the pentose phosphate pathway (Rennie et al., 2015) – see Figure 9.3. In addition, it serves as a coenzyme in the generation of many important proteins involved in cell survival (sirtuins) and DNA repair (PARPs). Vitamin B3 deficiency has both direct and indirect impacts on the brain. Directly, it reduces neuroprotection and neurogenesis by increasing competition for NAD between different protein-manufacturing operations in the cell, resulting in a reduction in proteins involved in neuronal cell survival, DNA repair and inflammation (Lautrup et al., 2019). Indirectly, it alters the kynurenine pathway so that tryptophan gets preferentially converted into NAD. This has the effect of generating neurotoxic by-products, reducing production of kynurenic acid that inhibits glutamate, and reducing production of monoamine neuro-transmitters (Badawy, 2014; Brown, 2010). Behaviourally, these alterations to brain function result in a form of delirium that is characterised by confusion, hallucinations, tremor, ataxia, incontinence, insomnia and less commonly by seizures, anxiety and depression (Cook et al., 1998). These symptoms can be reversed by administration of vitamin B3, but otherwise result in coma and death.

The apparent parallel between the delirium observed in pellagra and the dementia and decline of old age led to an interest in whether vitamin B3 deficiency could be a cause of, and its supplementation a potential treatment, for Alzheimer's disease and age-related cognitive decline. Some animal data have suggested that B3 may be beneficial in mouse models of dementia (slowing cognitive decline), and tissue culture studies of beta amyloid neurotoxicity indicate it is lessened by the presence of additional NAD (Gasperi et al., 2019). Human studies have been limited, and while there is general agreement that cerebral metabolism is reduced in AD, as are neural concentrations of NAD, there is no consistent evidence as yet (several clinical trials are underway; Lautrup et al., 2019) that B3 may serve as a treatment for Alzheimer's dementia (Gasperi et al., 2019; Song et al., 2019).

Age-related cognitive decline seems to have many of the same biochemical characteristics that occur during B3 deficiency – inflammation, impaired neurogenesis, increased oxidative stress – as well as lower levels of NAD (Gasperi et al., 2019). However, age-related cognitive decline is not ameliorated by vitamin B3 supplementation, as indicated by a well-powered study exploring its impact in elderly Australians (Martin, Dhillon, & Vardy, 2019). While there is a growing body of evidence to suggest that B3 may be an effective neuroprotectant following ischaemic injury to the brain (Gasperi et al., 2019), and possibly as an adjunct treatment in some people with Parkinson's disease (Belarbi et al., 2017), its role as an agent and treatment in other conditions (Huntington's disease, schizophrenia, migraine, ALS) is still being explored (Gasperi et al., 2019).

9.2.5   Vitamin B5 (Phosphopantetheine)

Vitamin B5 is found in many foodstuffs in the form of phosphopantetheine, with the richest sources being animal foods such as offal, beef and chicken, as well as peanuts, almonds and cheese (Kelly, 2011). Hypovitaminosis B5 may occur in the elderly, in the young and in pregnant women, generally through inadequate dietary intake. Vitamin

B5 is absorbed in the small intestine and actively transported across the blood-brain barrier by the sodium-dependent multivitamin transporter. The synthesis of coenzyme A (CoA) and Acyl Carrier Protein (ACP) are both dependent on an adequate supply of vitamin B5. CoA is necessary for the Krebs cycle, as well as serving as a coenzyme in multiple biochemical reactions, including key products necessary for brain function such as acetylcholine, steroid hormones and phospholipids. Deficiency states have been examined in both animals and humans, with similar consequences. Human studies have utilised a B5-deficient diet in addition to the administration of a drug to block vitamin B5's action (Kelly, 2011). This takes about 6 weeks to produce the deficiency syndrome, which is characterised by fatigue, headache, gastrointestinal disturbances, sleep impairment, personality changes, motor abnormalities and paraesthesia (e.g., burning hands and feet). There is considerable individual variation in symptom presentation, but it is accompanied by distinctive hypertrophy of the adrenal and thymus glands.

The neurological features of B5 deficiency are especially apparent in a related genetic disorder, called Hallervorden–Spatz syndrome. This syndrome is caused by a dysfunction of the enzyme pantothenic acid kinase, which forms the first part of the synthesis pathway of CoA. While the enzyme is present in the cytosol, it fails to transfer to mitochondria, where it is required (Johnson, Kuo, & Westaway, 2004). This leads to initial motor abnormalities that progressively worsen into a dementia-like state, coma and death, with median onset in late adolescence (Dooling, Schoene, & Richardson, 1974). The dementia-like state observed in Hallervorden–Spatz syndrome has (again) stimulated interest in whether B5-related processes may be abnormal in other forms of dementia. Examination of the brains of people with Alzheimer's disease indicate that they have vitamin B5 levels some 30–50% lower than healthy control brains, with the most notable reduction in areas strongly linked to disease onset (i.e., hippocampus, entorhinal cortex). In addition, a small proportion of people with Alzheimer's disease also possess auto-antibodies to pantothenic acid kinase, suggesting that disruption of the synthesis of CoA may sometimes participate in the origin of this disorder (Wang et al., 2020).

9.2.6 Vitamin B6 (Pyridoxal 5'-Phosphate)

Vitamin B6 comprises a number of biochemicals that can be interconverted to form pyridoxal 5'-phosphate. This micronutrient is widely available in plant and animal foods, being most concentrated in pork and other meats, wholegrains, bananas and eggs, and also in fortified foods (e.g., breakfast cereals). Vitamin B6 passively diffuses across the gut wall as well as being actively transported. In the liver it is phosphorylated and circulates in this form, but it requires dephosphorylation before it can cross the blood-brain barrier. As vitamin B6 levels are higher in the brain than in plasma, it would seem likely that some form of active transport ensures this gradient, but the specific transporter mechanism is not known (Tiani et al., 2019).

Functionally, vitamin B6 is involved as a coenzyme in more than 100 biochemical reactions. The deficiency state, which is better studied in animals than in people, includes anaemia, seizures, peripheral neuropathies, immune depression and an elevated risk of certain cancers (Spinneker, Sola, & Lemmen, 2007). In the brain, vitamin B6 serves as a coenzyme in the production of the neurotransmitters GABA, serotonin, dopamine, histamine, glycine and D-serine, in addition to its roles in nucleic acid synthesis, production of phospholipids and myelin (Sato, 2018; Spinneker et al., 2007).

Hypovitaminosis B6 has been documented in certain subgroups in US surveys, notably young women, women using the contraceptive pill, smokers, African Americans and the elderly. In the UK, hypovitaminosis B6 has been estimated to occur in 10% of children and in up to a quarter of adults, with lower levels common in the elderly and in the third trimester of pregnancy (Deijen et al., 1992; van de Rest, Van Hooijdonk, & Doets, 2012). Where there are problems eating food or in absorbing nutrients, hypovitaminosis becomes more likely.

Given the relative commonness of hypovitaminosis B6, there have been both animal and human investigations of whether supplementation may benefit cognition. In animals, supplementation in mice leads to improved memory performance, in addition to changes in neurotransmitter levels in the hippocampus (Jung, Kim, & Nam, 2017). Similar effects have been claimed in humans. Deijen et al. (1992) recruited healthy elderly participants who completed a neuropsychological test battery prior to and after 3 months of either vitamin B6 or placebo supplementation. There were some small improvements in both short-term and long-term memory performance, but with its modest sample size (n = 38 per group) the study may have been underpowered. A larger longitudinal study was reported by Hughes, Ward, and Tracey (2017) who followed a group of 155 healthy elderly participants to determine if B-group vitamins measured in bloods at baseline could predict subsequent cognitive decline (using the mini-mental state exam). After controlling for vitamins B3, B9 and B12 and an extensive range of demographic factors, vitamin B6 was the only significant predictor of cognitive decline. The same result was obtained when vitamin levels were estimated from dietary intake at baseline rather than from bloods. While these findings are favourable, there are several cross-sectional and longitudinal studies that have not found this type of relationship, and evidence from interventional studies is still inconclusive (van de Rest et al., 2012).

9.2.7   Vitamin B7 (Biotin)

Vitamin B7 is found in most foods, but is particularly concentrated in egg yolk, offal, green leafy vegetables, avocado and cheese. In food it is found in a protein-bound form, which is broken down in the small intestine to biocytin. Transport across the gut wall and blood-brain barrier involves the same mechanisms as for vitamin B5. In the body, biocytin is converted into its active form biotin by the enzyme biotinidase. One of the main functions of biotin is to serve as a coenzyme for several carboxylase enzymes, which requires the involvement of a further enzyme holocarboxylase (Rosko et al., 2019; Zempleni, Wijeratne, & Hassan, 2009).

Vitamin B7 deficiency may occur in children in developing countries through dietary insufficiency (Leon-Del-Rio, 2019). Hypovitaminosis B7 can occur in people who consume excessive quantities of egg whites as part of fad diets, as these contain the protein avidin that binds biotin, preventing absorption. Hypovitaminosis has also been observed in smokers and pregnant women, who excrete biotin at higher rates than normal, and in people taking certain medications, notably anti-convulsants (Zempleni et al., 2009).

Biotin deficiency manifests as dermatitis, conjunctivitis and alopecia, followed by the neurological symptoms of ataxia, hypotonia and seizures. If untreated, coma and death can occur. The neurological symptoms are delayed because the brain defends its biotin supplies. Biotin has seen use as a treatment in two neurological disorders. It has been suggested as a treatment in MS, as it is known to promote myelin synthesis (Rosko et al., 2019), and while some trials have been favourable, more recent studies have not been supportive (Leon-Del-Rio, 2019). Biotin has also been used in conjunction with thiamine to treat a rare genetic disorder resulting from a mutation in a thiamine transporter gene. It is unclear why biotin is able to assist in remediating the effects of a central thiamine deficiency (Tabarki, Al-Shafi, & Al-Shahwan, 2013).

9.2.8   Vitamin B9 (Folate)

Vitamin B9 refers to the folate family, a group of related organic molecules that come either from naturally occurring folates in nuts and green vegetables or from folic acid supplementation of bread, rice or maize. Insufficient folate during pregnancy raises the risk of neural tube and heart defects, a major motivator for deliberate dietary supplementation. Folate deficiency in adults manifests medically as megaloblastic anaemia, because inadequate supply of folate hinders cell division and hence the generation of new red blood cells (Alpert & Fava, 1997). The impacts extend beyond this, as folate is critical for more than 30 biochemical reactions that require transmethylation, including the production of several neurotransmitters. It is not surprising then that folate deficiency impacts brain function. Before turning to examine the neurocognitive impacts of folates, it is important to note that several other B-group vitamins are involved in both the synthesis of 5-methyltetrahydrofolate and its deployment in transmethylation (especially B12, but also B6 and B3). It is for this reason that many studies exploring the impacts of folate deficiency also concurrently measure other B-group vitamins, and notably B12 (folate can mask B12 deficiency).

Folate deficiency can arise in several different ways, including damage to the gut wall in conditions like Crohn's disease, inadequate dietary consumption, alcoholism, and from a number of commonly used drugs (e.g., certain oral contraceptives), some of which target or affect folate metabolism (e.g., methotrexate, valproic acid). Folate hypovitaminosis may be quite common.

The impact of folate deficiency on the brain seems to have been first noted by Herbert (1961), who subjected himself to a largely folate-free diet for 4 months to understand its effects. The neurocognitive impacts were insomnia, irritability, fatigue and forgetfulness, which agree with more contemporary understanding of its putative consequences: depression, cognitive impairment and dementia (Alpert & Fava, 1997; Miller, 2004). For depression, a number of cross-sectional studies have linked low folate levels with depression (e.g., Pan, Chang, & Yeh, 2012). Folate may enhance the effectiveness of serotonin-selective reuptake inhibitors such as fluoxetine, but clinical trials using folate as a primary treatment for depression have not produced a clear picture (Miller, 2004).

Findings on the cognitive profile of folate deficiency are more consistent, notably hippocampal-dependent learning and memory impairments, which have also been suggested by animal models (Kruman et al., 2005). Elderly participants with low folic acid levels (and with no related impact from B12 levels) have been found to have poorer verbal and object recall (with intact recognition; Hassing et al., 1999). Longitudinal evidence has also been obtained, with Qin, Xun, and Jacobs (2017) reporting on follow-up testing of CARDIA study participants (Coronary Artery Risk Development in Young Adults). Baseline levels of folate were independently (from B3, B6 and B12) predictive of memory performance (delayed verbal memory), in addition to two other tests (Stroop, digit symbol substitution test) conducted 25 years later. These analyses controlled for an extensive array of covariates, suggesting folate levels as one predictor, and B3, B6 and B12 as other independent predictors of long-term cognitive function. Where the folate deficiency is sufficient to produce overt medical symptoms (i.e., anaemia) it may impair performance on general intelligence tests and result in cerebral atrophy on MRI, both of which improve following folate supplementation (Botez, Botez, & Maag, 1984).

The cross-sectional evidence favouring a link between Alzheimer's disease and low folate levels is well established, finding in addition (and independently of folate) that low levels of vitamins B9 and B12 are similarly linked (Vogel et al., 2009). A consistent biochemical observation in people with Alzheimer's disease is elevated levels of the amino acid homocysteine (Hinterberger & Fischer, 2013). One cause for this is folate deficiency, which is involved in the transmethylation of homocysteine into methionine, a process that also requires vitamin B12 as an enzymatic co-factor. Homocysteine is one putative pathway to neural damage as it is pro-inflammatory and causes oxidative stress (Hinterberger & Fischer, 2013). However, the relationship between folate levels and Alzheimer's disease also seems to be independent of homocysteine levels, suggesting that other biochemical pathways mediate this relationship (Ma, Wu, & Zhao, 2017; Ramos, Allen, & Mungas, 2005).

Longitudinal findings have been more equivocal. Data from the Framingham study was used to examine if change in cognitive function (mini-mental state exam) over an 8-year period were predicted by folate and B12 levels at baseline (Morris, Selhub, & Jacques, 2012). The key observation was that an interaction between folate and B12 was predictive of the most rapid cognitive decline. Nonetheless, it still unclear if folate specifically is a direct contributor to Alzheimer's disease or if abnormal folate metabolism is a consequence. Similar uncertainty surrounding its links to cognition and depression.

9.2.9   Vitamin B12 (Cobalamin)

The main source of cobalamin (vitamin B12) is meat and dairy products. Following proteolysis in the stomach, cobalamin binds to intrinsic factor secreted by gastric parietal cells. This complex is then transported across the gut wall by the cubam receptor and then into the bloodstream via the MDR1 receptor. In the blood it binds with the transcobalamin carrier to form holotranscobalamin (Green, Allen, & Bjørke-Monsen, 2017). This is then taken up into cells around the body where it participates as a coenzyme in two key processes, the conversion of homocysteine to methionine (which importantly requires vitamin B9) and of methylmalonyl-coenzyme A to succinyl-coenzyme A. The former is necessary for the synthesis of thymidine (for DNA replication/repair) and the latter for a major metabolic pathway – the Krebs cycle (Green et al., 2017). It is not currently understood how vitamin B12 crosses the blood-brain barrier (Tiani et al., 2019); however, two things that have come to light are particularly important for considering the human literature on vitamin B12 and brain function. The first is that there may be no correlation between plasma-based measures of vitamin B12 (of which there are several) and levels of B12 in the brain (Tiani et al., 2019). The second is that there is likely to be some form of interaction with B9 levels, and there is some evidence that high levels of folate combined with low levels of B12 may be particularly deleterious for cognition in the elderly (Moore, Ames, & Mander, 2014).

The classic deficiency disease in which vitamin B12 is a significant cause is pernicious anaemia, which is an autoimmune condition. In pernicious anaemia, the immune system causes atrophic gastritis. One consequence of this is that gastric parietal cells no longer secrete intrinsic factor, which results in no absorption of vitamin B12 by the gut. The anaemia arises in much the same way as it does in vitamin B9 deficiency (folic acid), as impaired DNA replication leads to the production of large numbers of immature red blood cells, which are inefficient at carrying oxygen (Stabler, 2013).

Pernicious anaemia is accompanied by a variety of neurological manifestations (Gupta, Gupta, & Gupta, 2016; Sharrief, Raffel, & Zee, 2012). These include neuropathy, myelopathy, extra-pyramidal signs, sensory disturbances and impaired cognition (reductions in measures of general intelligence, memory and attention; Gupta et al., 2016; Sharrief et al., 2012). Imaging suggests widespread damage to the brain and spinal cord, notably with demyelination of white matter tracts, caused by B12 deficiency. While supplementation produces significant improvement in function, imaging suggests that the damage associated with B12 deficiency is still evident at least a year later (Sharrief et al., 2012).

There are somewhere between 50–4,000 cases of atrophic gastritis, and resultant pernicious anaemia, per 100,000 people. (Stabler, 2013). It occurs in all age groups but is far more common in the elderly, with a prevalence of up to 20% in those aged 70+ and is more frequent in people of Caucasian and African descent. The elderly may be susceptible to some level of vitamin B12 deficiency through age-related reductions in gut absorptive capacity and because the multiple pharmaceuticals they may be taking can also interfere with absorption (Pfisterer et al., 2016). Pfisterer et al. (2016) examined plasma levels of vitamin B12 in elderly care home residents, finding 14% with a deficiency, and 40% with a hypovitaminosis for B12. Another at-risk group are vegans who do not consume meat, dairy or eggs, and some vegetarians, and especially children raised on vegan diets who have unfortunately supplied important data on the effects of B12 deficiency on cognitive development (see Chapter 2).

More than 50 years of research has linked hypovitaminosis B12 to cognitive decline in the elderly (O'Leary et al., 2012). This can occur via a number of causal pathways: (1) reductions in DNA synthesis with its multiple knock-on consequences for brain function and metabolism; (2) the accumulation of homocysteine and methylmalonic acid (MMA) from reduced synthesis – noting that MMA is a neurotoxin – and the adverse effects of homocysteine on vascular health; and (3) the white matter damage characteristic of B12 deficiency states. While there seem to be good biochemical grounds for an effect, the evidence is not that support- ive. Some studies find that *elevated* B12 levels are linked to cognitive decline and higher rates of mortality (Cappello, Cereda, & Rondanelli, 2017; da Rosa, Beck, & Colonetti, 2019), others find little support for slowing cognitive decline with vitamin supplementation (van der Zwaluw, Brouwer-Brolsma, & van de Rest, 2017) and still others report cognitive benefits (Smith, Smith, & de Jager, 2010; Tangney, Aggarwal, & Li, 2011).

Early systematic reviews of this literature were ambivalent as to the benefits of B12 supplementation in the elderly, MCI or Alzheimer's disease groups (Balk, Raman, & Tatsioni, 2007; O'Leary et al., 2012). The most recent systematic review concludes that B12 (and B6 and B9) supplementation has no significant benefit in either the cognitively intact or impaired elderly (Ford & Almeida, 2019). While this is a disappointing conclusion to a large body of work, it is important to bear in mind the caveats noted earlier about B-group vitamin interactions and the apparent absence of a correlation between brain and plasma vitamin B12 levels. It may be that only a subset of the elderly actually have low brain levels of B12, as a reliance on plasma levels may be misleading.

9.2.10   Vitamin C (Ascorbic Acid)

Vitamin C refers to the lactone ascorbic acid, which is a water-soluble micronutrient that cannot be synthesised by humans, other primates or guinea pigs. The main dietary source of vitamin C is fresh fruit, especially citrus and some berries and potatoes, tomatoes and some green vegetables. Ascorbic acid is absorbed by the gut, with this process decreasing in efficiency as the amount of glucose present increases. As with the other micronutrients, there is a gradient from deficiency to hypovitaminosis through into the normal range. It is estimated that 10–15% of adults in Westernised countries have hypovitaminosis C, making this the fourth most prevalent nutritional deficiency in the United States (Brown, 2015; Travica, Ried, & Sali, 2019). Certain groups have far higher rates of hypovitaminosis C, including the elderly (estimated to be around 25% with hypovitaminosis), low SES groups and people in developing countries, primarily as their diet may be insufficient in this vitamin. Pregnant women are at risk through having to supply this vitamin for their foetus. Smokers have been consistently found to have higher rates of hypovitaminosis C, as do people with gut disorders (absorption problems), and alcoholics (Hansen, Tveden-Nyborg, & Lykkesfeldt, 2014).

The classic deficiency state for vitamin C is scurvy (see Figure 9.4). This is characterised by joint pain, tiredness, low mood and slow wound healing, and as it worsens, bleeding from the skin and gums, usually followed by death from infection. Studies on conscientious objectors in World War II and of prisoners exposed to vitamin C-deficient diets, indicate that around 4–6 weeks is needed before the first symptoms emerge (Brown, 2015). The earliest signs are neuropsychiatric – apathy, irritability, psychomotor slowing, nervousness and depression. A spectrum of extra-pyramidal symptoms is also observed, with psychomotor slowing the commonest, extending to resting tremor and dyskinesia. While these effects are reversible following vitamin C supplementation, deficiency during pregnancy (see Chapter 2), especially at the severe end, is often fatal (Hansen et al., 2014).

Vitamin C is involved in a range of different brain functions, with most data coming from animal studies. It enters the brain by utilising both a

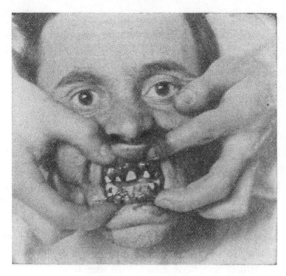

Figure 9.4   The gums of a person with scurvy

special active transporter (SDVC-2) and glucose transporters, with the brain maintaining levels of vitamin C up to 20–30 times that of plasma levels (e.g., Paidi et al., 2014). The brain is also able to recycle some of its vitamin C and brain levels remain well above plasma levels even during deficiency. Vitamin C serves as a co-factor for several enzymes used in neurotransmitter synthesis (e.g., norepinephrine), it has neuromodulatory functions (especially for glutamate) and it induces neurotrophin production (Travica, Ried,, & Sali, 2017, 2019). Vitamin C is also necessary to synthesise carnitine, which itself has several brain functions (e.g., GABA and glutamate synthesis, neuronal uptake of choline). Of all vitamin C's roles, its use as an antioxidant (i.e., regulating oxidative stress) is perhaps the most well known, with this being critical in highly metabolically active tissues such as the brain. In addition, vitamin C is necessary for the production of collagen and it is the failure of this pathway which produces many of the physical signs of scurvy (i.e., bleeding gums and skin). Collagen is also required for angiogenesis in the brain, and so deficiency is suspected to impact regions with high neuronal growth (and hence extension of the vasculature), such as the hippocampus.

Animal studies suggest that reduced or absent vitamin C during adulthood can lead to the sort of changes observed during Alzheimer's disease – increased oxidative stress, beta amyloid production, deposition and oligomerisation (e.g., Dixit, Bernardo, & Walker, 2015). While vitamin C levels do appear to be lower in people with Alzheimer's disease (Travica et al., 2017), there is mixed support for whether vitamin C supplementation can improve cognition – with a similarly mixed picture in animal models too (Hansen et al., 2014).

In healthy elderly participants (and possibly younger samples too; Travica et al., 2019), there is fairly consistent evidence of a link between plasma vitamin C and better performance across a range of different neurocognitive domains (e.g., short-term memory, working memory, information processing, abstract thinking; Travica et al., 2017). For example, a New Zealand study on aging contrasted a group with hypovitaminosis C with normal controls. The hypovitaminosis group were more likely to be male, smokers and those with a lower SES, a higher BMI and poorer regulation of blood glucose. They also performed more poorly on a cognitive screening test, even after controlling for these other factors. Interventional studies are now needed to see if maintaining adequate vitamin C levels is usefully protective against cognitive decline in aging.

9.2.11   Vitamin D (Calcitriol)

Vitamin D refers to a group of related secosteroids (notably ergocalciferol, cholecalciferol, calcitriol) that can only be synthesised either via skin exposure to ultraviolet light or obtained from food (McCann & Ames, 2008). The main natural dietary sources are fatty fish, eggs and mushrooms, but several countries (e.g., United States, Finland) fortify milk or other foods to ameliorate deficiencies (Chiang, Natarajan, & Fan, 2016). Deficiency states are common. Worldwide, around one billion people have some degree of deficiency for vitamin D, with the most visible consequence being the bowed legs from bone softening in children called rickets (Annweiler, Dursun, & Feron, 2015). Deficiency is more commonly observed in the elderly, in pregnant women (where the foetus is reliant on maternal vitamin D), in people with less access to sun exposure, and also in those from the tropics who migrate to more northerly or southerly regions (e.g., Hayden, Sandle, & Berry, 2015; McCann & Ames, 2008).

Vitamin D is primarily associated with the regulation of calcium and phosphate metabolism (and hence its impact on bone health), immune function and foetal brain development; see Chapter 2 (Bivona, Gambino, Iacolino, & Ciaccio, 2019). Vitamin D achieves these effects by binding to its receptor located in the cell nucleus. A vitamin D precursor can pass into the brain via passive diffusion, where it is metabolised in neurons and glial cells into its active form – calcitriol (Anjum et al., 2018). Vitamin D receptors are very widely expressed in the animal brain (and presumably in ours too), where they modulate neurotrophin production, calcium binding and calcium channel proteins, and enzymes involved in neurotransmitter synthesis (McCann & Ames, 2008). Many of these functions serve a neuroprotective role, in addition to fostering synaptic plasticity (Bivona et al., 2019). Together, this would imply that vitamin D deficiency should have consequences for neural function and behaviour.

Several animal deprivation models have been studied. For rats, 4–6 weeks of vitamin D-deficient diet increases impulsiveness and reduces performance on tests of hippocampal-dependent learning and memory, while for mice, they demonstrate hyperlocomotion and sensory abnormalities (e.g., increased pain sensitivity, startle; Overeem et al., 2016). These effects are reversible, and at least in older rats, additional vitamin D seems to protect against the typical age-related decline in hippocampal-dependent learning and memory. This is consistent with cell culture studies that indicate vitamin D protects hippocampal tissue from excitotoxic insult (Cui, Gooch, & Groves, 2015). An important caveat with these rodent findings are there generalisability to humans – as little is known about the direct effects of vitamin D deficiency on human brain function. Rodents are nocturnal (i.e., reduced opportunity for UV exposure) and they can also rely upon another secosterol not available to humans, allowing them to mitigate some vitamin D deficiency effects (but which is not known).

Research on the effects of hypovitaminosis for vitamin D has examined its relationship with depression, with little favourable evidence as either a cause or treatment (Gowda et al., 2015; Okereke, Reynolds, & Mischoulon, 2020). The impact of hypovitaminosis D on cognition in the elderly has also been explored. Cross-sectional studies suggest that reduced sun exposure and lower vitamin D levels in older people are linked to poorer performance on general tests like the mini-mental state exam (Annweiler, Allali, & Allain, 2009), and on more specific tests such as those for episodic memory (i.e., hippocampal dependent), set-shifting and processing speed (Brouwer-Brolsma & de Groot, 2015). Some, but not all, longitudinal studies indicate that lower vitamin D levels are predictive of poorer cognitive outcomes. Some cross-sectional designs have also used neuroimaging, linking these results to vitamin D levels. These reveal brain atrophy in the parietal and occipital regions, the precuneus and prefrontal cortices, vascular abnormalities, larger ventricles and smaller medial temporal lobe structures in elderly people with lower relative to higher vitamin D levels (Brouwer-Brolsma & de Groot, 2015).

These findings have led to the question of whether vitamin D deficiency may be a risk factor for Alzheimer's disease. There is good evidence that lower vitamin D levels occur in people with Alzheimer's disease, and that lower vitamin D levels are a risk factor for dementia (Balion, Griffith, & Strifler, 2012). However, there is as yet no consensus as to whether these relationships indicate a causal role for vitamin D in cognitive decline and dementia. Indeed, a metanalysis of interventional studies, looking at healthy aged participants and those with minimal cognitive impairment, failed to find any global cognitive benefit of vitamin D supplementation (Suh, Kim, & Han, 2020).

9.2.12   Vitamin E (α-Tocopherol)

Vitamin E is found in a wide variety of foods, but especially in nuts, seeds and vegetable oils (olive, sunflower and safflower). Six different compounds form the vitamin E family, namely α-tocopherol, β-tocopherol, γ-tocopherol, α-tocotrienol, β-tocotrienol and γ-tocotrienol. While γ-tocopherol is the commonest by quantity in food, α-tocopherol is the main active form of the vitamin (Lee & Ulatowski, 2019) and reference to vitamin E refers to this form. During digestion, tocopherols and tocotrienols pass through the gut wall both by passive diffusion and via several different trans-membrane proteins (Reboul, 2018). These are then packaged into chylomicrons for transit via the hepatic portal vein to the liver. Hepatic cells then selectively move the α-tocopherol into very-low-density lipoproteins, which act to carry the vitamin to different cells in the body. This packaging process is undertaken by the enzyme α-tocopherol transporter protein (TTP), which is expressed most in hepatic cells (Copp, Wisniewski, & Hentati, 1999; Ulatowski & Manor, 2015). Once the blood-brain barrier is reached, transfer across is undertaken by receptor-mediated transcytosis, involving both SRB1 and afamin systems (Tiani, Stover, & Field, 2019). Vitamin E is then moved into specialised astrocytes, and through a process that is not fully understood, the vitamin is found to be more concentrated in some brain regions than others (Lee & Ulatowski, 2019).

Vitamin E has a number of functions, including in the regulation of gene expression, but its primary role is in limiting the damage caused by lipid peroxidation (Ulatowski & Manor, 2015). Reactive oxygen species interact with the fatty acid tails in the lipid bilayer that forms the membrane of every cell in the body. This creates a cascade of reactions, which both damage the integrity of the lipid bilayer by deforming the fatty acid tails and generate a range of breakdown products (4-hydroxy-2,3-nonenal (HNE), malondialdehyde (MDA), acrolein, F2-isoprostanes), which are in some cases toxic and mutagenic, especially at higher concentrations. The body has an array of enzymes to deal with this, such as superoxide dismutase, catalase and glutathione peroxidases, as well as antioxidants derived from foods, such as polyphenols and catechins. Of the latter food-based antioxidants, vitamin E is particularly important because it locates into the lipid bilayer to limit peroxidation occurring. While this is important for all cells, it is especially so for neurons, which are vulnerable to lipid peroxidation due to their high lipid content and sometimes extensive cell membranes. Consequently, a deficit in vitamin E should adversely affect the nervous system.

Most American adults, and particularly the obese, do not meet the recommended dietary intake for vitamin E, but do not seem to show any obvious consequences from this (Traber, 2014). Nonetheless, adult animals exposed to a vitamin E-deficient diet demonstrate increased anxiety (Desrumaux, Mansuy, & Lemaire, 2018) plus evidence of poorer hippocampal function, effects that have been attributed to oxidative stress (Fukui, Nakamura, & Shirai, 2015). Oxidative stress is also thought to have a central role in degenerative brain disorders such as Alzheimer's, Parkinson's, amyotrophic lateral sclerosis (ALS), in the secondary effects resulting from an initial brain injury and in depression. There is clear evidence that serum levels of vitamin E are reduced in Alzheimer's disease and in age-related cognitive degeneration (Ashley, Bradburn, & Murgatroyd, 2019). These observations, combined with the functions of vitamin E in the brain, have led to interest in using it as a treatment. While animal data have been supportive (Ricciarelli et al., 2007), human trials have not. Supplementary vitamin E neither slows nor ameliorates Alzheimer's disease (Ashley et al., 2019; Jia, McNeill, & Avenell, 2008). Although there has been less work, a similar conclusion has emerged for ALS, Parkinson's disease and the secondary consequences of brain injury (Dobrovolny, Smrcka, & Bienertova-Vasku, 2018). Finally, for depression, there is evidence of lower serum vitamin E levels in people with this disease, relative to controls, but the evidence is equivocal for supplementation assisting recovery or aiding prevention (Islam, Ali, & Karmoker, 2020).

9.2.13   Choline (Vitamin J or B Group)

Choline, also known as vitamin J and considered by some more properly part of the vitamin B group, was designated an essential nutrient in 1998 by the Institute of Medicine. It is found in several different available forms (e.g., sphingomyelin, phosphocholine) in many animal and plant foods, but especially rich sources are liver, eggs and wheat germ (Zeisel, 2006). Choline can be synthesised de novo by the body, but the amounts generated are insufficient to meet requirements. However, unlike the other essential nutrients, variation in the capacity to absorb, process and synthesise choline is marked. First, pre-menopausal women are able to synthesise choline to a far greater extent than men or post-menopausal women, due to oestrogen facilitating the synthesis pathway (da Costa, Kozyreva, & Song, 2006). This ability has probably been favoured by evolution, because pregnancy requires a major upswing in the amount of choline needed for foetal development, with failure to provide this risking foetal viability – see Chapter 2 (Korsmo, Jiang, & Caudill, 2019). Second, up to half of Western European descendants may have genetic polymorphisms that impairs their capacity to use or process choline effectively, meaning they require far more via diet than the guidelines would suggest (da Costa et al., 2006; Kohlmeier et al., 2005). Third, low intakes or levels of choline are observed in athletes, vegetarians/vegans, drug-users, alcoholics and in people in developing countries (Biasi, 2011).

Following absorption in the gut, transport to the liver depends on solubility. Water-soluble forms (e.g., choline) are carried directly in blood, and lipid-soluble forms are moved in chylomicrons (e.g., sphingomyelin). The liver is the main processing hub for choline, which is why deficiency particularly impacts this organ. Choline is moved into cells and relatedly across the blood-brain barrier, via one of three different families of choline transporters, which differ in their affinity for this nutrient (Fagerberg, Taylor, & Distelmaier, 2020). There are then three main biochemical fates for choline. The first, which is reversible, is the transformation of choline into the neurotransmitter acetylcholine, which utilises only a small fraction of available supply. The second, which is also reversible, is the synthesis of specific lipids for use in cell membranes and for the formation of myelin sheaths on certain nerve cells. The third, which is irreversible, is the generation of betaine, which then feeds into the regeneration of methionine. Choline is the single largest source of methyl groups for feeding into the methionine regeneration cycle, and as this involves other B vitamins, it was for this reason once considered a possible B-group member. Betaine is also available from dietary sources (e.g., prawns) and increasing intake of this nutrient reduces need for dietary choline.

In human adults, deficiency states have been experimentally produced by placing subjects on 7 weeks of a low-choline diet. The impacts can be detected biochemically, mainly on the liver, muscles and kidneys (da Costa et al., 2006), but it does not seem to cause any harm to the central nervous system, unlike in animals where it impacts hippocampal-dependent learning and memory (Biasi, 2011). Adult supplementation with choline has been found to aid learning and memory, plus improving other cognitive domains, however there are as many studies that find no effects. A similarly equivocal picture emerges in its use as a treatment or disease-slowing agent, in Alzheimer's disease (Biasi, 2011; Korsmo, Jiang, & Caudill, 2019; Zeisel, 2006).

9.2.14 Vitamin K (Phylloquinone)

Vitamin K is composed of a group of lipid-soluble vitamers. These are phylloquinone (vitamin K1), the menaquinones, which vary in the number of isoprenoid side chains (together, vitamin K2; but also MQ1–9 (sometimes MK1–9) depending on the number of side chains), and several synthetic forms (e.g., K3, menadione; Booth, 2009). The principal dietary source of K1 is green leafy vegetables. For K2, with the exception of MQ4, which is synthesised from K1 by an unknown pathway in the body, the remainder are obtained from gut bacterial processing of K1, and indirectly from consumption of fermented foods (i.e., from bacteria again). The principal function of vitamin K concerns blood coagulation, where it serves as an enzyme co-factor, but it also has roles in calcium metabolism and vascular function, and it has anti-inflammatory properties, as well as being protective against type II diabetes (Booth, 2009). It is also recognised as having several roles in brain function.

The form of vitamin K found in the brain (or at least the rodent brain, with the assumption this also applies to humans) is MQ4. This has its highest concentration in the midbrain, pons and medulla, and its lowest concentration in the cerebellum, olfactory bulb, thalamus, hippocampus and striatum (Ferland, 2012). It is unclear what this pattern of distribution means, how it is maintained, how (and if) it is synthesised in the brain and how it is transported. MQ4 has several functions. First, it serves as a co-factor for the enzyme coded for by growth arrest-specific gene 6 (Gas6). Gas6 has many roles in neurons and glia (e.g., cell survival, mitogenesis, cell signalling), and is expressed in multiple brains areas, but especially the cerebellum (perhaps the low levels of MQ4 here (see earlier) reflect high utilisation). Expression of Gas6 declines with age, and especially so in the hippocampus and frontal cortex. A second role for MQ4 is as a co-factor for the enzyme Protein S, which is normally involved in clotting. In the brain Protein S seems to be a neuroprotectant against the effects of ischaemic or hypoxic damage. Finally, MQ4 acts to promote sphingolipid metabolism, although this may be via Gas6.

Vitamin K's importance in brain function is suggested by the impacts of warfarin, which interferes with vitamin K metabolism and so impairs blood coagulation. Foetal exposure to warfarin causes multiple structural defects in the brain (ventricular enlargement, microencephalopathy) with related functional abnormalities (mental retardation, blindness), suggesting that vitamin K is involved in development (Alisi, Cao, & de Angelis, 2019). In adults, animal studies indicate that warfarin causes cognitive impairments in hippocampal-dependent learning and memory, as well as increasing anxiety as measured by the open field test (e.g., Tamadon-Nejad et al., 2018). In humans, warfarin reduces the risk of Alzheimer's disease because it decreases the likelihood of ischaemic events. However, there are indications that it also impairs hippocampal-dependent learning and memory (Ferland, Feart, & Presse, 2016), and that it is associated with reductions in grey and white matter volume on the right side of the brain (Alisi et al., 2019). The cognitive impacts of taking anticoagulants seem to be somewhat reduced if they do not affect vitamin K metabolism.

Animal data suggests that both MQ4 levels and Gas6 expression is reduced in the aging brain. This also seems to be the case in humans, and especially so in Alzheimer's disease, where it has been suggested that vitamin K may be protective. Gas6 seems to impair the capacity of beta amyloid to kill brain cells, while as noted earlier, protein S may be neuroprotective during ischaemic events (i.e., with relevance to multi-infarct dementia). It is, however, unlikely that vitamin K will serve as an effective treatment, because its effects may be protective rather than restorative – but this remains to be established. There is, however, cross-sectional evidence indicating a protective role of vitamin K both in healthy aging and in people with cognitive impairment. This has been observed with multiple cognitive measures and in many diverse populations (e.g., Chouet, Ferland, & Féart, 2015; Soutif-Veillon, Ferland, & Rolland, 2016). Unfortunately, the only longitudinal prospective trial found no benefit of higher vitamin K levels (Alisi et al., 2019).

9.3   Minerals

9.3.1   Iodine

Iodine is present in low concentrations in vegetable and animal foods, with seafood and seaweed being rich sources. Iodine levels in vegetable and animal foods depend upon the quantity of iodine in the soil. Certain regions are known to have low soil iodine levels and these are called 'goitre-belts' after the characteristic thickening of the neck seen in chronic iodine deficiency. Notorious goitre-belts are in midwestern United States, south Australia, the Alps, the Apennine mountains in the United States, and inland UK and Wales (Zimmerman & Boelaert, 2015). Other factors also contribute to iodine deficiency. Certain chemicals in food can affect the bioavailability of iodine, and these are termed goitrogens of which there are many (Delange, 1994). The genus *Brassica* (e.g., cabbage, broccoli, brussels sprouts) and staple crops such as cassava, sweet potato and lima beans contain, respectively, thioglucosides and cyanglucosides, which impair the ability to utilise dietary iodine. Iodine utilisation is also impaired by other nutritional deficiencies, notably iron, selenium and folate (Zimmerman, 2009).

Once iodine is consumed, it is actively extracted from the luminal content in the small intestine. From the bloodstream it is taken up by the thyroid gland, where it is used to produce two of the three hormones made by this structure. The largest proportional hormone product of the thyroid is thyroxine (T4), with smaller quantities of the main bioactive form triiodothyronine (T3) also produced (Chiovato, Magri, & Carlé, 2019). These are then released into the bloodstream in protein-bound form, and both T3 and T4 are actively transported into the brain using at least two different transporters across the blood-brain barrier. The regulation of T3/4 is carefully controlled. First, if T3/4 levels fall, the pituitary gland in the brain secretes thyroid-stimulating hormone (TSH), which among other effects increases the efficiency with which the thyroid extracts iodine from the blood. Second, T3/4 levels are controlled by a series of enzymes (deiodinases), which serve to convert the less-active T4 into T3 (type-2 deiodinase found in glia and astrocytes), and to convert both T3/4 into a temporarily inactive form (type-3 deiodinase found in neurons). These enzymes provide tight control of T3/4 across the brain, allowing greater expression in some areas over others (Bunevičius & Prange, 2010). The brain and the body also possess multiple types of thyroid receptors

(TRs), and while there are two main ones, each has several isoforms. The TRs serve to regulate the expression of particular genes, with T3 needed to switch them on and off. The proteins regulated in this way are critical both for brain development (and T3/4 have further roles too) and for neural plasticity. Not surprisingly, iodine deficiency has catastrophic effects on brain development in the foetus (see Chapter 2), as well as impairing learning and memory in children, adolescents and adults who are exposed to iodine-deficient diets (Leach & Gould, 2015).

Iodine deficiency has and continues to be a major public health problem. In the 1980s the WHO estimated that somewhere between 20% and 60% of the world's populace was iodine deficient (Zimmerman, 2009). With the widespread adoption of iodisation of salt, there has been major improvements in this regard. In 2014, 29 countries were deemed to have insufficient intake (112 countries with adequate intake; Zimmerman & Boelaert, 2015), and more recent estimates indicate 8.5% of the world's population are deficient, with around 5% in Europe (Chiovato et al., 2019; Eveleigh et al., 2020). Countries that are currently identified as having an iodine deficiency problem are Ethiopia, Morocco, Mozambique, Russia, Ukraine, Denmark, Italy and the UK.

Iodine deficiency in adults produces a range of biological effects, the most visible being swelling of the neck as the thyroid gland increases in size in response to the deficiency – goitre. Deficiency also manifests with impaired cognition and apathy (and possibly depression, but the link here is less certain), but these impacts are not in any way as severe as during brain development, and seem to be largely reversible when dietary iodine levels increase (Cooke et al., 2014; Leach & Gould, 2015). Some of the effects of iodine deficiency on the adult human brain can be inferred from the more detailed studies undertaken of other causes of hypothyroidism (e.g., autoimmune diseases) as well as from the large animal literature.

The animal findings point to a clear and consistent impact on the hippocampus, manifesting as impaired learning and memory. At the physiological level, this results from dysfunctional long-term potentiation (LTP). The cellular basis for this deficit results from the fact that thyroid hormones are needed to turn on genes for protein synthesis that support LTP and hence learning (Leach & Gould, 2015). In addition, lower T3/T4 levels act to reduce brain monoamines and slow hippocampal neurogenesis. These effects are reversed in animal models by administering synthetic thyroid hormones.

Adult humans with hypothyroidism are poorer on hippocampal-dependent learning and memory tasks. The neural impacts though seem to be wider than just the hippocampus, as neuroimaging indicates overall reductions in brain size and ventricular enlargement, which is reversible with thyroid hormone medication. More specific MRI examinations have found evidence of volume reductions in the hippocampus, which exceed the overall volume reductions in brain size (Cooke et al., 2014). The sensitivity of the hippocampus in both animal studies and human findings has led to interest in whether thyroid hormones play any role in the development of Alzheimer's disease (noting that this disease is also linked to other hormonal insufficiencies – insulin, cortisol, gonadal hormones). There is cross-sectional evidence for higher rates of Alzheimer's disease in people with hypothyroidism (2× greater risk), as well as some evidence that synthetic thyroid hormones can improve cognition in this disease (Bavarsad et al., 2018).

9.3.2 Iron

Dietary iron comes in two forms, heme and non-heme, with the former providing around 15% of intakes and the latter around 85%. Heme iron comes from meat (red and poultry), and non-heme iron from plant sources, with bioavailability improved with co-consumption of fermented foods and those rich in vitamin C and impaired by soy protein, and polyphenols (Hallberg, 2001). Heme iron is captured by a special gut receptor and its iron is made available alongside that from non-heme sources, to form an iron pool stored as a protein complex called ferritin. Iron is liberated from gut cells into the bloodstream via the ferroportin transporter, where it is immediately bound to a transferrin molecule. Transferrin delivers iron to various tissues, including the brain, where iron is moved across the blood-brain barrier via a receptor-mediated transporter. Apart from its specific roles in the brain, iron is a vital molecular component of haemoglobin (hence anaemia with severe iron deficiency), for immune function and as a co-factor for multiple enzymes (notably energy regulation, DNA synthesis). Unlike other micronutrients, the body's iron economy is regulated by absorption, as there is only very limited capacity for active excretion.

An iron concentration below that required for healthy functioning is the commonest adult deficiency disorder (Hallberg, 2001). Around half of all women of reproductive age are iron deficient, and even in developed countries such as the United States, 10–20% of menstruating women have insufficient levels, and even more so among adolescent girls (Beard & Connor, 2003; Bruner et al., 1996; Scott & Murray-Kolb, 2016). While consumption of less dietary iron than needed is one factor in the far higher rates of women with low iron (Farhat et al., 2019), the other is the loss of blood associated with menstruation. In addition, pregnancy and lactation impose further high demands for iron, and as discussed in Chapter 2, foetal iron deficiency – even if treated in infancy – has lifelong impacts on the brain and cognition (Algarin et al., 2017). Adolescence is another period where iron demands are high, and in fact these exceed requirements for adult menstruating women.

Iron is involved in a number of roles in the brain. As with other tissues, it serves as a co-factor for enzymes utilised in energy metabolism. One characteristic feature of iron deficiency is elevated blood glucose, and alterations in glucose transport into the brain. In animal models, three months of iron-deficient diet in adult rats produces significant changes in the proteome, especially relating to energy metabolism (Pino, Nishiduka, & da Luz, 2020). These changes occur even in the absence of anaemia, as the body recycles much of the iron used in red blood cells, as well as having a sophisticated response system to preserve oxygen delivery to tissues in the event of low iron availability (Hallberg, 2001). In addition to metabolic functions, iron serves as a co-factor for enzymes involved in dopamine and serotonin synthesis, and for the production of myelin by oligodendrocytes (Beard & Connor, 2003; Larsen, Bourque, & Moore, 2020). The distribution of iron in the brain is not homogenous, with high concentrations in the basal ganglia (Larsen et al., 2020), deep cerebellar nuclei, red nucleus and certain parts of the hippocampus. At least some of this heterogeneity is linked to dopamine metabolism (e.g., basal ganglia).

Perhaps not surprisingly, iron deficiency has been linked to cognitive impairment in both animal and human studies – although the findings are inconsistent – until one takes into account age and the magnitude of the deficiency. The clearest cognitive deficits emerge with anaemia, where iron levels are so low that haemoglobin concentration and adequate oxygen supply are compromised. Here fatigue and impaired ability to work are prominent symptoms, along with cold intolerance and problems concentrating. Khedr, Hamed, and Elbeih (2008) compared a group of young adult anaemics, with healthy controls. The anaemic group's iron deficiency stemmed primarily from chronic blood loss (heavy periods, nose bleeds, piles, parasites), and when they were tested on the Weschler memory and intelligence scales, they performed more poorly on nearly all measures, having a lower IQ and reduced mini-mental state score. Following iron supplementation, there was a significant improvement in IQ, and on some domains on the Weschler memory scale. These cognitive improvements were primarily correlated with increases in haemoglobin levels.

Apart from severity, the other factor that seems to be important is age. Bruner et al. (1996) noted improvements in hippocampal-dependent learning and memory (but not on tests of attention) in adolescents who had iron deficiency, but without any anaemia, following iron supplementation. As noted earlier, adolescents have high dietary needs for iron, and the brain is still actively increasing iron concentrations during this period (Larsen et al., 2020).

Studies in healthy adults are more mixed. Scott and Murray-Kolb (2016) examined for relationships between iron levels and cognitive performance in a non-anaemic cross-sectional sample of young women. Attention, inhibitory control and planning were better in women with higher iron levels (using multiple markers), while working memory was poorer (a number of other cognitive domains were not related to iron levels). Blanton et al. (2014) examined iron supplementation in healthy non-anaemic females via providing three beef meals a week (vs a control group with non-beef lunches) for 16 weeks. While biomarkers indicated an increase in iron levels in the treatment group, the lunch manipulation had no effect on cognitive performance (some positive cross-sectional findings were also obtained).

Finally, a large longitudinal study of late middle-aged adults (Andreeva, Galan, & Arnaud, 2013) examined whether baseline iron (ferritin) levels predicted cognition 6 years later. There were few effects, and none in men. Indeed, in the three significant relationships uncovered in this study – all in women – there were negative correlations, suggesting that higher iron levels were linked to poorer cognition (phonemic fluency, digit span, overall cognition). The tentative conclusion here is that while in adolescent samples deficiency may impair cognition, in older samples high iron levels may be associated with impairment. Notably, raised brain iron levels have been observed in Alzheimer's, Parkinson's and Huntington's disease (Larsen et al., 2020).

9.3.3   Zinc

Zinc can be obtained from foods that are rich in iron, notably beef (Sandstead, 2000). Certain diets predispose to zinc deficiency, where there is low red meat and seafood intake, with high consumption of unrefined cereals. Not only are unrefined cereals relatively low in zinc content, the phytic acid they contain binds zinc (and iron and calcium), lowering bioavailability (Warthon-Medina, Moran, & Stammers, 2015). Zinc deficiency is common, with around 20% of the world's population consuming less than the recommended daily intake (RDI). This is the case even in wealthier countries, with earlier dietary surveys suggesting that many Americans ate less than the RDI (Sandstead, 2000). The impacts of more severe zinc deficiency are profound. Worldwide, it is estimated to be responsible for 20% of perinatal deaths, 500,000 deaths in under 5s, and 800,000 deaths annually (Hagmeyer, Haderspeck, & Grabrucker, 2015). As this suggests, zinc deficiency is more common in infants and children (and more so in boys), in women, and in the elderly. This reflects diet, differing bodily needs (growth requiring increased zinc) and the bodies capacity to absorb zinc in the gut (especially in the elderly).

The body has an intricate set of systems to ensure zinc homeostasis, with the brain having a slower rate of zinc turnover and being more resistant to changes in zinc levels than the body (Takeda, 2001). Zinc is regulated in three main ways (Bitanihirwe & Cunningham, 2009). Its import into cells, including those of the gut, bodily cells, the blood-brain barrier, neurons and glia, is controlled by the Zrt and Irt-like protein transporters (collectively ZIPs), of which there are 15 different types. Once inside a cell, zinc has to be sequestered and stored, which is undertaken in two ways. First, all cells contain metallothioneins (of which there are four types, with multiple isoforms) which are capable of temporarily holding zinc and other biological and non-biological metals. Second, certain types of brain neurons have vesicles that specifically hold zinc. Its export from any cell type is regulated by the zinc transporters (ZnT), of which there are 10 different types (Hagmeyer et al., 2015). If zinc is exported into the bloodstream, it is carried bound to albumin.

Zinc has a number of general functions that are critical to all cells. It is a key structural component or co-factor to more than 300 enzymes, including ones involved in DNA transcription, and cellular metabolism for immune, hormonal and antioxidant functions (Bitanihirwe & Cunningham, 2009; Cuajungco & Lees, 1997; Takeda, 2001). In the brain, zinc is present in most regions, but concentration hotspots are found in the hippocampus, amygdala and neocortex. Zinc serves as a neuromodulator of GABAergic neurons and of certain glutaminergic neurons found in the hippocampus, amygdala and neocortex. In these zinc-containing glutaminergic neurons (called 'gluzinergic' or 'ZEN' (Zinc-enriched neuron)), zinc is concentrated in vesicles that are released into the synaptic cleft alongside glutamate following depolarisation. This may serve a number of roles, dampening excitability and reducing excitotoxicity, and facilitating neuronal structural changes that may underpin learning and memory. This is suggested by the effects of turning-off one of the brain's zinc transporters (ZnT3), which acts to increase seizure proneness in mice, and to impair learning and memory (Bitanihirwe & Cunningham, 2009; Hagmeyer et al., 2015). Additional learning- and memory-related functions have also been identified, with zinc activating cell signalling molecules, secondary messenger signalling, and facilitating neurogenesis in the hippocampus (via its role in transcription factors).

In adult humans, zinc deficiency has a number of symptoms (Hagmeyer et al., 2015; Sandstead, 2003). Skin lesions and hair loss are common, reflecting zinc's role in DNA transcription in tissues with a high cell turnover. There is also immune suppression and slowed wound healing. Almost all of the other symptoms relate to the central nervous system, including loss of appetite, sensory impairment (taste and smell probably due to high cell turnover), seizure susceptibility, visual problems, depression, irritability, anxiety, aggression and neuropsychological impairments (learning and memory, attention). In animal models of zinc deficiency, appetite loss appears rapidly following the onset of a zinc-deficient diet in initially healthy adult animals, and this may be due to another consequence of zinc deficiency, which is to induce corticosterone release, which can impair appetite (Takeda & Tamano, 2009).

Animal models suggest that 4 weeks of dietary deficiency is necessary to shift brain zinc levels. A notable effect is depression, which has been widely detected using behavioural tests in zinc-deficient animals (e.g., Tassebehji et al., 2008). There is also some interest in whether zinc deficiency may have a role in human depression. Cross-sectional data indicates low zinc levels in depressed participants, which normalises following anti-depressant treatment. Zinc can also function as an anti-depressant in animal models of depression and at least some of its effects in the brain impact systems implicated in causing depression (e.g., suppressed hippocampal neurogenesis; Szewczyk, Kubera, & Kowak, 2011).

Another related finding from animal models, and from human cross-sectional data, is the adverse impact on hippocampal-dependent learning and memory of zinc deficiency (Cuajungco & Lees, 1997; Penland, 2000). This has led to interest in the role of zinc in age-related cognitive decline and Alzheimer's disease. For age-related decline, the ZENITH trial conducted a well-powered placebo-controlled zinc supplementation study in healthy elderly adults, but found little cross-sectional or interventional support for a beneficial effect of zinc (Maylor, Simpson, & Secker, 2006). In Alzheimer's disease, some post mortem studies have found reduced levels of zinc in the hippocampus, while others have reported elevated zinc levels, linking this to beta amyloid plaque formation, oxidative stress, excitotoxicity and cell death (Bitanihirwe & Cunningham, 2009; Cuajungco & Lees, 1997). Abnormal zinc metabolism has also been reported in schizophrenia, autism spectrum disorder and ALS, and it is plausible that both low or high levels of zinc may exert similarly deleterious effects on brain function (Bitanihirwe & Cunningham, 2009).

9.3.4   Copper

The copper content of food is variable as it reflects the concentration of the water or soil in which it was grown. Foods with typically the highest copper content are organ meats, oysters and chocolate, but drinking water can also be an excellent source dependent upon having copper pipes and appropriate water pH (Olivares & Uauy, 1996). There is some disagreement over how many people have inadequate copper intake because there is no well-established biomarker to assess this (Freeland-Graves et al., 2020). Concerns have been raised that Western-style diets, which may be lower in copper than traditional diets, combined with the effects of modern agricultural practices that lead to reduction in soil copper levels, may result in many people in developed countries not consuming sufficient amounts (Freeland-Graves et al., 2020; Klevay, 2011). Deficiency states for copper have been reportedly documented amongst malnourished children, in premature infants, in people receiving enteral or parenteral feeding without adequate copper supplementation, people with celiac disease or gut malabsorption disorders, and more recently in people who have undergone small intestine shortening as part of bariatric surgery (Gupta & Lutsenko, 2009; Olivares & Uauy, 1996).

Once copper is ingested, it is transported into the cells of the gut wall via the CTR1 high-affinity copper transporter. Inside the cell, copper is carefully chaperoned by a variety of agents, and exits the cell via the ATP7A transporter (Scheiber, Mercer, & Dringen, 2014). In the blood copper is mainly bound to ceruloplasmin, but the transportable form seems to be via albumin, histidine or other small proteins (Ahuja et al., 2015; Zatta & Frank, 2007). The liver is the main storage site for copper in the body with excess copper excreted in bile (Madsen & Gitlin, 2007). The brain is a major user of copper, which is transported over the blood-brain barrier and into astrocytes and neurons using the same set of cellular transporters, CTR1 and ATP7A (Scheiber et al., 2014). Distribution of copper in the brain is heterogenous, with higher concentrations reported in the basal ganglia, cerebellum, hippocampus, locus coeruleus and in grey matter (Madsen & Gitlin, 2007; Scheiber et al., 2014; Zatta & Frank, 2007). Particular cell types have also been found to have higher copper concentrations notably glia, cortical pyramidal and cerebellar granule cells.

Copper is necessary for mitochondrial metabolism, with it serving as a co-factor for cytochrome C oxidase. Further general functions pertain to its role in managing oxidative stress (superoxide dismutase) and iron metabolism (ceruloplasmin). While both of these are generic to all bodily systems, copper deficiency may make the brain more susceptible to oxidative stress and dysregulation of brain iron metabolism has its own negative consequences on function (see above). More specific roles in the brain include neurotransmitter synthesis, with copper catalysing the production of noradrenalin, the amidation of neuropeptides, and the modulation of long-term potentiation in the hippocampus by release of vesicular copper (Madsen & Gitlin, 2007; Scheiber et al., 2014). Copper also serves non-enzymatic roles in angiogenesis, myelination and the action of endorphins (Zatta & Frank, 2007).

With these various functions, copper deficiency would be expected to cause neurocognitive problems. It certainly does during development, but in adulthood neurocognitive symptoms as a consequence of copper deficiency are rare. Rather than central deficits, the consequences are severe but localised to the peripheral nervous system and spinal cord, generating a reversible myeloneuropathy, which is also seen in ruminants grazed on copper-deficient soils (Madsen & Gitlin, 2007; Zatta & Frank, 2007). In fact, there is more evidence that higher intakes of copper may be more harmful to the brains of adults, than deficiencies (Takeuchi, Taki, & Nouchi, 2019).

9.3.5 Selenium

Selenium is obtained in two main forms, as selenomethionine in Brazil nuts, grains and legumes, and as methylselenocysteine in onion, garlic and leeks, and members of the genus *Brassica* (e.g., broccoli, cabbage; Whanger, 2001). It has been estimated that up to half a billion people worldwide may obtain less dietary selenium than they require (Gashu, Stoecker, & Bougma, 2016), with many also in developed countries and with deficiency more apparent with aging and in Alzheimer's disease (Cardoso, Ong, & Jacob-Filho, 2010). Selenium requirements fall into quite a narrow window, with too much being highly toxic and with too little producing deficiency states as described later.

After absorption, selenium is primarily stored and processed in the liver into an exportable form found in plasma, called selenoprotein P (SeP). Around 70% of plasma selenium is in this form, and it is the main vehicle for delivery of selenium to the brain, where it is moved across the blood-brain barrier by the ApoER2 and LRP8 transporters (Saito, 2020). SeP is then used to deliver selenium to various brain structures, with concentrations being highest in the cortex, cerebellum, pons, substantia nigra and hippocampus (Zhang et al., 2019). Selenium plays an important role in the management of oxidative stress, in both the body and brain. Humans have 25 selenoproteins, of which 5 are glutathione peroxidases (GPxs) and 3 thioredoxin reductases (TrxRs), all of which are neuroprotective antioxidants. In addition, there are three selenoprotein thyroid hormone deiodinases, which are necessary for normal thyroid function, but which do not seem to contribute to thyroid deficiency states (Arthur, Beckett, & Mitchell, 1999).

The brain is well defended against mild to moderate selenium deficiency, with bodily systems affected first (Berr, Arnaud, & Akbaraly, 2012). This is evident in Keshan disease, which was prevalent in China during the 1970s. The disease is an interaction between selenium deficiency and infectious disease. The high levels of oxidative stress resulting from a selenium-deficient diet provide an environment that facilitates an infectious coxsackie virus to mutate into a more virulent form resulting in severe and sometimes fatal damage to the heart. Keshan disease is not associated with any known neurological signs, suggesting the deficiency is not sufficient to affect brain concentrations of selenium (Berr et al., 2012). However, there is evidence that selenium deficiency can adversely affect brain function. Knockout mice that are unable to metabolise selenium do not live to term, and those with partial selenium deficiencies show neurological dysfunction (progressive spasticity) when exposed to a selenium-deficient diet (Saito, 2020). Effects are also detectable in healthy adult rats placed on a 3-week selenium-deficient diet, with impairments on hippocampal-dependent learning and memory, resulting from impaired long-term potentiation (Babur, Tan, & Yousef, 2019).

Apart from some rare genetic diseases affecting selenium metabolism that result in severe neurological symptoms (Zhang et al., 2019), significant deficits have only been observed in people on long-term total parenteral nutrition (TPN). Oguri, Hattori, and Yamawaki (2012) describe the case of a person on TPN because of a large resection of their small intestine for Crohn's disease. They developed visual loss, slurred speech and staggering gait over a 2-month period. This was identified as a selenium deficiency on the basis of blood tests and the absence of selenium in the TPN feed. Selenium replacement stopped progression of the neurological symptoms but did not reverse them.

Selenium dietary insufficiency can also affect cognitive function. Berr et al. (2012) reported a large cross-sectional and longitudinal study of elderly French participants, who undertook cognitive testing at baseline and then 9 years later, along with baseline bloods, including measurement of selenium. The most interesting finding was that after controlling for other risk factors, an initially lower level of selenium at baseline was predictive of cognitive decline on the MMSE across the 9 years of the study. The authors suggest this may be due to the effects of greater oxidative stress. A number of other studies have looked for a similar effect in elderly participants, but have not found it, perhaps because the levels of selenium were much lower in the Berr et al. (2012) study than in the later ones (Cardoso, Szymlek-Gay, & Roberts, 2018).

9.3.6 Electrolyte Disturbances

While the vitamin and mineral deficiencies examined so far arise primarily from dietary insufficiency and then other causes, for the electrolyte disturbances the primary cause is rarely a diet missing a specific nutrient – although calcium deficiency can be a consequence of vitamin D deficiency and hypothyroidism. Electrolyte disturbances generally result from medical conditions (e.g., burns, starvation, kidney disease, shock) which then lead to abnormally low plasma levels of one or more of the following minerals: calcium (hypocalcaemia), magnesium (hypomagnesemia), phosphorous (hypophosphatemia), sodium (hyponatremia), chlorine (hypochloremia) and potassium (hypokalemia). With the exception of hypokalemia (it is associated with paralysis), all of these electrolyte disturbances have common neurological sequelae starting with fatigue and mental dulling (obtundation), and ending in convulsions, coma and death (e.g., Hurley & Johnson, 2015; Rude, 1998; Whang, Hampton, & Whang, 1994). There is one additional observation here, regarding consistently low magnesium and/or calcium levels that do not reach the threshold for hypomagnesemia and hypocalcaemia. Several studies have suggested an association with depression, with this supported by a recent meta-analysis (Li et al., 2017).

Sodium deficiency deserves a special mention because the body has developed a system to identify environmental sources of sodium (i.e., tongue-based salt and monosodium glutamate receptors), and a carefully orchestrated physiological response to sodium depletion – the central and peripheral renin-angiotensin systems (Hurley & Johnson, 2015). Reductions in plasma sodium, from sweat or blood loss, for example, results in a salt appetite, which has both motivational and sensory consequences. Motivationally, hyponatremia activates the mesolimbic dopaminergic pathways, incentivising the pursuit of salt. Hyponatremia also has the effect of suppressing signals from the chorda tympani nerve (i.e., taste signals from the tongue) at the nucleus of the solitary tract, such that higher concentrations of salt are necessary to generate the same sensory signal as would occur normally for a lower concentration of salt. A much higher concentration of salt can then be consumed, allowing a speedier return to normal sodium levels.

9.3.7   Other Minerals

There are several other minerals that have not been mentioned. There are three reasons for this: (1) little data regarding their impact on the brain, in the case of manganese, molybdenum and sulphur; (2) linkages to other deficiency states, with this being the case for cobalt, where its main occurrence is in vitamin B12 [cobalamin] – so arguably the body does not need to consume cobalt per se; and (3) disagreement over whether a mineral is or is not essential, as with fluorine and chromium. Apart from evidence indicating the necessity of adequate manganese and molybdenum for neurodevelopment (from rare genetic disorders), only molybdenum deficiency in adulthood seems to be linked to neurocognitive problems, in the form of delirium and coma (Bayram, Topcu, & Karakaya, 2013).

9.4   Macronutrients

9.4.1   Essential and Conditionally Essential Fatty Acids

There are two families of polyunsaturated fatty acids (PUFA) that are essential for bodily function, and which need to come from our diet. One is the omega-3 fatty acid family and the other the omega-6 fatty acid family. As can be seen in Figure 9.5, for the omega-3 fatty acid family, alpha-linolenic acid can be used to synthesise two PUFAs that are critical to brain function and development (see Chapter 2), eicosapentaenoic acid (EPA) and docosahexaenoic acid (DHA). The omega-3 fatty acid synthesis pathway illustrated in Figure 9.5 is quite inefficient and it probably does not make much of the EPA and DHA required by the brain and body.

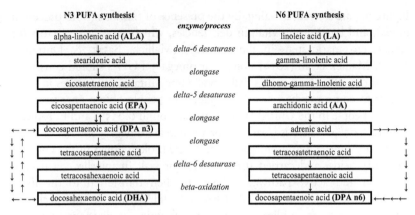

Figure 9.5   The omega-3 and -6 fatty acid synthesis pathways

Alpha-linolenic acid cannot be synthesised at all, and so is an essential nutrient (EFSA, 2010), and most of the required EPA and DHA must also be sourced from diet (although vegans and vegetarians may have some additional capacity to produce these fatty acids). Alpha-linolenic acid is found in some seeds (canola, flax) and nuts (walnuts) and the oils and margarines they are used in, and the main sources of EPA and DHA are from seafood, but also from grass-fed herbivores. Next, the omega-6 fatty acid family: Figure 9.5 indicates that linoleic acid can be used to synthesise arachidonic acid (ARA), a further PUFA critical to brain function and development (see Chapter 2). As with the omega-3 synthesis pathways, the omega-6 one is also inefficient, as both share a number of common enzymatic steps. Linoleic acid cannot be synthesised and so must come from food (EFSA, 2010), as must most ARA. Linoleic acid is found in many types of seeds used for making cooking oils (e.g., sunflower oil) and ARA is found in meat and eggs.

It has been suggested that many people in developed countries may be deficient in their intake of omega-3 PUFAs (Melo, Santos, & Ferreira, 2019). Historically, human diet probably consisted of a 1:1 ratio of omega-6 to omega-3 PUFAs. Currently, this ratio may sit anywhere between 10:1 and 20:1, with omega-6 PUFAs far outweighing intake of omega-3s (Liu, Zhao, & Reyes, 2015), with this driven by a reduction in dietary intake of omega-3s and concomitant increase in omega-6s (Melo et al., 2019). As the synthesis pathways (see Figure 9.5) share the same enzymes, the more plentiful linoleic acid dominates, compounding lower dietary intake of omega-3 PUFAs. Synthesis along both pathways is illustrated in

Figure 9.5 are slowed, in aging, by the presence of transfats (from processed foods), and by B-group vitamin deficiencies, which serve as co-factors for certain enzymatic steps in the pathways (Mallick, Basak, & Duttaroy, 2019). Mallick et al. (2019) notes that omega-3 PUFAs should constitute around 0.5–2% of a person's daily total energy intake, but intakes in most countries come nowhere near this. Japanese people obtain an average of 0.15%, people in the United States/Canada around 0.055% and Europeans around 0.05%. There is clearly scope to increase omega-3 intakes.

Dietary omega-3 and omega-6 PUFAs are broken down in the gut into free fatty acids, and carried through the gut wall in micelles via passive diffusion and active pathways. They are then transferred to the liver, probably the major site of ARA, EPA and DHA synthesis, and packaged into lipoprotein assemblies or bound to albumin for distribution to the body and brain. Entry into the brain is via multiple active pathways, with blood-brain barrier endothelial cells and astrocytes serving as further locations for synthesis of ARA, EPA and DHA (Liu et al., 2015). Just over a third of brain lipids are PUFAs, and of this fraction, 50% is AA and 40% DHA, with the remainder composed of other PUFA forms, most notably EPA. Adult animal models of deficiency, involving dietary exclusion of either alpha-linolenic acid or linoleic acid, are slow to effect respective levels of omega-3 and 6 in the brain. Three to four months of deficiency causes a 30% reduction of each respective PUFA family. Animals subjected to omega-3 deficiency regimens demonstrate an increase in depressive and anxiety-related behaviours, alterations in monoamine neurotransmitter metabolism and an exaggerated hypothalamic–pituitary–adrenal axis response to stress (Bazinet & Laye, 2014). It is unclear if something similar is happening to adults in developed countries. However, it has been suggested that increases in depression and anxiety may in part arise from the alteration in intake ratios between omega-6 and omega-3 PUFAs that has taken place over the last century (Melo et al., 2019).

Omega-3 and omega-6 PUFAs have several key roles in brain function. The most important is the part they play in maintaining cell membrane function, where they alter the fluid characteristics of the lipid bilayer. This in turn has an impact on all of the processes that require transmission of chemical or electrical signals across the membrane. In addition to roles in cellular energy metabolism and cell signalling, omega-3 and omega-6 PUFAs exert effectively opposite effects on neuro-immune function. An inflammatory stimulus leads to the cleaving of phospholipids from the cell membrane and the release of ARA. ARA forms the input to the production of a whole range of pro-inflammatory mediators: prostaglandins, thromboxanes and leukotrienes (Melo et al., 2019). In contrast, omega-3 PUFAs can inhibit microglial activity (notably EPA), shift cells to a neuroprotective posture and modulate the neuro-immune response (DHA). The importance of these processes is illustrated by the fact that mood stabilisers such as lithium exert some of their effects on the omega-6 pro-inflammatory process.

As the diets of many people in the developed world may be deficient in omega-3 PUFAs, there has been much interest in their role in mood disorders, mental health more generally, and whether they may play a role in age-related degenerative diseases. Studies conducted on living people often find that plasma DHA levels are reduced in several disorders, notably of mood, Alzheimer's and Parkinson's disease (Dyall, 2015), schizophrenia (Bazinet & Laye, 2014) and attention-deficit hyperactivity disorder (Morgese & Trabace, 2016), as well as in some studies of normal aging (Solfrizzi, Agosti, & Lozupone, 2018). The assumption in all of these cases is that plasma DHA reflects what is happening with DHA in the brain, such that a plasma reduction equates to a central reduction. This assumption may be incorrect. Plasma levels may not correlate with brain levels, at least when the brain samples are obtained post mortem from people with Alzheimer's disease, in minimal cognitive impairment and in healthy controls (Dyall, 2015).

Reductions in omega-3 fatty acids have also been observed in post mortem brain samples obtained from people with Alzheimer's and Parkinson's disease, mood disorders and schizophrenia, which provides much stronger support for a potential causative role (Bazinet & Laye, 2014; Dyall, 2015). Unfortunately, attempts to follow this up by examining whether supplementation may ameliorate disease-related deficits have generally been disappointing, most notably in Alzheimer's disease (Solfrizzi et al., 2018). However, as Dyall (2015) notes, there may be marked individual differences in response to supplementation, and the nature of the supplement (e.g., alpha-linolenic acid vs DHA) and the dose vary considerably between studies. There may be some instances where supplementation could be effective. In people who are at risk of developing schizophrenia, omega-3 supplementation may reduce the risk of a first episode psychosis (Bazinet & Laye, 2014). Indeed, one of the susceptibility genes for schizophrenia codes for a neuronal PUFA transporter. There is also some evidence that people with severe depression who are medicated may respond better when they are supplemented (Bazinet & Laye, 2014). Finally, animal data seemed to provide promising support for the idea that omega-3 supplementation during aging might ameliorate age-related cognitive decline – but human studies, including of younger people, present a mixed picture, with no clear indication of a cognitive or mood-related benefit (Cutuli, 2017).

9.4.2 Essential and Conditionally Essential Amino Acids

Of the around 300 amino acids (AAs) identified, only 21 are used to make proteins in the human body. Of these, many cannot be synthesised (those that can utilise glucose or other AAs as their starting point) and so they have to be obtained from diet (Metges, Petzke, & Young, 1999; Visek, 1984; see Table 9.2). The use of 'many' is deliberately vague, because membership of the three categories of essential, conditionally essential and non-essential AA vary according to bodily needs (e.g., injury, growth, availability of other AAs; Reeds, 2000). The focus here is on the essential and conditionally essential AAs.

AAs come from dietary protein, which is broken down in the stomach and small intestine to yield free AAs. These are absorbed across the gut wall, and travel in the blood to the liver or for direct uptake by cells in the body. AAs are actively transported across the blood-brain barrier so as to be available to neurons and glia, with AAs being utilised for protein synthesis and for energy metabolism (Massey, Blakeslee, & Pitkow, 1998). While the body has a substantial pool of protein, at around 12 kg in an adult man, the pool of free AAs is small at around 100 g. If an essential AA is missing, the consequences become apparent very quickly due to the small size of this free AA pool, and if the body is not able to source the missing AA by altering diet (more below), it has to scavenge it from existing protein resources within the body (i.e., via catabolism).

Table 9.2. *Human amino acids*

Essential	Conditionally essential	Non-essential
Lysine	Histidine	Asparagine
Tryptophan	Arginine	Alanine
Phenylalanine	Cysteine	Serine
Leucine	Glutamine	Aspartic acid
Isoleucine	Proline	Selenocysteine
Valine	Tyrosine	
Threonine	Glycine	
Methionine	Glutamic acid	

Animals, and seemingly humans too, are sensitive to both the protein content of their diet, and to the absence of essential AAs. Three types of behaviour have been documented. If a food is deficient in an essential AA, a loss of appetite for it will develop while it is still being eaten. The food will also be avoided in the future. Normal appetite does not return until another food source that provides a comprehensive set of essential AAs is eaten (Gietzen & Rogers, 2006). If a food is just generally low in protein (around 8–10%), this causes hyperphagia if no alternative food source is available (Heeley & Blouet, 2016). If the food is even lower in protein – less than 5–6% – animals will not continue to eat it. In all cases, if a more proteinaceous alternative is available, animals will choose this option over the protein-poor food. If a food is excessively high in protein (75%+), this suppresses food intake and the food is avoided (Gietzen & Aja, 2012). A considerable amount is known about the mechanism behind the essential AA sensing and response, but far less is known about general protein level sensing in foods.

In animal models, presenting a food for the first time that is deficient in any one of the essential AAs has the same effect: the animal becomes anorexic if the deficient food is repeatedly presented, it refrains from drinking, and its body weight starts to fall with this coming especially from muscle loss (Kamata, Yamamoto, & Kamijo, 2014; Zhu, Krasnow, & Roth-Carter, 2012). This same pattern was observed in a pioneering series of human studies in the 1940s and 1950s by the nutritional scientist William Rose (Rose, 1968). Over a 20–30-year period, he and his students identified many of the essential AAs by providing healthy participants with diets deficient in just a single target AA. As in animal models the effects were generally rapid, and they occurred even when the participant had no idea that the diet had a specific deficiency. There was a loss of appetite for the food, extreme fatigue and irritability, and these deficiency symptoms very rapidly disappeared when the deficiency was remedied. (e.g., Rose, Haines, & Warner, 1954).

In an extensive series of studies by Gietzen et al., it is now known that the brain itself serves as the primary sensor for essential AA deficiencies (Rudell, Rechs, & Kelman, 2011). Sensing occurs in the anterior piriform cortex, which is normally considered primary olfactory cortex (Gietzen & Aja, 2012). Detection seems to occur in the following manner. Each amino acid has one or more dedicated form of transfer RNA (tRNA), which collects its particular AA as part of the process of protein manufacture within the cell. As protein synthesis is on-going, if a particular AA is missing, its dedicated form of tRNA starts to build up rapidly – within the timeframe of a meal (Gietzen & Aja, 2012). This results in a biochemical cascade leading to the activation of anterior piriform neurons. These neurons project to three brain areas that seem important in rectifying the deficient diet (Gietzen, Hao, & Anthony, 2007): first, to the hypothalamus, presumably to supress further food intake and to initiate foraging for other food sources; second, to the amygdala, to generate a conditioned taste aversion to the flavour of the deficient food; and third, to the hippocampus, to encode into memory the more general context in which the deficient food was encountered. The consequences of these steps is to avoid the deficient food and to seek out other food sources that provide a comprehensive set of essential AAs.

9.5   Conclusion

A summary of the findings from this chapter are presented in Table 9.3. Paralleling the previous chapter on starvation, depression features as consequence of diverse specific deficiencies – thiamine, folate, ascorbic acid, iodine, zinc, amongst several others. This commonality of outcome is not well explained, and perhaps equally puzzling, it seems to have no obvious functional benefit. If a deficiency is sufficiently bad so as to be affecting the brain (i.e., the central organiser of feeding behaviour), it would seem more appropriate for the organism to forage and eat, in the hope of consuming *something* that might ameliorate the deficiency state. Yet the brain's reaction is often similar to that of acquiring an infectious disease, but at least with infection, inactivity may be beneficial by allowing the body to recover. Dietary deficiency seems to require a different response – activity and feeding – but puzzlingly this does not seem to occur.

There is a clear tendency with advancing age for lower levels of many micronutrients, and at least some of the causes of this have been identified – notably poorer absorption in the gut. Levels of many micronutrients become even more reduced in Alzheimer's disease, this being the case for most vitamins and minerals, with the possible exception of iron. The generality of this finding suggests either a worsening of age-related causes (e.g., gut absorption) and/or the presence of another problem affecting the supply of nutrients to the brain. The transport and retention of micronutrients to the brain requires an intact blood-brain barrier. A weakening of the blood-brain barrier may be an early event in the longer-term cascade of changes that ultimately ends in neurodegeneration (e.g., Hsu & Kanoski, 2014). This possibility raises two issues. First, does a slow failure of the blood-brain barrier explain any of the hypovitaminosis and mineral

Table 9.3. *Summary of brain-related findings for essential micronutrient and indispensable macronutrients deficiencies (– = no data)*

Agent (name)	Deficiency state name(s)	Impairment summary drawn from animal and human data	Investigated in relation to: Depression	Investigated in relation to: Aging	Investigated in relation to: Alzheimer's
Vitamins					
A (retinoic acid)	–	Learning, memory	Yes	–	–
B1 (thiamine)	Dry beriberi	Ophthalmoplegia, ataxia, confusion, memory, confabulation			
(Korsakoff's syndrome, Wernicke's encephalopathy)	Yes	Yes	Yes		
B2 (riboflavin)	–	Peripheral nerve function	–	Yes	–
B3 (NAD)	Pellagra	Delirium	–	Yes	Yes
B5 (phosphpanteitheine)	–	Motor, sleep fatigue, personality change	–	–	Yes
B6 (pyridoxal 5'-phosphate)	–	Seizures, peripheral neuropathy	–	–	–
B7 (biotin)	–	Ataxia, hypotonia, seizures	–	–	–
B9 (folate)	Anaemia	Depression, cognition, dementia	Yes	–	Yes
B12 (cobalamin)	Pernicious anaemia	Cognition, extra-pyramidal signs	–	Yes	Yes
C (ascorbic acid)	Scurvy	Depression, extra-pyramidal signs	Yes	–	Yes
D (calcitriol)	–	Learning, memory	Yes	Yes	Yes
E (α-tocopherol)	–	Anxiety, learning, memory	Yes	–	Yes
J (choline)	–	Learning, memory	–	–	Yes
K (phylloquinone)	–	Learning, memory	–	–	Yes

Table 9.3. (*cont.*)

Agent (name)	Deficiency state name(s)	Impairment summary drawn from animal and human data	Investigated in relation to:		
			Depression	Aging	Alzheimer's
Minerals					
Iodine (I)	Goitre	Cognition, apathy	Yes	–	Yes
Iron (Fe)	Anaemia	Cognition, apathy	–	–	Yes
Zinc (Zn)	–	Appetite, smell/taste, seizures, cognition	Yes	Yes	Yes
Copper (Cu)	–	Peripheral nerve function	–	–	–
Selenium (Se)	–	Blindness, ataxia, dysarthria	–	–	Yes
Ca, Mg, P, Na, Cl, K	Electrolyte imbalance	Delirium, convulsions, coma	Yes	–	–
Macronutrients					
Indispensable fatty acids	–	Depression, anxiety, stress response	Yes	–	Yes
Indispensable amino acids	–	Appetite, fatigue, irritability	–	–	–

354

deficiencies of old age? Second, if a slow failure of the blood-brain barrier does ultimately result in Alzheimer's disease by – in part – preventing many key antioxidant functioning vitamins and minerals from reaching their usual targets, could broad supplementation *starting in early middle age* delay onset at the population level?

Although there are studies that have looked at multiple micronutrient effects on brain function, the majority have focussed on single nutrients. This is particularly problematic with the B-group vitamins, because their biochemistry is closely interlinked (e.g., B3, B9 and B12; B6 and B2). There are also B-group interactions with choline, magnesium, with some of the essential fatty acids, and with iodine metabolism. Selenium is also necessary for the utilisation of iodine by the thyroid gland, as is iron – and copper is linked to iron metabolism – and these are just some of the more well-known interactions. Particularly in aging, where poor gut absorption may be a problem for multiple micronutrients, and in dietary deficiency generally (malnourishment from whatever cause), examining for multiple micronutrient deficiencies is probably a necessity. This would allow an accurate picture of which pattern of deficiencies and their interactions, are linked to particular neurocognitive profiles.

CHAPTER 10

Implications and Conclusions

10.1 Introduction

This final chapter has two goals. The first is to discuss what we regard as some of the interesting findings and themes that emerge from the various chapters of this book, and the research agendas or implications that flow from them. The second is to examine some of the approaches that may be important for shaping future advances in our field.

10.2 Interesting Findings and Themes from Chapters 2 to 9

Chapter 2 focussed on pregnancy and breastfeeding. While there are probably some benefits to physical development from breastfeeding, especially in developing countries where sterile water to make formula is not available, the cognitive benefits of breastfeeding seem limited. Observational studies seem to overestimate the cognitive benefits of breastfeeding due to the confounding of this behaviour with parental characteristics that are themselves correlates of intelligence. Where such confounds are avoided (e.g., within family studies), the cognitive benefits of breastfeeding diminish, so that at an individual level the effects of breastfeeding versus bottle-feeding are probably minimal. As we noted in Chapter 2, this is actually reassuring, because many mothers find it difficult to breastfeed and come under quite intense pressure to try and do so. Part of this pressure are the continuous assertions about the benefits of breastfeeding, including for cognitive development and the future mental health of the child. This is not a very helpful strategy, especially as the evidence for the cognitive and mental health benefits is weak and the effect size at best is negligible.

Chapter 3 explored the effects of acute food intake on brain and mind. Two broader issues were raised by the research featured in this chapter. The first concerns inconsistent findings, which form part of an even wider issue that comes across in this book about the often-poor reproducibility of research on diet, brain and mind – an issue that is directly addressed in Section 10.3. One aspect of the reproducibility problem in our field is probably the very diverse range of neuropsychological tests that are presumed to measure the same underlying construct (e.g., attention, vigilance, executive function). Just because something is labelled as a test of executive function does not automatically mean that it measures the same thing as another test that shares the same label. This results in two problems. Literature reviews and meta-analyses (and at some points the authors of this book) often combine results from different neuropsychological tests that purportedly measure the same cognitive trait – a generally untested assumption. The groupings under which they are combined often vary markedly between different reviews/meta-analyses –there being no agreed system of classification. One solution is to suggest some agreed standards in the discipline: (1) to aim for increasing convergence between studies in their selection of neuropsychological tests perhaps from an agreed pool, (2) agreement about what a minimal set of cognitive categories might look like and their theoretical and empirical basis and (3) agreement about which tests belong in which cognitive categories, again with theoretical and empirical verification. This would probably work to reduce between-study variation, and hence improve replicability.

A second issue to arise from Chapter 3, and one for which we have not been able to find a satisfactory answer, is a scientific problem. It seems to be broadly agreed that the brain has a special requirement for burning glucose as fuel, and that its only alternative, should this become unavailable, is to utilise ketone bodies. Why is this the case? One possibility that occurred to us was that allowing the brain to utilise fats and proteins for energy, as with other bodily tissues, might result in fatal self-cannibalism. That is, stripping fat from white matter or using protein destined to support learning and memory may permanently impair cognition, leaving the animal vulnerable to predation and starvation as it becomes unable to think and respond appropriately. In contrast, while depleting bodily fat stores or muscle bulk may be costly, it is easily replenished and not potentially fatal in the same way that it would be for the brain. This is of course entirely speculative, but it seems an interesting issue and one we could not find discussed in the many things we read in preparing this book.

Western-style diet and its various impacts were the main focus of Chapter 4. Two important issues were raised by this chapter. A recurring theme has been the contrast between studies that focus on single nutrients versus those that focus on patterns of dietary intake. There is a tension between these approaches. The single nutrient approach is highly reductionist at the expense of ecological validity, and seems to have as its role model behavioural pharmacology. There is a paradox here. If a food ingredient is pharmacologically potent, it is probably dangerous and so renders that substance a non-food (e.g., it would probably not be a good idea to include the heads of opium poppies as a vegetable in your casserole). So, is it wise to use a pharmacologically based paradigm?

Clearly the constituents of food are biologically active, but they are probably synergistic, with low potency, and their effects manifest generally quite slowly over longer periods of time. As we discuss further in the next section, the failure to find consistent effects with single nutrients like resveratrol and curcumin for example, is perhaps because we are using the wrong paradigm to explore the beneficial effects of foods. In contrast to the single nutrient approach, the focus on dietary patterns has a much stronger claim for ecological validity, but at the expense of specifying exactly what elements of that 'pattern' are responsible for its effects. And while we are disposed to the pattern approach because this is how people seem to eat, it is very important to acknowledge that the reductionist approach has allowed us to identify the vitamins and other micronutrients, and their impacts on brain and mind. A reductionist approach just has its limits, and one of those may be in trying to identify individual agents, when in fact many effects in our field arise from the synergistic action of multiple low-potency biologically active compounds, which work together slowly and subtly over longer periods of time.

Obesity is generally considered to be the product of genetic dispositions that favour eating (e.g., poor self-control) and metabolic adaptations for fat storage, etc., combined with an obesogenic environment. A new, 'third way' explanation is arising, driven by the work of people like Winocur, Small, Davidson, Gomez-Pinilla, Parent, Morris, Westbrook and Kanoski, whereby the food that constitutes the modern (or Western-style diet) actively damages brain functions involved in appetite regulation. This really represents a new take on obesity, and whether it comes to be seen as a critical aspect of the weight-gain process is something that translational work will decide. This is because much of the key work so far has been completed in animals, and so human work remains to be done.

Another focus of Chapter 4 concerned interactions between diet, gut, brain and mind. Out of all of the areas that this book has covered, this somehow seems one of the most exciting. There is not a lot known at the moment, but what there is suggests some interesting ways that diet can impact brain function, through its effects on the gut microbiome. The important findings here seem to be shifts in the microbiome that favour a leaky gut, with its possible implications of inflammatory effects on the brain and of the release of beta-amyloid into the blood stream, but also the production of anti-inflammatory agents (e.g., short-chain fatty acids) and the intriguing work linking gut microbiome to obesity. The development of kits to collect human faeces without need for refrigeration is an important step forward as it gets over the disgust factor of participants having to keep samples in their own fridge before returning them to the laboratory. Lower unit costs of the assays will also be an important development (allowing larger sample sizes with more power), alongside an opening up of collaborations between microbiologists and experts in our own fields – who have not traditionally worked together.

Chapter 5 reviewed the diverse literature on acute and chronic dietary neurotoxins. Several substantive issues arose. It is apparent that misfolded prion proteins gain their initial point of access to the brain via the gut. There is circumstantial evidence that the abnormal form of the alpha-synuclein protein may also gain access to the brain in the same manner. Exploring this possibility would seem particularly interesting. A second issue concerns the synergistic effects of dietary neurotoxins. Most of the studied effects have focussed on single toxins and their impacts, but there are a few reports that examine, for example, the impact of toxins in the context of malnutrition (e.g., poor cassava processing and thiamine deficiency), but not multiple toxin effects. And yet such multiple toxin effects are probably important, particularly with low-potency endocrine-affecting agents, and with exposure to micro-plastics, whose impacts are largely unknown.

Chapter 6 explored the effects of different forms of dietary intervention, both at the supplement level and at that of the dietary pattern. A growing area of interest is in the use of various twists of the Mediterranean diet, as a treatment for and as a preventative factor against depression. There is a growing body of favourable clinical data, but two major questions remain to be addressed. The first is whether any other mental health conditions might be preventable by or responsive to whole diet manipulations. The low hanging fruit would be to explore impacts of the Mediterranean diet on stress and anxiety, as there is some evidence already that this *might* be beneficial. It is also unclear at the moment who might best benefit from using something like the Mediterranean diet as an intervention – the level of depression, the type, the person's age, whether they have existing poor diet – there are many such individual factors that might be important in determining treatment success with this approach. The second and particularly important issue concerns the choice of control arm. A general weakness of lifestyle interventions is that it is not generally possible to blind participants in the treatment and control arms, and as people clearly have strong expectancies about the benefits of fresh fruit and vegetables, regular exercise, meditation, etc., these may inflate the apparent potency of the treatment effect (i.e., a placebo effect). Designing better control conditions is important for determining actually how much of the diet intervention effects are placebo and how much are actual biological effects.

The focus of Chapter 7 was alcohol, caffeine and food addiction. There were two things that seemed important to discuss from this chapter. The first is the interesting possibility that caffeine may potentiate the rewarding effects of sweeteners in many popular drinks. This is suggested by the ability of caffeine to directly and indirectly affect dopamine release and binding to the D2 receptor. While caffeine does not have the abuse potential of many agents that directly affect dopamine and the D2 receptor, its potential to indirectly affect the rewarding properties of other drugs, and natural rewards like sugar, have not been well explored. A second issue is food addiction, which seems to be accepted as a fact by many laypeople. There is also a growing scientific literature, especially that built around time-limited exposure to sucrose in rodents. There are a lot of problems with a general food addiction model, not least that the characteristics of 'food addiction' seem a long way from the harms that are linked to behavioural addictions like gambling or substance abuse disorders. As it currently stands, the literature would seem to suggest that certain people may have a propensity to overeat particular types of food, but this notion is at least partially captured already by the binge-eating disorder category in DSM-V.

Chapter 8 dealt with starvation and calorie restriction in adults. From the starvation literature two particularly interesting observations emerged, which do not seem to have been given the scrutiny that they deserve. Starvation, and it seems intermittent bouts of hunger, seem linked to immorality. Put more bluntly, restriction of energy intake, chronically or intermittently, results in people doing things to obtain food (directly and indirectly) that even by the standards of desperation (e.g., many people would probably countenance shoplifting for food if the need was urgent) would be considered by many as shameful (e.g., stealing from family and friends). There is no surprise when this type of behaviour is observed for people with drug dependence, and it is now well established that eliminating their drug cravings by using things like methadone in opiate dependence is an excellent way to reduce property crime. There does not, however, seem to be the same appreciation that the biology of drug dependence hijacks extant reward systems used primarily for food, and that this might too be similarly expected to bring about a marked decline in moral behaviour. The full extent of the effects of hunger on delinquency have not been explored, and they deserve to be.

The starvation literature yielded another interesting observation. It seems that obese and normal-weight people may respond quite differently to periods of energy deprivation. A number of studies, especially in the 1960s and 1970s seemed to imply that obese people could go on starvation diets to lose weight, without apparently reporting markedly increased levels of hunger. In contrast, almost all reports of starvation in normal-weight people are dominated by hunger, and the intrusive nature of hunger impacts on every aspect of their personal lives. Why this difference should exist, if in fact it is a real effect, would be intriguing to understand, especially if it were to yield some means of effectively controlling hunger and thus aiding weight loss.

Based on the well-documented finding that calorie restriction increases lifespan and well-span in many animals, there has been much interest in whether this could be extended to humans. The human literature is really disappointing. Benefits – at least as currently understood – do not seem to extend much beyond those that come from maintaining a normal body weight (e.g., avoiding metabolic disease, high blood pressure, etc.) and there seem to be good theoretical evolutionary reasons for thinking that calorie restriction will probably not act to increase lifespan in people. Nonetheless, there is not a lot of high-quality human research (much has been completed in older people and often with some degree of existing metabolic problems) and it would be premature to right this field off before a proper examination has been conducted (i.e., starting in young healthy people).

Finally, Chapter 9 examined micronutrient deficiencies and their impacts on brain and mind. This is the chapter where the reductionist case is probably strongest and most appropriate, but then this has to be balanced with the many contradictory findings that emerge in exploring the role of micronutrients in neurodegenerative and mental health disorders. Here the literature is a real mess of conflicting reports and some of the reasons for this are discussed in Section 10.3. One finding that is particularly intriguing and seems to be robust is the emergence of depression as a common consequence of many deficiency states (e.g., thiamine, folate, vitamin C, iodine, zinc). Depression seems an odd response to a nutritional deficiency. Rather, one would expect behavioural activation and appetite, to try and consume something to ameliorate the deficit, but this does not appear to be the case. There just seems no obvious functional benefit from a depressive response to deficiency, unless it reflects an incapacity by bodily systems to distinguish between pathogen infection, where rest and withdrawal (i.e., apathy) may be appropriate responses, and dietary deficiency, where they are not.

10.3   Future Developments

10.3.1   Improving Dietary Recording

While the mainstay dietary recording methods of 24-hour recall, diet diaries and food frequency questionnaires can give us a reliable indication of diet, they are far from perfect. Many authors have noted that improved methods of diet recording are needed (e.g., Alshurafa et al., 2019; Gemming, Utter, & Mhurchu, 2015; Willis et al., 2020), which would make detecting linkages between diet and brain and mind more reliable and more sensitive. All of the current techniques share similar problems. They are time consuming for participants and for researchers who have to code their responses (Willis et al., 2020). Compliance is probably an issue, but this in itself is difficult to measure, which is an additional concern (Stumbo, 2013). There are well-established problems with memory (i.e., not recalling all that was eaten or what or how much), and also with the demand-related characteristics of the task, especially if an obese person has to report eating nutritionally poor-quality food to a person in a 'white coat' – dietician, doctor or researcher (Soldevila-Domenech et al., 2019). However, the most frequently identified problem is that of under-reporting, which across all three major methods varies between 3 and 40% of daily energy intake (Burrows et al., 2019).

Four major approaches have emerged to tackle these various problems. The first, which has been around for a while, but is evolving into something progressively more powerful, is the use of biomarkers, typically now from urine. Urine is advantageous to collect as it is less off-putting for participants than collecting saliva, blood or faeces, and it provides a record of the last few hours of diet as excreted metabolites (Willis et al., 2020). The biomarker approach can be divided into three main classes – the measurement of major nutrients like nitrogen intake, the measurement of food groups, and the measurement of single specific foods (Garcia-Aloy et al., 2017; McNamara et al., 2021; Willis et al., 2020). Measurement of the major nutrients is still not fully worked out. It is possible to get a good measure of protein intake and an adequate measure of certain aspects of carbohydrate intake, but fat-related data is the most problematic, with it being the ratio between fat types rather than absolute quantity of each. Indeed, it would be hard to calculate overall energy intake based solely on urinary metabolites and, similarly, the quantity consumed of specific foods or food groups.

The major advance in recent years is the steadily growing database listing biomarkers (typically from urine) for different specific foods and food groups. For specific foods, measures have been obtained for red meat, beer, wine and bananas, and for broader categories, curry (e.g., eugenol), toasted foods (e.g., furoyglycines), low-calorie drinks (e.g., acesulfame potassium), legumes (e.g., pyrogallol sulphate), berry fruits (e.g., furaneols), citrus fruit (e.g., proline betaine), bread, cocoa and cruciferous vegetables (e.g., sulforaphane; Garcia-Aloy et al., 2017; Willis et al., 2020). Certainly, at the moment specific single food markers are likely to be less reliable than composite measures, which better discriminate between foods that share certain common metabolites (e.g., ellagitannins in many fruits and walnuts, proline betaine in citrus fruits and rye bran, chlorogenic acid in coffee and legumes; Garcia-Aloy et al., 2017). Not only should it be possible in the future to use nuclear magnetic spectroscopy to identify a broad range of dietary biomarkers (from the building of libraries, which is currently taking place), but there may also be wearable devices that monitor sweat-related biomarkers in real time – although these are impractical at the moment (Alshurafa et al., 2019).

The second approach has been a gradual refinement in the collection of food-based images as people go about their day-to-day lives (Alshurafa et al., 2019). These methods are not new, but the technology has improved markedly especially with most people now routinely carrying a powerful small computer/camera in the form of their smartphone. There are two basic distinctions when it comes to image-based collection. One is active collection, which is what we have been referring to so far, in which a person with a smartphone takes a picture of their meal. The other, which is more the emerging technology, is passive image acquisition, in which an ear or neck pendant-mounted camera automatically records all of the time it is turned on, thus capturing each bout of feeding (Gemming et al., 2015).

Each of these approaches has its strengths and weaknesses. The active approach can probably better ensure that the food is in the picture, but critically the participant has to actually remember to take the photograph (Vu et al., 2017). If only a picture is taken, then multiple problems arise in relation to its utility. First, how big a portion is it? This can be assisted by placing a standard object in the picture (e.g., a pen) but again the person has to remember to do this. Second, a plate of food will often have multiple foods on it, in which case how is the image to be segmented into its different foods and a portion size for each calculated? This problem, which may be solvable using artificial intelligence techniques, is not currently resolved (Zhao et al., 2021). Third, unless the person provides additional details about the food, it may be difficult to ascertain its nutritional value (e.g., was it boiled or fried? Any hidden ingredients, like cream in soup?).

All of these three problems apply with equal force to food images captured passively, but with some additional problems too. As images may be collected continuously it is a labour-intensive job to separate food from non-food images, although a recent paper describes an artificial intelligence tool that can aid this process (Jia et al., 2019). Image quality may be a problem. For example, if a person is eating at the computer, the food may be on the side, while they are facing the computer, meaning that only fragments of the food are recorded. Then there is the privacy-related problem of other people being caught on camera without their consent and the possibility that wearing the camera alters behaviour (although this may apply to any diet recording technique). There are solutions of course. It is possible to have devices that turn the camera on when it detects the person is eating, but this usually means wearing some form of sensor which may be uncomfortable and intrusive, thereby reducing compliance (Vu et al., 2017). It is also likely that as wearable devices improve in size and sensitivity and that as databases of food-related images grow and artificial intelligence algorithms develop, this will allow for real-time identification of food and portion size, and the context in which eating is occurring.

The final two approaches integrate with image-based collection. New techniques have emerged that allow real-time detection of when a person is eating (Vu et al., 2017). This can include inertial devices such as particular movements of the wrist, acoustic devices to detect the sound of chewing or swallowing and skin-based sensory devices to measure muscle movement or electrical impulses connected with jaw movements or swallowing. These methods have the potential to be synchronised with automatic image-based capture of food, so that recording only takes place during eating, but some of these approaches can collect additional information. For example, as 'mouthfuls of food' tend to be relatively constant in size, it is possible to measure total number of mouthfuls per snack, meal and per day, providing a rough estimate of energy intake (Alshurafa et al., 2019). Similarly, there is data now to indicate that chewing noise can be used to identify up to 19 different foods (Vu et al., 2017) – and again, with the use of artificial intelligence approaches this type of auditory data collection may prove a useful addition to image-based capture. Finally, all of the methods outlined here can be combined with the traditional methods of dietary data collection, hopefully improving upon the shortcomings that were identified in the opening paragraph of this section. However, at least the early attempts to include image-based approaches with the traditional methods do not seem to have radically altered the problem of under-reporting (Burrows et al., 2019). Indeed, the way forward may be to try and minimise the involvement of the participant in diet data collection.

10.3.2 Nutraceuticals and Nutrigenomics

Starting with nutraceuticals or functional foods, these have been defined in several related ways (Kaur et al., 2020; Rana et al., 2016). The National Academy of Sciences define them as 'any modification of food or ingredients of food that is beneficial in providing health benefits beyond any traditional use'. The American Dietetic Association defines them as 'fortified, enriched, enhanced and whole foods' and the Institute of Medicine as 'any food or food component that may provide health benefits beyond the traditional nutrients it contains'. The spectrum of chemical agents referred to as nutraceuticals often extends well beyond what would be traditionally termed a food or food component, to include things like traditional medicines (e.g., ginseng), but definitely includes: (1) probiotics (microorganisms found often in fermented food), prebiotics (agents that promote gut microorganisms) and synbiotics (the combination of the latter; Tong, Satyanarayanana, & Su, 2020); (2) vitamins and micronutrients – some 60 or so agents; (3) plant phytochemicals found in foods and spices, perhaps constituting 5,000 known agents of which around 1,000 have been studied to some degree (Williams, Mohanakumar, & Beart, 2015); and (4) chemical agents derived from fungi and marine sources (Talebi et al., 2021). Together, this yields a sizeable array of diverse chemical agents, although only a small handful have been studied in depth (e.g., resveratrol, curcumin, crocin, certain berry flavonoids; see Chapter 6).

Based on the sales of supplements – essentially the four sets of chemical agents listed at the end of the last paragraph – the public clearly believe in their efficacy, with sales around 40 billion US dollars per year attesting to this fact. The public also seems to hold the general view that many of these supplements exert beneficial effects on brain function and cognition. For example, the 'Healthline' website lists 11 'brain boosting foods' many of which the reader, and the lay public, would readily identify as such, namely – fatty fish, coffee, blueberries, turmeric, broccoli, pumpkin seeds, dark chocolate, nuts, oranges, eggs and green tea. In the scientific literature, many of the same supplements crop up again and again, with claims made for potential benefits to gut integrity (Chen et al., 2021), the gut microbiome (and hence to brain and mental health; Tong et al., 2020), reducing the impact of acute traumatic brain injury (McCarty & Lerner, 2021), treating Alzheimer's disease, neurodegenerative disease and age-related decline (Talebi et al., 2021; Virmani et al., 2013) and enhancing cognition in healthy people (Williams, Mohanakumar, & Beart, 2016). These putative benefits typically derive from in vitro studies and animal models, with a smaller body of human data (again see Chapters 6 and 9).

Currently, the evidence for any beneficial effect on brain and mind seems very limited, with no supplement really able to provide a consistent level of support from human clinical trials. That's not to say there are not positive findings; there are, but there are probably as many negative ones or those offering partial support to make the whole picture inconclusive. Indeed, focussing on perhaps two of the most studied supplements, resveratrol and curcumin, there is actually very little evidence that they have any beneficial effect on human health (Nelson et al., 2017). There may be several reasons for this lack of any clear findings. First, sales of these agents are unregulated and there is little motivation to conduct large-scale clinical trials that are probably needed to establish efficacy (Williams et al., 2015). Second, running a clinical trial does not necessarily provide *useful* evidence, especially if it is underpowered, poorly controlled, not of sufficient length, etc. Third, there is often conflation between particular single agents studied in clinical trials and the foods they are derived from, good examples being resveratrol and red wine, and curcumin and turmeric. In fact, most foods contain a large number of low-potency bioactive compounds – including red wine and turmeric – and it is possible (probable) that there are synergistic effects between agents that render the whole food healthful in a way that individual agents may not be. Moreover, there may be individual components that are singularly or jointly active, but that just have not been identified as yet (Neale et al., 2012; Williams et al., 2016). Fourth, there are often problems generalising across studies that purport to examine the same agent, and variations in chemical formulation may significantly impact dosing and timing of impacts (Neale et al., 2012). There are a lot of unknowns in this type of research, including interactions with the participants diet and other individual differences, all of which may contribute to inconsistencies across studies.

There are several steps that could be taken to improve things. The first concerns considering individual differences in biology, which may be a significant factor in whether a supplement exerts an effect or not – nutrigenomics (Vergeres, 2013). The second is to pay more attention to the nature of clinical trials used for supplements. This includes consideration of who funds the research, adequate sample size, pre-registration as a clinical trial with an analysis plan and clear primary and secondary outcomes, and the utilisation of new methods to explore the myriad potential bioactive chemical agents in food using N-of-1 trials (Soldevila-Domenech et al., 2019). The third is to be clearer in general about what this whole literature is actually trying to do. Is it trying to identify biologically active molecules for drug development and if not, what is the point of focussing on developing a new supplement other than the profit motive? And while both drug development and supplements make people and businesses money, only pharmaceuticals tend to be subsidised by the state for treating medical conditions, surely making this the more humanitarian goal. The fourth is to reiterate the comment made in the preceding section, namely that food effects on health almost certainly reflect multiple low-potency agents, with complex synergistic interactions, exerting effects slowly over long periods of time. These type of effects may just not be suited to a reductionist approach based around the behavioural pharmacology model.

While we have 30 or 40 years of nutraceutical study, nutrigenomics is relatively new. It can be defined broadly as the convergence of nutrition and individual biology in the treatment and prevention of disease and the maintenance of health (Rana et al., 2016; Sikalidis, 2019; Vergeres, 2013). In practical terms this would mean identifying what diet or supplements might actually best benefit a given health condition for a given person, or help a given person from developing a particular health condition. The type of information that is potentially available about a person's individual biology spans from their genome (DNA), including epigenetic factors (methylation patterns, chromatin structure, histone codes, non-coding small RNAs), their transcriptome (RNA), their proteome (proteins) and their metabolome (metabolites and metabolic pathways; Kussmann, Krouse, & Siffert, 2010).

At present there are relatively few examples of how this might practically work. One example concerns high blood pressure. People who have a certain mutation of the ANG gene do not appear to benefit as much from adopting a DASH-type diet designed to lower their blood pressure (Sikalidis, 2019). Another concerns serum vitamin C levels in healthy young people, with those manifesting deficient levels having markedly different polymorphisms for various aspects of vitamin C metabolism than those with adequate serum levels (Vergeres, 2013). There are also conflicting reports about the impact of undernutrition during human pregnancy on the epigenome of offspring, and in turn, their offspring, with either favourable or unfavourable impacts on metabolic-related disorders (Vergeres, 2013). The application of nutrigenomics to animal diet studies is also a developing area, with, for example, high fructose diets in rodents found to alter the transcriptome and induce epigenetic changes to genes known to be involved in several human diseases, including psychiatric illnesses (Meng et al., 2016). As the costs of establishing an individual's genome, transcriptome, proteome and metabolome drop, it is likely that there will be a lot of research trying to identify who will most benefit from particular foods and supplements, especially relating to brain-related disease, weight loss, diabetes and enhancing cognitive function. This is an emerging field to watch, because its focus on individual differences offers yet another potential solution as to why there is so often a confusing pattern of outcomes in diet-brain-behaviour studies.

10.3.3   Lost in Translation

A number of authors have made the claim that there is a translational 'crisis' in the biomedicine field (Hentze & Ibsen, 2019; Schulz, Cookson, & Hausmann, 2016). Schulz et al. (2016) put it like this: '. . .to date no disease modifying treatment has been clinically validated for common neurodegenerative disorders, despite an enormous amount of published preclinical research data on disease models in animals and cell culture' (p. 256, ibid). It seems a fair question to ask whether this also includes some of the research featured in this book, although of course much of our focus has been on humans, rather than on animal models and cell cultures. We would suggest there is a case to answer. Chapter 3 (acute effects of food intake), Chapter 6 (diet or dietary components as an intervention) and Chapter 9 (micronutrient deficiencies), all provide some grounds for concern. Take Chapter 9 as a specific example. Here, most vitamins have been explored as a possible correlate or treatment for dementia, with in most cases some favourable findings and an almost equal number of unfavourable ones too. A careful inspection of even 'favourable' findings often reveals an incomplete picture, with one variable finding an effect but not another. The overall picture is often one of confusion, with no clear answer. Indeed, this also holds for much of the work reported in Chapter 3, and as discussed in the previous section (and see Chapter 6), for well-tested individual food components such as resveratrol and curcumin (Nelson et al., 2017). Some see this type of uncertainty and poor reproducibility across studies as part of a broader malaise in science, which has been termed the reproducibility crisis (Baker, 2016). A survey conducted by *Nature* reported that many biomedical scientists had tried and failed to replicate other biomedical scientists' results, a finding that has been widely cited to support the idea of a crisis (Baker, 2016). There are also sceptical voices, who point to various pieces of evidence indicating the robustness of the literature, the good faith of most scientists and that such 'crises' have been reported many times before in the history of science (Fanelli, 2018). We agree with Fanelli (2018) that there is much that is good, but a critical look and possible revision of our processes would seem wise.

A list of potential problems with the way that we currently conduct ourselves is not hard to find. There are several problem areas. The first concerns animal models, and how these can be either poor models of human disease or because of cross-species differences in biology may not offer an ideal mirror of what happens in human biology (Franca & Monserrat, 2018; Schulz et al., 2016). For the study of diet, brain and mind, this is worrying, because animal studies are an important bedrock because we can be sure that the animals have exactly followed the dietary modification – something that is typically difficult to establish in humans. The lesson here is to question and test *assumptions* about the translatability of animal findings and to improve diet validation techniques for human dietary interventions. Both of these seem achievable, and the latter was the focus of an earlier discussion in this chapter.

A second issue concerns various forms of biases that occur during a study (Schulz et al., 2016). The most relevant for our field would seem to be attrition and reporting biases. Studies that involve an experimental alteration of diet versus a control group that does not are likely to suffer greater attrition in the experimental arm than in the control arm, producing non-random differences between groups. Dropout rates are significant issues in many nutrition studies. A more pressing concern though is reporting bias. This covers a range of ills, including inadequate details about randomisation, blinding, attrition, incomplete reporting of all study components and most importantly of all, alteration of the study aims such that if the original focus 'doesn't work' then the study is re-tasked in a new direction. Much of the motivation for the last-mentioned manifestation for bias comes from the all too well-known incentives in science, which favour publication of positive findings and the non-publication of null results.

Many studies in our field are also paid for from funders who sometimes have vested interests in positive outcomes. If a supplement producer provides money to test the effects of a supplement on a particular problem, there is a clear but unspoken expectation of a finding consistent with this expectation. Such expectancy effects are powerful and their impact in clinical medicine has been known about for years, with industry-funded studies more likely to report favourable results and less likely to publish unfavourable ones, relative to publicly funded research (e.g., Bourgeois, Murthy, & Mandl, 2010; Perlis et al., 2005). There is of course increasing awareness of this form of bias, and it is now routine to declare conflicts of interest. However, such declarations may simply make the effects of this form of bias detectable rather than eliminating it as a problem.

The final issue, and in our minds perhaps the most pressing of all, is low sample size (Bespalov & Steckler, 2018; Franca & Monserrat, 2018). In animal research, the cost of housing and maintenance of a colony is substantial, putting downward pressure on sample size, but the most significant downward pressure comes from animal ethics committees, who want to minimise animal suffering and thus reduce usage to the lowest levels possible (Bespalov & Steckler, 2018). The effect of these financial and ethical contingencies is probably to make animal investigators more optimistic about probable effect sizes than is realistic, with the result that many preclinical studies, including in our field, are often very underpowered. This works against replicability and robustness of the literature.

This problem is not restricted to the animal literature. It is often difficult and expensive to recruit and keep human participants particularly in experimental or longitudinal studies (Franca & Monserrat, 2018). And the problem is real. We examined a leading academic publication in our field, searching back over the last 70 issues. This revealed 43 human experimental studies, of which 20 used a between-subject design and 23 a within design. For the between designs, which might compare the effects say of a nutritional intervention on some brain/mind-dependent variable versus a non-interventional control, the median sample size was 25 per group (range 10–76). Twenty-five per group is capable of detecting a large effect size (Cohen's $d = 0.8$) 80% of the time if Ho is false – but how often might we reasonably expect this magnitude of effect? A more reasonable expectation is small-to-medium effect sizes (d's around 0.35), which require 128/group with an 80% power of correctly rejecting the null if it is false. There is a big gap between 24 and 128 participants. For within-subject designs, the median sample size is 24 (range 6–84), which provides 80% power of detecting medium-to-large effect sizes (i.e., d = 0.6). Again, for detection of small-to-medium effect sizes (d's around 0.35) requires 64 participants – well below the number typically reported in this journal. Larger sample sizes would aid reproducibility by making chance findings resulting from small sample sizes less likely, and provide a more robust basis for evaluating whether an effect is real or noise.

The remedies for many of these problems have been the source of a very active debate over the last decade. One widely favoured solution is to pre-register the design and analysis (Gorgolewski & Poldrack, 2016; Gosselin, 2020; Maizey & Tzavella, 2019). This approach means that the primary aims of the study are set in stone before data collection begins, and so when it is complete the reader can readily differentiate between planned analyses (what was expected to be tested) and explorative analyses (seren-dipity, etc.). Clearly, when a paper is read in this way, planned analyses carry more weight because there was an a priori expectation of finding a particular outcome, while post hoc analyses can be treated with more suspicion as they were unanticipated and so more likely to be the product of chance. This approach does not negate data exploration, it just makes it clear which is which.

An additional benefit of pre-registration is that appropriate details of the study can be ensured as valid, as the registration process may involve peer review – adequate statistical power, randomisation, blinding – and relat-edly there can be no omission of study components or tests if they prove 'recalcitrant'. A number of journals now offer pre-registration and guaran-tee publication even if there is a null result, ensuring that the literature reflects findings as they are. This process also involves data availability, allowing other researchers to use existing findings (Gorgolewski & Poldrack, 2016). As with any significant change in how things work, it will take a while to adjust. There is substantially increased workload for pre-registration of studies and this needs to be considered by funding bodies and employers. It is also very important to preserve the investiga-tor's ability to undertake exploratory analyses. If pre-registration simply results in a straightjacket of pre-planned analyses, science will be the poorer – that is our fear – but if pre-registration simply allows the flagging of planned versus unplanned analyses, this will very likely improve the quality and reproducibility of the literature.

10.4 General Conclusion

The aim of this book has been to provide a comprehensive account of the acute and chronic impacts of diet on the human brain and mind. Studying these interactions is an important endeavour because every single one of us eats, and our food choices in turn impact our brain and behaviour, and our long-term health and well-being. We hope this book inspires a new generation of scientists to continue this interesting and important research endeavour.

References

Abbott, K. N., Arnott, C. K., Westbrook, R. F., & Tran, D. M. D. (2019). The effect of high fat, high sugar, and combined high fat-high sugar diets on spatial learning and memory in rodents: A meta-analysis. *Neuroscience & Biobehavioral Reviews*, 107, 399–421.

Abbott, R. D., Webster Ross, G., White, L. R., Sanderson, W. T., Burchfiel, C. M., Kashon, M., & Petrovitch, H. (2003). Environmental, life-style, and physical precursors of clinical Parkinson's disease: Recent findings from the Honolulu-Asia Aging Study. *Journal of Neurology*, 250, 30–39.

Abdelwahab, M. G., Fenton, K. E., Preul, M. C., Rho, J. M., Lynch, A., Stafford, P., & Scheck, A. C. (2012). The ketogenic diet is an effective adjuvant to radiation therapy for the treatment of malignant glioma. *PLoS One*, 7, e36197.

Abdelwahab, M. G., Preul, M. C., Rho, J. M., & Scheck, A. C. (2010). The ketogenic diet reverses gene expression patterns and reduces reactive oxygen species levels when used as an adjuvant therapy for glioma. *Nutrition & Metabolism*, 7, Article 74.

Accurso, E. C., Ciao, A. C., Fitzsimmons-Craft, E. E., Lock, J. D., & Grange, D. L. (2014). Is weight gain really a catalyst for broader recovery? The impact of weight gain on psychological symptoms in the treatment of adolescent anorexia nervosa. *Behaviour Research & Therapy*, 56, 1–6.

Adamolekun, B. (1993). *Anaphe venata* entomophagy and seasonal ataxic syndrome in southwest Nigeria. *The Lancet*, 341, 629.

(2011). Neurological disorders associated with cassava diet: A review of putative etiological mechanisms. *Metabolic Brain Disease*, 26, 79–85.

Adamse, P., van Egmond, H. P., Noordam, M. Y., Mulder, P. P., & de Nijs, M. (2014). Tropane alkaloids in food: Poisoning incidents. *Quality Assurance and Safety of Crops and Foods*, 6, 15–24.

Adolphus, K., Lawton, C. L., Champ, C. L., & Dye, L. (2016). The effects of breakfast and breakfast composition on cognition in children and adolescents: A systematic review. *Advances in Nutrition*, 7, 590S–612S.

Advani, S. M., Advani, P. G., VonVille, H. M., & Jafri, S. H. (2018). Pharmacological management of cachexia in adult cancer patients: A systematic review of clinical trials. *BMC Cancer*, 18, 1174.

Agim, Z. S., & Cannon, J. R. (2015). Dietary factors in the etiology of Parkinson's disease. *BioMed Research International*, Article 672838.

Agrawal, R., & Gomez-Pinilla, F. (2012). 'Metabolic syndrome' in the brain: Deficiency in omega-3 fatty acid exacerbates dysfunctions in insulin receptor signalling and cognition. *Journal of Physiology*, 590, 2485–2499.

Aguzzi, A., Baumann, F., & Bremer, J. (2008). The prion's elusive reason for being. *Annual Review of Neuroscience*, 31, 439–477.

Ahmad, M. (2013). Protective effects of curcumin against lithium-pilocarpine induced status epilepticus, cognitive dysfunction and oxidative stress in young rats. *Saudi Journal of Biological Sciences*, 20, 155–162.

Ahuja, A., Dev, K., Tanwar, R. S., Selwal, K. K., & Tyagi, P. K. (2015). Copper mediated neurological disorder: Visions into amyotrophic lateral sclerosis, Alzheimer and Menkes disease. *Journal of Trace Elements in Medicine and Biology*, 29, 11–23.

Ajith, T. A. (2018). A recent update on the effects of omega-3 fatty acids in Alzheimer's disease. *Current Clinical Pharmacology*, 13, 252–260.

Al Bulushi, I., Poole, S., Deeth, H. C., & Dykes, G. A. (2009). Biogenic amines in fish: Roles in intoxication, spoilage, and nitrosamine formation – A review. *Critical Reviews in Food Science & Nutrition*, 49, 369–377.

Alaimo, K., Olson, C. M., & Frongillo, E. A. (2002). Family food insufficiency, but not low family income, is positively associated with dysthymia and suicide symptoms in adolescents. *Journal of Nutrition*, 132, 719–725.

AlAmmar, W. A., Albeesh, F. H., Ibrahim, L. M., Algindan, Y. Y., Yamani, L. Z., & Khattab, R. Y. (2021). Effect of omega-3 fatty acids and fish oil supplementation on multiple sclerosis: A systematic review. *Nutritional Neuroscience*, 24, 569–579.

Alamy, M., & Bengelloun, W. (2012). Malnutrition and brain development: An analysis of the effects of inadequate diet during different stages of life in rat. *Neuroscience & Biobehavioral Reviews*, 36, 1463–1480.

Alaverdashvili, M., Hackett, M. J., Caine, S., & Paterson, P. G. (2017). Parallel changes in cortical neuron biochemistry and motor function in protein-energy malnourished adult rats. *NeuroImage*, 149, 275–284.

Alaverdashvili, M., Li, X., & Paterson, P. G. (2015). Protein-energy malnutrition causes deficits in motor function in adult male rats. *Journal of Nutrition*, 145, 2503–3511.

Alcalay, R. N., Gu, Y., Mejia-Santana, H., Cote, L., Marder, K. S., & Scarmeas, N. (2012). The association between Mediterranean diet adherence and Parkinson's disease. *Movement Disorders*, 27, 771–774.

Algarin, C., Karunakaran, K. D., Reyes, S., Morales, C., Lozoff, B., Peirano, P., & Biswal, B. (2017). Differences on brain connectivity in adulthood are present in subjects with iron deficiency anemia in infancy. *Frontiers in Aging Neuroscience*, 9, 54.

Algarin, C., Nelson, C. A., Peirano, P., Westerlund, A., Reyes, S., & Lozoff, B. (2013). Iron-deficiency anemia in infancy and poorer cognitive inhibitory control at age 10 years. *Developmental Medicine & Child Neurology*, 55, 453–458.

Alisi, L., Cao, R., & de Angelis, C. (2019). The relationships between vitamin K and cognition: A review of current evidence. *Frontiers in Neurology*, 10, 239.

Aliu, E., Kanungo, S., & Arnold, G. L. (2018). Amino acid disorders. *Annals of Translational Medicine*, 6, 471.

Allen, V. J., Methven, L., & Gosney, M. A. (2013). Use of nutritional complete supplements in older adults with dementia: Systematic review and meta-analysis of clinical outcomes. *Clinical Nutrition*, 32, 950–957.

Almaas, A. N., Tamnes, C. K., Nakstad, B., Henriksen, C., Walhovd, K. B., Fjell, A. M., & Iversen, P. O. (2015). Long-chain polyunsaturated fatty acids and cognition in VLBW infants at 8 years: An RCT. *Pediatrics*, 135, 972–980.

Al-Naama, N., Mackeh, R., & Kino, T. (2020). C_2H_2-type zinc finger proteins in brain development, neurodevelopmental, and other neuropsychiatric disorders: Systematic literature-based analysis. *Frontiers in Neurology*, 11, 32.

Alpert, J. E., & Fava, M. (1997). Nutrition and depression. *Nutrition Reviews*, 55, 145–149.

Alshurafa, N., Lin, A. W., Zhu, F., Ghaffari, R., Hester, J., Delp, E., Rogers, J., & Spring, B. (2019). Counting bites with bits: Expert's workshop addressing calorie and macronutrient intake monitoring. *Journal of Medical Internet Research*, 21, e14904.

Alsiö, J., Olszewski, P. K., Levine, A. S., & Schiöth, H. B. (2012). Feed-forward mechanisms: Addiction-like behavioral and molecular adaptations in overeating. *Frontiers in Neuroendocrinology*, 33, 127–139.

Altmann, P., Cunningham, J., & Dhanesha, U. (1999). Disturbances of cerebral function in people exposed to drinking water contaminated with aluminium sulphate: Retrospective study of the Camelford water incident. *British Medical Journal*, 319, 807–811.

Al-Zubaidi, A., Heldmann, M., Mertins, A., Jauch-Chara, K., & Münte, T. F. (2018). Influences of hunger, satiety, and oral glucose on functional brain connectivity: A multimethod resting-state fMRI study. *Neuroscience*, 382, 80–92.

Amani, R., Tabmasebi, K., & Nazari, Z. (2019). Association of cognitive function with nutritional zinc status in adolescent female students. *Progress in Nutrition*, 21, 86–93.

Amenta, F., & Tayebati, S. K. (2008). Pathways of acetylcholine synthesis, transport and release as targets for treatment of adult-onset cognitive dysfunction. *Current Medicinal Chemistry*, 15, 488–498.

Amin, S. B., Orlando, M., Eddins, A., MacDonald, M., Monczynski, C., & Wang, H. (2010). In utero iron status and auditory neural maturation in premature infants as evaluated by auditory brainstem response. *Journal of Pediatrics*, 156, 377–381.

Amissah, E. A., Brown, J., & Harding, J. E. (2018). Protein supplementation of human milk for promoting growth in preterm infants. *Cochrane Database of Systematic Reviews*, CDD000433.

Anderson, C., Checkoway, H., & Franklin, G. M. (1999). Dietary factors in Parkinson's disease: The role of food groups and specific foods. *Movement Disorders*, 14, 21–27.

Anderson, G., Berk, M., Dean, O., Moylan, S., & Maes, M. (2014). Role of immune-inflammatory and oxidative and nitrosative stress pathways in the etiology of depression: Therapeutic implications. *CNS Drugs*, 28, 1–10.

Anderson, R. M., Donnelly, C. A., & Ferguson, N. M. (1996). Transmission dynamics and epidemiology of BSE in British cattle. *Nature*, 382, 779–788.

Andrade, J. P., Madeira, M. D., & Paula-Barbosa, M. M. (1995a). Evidence of reorganisation in the hippocampal mossy fiber synapses of adult rats rehabilitated after prolonged undernutrition. *Experimental Brain Research*, 104, 249–261.

(1995b). Effects of long-term malnutrition and rehabilitation on the hippocampal formation of the adult rat: A morphometric study. *Journal of Anatomy*, 187, 379–393.

Andreeva, V. A., Galan, P., & Arnaud, J. (2013). Midlife iron status is inversely associated with subsequent cognitive performance, particularly in perimenopausal women. *Journal of Nutrition*, 143, 1974–1981.

Angulo-Barroso, R. M., Li, M., Santos, D. C., Bian, Y., Sturza, J., Jiang, Y., & Lozoff, B. (2016). Iron supplementation in pregnancy or infancy and motor development: A randomized controlled trial. *Pediatrics*, 137, 4.

Anjum, I., Jaffery, S. S., Fayyaz, M., Samoo, Z., & Anjum, S. (2018). The role of vitamin D in brain health: A mini literature review. *Cureus*, 10, e2960.

Annweiler, C., Allali, G., & Allain, P.(2009). Vitamin D and cognitive performance in adults: A systematic review. *European Journal of Neurology*, 16, 1083–1089.

Annweiler, C., Dursun, E., & Feron, F.(2015). Vitamin D and cognition in older adults: Updated international recommendations. *Journal of Internal Medicine*, 277, 45–57.

Anton, K., Baehring, J. M., & Mayer, T. (2012). Glioblastoma multiforme: Overview of current treatment and future perspectives. *Hematology/ Oncology Clinics*, 26, 825–853.

Anton, S. D., Han, H., & York, E. (2009). Effect of calorie restriction on subjective ratings of appetite. *Journal of Human Nutrition and Dietetics*, 22, 141–147.

Aoki, Y. (2001). Polychlorinated biphenyls, polychlorinated dibenzo-p-dioxins, and polychlorinated dibenzofurans as endocrine disrupters: What we have learnt from Yusho disease. *Environmental Research Section*, 86, 2–11.

Appelberg, K. S., Hovda, D. A., & Prins, M. L. (2009). The effects of a ketogenic diet on behavioral outcome after controlled cortical impact injury in the juvenile and adult rat. *Journal of Neurotrauma*, 26, 497–506.

Arab, A., Khorvash, F., Kazemi, M., Heidari, Z., & Askari, G. (2021). Effects of the dietary approaches to stop hypertension (DASH) diet on clinical, quality of life, and mental health outcomes in women with migraine: A randomised controlled trial. *British Journal of Nutrition*, 1–28.

Armario, A., Montero, J. L., & Jolin, T. (1987). Chronic food restriction and the circadian rhythms of pituitary-adrenal hormones, growth hormone and thyroid-stimulating hormone. *Annals of Nutrition & Metabolism*, 31, 81–87.

Armony-Sivan, R., Eidelman, A. I., Lanir, A., Sredni, D., & Yehuda, S. (2004). Iron status and neurobehavioral development of premature infants. *Journal of Perinatology*, 24, 757–762.

Arnulf, I., Quintin, P., & Alvarez, J. C. (2002). Mid-morning tryptophan depletion delays REM sleep onset in healthy subjects. *Neuropsychopharmacology*, 27, 843–851.

Arranz, S., Chiva-Blanch, G., Valderas-Martínez, P., Medina-Remón, A., Lamuela-Raventós, R. M., & Estruch, R. (2012). Wine, beer, alcohol and polyphenols on cardiovascular disease and cancer. *Nutrients*, 4, 759–781.

Arthur, J. R., Beckett, G. J., & Mitchell, J. H. (1999). The interactions between selenium and iodine deficiencies in man and animals. *Nutrition Research Reviews*, 12, 55–73.

Arts, N. J. M., Walvoort, S. J. W., & Kessels, R. P. C. (2017). Korsakoff's syndrome: A critical review. *Neuropsychiatric Disease & Treatment*, 13, 2875–2890.

Ashley, S., Bradburn, S., & Murgatroyd, C. (2019). A meta-analysis of peripheral tocopherol levels in age-related cognitive decline and Alzheimer's disease. *Nutritional Neuroscience*, 10.1080/1028415X.2019.1681066

Attuquayefio, T., & Stevenson, R. J. (2015). A systematic review of longer-term dietary interventions on human cognitive function: Emerging patterns and future directions. *Appetite*, 95, 554–570.

Attuquayefio, T., Stevenson, R. J., Boakes, R. A., Oaten, M. J., Yeomans, M. R., Mahmut, M., & Francis, H. M. (2016). A high-fat high-sugar diet predicts poorer hippocampal related memory and a reduced ability to suppress wanting under satiety. *Journal of Experimental Psychology: Animal Learning & Cognition*, 42, 415–428.

Attuquayefio, T., Stevenson, R. J., Oaten, M. J., & Francis, H. M. (2017). A four-day Western-style dietary intervention causes reductions in hippocampal-dependent learning and memory and interoceptive sensitivity. *PLoS One*, 12, e0172645.

Authority, E. F. S. (2004). Opinion of the scientific panel on dietetic products, nutrition and allergies [NDA] related to the tolerable upper intake level of boron (sodium borate and boric acid). *EFSA Journal*, 2, 80.

Auvinen, H. E., Romijn, J. A., Biermasz, N. R., Pijl, H., Havekes, L. M., Smit, J. W., & Pereira, A. M. (2012). The effects of high fat diet on the basal activity of the hypothalamus-pituitary-adrenal axis in mice. *Journal of Endocrinology*, 214, 191–197.

Avena, N. M., Rada, P., & Hoebel, B. G. (2009). Sugar and fat bingeing have notable differences in addictive-like behavior. *The Journal of Nutrition*, 139, 623–628.

Avitzur, Y., & Courtney-Martin, G. (2016). Enteral approaches in malabsorption. *Best Practice & Research Clinical Gastroenterology*, 30, 295–307.

Azary, S., Schreiner, T., Graves, J., Waldman, A., Belman, A., Guttman, B. W., & Waubant, E. (2018). Contribution of dietary intake to relapse rate in early paediatric multiple sclerosis. *Journal of Neurology Neurosurgery & Psychiatry,* 89, 28–33.

Babur, E., Tan, B., & Yousef, M. (2019). Deficiency but not supplementation of selenium impairs the hippocampal long-term potentiation and hippocampus-dependent learning. *Biological Trace Element Research,* 192, 252–262.

Bachar, E., Canetti, L., & Berry, E. M. (2005). Lack of long-lasting consequences of starvation on eating pathology in Jewish Holocaust survivors of Nazi concentration camps. *Journal of Abnormal Psychology,* 114, 165–169.

Badawy, A. A. (2014). Pellagra and alcoholism: A biochemical perspective. *Alcohol & Alcoholism,* 49, 238–250.

Baggott, M. J., Childs, E., Hart, A. B., de Bruin, E., Palmer, A. A., Wilkinson, J. E., & de Wit, H. (2013). Psychopharmacology of theobromine in healthy volunteers. *Psychopharmacology,* 228, 109–118.

Bailes, J. E., & Mills, J. D. (2010). Docosahexaenoic acid reduces traumatic axonal injury in a rodent head injury model. *Journal of Neurotrauma,* 27, 1617–1624.

Baker, L. B., Nuccio, R. P., & Jeukendrup, A. E. (2014). Acute effects of dietary constituents on motor skills and cognitive performance in athletes. *Nutrition Reviews,* 72, 790–802.

Baker, M. (2016). Is there a reproducibility crisis? *Nature,* 533, 452–454.

Bakir, F., Damluji, S. F., & Amin-Zaki, L. (1973). Methylmercury poisoning in Iraq. *Science,* 181, 230–241.

Balion, C., Griffith, L. E., & Strifler, L. (2012). Vitamin D, cognition, and dementia: A systematic review and meta-analysis. *Neurology,* 79, 1397–1405.

Balk, E. M., Raman, G., & Tatsioni, A. (2007). Vitamin B6, B12, and folic acid supplementation and cognitive function: A systematic review of randomized trials. *Archives of Internal Medicine,* 167, 21–30.

Bambini-Junior, V., Zanatta, G., Della Flora Nunes, G., Mueller de Melo, G., Michels, M., Fontes-Dutra, M., & Gottfried, C. (2014). Resveratrol prevents social deficits in animal model of autism induced by valproic acid. *Neuroscience Letters,* 583, 176–181.

Banji, D., Banji, O. J., Abbagoni, S., Hayath, M. S., Kambam, S., & Chiluka, V. L. (2011). Amelioration of behavioral aberrations and oxidative markers by green tea extract in valproate induced autism in animals. *Brain Research,* 1410, 141–151.

Banks, W. A., Owen, J. B., & Erickson, M. A. (2012). Insulin in the brain: There and back again. *Pharmacology & Therapeutics,* 136, 82–93.

Barbano, M. F., & Cador, M. (2007). Opioids for hedonic experience and dopamine to get ready for it. *Psychopharmacology,* 191, 467–506.

Barceloux, D. G., Bond, G. R., Krenzelok, E. P., Cooper, H., & Vale, J. A. (2002). American Academy of Clinical Toxicology practice guidelines on the treatment of methanol poisoning. *Journal of Toxicology: Clinical Toxicology,* 40, 415–446.

Barichella, M., Cereda, E., Cassani, E., Pinelli, G., Iorio, L., Ferri, V., & Pezzoli, G. (2017). Dietary habits and neurological features of Parkinson's disease patients: Implications for practice. *Clinical Nutrition, 36,* 1054–1061.

Barona, M., Brown, M., & Clark, C. (2019). White matter alterations in anorexia nervosa: Evidence from a voxel-based meta-analysis. *Neuroscience & Biobehavioral Reviews,* 100, 285–295.

Barra, R., Morgan, C., Saez-Briones, P., Reyes-Parada, M., Burgos, H., Morale, B., & Hernandez, A. (2018). Facts and hypotheses about the programming of neuroplastic deficits by prenatal malnutrition. *Nutrition Review,* 77, 65–80.

Barrientos, R. M., Higgins, E. A., Biedenkapp, J. C., Sprunger, D. B., Wright-Hardesty, K. J., Watkins, L. R., & Maier, S. F. (2006). Peripheral infection and aging interact to impair hippocampal memory consolidation. *Neurobiology of Aging,* 27, 723–732.

Barros, A. S., Crispim, R. Y. G., Cavalcanti, J. U., Souza, R. B., Lemos, J. C., Cristino Filho, G., & Aguiar, L. M. V. (2017). Impact of the chronic omega-3 fatty acids supplementation in hemiparkinsonism model induced by 6-hydroxydopamine in rats. *Basic Clinical Pharmacology & Toxicology,* 120, 523–531.

Barrow, M. V., Simpson, C. F., & Miller, E. J. (1974). Lathyrism: A review. *Quarterly Review of Biology,* 49, 101–128.

Başoğlu, M., Yetimalar, Y., & Gürgör, N.,(2006). Neurological complications of prolonged hunger strike. *European Journal of Neurology,* 13, 1089–1097.

Basu, S., McKee, M., Galea, G., & Stuckler, D. (2013). Relationship of soft drink consumption to global overweight, obesity, and diabetes: A cross-national analysis of 75 countries. *American Journal of Public Health,* 103, 2071–2077.

Bavarsad, K., Hosseini, M., Hadjzadeh, M. A. R., & Sahebkar, A. (2018). The effects of thyroid hormones on memory impairment and Alzheimer's disease. *Journal of Cellular Physiology,* 234, 14633–14640.

Bayer-Carter, J. L., Green, P. S., Montine, T. J., VanFossen, B., Baker, L. D., Watson, G. S., & Craft, S. (2011). Diet intervention and cerebrospinal fluid biomarkers in amnestic mild cognitive impairment. *Archives of Neurology,* 68, 743–752.

Bayes, J., Schloss, J., & Sibbritt, D. (2020). Effects of polyphenols in a Mediterranean diet on symptoms of depression: A systematic literature review. *Advances in Nutrition,* 11, 602–615.

Bayram, E., Topcu, Y., & Karakaya, P. (2013). Molybdenum cofactor deficiency: Review of 12 cases (MoCD and review). *European Journal of Paediatric Neurology,* 17, 1–6.

Bazinet, R. P., & Laye, S. (2014). Polyunsaturated fatty acids and their metabolites in brain function and disease. *Nature Reviews Neuroscience,* 15, 771–785.

Beard, J. L., & Connor, J. R. (2003). Iron status and neural functioning. *Annual Review of Nutrition,* 23, 41–58.

Beard, J., Erikson, K. M., & Jones, B. C. (2003). Neonatal iron deficiency results in irreversible changes in dopamine function in rats. *Journal of Nutrition,* 133, 1174–1179.

Beasley, A. N. (2012). Tensions in the field: The politics of researching kuru in New Guinea. *History & Anthropology,* 23 63–89.

Becker, C. B., Middlemass, K., Taylor, B., Johnson, C., & Gomez, F. (2017). Food insecurity and eating disorder pathology. *International Journal of Eating Disorders,* 50, 1031–1040.

Beilharz, J. E., Kaakoush, N. O., Maniam, J., & Morris, M. J. (2016a). The effect of short-term exposure to energy-matched diets enriched in fat or sugar on memory, gut microbiota and markers of brain inflammation and plasticity. *Brain Behavior & Immunity,* 57, 304–313.

(2018). Cafeteria diet and probiotic therapy: Cross talk among memory, neuroplasticity, serotonin receptors and gut microbiota in the rat. *Molecular Psychiatry,* 23, 351–361.

Beilharz, J. E., Maniam, J., & Morris, M. J. (2016b). Short-term exposure to a diet high in fat and sugar, or liquid sugar, selectively impairs hippocampal-dependent memory, with differential impacts on inflammation. *Behavioural Brain Research,* 306, 1–7.

Belarbi, K., Cuvelier, E., Destée, A., Gressier, B., & Chartier-Harlin, M. C. (2017). NADPH oxidases in Parkinson's disease: A systematic review. *Molecular Degeneration,* 12, 84.

Belfort, M., Anderson, P., Nowak, V., Lee, K., Molesworth, C., Thompson, D., Doyle, L., & Inder, T. (2016). Breast milk feeding, brain development and neurocognitive outcomes: A 7-year longitudinal study in infnts born at less than 30 weeks. *Journal of Pediatrics,* 177, 133–139.

Bellinger, F. P., Madamba, S. G., Campbell, I. L., & Siggins, G. R. (1995). Reduced long-term potentiation in the dentate gyrus of transgenic mice with cerebral overexpression of interleukin-6. *Neuroscience Letters,* 198, 95–98.

Benarroch, E. E. (2014). Brain glucose transporters: Implications for neurologic disease. *Neurology,* 82, 1374–1379.

Benau, E. M., Orloff, N. C., Janke, E. A., Serpell, L., & Timko, C. A. (2014). A systematic review of the effects of experimental fasting on cognition. *Appetite,* 77, 52–61.

Benitez-Bribiesca, L., De la Rosa-Alvarez, A., & Mansilla-Olivares, A. (1999). Debdritic spine pathology in infants with severe protein-calorie malnutrition. *Pediatrics,* 104, e21.

Bent, S., Bertoglio, K., & Hendren, R. L. (2009). Omega-3 fatty acids for autistic spectrum disorder: A systematic review. *Journal of Autism & Developmental Disorders,* 39, 1145–1154.

Benton, D. (2007). The impact of diet on anti-social, violent and criminal behaviour. *Neuroscience & Biobehavioral Reviews,* 31, 752–774.

(2008a). Micronutrient status, cognition and behavioral problems in child-hood. *European Journal of Nutrition,* 47, 38–50.

(2008b). Sucrose and behavioral problems. *Critical Reviews in Food Science & Nutrition*, 48, 385–401.

(2012). Symposium 1: Vitamins and cognitive development and performance : Vitamins and neural and cognitive development outcomes in children. *Proceedings of the Nutrition Society*, 71, 14–26.

Benton, D., & Brock, H. (2010). Mood and the macro-nutrient composition of breakfast and the mid-day meal. *Appetite*, 55, 436–440.

Benton, D., & Donohoe, R. (1999). The effects of nutrients on mood. *Public Health Nutrition*, 2, 403–409.

Benton, D., Slater, O., & Donohoe, R. T. (2001). The influence of breakfast and a snack on psychological functioning. *Physiology & Behavior*, 74, 559–571.

Berding, K., Vlckova, K., Marx, W., Schellekens, H., Stanton, C., Clarke, G, Jacka, F., Dinan, T. G., & Cryan, F. J. (2021). Diet and the microbiota-gut-brain axis: Sowing the seeds of good mental health. *Advances in Nutrition*, 12, 1239–1285.

Berendsen, A. A., Kang, J. H., van de Rest, O., Feskens, E. J., de Groot, L. C., & Grodstein, F. (2017). The dietary approaches to stop hypertension diet, cognitive function, and cognitive decline in American older women. *Journal of the American Medical Directors Association*, 18, 427–432.

Bergami, M., Rimondini, R., Santi, S., Blum, R., Gotz, M., & Canossa, M. (2008). Deletion of TrkB in adult progenitors alters newborn neuron integration into hippocampal circuits and increases anxiety-like behavior. *Proceedings of the National Academy of Sciences of the United States of America*, 105, 15570–15575.

Berglund, S. K., Chmielewska, A., Starnberg, J., Westrup, B., Hagglof, B., Norman, M., & Domellof, M. (2018). Effects of iron supplementation of low-birth-weight infants on cognition and behavior at 7 years: A randomized controlled trial. *Pediatric Research*, 83, 111–118.

Bernal, J. (2007). Thyroid hormone receptors in brain development and function. *Nature Clinical Practice Endocrinology & Metabolism*, 3, 249–259.

Berr, C., Arnaud, J., & Akbaraly, T. N. (2012). Selenium and cognitive impairment: A brief-review based on results from the EVA study. *Biofactors*, 38, 139–144.

Bertolino, B., Crupi, R., Impellizzeri, D., Bruschetta, G., Cordaro, M., Siracusa, R., & Cuzzocrea, S. (2017). Beneficial effects of co-ultramicronized palmitoylethanolamide/luteolin in a mouse model of autism and in a case report of autism. *CNS Neuroscience Therapeutics*, 23, 87–98.

Bespalov, A., & Steckler, T. (2018). Lacking quality in research: Is behavioral neuroscience affected more than other areas of biomedical science? *Journal of Neuroscience Methods*, 300, 4–9.

Besson, A., Lagisz, M., Senior, A., Hector, K., & Nakagawa, S. (2016). Effect of maternal diet on offspring coping styles in rodents: A systematic review and meta-analysis. *Biological Review*, 91, 1065–1080.

Bhandari, R., & Kuhad, A. (2017). Resveratrol suppresses neuroinflammation in the experimental paradigm of autism spectrum disorders. *Neurochemical International*, 103, 8–23.

Biasi, E. (2011). The effects of dietary choline. *Neuroscience Bulletin*, 27, 220–342.

Biasini, A., Neri, C., China, M. C., Monti, F., Di Nicola, P., & Bertino, E. (2012). Higher protein intake strategies in human milk fortification for preterm infants feeding. Auzological and neurodevelopmental outcome. *Journal of Biological Regulators & Homeostatic Agents*, 26, 43–47.

Biggio, G., Porceddu, M. L., & Gessa, G. L. (1976). Decrease of homovanillic, dihydroxyphenylacetic acid and cyclic adenosine-3', 5'-monophosphate content in the rat caudate nucleus induced by the acute administration of an amino acid mixture lacking tyrosine and phenylalanine. *Journal of Neurochemistry*, 26, 1253–1255.

Birch, E. E., Garfield, S., Castaneda, Y., Hughbanks-Wheaton, D., Uauy, R., & Hoffman, D. (2007). Visual acuity and cognitive outcomes at 4 years of age in a double-blind, randomized trial of long-chain polyunsaturated fatty acid-supplemented infant formula. *Early Human Development*, 83, 279–284.

Bisanz, J. E., Upadhyay, V., Turnbaugh, J. A., Ly, K., & Turnbaugh, P. J. (2019). Meta-analysis reveals reproducible gut microbiome alterations in response to a high-fat diet. *Cell Host and Microbe*, 26, 265–272 e264.

Bitanihirwe, B. K. Y., & Cunningham, M. G. (2009). Zinc: The brain's dark horse. *Synapse*, 63, 1029–1049.

Bivona, G., Gambino, C. M., Iacolino, G., & Ciaccio, M. (2019). Vitamin D and the nervous system. *Neurological Research*, 41, 827–835.

Bjork, J. M., Grant, S. J., Chen, G., & Hommer, D. W. (2014). Dietary tyrosine/phenylalanine depletion effects on behavioural and brain signatures of human motivational processing. *Neuropsychopharmacology*, 39, 595–604.

Blaak, E. E., Antoine, J. M., & Benton, D. (2012). Impact of postprandial glycaemia on health and prevention of disease. *Obesity Reviews*, 13, 923–984.

Black, R., Allen, L., Bhutta, Z., Caulfield, L., de Onis, Ezzat, M., Mathers, C., Rivera, J., for the Maternal and Child Undernutrition Study Group. (2008). Maternal and child undernutrition: Global and regional exposures and health consequences. *The Lancet*, 371, 243–260.

Blaise, S. A., Nedelec, E., Schroeder, H., Alberto, J. M., Bossenmeyer-Pourie, C., Gueant, J. L., & Daval, J. L. (2007). Gestational vitamin B deficiency leads to homocysteine-associated brain apoptosis and alters neurobehavioral development in rats. *American Journal of Pathology*, 170, 667–679.

Blandina, P., Munari, L., Provensi, G., & Passani, M. B. (2012). Histamine neurons in the tuberomamillary nucleus: A whole center or distinct subpopulations? *Frontiers in Systems Neuroscience*, 6, 33.

Blanton, C. (2014). Improvements in iron status and cognitive function in young women consuming beef or non-beef lunches. *Nutrients*, 6, 90–110.

Bloemendaal, M., Froböse, M. I., & Wegman, J., (2018). Neuro-cognitive effects of acute tyrosine administration on reactive and proactive response inhibition in healthy older adults. *eNeuro*, 5, 1–18.

Blumenthal, J. A., Smith, P. J., Mabe, S., Hinderliter, A., Lin, P. H., Liao, L., & Sherwood, A. (2019). Lifestyle and neurocognition in older adults with cognitive impairments: A randomized trial. *Neurology*, 92, e212–e223.

Blusztajn, J. K., & Wurtman, R. J. (1983). Choline and cholinergic neurons. *Science*, 221, 614–620.

Boggiano, M. M., Turan, B., Maldonado, C. R., Oswald, K. D., & Shuman, E. S. (2013). Secretive food concocting in binge eating: Test of a famine hypothesis. *International Journal of Eating Disorders*, 46, 212–225.

Boivin, M. J., Okitundu, D., & Makila-Mabe Bumoko, G. (2013). Neuropsychological effects of konzo: A neuromotor disease associated with poorly processed cassava. *Pediatrics*, 131, e1231–e1239.

(2017). Cognitive and motor performance in Congolese children with konzo during 4 years of follow-up: A longitudinal analysis. *The Lancet Global Health*, 5, e936–e947.

Bolton, H. M., Burgess, P. W., Gilbert, S. J., & Serpell, L. (2014). Increased set shifting costs in fasted healthy volunteers. *PLoS One*, 9, e101946.

Bond, L., Mayerl, C., Stricklen, B., German, R., & Gould, F. (2020). Changes in the coordination between respiration and swallowing from suckling through weaning. *Biology Letters*, 16, 20190942.

Bondy, S. C. (2010). The neurotoxicity of environmental aluminium is still an issue. *Neurotoxicity*, 31, 575–581.

(2016). Low levels of aluminium can lead to behavioral and morphological changes associated with Alzheimer's disease and age-related neurodegeneration. *NeuroToxicology*, 52, 222–229.

Bonello, M., & Ray, P. (2016). A case of ataxia with isolated vitamin E deficiency initially diagnosed as Friedreich's ataxia. *Case Reports in Neurological Medicine*, 2016, 8342653.

Boonstra, E., de Kleijn, R., Colzato, L. S., Alkemade, A., Forstmann, B. U., & Nieuweenhuis, S. (2015). Neurotransmitters as food supplements: The effects of GABA on brain and behaviour. *Frontiers in Psychology*, 6, 1520.

Booth, S. L. (2009). Roles for vitamin K beyond coagulation. *Annual Review of Nutrition*, 29, 89–110.

Borea, P. A., Gessi, S., Merighi, S., Vincenzi, F., & Varani, K. (2018). Pharmacology of adenosine receptors: The state of the art. *Physiological Reviews*, 98, 1591–1625.

Borge, T., Aase, H., Brantsaeter, A., & Biele, G. (2017). The importance of maternal diet quality during pregnancy on cognitive and behavioural outcomes in children: A systematic review and meta-analysis. *BMJ Open*, 7, e016777.

Borghammer, P. (2018). How does Parkinson's disease begin? Perspectives eon neuroanatomical pathways, prions, and histology. *Movement Disorders*, 33, 48–57.

Borowitz, S. (2021). First bites – Why, when and what solid foods to fee infants. *Frontiers in Pediatrics*, 9, 654171.

Boswell, R. G., & Kober, H. (2016). Food cue reactivity and craving predict eating and weight gain: A meta-analytic review. *Obesity Reviews*, 17, 159–177.

Botez, M. I., Botez, T., & Maag, U. (1984). The Weschler subtests in mild organic brain-damage associated with folate-deficiency. *Psychological Medicine*, 14, 431–437.

Bouayed, J., Rammal, H., Dicko, A., Younos, C., & Soulimani, R. (2007). Chlorogenic acid, a polyphenol from Prunus domestica (Mirabelle), with coupled anxiolytic and antioxidant effects. *Journal of the Neurological Sciences*, 262, 77–84.

Bough, K. J., Wetherington, J., Hassel, B., Pare, J. F., Gawryluk, J. W., Greene, J. G., & Dingledine, R. J. (2006). Mitochondrial biogenesis in the anticonvulsant mechanism of the ketogenic diet. *Annals of Neurology*, 60, 223–235.

Boukouvalas, G., Gerozissis, K., & Kitraki, E. (2010). Adult consequences of post-weaning high fat feeding on the limbic-HPA axis of female rats. *Cellular & Molecular Neurobiology*, 30, 521–530.

Bourg, E. L. (2018). Does calorie restriction in primates increase lifespan? Revisiting studies on macaques (*Macaca mulatta*) and mouse lemurs (*Microcebus murinus*). *BioEssays*, 40, 1800111.

Bourgeois, F. T., Murthy, S., & Mandl, K. D. (2010). Outcome reporting among drug trials registered in ClinicalTrials.gov. *Annals of Internal Medicine*, 153, 158–166.

Boyle, N. B., Lawton, C. L., Allen, R., Croden, F., Smith, K., & Dye, L. (2016). No effects of ingesting or rinsing sucrose on depleted self-control performance. *Physiology & Behavior*, 154, 151–160.

Boyle, N. B., Lawton, C. L., & Dye, L. (2018). The effects of carbohydrates, in isolation and combined with caffeine, on cognitive performance and mood–current evidence and future directions. *Nutrients*, 10, 192.

Bradley, S. J., Taylor, M. J., & Rovet, J. F. (1997). Assessment of brain function in adolescent anorexia nervosa before and after weight gain. *Journal of Clinical and Experimental Neuropsychology*, 19, 20–33.

Bragg. C., Desbrow, B., Hall, S., & Irwin, C. (2017). Effect of meal glycemic load and caffeine consumption on prolonged monotonous driving performance. *Physiology & Behavior*, 181, 110–116.

Brands, A. M. A., Biessels, G. J., de Haan, E. H. F., Kappelle, L. J., & Keessels, R. P. C. (2005). The effects of type 1 diabetes on cognitive performance. *Diabetes Care*, 28, 726–735.

Brandt, K. R. (2015). Effects of glucose administration on category exclusion recognition. *Journal of Psychopharmacology*, 29, 777–782.

Brenner, E. D., Stevenson, D. W., & Twigg, R. W. (2003). Cycads: Evolutionary innovations and the role of plant-derived neurotoxins. *Trends in Plant Science*, 8, 446–452.

Brickman, A. M., Khan, U. A., Provenzano, F. A., Yeung, L. K., Suzuki, W., Schroeter, H., & Small, S. A. (2014). Enhancing dentate gyrus function with dietary flavanols improves cognition in older adults. *Nature Neuroscience*, 17, 1798–1803.

Brock, J. W., & Prasad, C. (1992). Alterations in dendritic spine density in the rat brain associated with protein malnutrition. *Developmental Brain Research*, 66, 266–269.

Brouwer-Brolsma, E. M., & de Groot, L. (2015). Vitamin D and cognition in older adults: An update of recent findings. *Current Opinion in Clinical Nutrition & Metabolic Care*, 18, 11–16.

Brown, J. M., Bland, R., Jonsson, E., & Greenshaw, A. J. (2019). The standardization of diagnostic criteria for Fetal Alcohol Syndrome Disorder (FASD): Implications for research, clinical practice and population health. *Canadian Journal of Psychiatry*, 64, 169–176.

Brown, K., DeCoffe, D., Molcan, E., & Gibson, D. L. (2012). Diet-induced dysbiosis of the intestinal microbiota and the effects on immunity and disease. *Nutrients*, 4, 1095–1119.

Brown, T. M. (2010). Pellagra: An old enemy of timeless importance. *Psychosomatics*, 51, 93–97.

(2015). Neuropsychiatric scurvy. *Psychosomatics*, 56, 12–20.

Brubacher, D., Monsch, A. U., & Stähelin, H. B. (2004). Weight change and cognitive performance. *International Journal of Obesity*, 28, 1163–1167.

Bruner, A. N., Joffe, A., Duggan, A. K., Casella, J. F., & Brandt, J. (1996). Randomised study of cognitive effects of iron supplementation in non-anaemic adolescent girls. *The Lancet*, 348, 992–996.

Bryan, J., Calvaresi, E., & Hughes, D. (2002). Short-term folate, vitamin B-12 or vitamin B-6 supplementation slightly affects memory performance but not mood in women of various ages. *Journal of Nutrition*, 132, 1345–1356.

Bryan, J., & Tiggemann, M. (2001). The effect of weight-loss dieting on cognitive performance and psychological well-being in overweight women. *Appetite*, 36, 147–156.

Budney, A. J., Lee, D. C., & Juliano, L. M. (2015). Evaluating the validity of caffeine use disorder. *Current Psychiatry Reports*, 17, 74.

Buffenstein, R., Karklin, A., & Driver, H. S. (2000). Beneficial physiological and performance responses to a month of restricted energy intake in healthy overweight women. *Physiology & Behavior*, 68, 439–444.

Bunevičius, R., & Prange, A. J. (2010). Thyroid disease and mental disorders: Cause and effect or only comorbidity? *Current Opinion in Psychiatry*, 23, 363–368.

Burger, G. C. E., Sandstead, H. R., & Drummond, J. (1945). Starvation in Western Holland: 1945. *The Lancet*, 2, 282–283.

Burger, K. S., & Stice, E. (2012). Frequent ice cream consumption is associated with reduced striatal response to receipt of an ice cream-based milkshake. *American Journal of Clinical Nutrition*, 95, 810–817.

(2014). Neural responsivity during soft drink intake, anticipation, and advertisement exposure in habitually consuming youth. *Obesity*, 22, 441–450.

Burkle, F. M., Chan, J. T. S., & Yeung, R. D. S. (2013). Hunger strikers: Historical perspectives from the emergency management of refugee camp asylum seekers. *Prehospital and Disaster Medicine*, 28, 625–629.

Burley, V. J., Kreitzman, S. N., Hill, A. J., & Blundell, J. E. (1992). Across-the-day monitoring of mood and energy intake before, during, and after a very-low-calorie diet. *The American Journal of Clinical Nutrition*, 56, 277S–278S.

Burrows, T. L., Ho, Y. Y., Rollo, M. E., & Collins, C. E. (2019). Validity of dietary assessment methods when compared to the method of doubly labelled water: A systematic review in adults. *Frontiers in Endocrinology*, 10, e00850.

Butterly, J., & Shepherd, J. (2010). *Hunger: The Biology and Politics of Starvation*. Lebanon, PA: Dartmouth College Press.

Cahill, G. F. (1970). Starvation in man. *New England Journal of Medicine*, 282, 668–675.

Callahan, L. S., Thibert, K. A., Wobken, J. D., & Georgieff, M. K. (2013). Early-life iron deficiency anemia alters the development and long-term expression of parvalbumin and perineuronal nets in the rat hippocampus. *Developmental Neuroscience*, 35, 427–436.

Calugi, S., Miniati, M., & Milanese, C. (2017). The Starvation Symptom Inventory: Development and psychometric properties. *Nutrients*, 9, 967.

Canda, E., Ucar, S. K., & Coker, M. (2020). Biotinidase deficiency: Prevalence, impact and management strategies. *Pediatric Health, Medicine & Therapeutics*, 11, 127–133.

Canhada, S., Castro, K., Perry, I. S., & Luft, V. C. (2018). Omega-3 fatty acids' supplementation in Alzheimer's disease: A systematic review. *Nutritional Neuroscience*, 21, 529–538.

Cannell, J. J. (2008). Autism and vitamin D. *Medical Hypotheses*, 70, 750–759.

Capewell, S., & Lloyd-Williams, F. (2018). The role of the food industry in health: Lessons from tobacco? *British Medical Bulletin*, 125, 131–143.

Cappelletti, S., Piacentino, D., Fineschi, V., Frati, P., Cipolloni, L., & Aromatario, M. (2018). Caffeine-related deaths: Manner of deaths and categories at risk. *Nutrients*, 10, 611.

Cappello, S., Cereda, E., & Rondanelli, M. (2017). Elevated plasma vitamin B12 concentrations are independent predictors of in-hospital mortality in adult patients at nutritional risk. *Nutrients*, 9, 1.

Cardoso, A., Castro, J. P., Pereira, P. A., & Andrade, J. P. (2013). Prolonged protein deprivation, but not food restriction, affects parvalbumin-containing interneurons in the dentate gyrus of adult rats. *Brain Research*, 1522, 22–30.

Cardoso, B. R., Ong, T. P., & Jacob-Filho, W. (2010). Nutritional status of selenium in Alzheimer's disease patients. *British Journal of Nutrition*, 103, 803–806.

Cardoso, B. R., Szymlek-Gay, E. A., & Roberts, B. R. (2018). Selenium status is not associated with cognitive performance: A cross-sectional study in 154 older Australian adults. *Nutrients*, 10, 1847.

Carlson, E. S., Stead, J. D., Neal, C. R., Petryk, A., & Georgieff, M. K. (2007). Perinatal iron deficiency results in altered developmental expression of genes mediating energy metabolism and neuronal morphogenesis in hippocampus. *Hippocampus*, 17, 679–691.

Carpenter, K. J. (2003). A short history of nutritional science: Part 1 (1795–1885). *Journal of Nutrition*, 133, 638–645.

Carr, K. D. (1996). Feeding, drug abuse, and the sensitization of reward by metabolic need. *Neurochemical Research*, 21, 1455–1467.

Carr, K. D., Park, T. H., Zhang, Y., & Stone, E. A. (1998). Neuroanatomical patterns of Fos-like immunoreactivity induced by naltrexone in food-restricted and ad libitum fed rats. *Brain Research*, 779, 26–32.

Carter, A., Hendrikse, J., Lee, N., Yücel, M., Verdejo-Garcia, A., Andrews, Z. B., & Hall, W. (2016). The neurobiology of 'food addition' and its implications for obesity treatment and policy. *Annual Review of Nutrition*, 36, 105–128.

Carter, E. C., Kofler, L. M., Forster, D. E., & McCullough, M. E. (2015). A series of meta-analytic tests of the depletion effect: Self-control does not seem to rely on a limited resource. *Journal of Experimental Psychology: General*, 144, 796–815.

Carter, R. C., Jacobson, J. L., Burden, M. J., Armony-Sivan, R., Dodge, N. C., Angelilli, M. L., & Jacobson, S. W. (2010). Iron deficiency anemia and cognitive function in infancy. *Pediatrics*, 126, e427–434.

Carvalho, K. M. B., Ronca, D. B., Michels, N., Huybrechts, I., Cuenca-Garcia, M., Marcos, A., & Carvalho, L. A. (2018). Does the Mediterranean diet protect against stress-induced inflammatory activation in European adolescents? The HELENA Study. *Nutrients*, 10, Article 1770.

Casadesus, G., Shukitt-Hale, B., Stellwagen, H. M., Zhu, X. W., Lee, H. G., Smith, M. A., & Joseph, J. A. (2004). Modulation of hippocampal plasticity and cognitive behavior by short-term blueberry supplementation in aged rats. *Nutritional Neuroscience*, 7, 309–316.

Casper, R. C., Voderholzer, U., Naab, S., & Schlegl, S. (2020). Increased urge for movement, physical and mental restlessness, fundamental symptoms of restricting anorexia nervosa. *Brain & Behavior*, 10, e01556.

Cassin, S. E., Buchman, D. Z., Leung, S. E., Kantarvoich, K., Hawa, A., Carter, A., & Sockalingam, S. (2019). Ethical, stigma, and policy implications of food addiction: A scoping review. *Nutrients*, 11, 710.

Castoldi, A. F., Johansson, C., & Onishchenko, N. (2008). Human developmental neurotoxicity of methylmercury: Impact of variables and risk modifiers. *Regulatory Toxicology & Pharmacology*, 51, 201–214.

Castro, K., Baronio, D., Perry, I. S., Riesgo, R. D. S., & Gottfried, C. (2017). The effect of ketogenic diet in an animal model of autism induced by prenatal exposure to valproic acid. *Nutritional Neuroscience*, 20, 343–350.

Ceccatelli, S., Bose, R., Edoff, K., Onishchenko, N., & Spulber, S. (2013). Long-lasting neurotoxic effects of exposure to methylmercury during development. *Journal of Internal Medicine*, 273, 490–497.

Cederholm, T., Salem, N., Jr, & Palmblad, J. (2013). ω-3 Fatty acids in the prevention of cognitive decline in humans. *Advances in Nutrition*, 4, 672–676.

Chae, J., Nahas, Z., & Lomarev, M. (2003). A review of functional neuroimaging studies of vagus nerve stimulation (VNS). *Journal of Psychiatric Research*, 37, 443–455.

Challa, S., Sharkey, J. R., Chen, M., & Phillips, C. D. (2007). Association of resident, facility, and geographic characteristics with chronic undernutrition in a nationally represented sample of older residents in U.S. nursing homes. *Journal of Nutrition Health and Aging*, 11, 179–184.

Chamari, K., Briki, W., & Farooq, A. (2016). Impact of Ramadan intermittent fasting on cognitive function in trained cyclists: A pilot study. *Biology of Sport*, 33, 49–56.

Champ, C. E., Palmer, J. D., Volek, J. S., Werner-Wasik, M., Andrews, D. W., Evans, J. J., & Shi, W. (2014). Targeting metabolism with a ketogenic diet during the treatment of glioblastoma multiforme. *Journal of Neurooncology*, 117, 125–131.

Chandrakumar, A., Bhardwaj, A., & Jong, G. W. (2019). Review of thiamine deficiency disorders: Wernicke encephalopathy and Korsakoff psychosis. *Journal of Basic and Clinical Physiology and Pharmacology*, 30, 153–162.

Chang, S., Zeng, L., Brouwer, I. D., Kok, F. J., & Yan, H. (2013). Effect of iron deficiency anemia in pregnancy on child mental development in rural China. *Pediatrics*, 131, e755–763.

Chaplin, K., & Smith, A. P. (2011). Breakfast and snacks: Associations with cognitive failures, minor injuries, accidents, and stress. *Nutrients*, 3, 515–528.

Chatzi, L., Papadopoulou, E., Koutra, K., Roumeliotaki, T., Georgiou, V., Stratakis, N., & Kogevinas, M. (2012). Effect of high doses of folic acid supplementation in early pregnancy on child neurodevelopment at 18 months of age: The mother-child cohort 'Rhea' study in Crete, Greece. *Public Health Nutrition*, 15, 1728–1736.

Cheatham, R. A., Roberts, S. B., & Das, S. K.(2009). Long-term effects of provided low and high glycemic load low energy diets on mood and cognition. *Physiology & Behavior*, 98, 374–379.

Chen, G., Li, Y., Li, X., Zhou, D., Wang, Y., Wen, X., Wang, C., Liu, X., Feng, Y., Li, B., & Li, N. (2021). Functional foods and intestinal homeostasis: The perspective of in vivo evidence. *Trends in Food Science & Technology*, 111, 475–482.

Chen, L. -Y., Liu, L. -K., & Hwang, A., -C. (2016). Impact of malnutrition on physical, cognitive function and mortality among older men living in veteran homes by minimum data set: A prospective cohort study in Taiwan. *Journal of Nutrition, Health & Aging*, 20, 41–47.

Chen, X., Liu, Z., Sachdev, P. S., Kochan, N. A., O'Leary, F., & Brodaty, H. (2021). Dietary patterns and cognitive health in older adults: Findings from the Sydney Memory and Ageing Study. *Journal of Nutrition Health & Aging*, 25, 255–262.

Chen, Y., & Xue, F. (2020). The impact of gestational hypothyroxinemia on the cognitive and motor development of offspring. *Journal of Maternal-Fetal & Neonatal Medicine*, 33, 1940–1945.

Chen, Y. X, Liu, Z. R., Yu, Y., Yao, E. S., Liu, X. H., & Liu, L. (2017). Effect of recurrent severe hypoglycaemia on cognitive performance in adult patients with diabetes: A meta-analysis. *Journal of Huazhong University of Science and Technology*, 37, 642–648.

Cherian, L., Wang, Y., Holland, T., Agarwal, P., Aggarwal, N., & Morris, M. C. (2020). DASH and Mediterranean-DASH intervention for neurodegenerative delay (MIND) diets are associated with fewer depressive symptoms over time. *Journals of Gerontology: Series A*, 76, 151–156.

Chesler, B. E. (2005). Implications of the Holocaust for eating and weight problems among survivors' offspring: An exploratory study. *European Eating Disorders Review*, 13, 38–47.

Chiang, M., Natarajan, R., & Fan, X. D. (2016). Vitamin D in schizophrenia: A clinical review. *Evidence-Based Mental Health*, 19, 6–9.

Chiovato, L., Magri, F., & Carlé, A. (2019). Hypothyroidism in context: Where we've been and where we're going. *Advances in Therapy*, 36, S47–S58.

Chiu, C., Liu, S., & Willett, W. C. (2011). Informing food choices and health outcomes by use of dietary glycemic index. *Nutritional Reviews*, 69, 231–242.

Choi, I. Y., Piccio, L., Childress, P., Bollman, B., Ghosh, A., Brandhorst, S., & Longo, V. D. (2016). A diet mimicking fasting promotes regeneration and reduces autoimmunity and multiple sclerosis symptoms. *Cell Reports*, 15, 2136–2146.

Choudhary, K. M., Mishra, A., Poroikov, V. V., & Goel, R. K. (2013). Ameliorative effect of Curcumin on seizure severity, depression like behavior, learning and memory deficit in post-pentylenetetrazole-kindled mice. *European Journal of Pharmacology*, 704, 33–40.

Chouet, J., Ferland, G., & Féart, C. (2015). Dietary vitamin K intake is associated with cognition and behaviour among geriatric patients: The CLIP study. *Nutrients*, 7, 6739–6750.

Chowdhury, R., Warnakula, S., Kenutsor, S., Crows, F., Ward. H. A., Johnson, L., Franco, O. H., Butterworth, A. S., Forouhi, N. G., Thompson, S. G., Khaw, K. -T., Mozaffarian, D., Danesh, J., & Di Angelantonio, E. (2014). Association of dietary, circulating, and supplement fatty acids with coronary risk: A systematic review and meta-analysis. *Annals of Internal Medicine*, 160, 398–406.

Christian, P., Murray-Kolb, L. E., Khatry, S. K., Katz, J., Schaefer, B. A., Cole, P. M., & Tielsch, J. M. (2010). Prenatal micronutrient supplementation and intellectual and motor function in early school-aged children in Nepal. *Journal of the American Medical Association*, 304, 2716–2723.

Chugh, G., Asghar, M., Patki, G., Bohat, R., Jafri, F., Allam, F., & Salim, S. (2013). A high-salt diet further impairs age-associated declines in cognitive, behavioral, and cardiovascular functions in male Fischer brown Norway rats. *Journal of Nutrition*, 143, 1406–1413.

Clark, I., & Landolt, H. P. (2017). Coffee, caffeine, and sleep: A systematic review of epidemiological studies and randomized controlled trials. *Sleep Medicine Reviews*, 31, 70–78.

Clarkson, T. W., & Magos, L. (2006). The toxicology of mercury and its chemical compounds. *Clinical Reviews in Toxicology*, 36, 609–662.

Cliff, J., Muquingue, H., Nhassico, D., Nzwalo, H., & Bradbury, J. H. (2011). Konzo and continuing cyanide intoxication from cassava in Mozambique. *Food and Chemical Toxicology*, 631–635.

Cliff, J., & Nicala, D. (1997). Long term follow-up on konzo patients. *Transaction of the Royal Society of Tropical Medicine & Hygiene*, 91, 447–449.

Cocco, S., Diaz, G., & Stancampiano, R. (2002). Vitamin A deficiency produces spatial learning and memory impairment in rats. *Neuroscience*, 115, 475–482.

Cogswell, M. E., Loria, C. M., Terry, A. L., Zhao, L., Wang, C. Y., Chen, T. C., & Appel, L. J. (2018). Estimated 24-hour urinary sodium and potassium excretion in US adults. *Journal of the American Medical Association*, 319, 1209–1220.

Cohen, J., Gorski, M., Gruber, S., Kurdziel, L., & Rimm, E. (2016). The effect of healthy dietary consumption on executive cognitive functioning in children and adolescents: A systematic review. *British Journal of Nutrition*, 116, 989–1000.

Colen, C. G., & Ramey, D. M. (2014). Is breast truly best? Estimating the effects of breastfeeding on long-term child health and wellbeing in the United States using sibling comparisons. *Social Science & Medicine*, 109, 55–65.

Collee, J. G., & Bradley, R. (1997). BSE: A decade on – Part 2. *The Lancet*, 349, 715–721.

Collie, A., Maruff, P., Darby, D., & McStephen, M. (2003). The effects of practice on the cognitive test performance of neurologically normal individuals assessed at brief test-retest intervals. *Journal of the International Neuropsychological Society*, 9, 419–428.

Collinge, J., Whitfield, J., & McKintosh, E. (2006). Kuru in the twenty-first century – An acquired human prion disease with very long incubation periods. *The Lancet*, 367, 2068–2074.

Collins, S. (1995). The limit of human adaptation to starvation. *Nature Medicine*, 1, 810–814.

Collins, S., Dash, S., Allender, S., Jacka, F., & Hoare, E. (2020). Diet and mental health during emerging adulthood: A systematic review. *Emerging Adulthood*, 10, 645–659.

Collins, S., Dent, N., Binns, P., Bahwere, P., Sadler, K., & Hallam, A. (2006). Management of severe acute malnutrition in children. *The Lancet*, 368, 1992–2000.

Colman, R. J., Anderson, R. M., & Johnson, S. C. (2009). Caloric restriction delays disease onset and mortality in rhesus monkeys. *Science*, 325, 201–204.

Colombo, J., Carlson, S. E., Cheatham, C. L., Fitzgerald-Gustafson, K. M., Kepler, A., & Doty, T. (2011). Long-chain polyunsaturated fatty acid supplementation in infancy reduces heart rate and positively affects distribution of attention. *Pediatric Research*, 70, 406–410.

Colombo, J., Carlson, S. E., Cheatham, C. L., Shaddy, D. J., Kerling, E. H., Thodosoff, J. M., & Brez, C. (2013). Long-term effects of LCPUFA supplementation on childhood cognitive outcomes. *American Journal of Clinical Nutrition*, 98, 403–412.

Coltheart, M. (2013). How can functional neuroimaging inform cognitive theories? *Perspectives on Psychological Science*, 8, 98–103.

Colzato, L. S., Steenbergen, L., de Kwaadsteniet, E. W., Sellaro, R., Liepelt, R., & Hommel, B. (2013). Tryptophan promotes interpersonal trust. *Psychological Science*, 24, 2575–2577.

Colzato, L. S., Steenbergen, L., Sellaro, R., Stock, A., Arning, L., & Beste, C. (2016). Effects of L-tyrosine on working memory and inhibitory control are determined by DRD2 genotypes: A randomized controlled trial. *Cortex*, 82, 217–224.

Combs, C. K. (2009). Inflammation and microglia actions in Alzheimer's disease. *Journal of Neuroimmune Pharmacology*, 4, 380–388.

Conner, K. R., Pinquart, M., & Gamble, S. A. (2008). Meta-analyses of depression and substance use among individuals with alcohol use disorders. *Journal of Substance Abuse Treatment*, 37, 127–137.

Conner, K.R., Pinquart, M., & Gamble S. (2009). Meta-analysis of depression and substance use among individuals with alcohol use disorders. *Journal of Substance Abuse and Treatment*, 37, 127–137.

Convit, A. (2005). Links between cognitive impairment in insulin resistance: An explanatory model. *Neurobiology of Aging*, 26, S31–S35.

Cook, C. C., Hallwood, P. H., & Thomson, A. D. (1998). B vitamin deficiency and neuropsychiatric syndromes in alcohol misuse. *Alcohol & Alcoholism*, 33, 317–336.

Cooke, G. E., Mullally, S., Correia, N., O'Mara, S. M., & Gibney, J. (2014). Hippocampal volume is decreased in adults with hypothyroidism. *Thyroid*, 24, 433–440.

Cooper, S. B., Bandelow, S., Nute, M. L., Morris, J. G., & Nevill, M. E. (2015). Breakfast glycaemic index and exercise: Combined effects of adolescents' cognition. *Physiology & Behavior*, 139, 104–111.

Copeland, J., Stevenson, R. J., Gates, P., & Dillon, P. (2007). Young Australians and alcohol: The acceptability of ready-to-drink (RTD) alcoholic beverages among 12-30-year-olds. *Addiction*, 102, 1740–1746.

Copp, R. P., Wisniewski, T., & Hentati, F. (1999). Localisation of alpha-tocopherol transfer protein in the brains of patients with ataxia with vitamin E deficiency and other oxidative stress related neurodegenerative disorders. *Brain Research*, 822, 80–87.

Corbit, L. (2016). Effects of obesogenic diets on learning and habitual responding. *Current Opinion in Behavioral Sciences*, 9, 84–90.

Cordain, L., Eaton, S. B., Sebastian, A., Mann, N., Lindeberg, S., Watkins, B. A., & Brand-Miller, J. (2005). Origins and evolution of the Western diet: Health implications for the twenty-first century. *American Journal of Clinical Nutrition*, 81, 341–354.

Cornu, C., Mercier, C., Ginhoux, T., Masson, S., Mouchet, J., Nony, P., & Revol, O. (2018). A double-blind placebo-controlled randomised trial of omega-3 supplementation in children with moderate ADHD symptoms. *European Child & Adolescent Psychiatry*, 27, 377–384.

Cova, I., Leta, V., Mariani, C., Pantoni, L., & Pomati, S. (2019). Exploring cocoa properties: Is theobromine a cognitive modulator? *Psychopharmacology*, 236, 561–572.

Covaci, A., Voorspoels, S., & Schepens, P. (2008). The Belgian PCB/dioxin crisis–8 years later: An overview. *Environmental Toxicology & Pharmacology*, 25, 164–170.

Cox, P. A., Davis, D. A. Mash, D. C., Metcalf, J. S., & Banack, S. A. (2016). Dietary exposure to an environmental toxin triggers neurofibrillary tangles and amyloid deposits in the brain. *Proceedings of the Royal Society B: Biological Sciences*, 283, 1–9.

Craciunescu, C. N., Brown, E. C., Mar, M. H., Albright, C. D., Nadeau, M. R., & Zeisel, S. H. (2004). Folic acid deficiency during late gestation decreases progenitor cell proliferation and increases apoptosis in fetal mouse brain. *Journal of Nutrition*, 134, 162–166.

Craft, S., Murphy, C., & Wemstrom, J. (1994). Glucose effects on complex memory and nonmemory tasks: The influence of age, sex, and glucoregulatory response. *Psychobiology*, 22, 95–105.

Craig, A., Baer, K., & Diekmann, A. (1981). The effects of lunch on sensory-perceptual functioning in man. *International Archives of Occupational & Environmental Health*, 49, 105–114.

Craig, A., & Richardson, E. (1989). Effects of experimental and habitual lunch-size on performance, arousal, hunger, and mood. *International Archives of Occupational & Environmental Health*, 61, 313–319.

Crook, W. G. (1974). Letter: An alternate method of managing the hyperactive child. *Pediatrics*, 54, 656.

Cryan, J. F., O'Riordan, K. J., Sandhu, K., Peterson, V., & Dinan, T. G. (2020). The gut microbiome in neurological disorders. *The Lancet Neurology*, 19, 179–194.

Cuajungco, M. P., & Lees, G. J. (1997). Zinc metabolism in the brain: Relevance to human neurodegenerative disorders. *Neurobiology of Disease*, 4, 137–169.

Cubo, E., Rivadeneyra, J., Armesto, D., Mariscal, N., Martinez, A., Camara, R. J., & Spanish members of the European Huntington Disease Network. (2015). Relationship between nutritional status and the severity of Huntington's disease. A Spanish multicenter dietary intake study. *Journal of Huntington's Disease*, 4, 78–85.

Cucarella, J. O., Tortajada, R. E., & Moreno, L. R. (2012). Neuropsychology and anorexia nervosa: Cognitive and radiological findings. *Neurología*, 27, 504–510.

Cui, X. Y., Gooch, H., & Groves, N. J. (2015). Vitamin D and the brain: Key questions for future research. *Journal of Steroid Biochemistry & Molecular Biology*, 148, 305–309.

Cusick, K. D., & Sayler, G. S. (2013). An overview on the marine neurotoxin, saxitoxin: Genetics, molecular targets, methods of detection, and ecological functions. *Marine Drugs*, 11, 991–1018.

Cutuli, D. (2017). Functional and structural benefits induced by omega-3 polyunsaturated fatty acids during aging. *Current Neuropharmacology*, 15, 534–542.

Czeizel, A. E., & Dudas, I. (1992). Prevention of the first occurrence of neural-tube defects by periconceptional vitamin supplementation. *New England Journal of Medicine*, 327, 1832–1835.

D'Amour-Horvat, V., & Leyton, M. (2014). Impulsive actions and choices in laboratory animals and humans: Effects of high vs. low dopamine states produced by systemic treatments given to neurologically intact subjects. *Frontiers in Behavioral Neuroscience*, 8, Article 432.

da Costa, K. -A., Kozyreva, O. G., & Song, J. (2006). Common genetic polymorphisms affect the human requirement for the nutrient choline. *FASEB Journal*, 20, 1336–1344.

da Rosa, M. I., Beck, W. O., & Colonetti, T. (2019). Association of vitamin D and vitamin B-12 with cognitive impairment in elderly aged 80 years or older: A cross-sectional study. *Journal of Human Nutrition & Dietetics*, 32, 518–524.

da Silva, T. M., Munhoz, R. P., Alvarez, C., Naliwaiko, K., Kiss, Á., Andreatini, R., & Ferraz, A. C. (2008). Depression in Parkinson's disease: A double-blind, randomized, placebo-controlled pilot study of omega-3 fatty-acid supplementation. *Journal of Affective Disorders*, 111, 351–359.

Dang, J. (2016). Testing the role of glucose in self-control: A meta-analysis. *Appetite*, 107, 222–230.

Danzer, S. C., Kotloski, R. J., Walter, C., Hughes, M., & McNamara, J. O. (2008). Altered morphology of hippocampal dentate granule cell presynaptic and postsynaptic terminals following conditional deletion of TrkB. *Hippocampus*, 18, 668–678.

Davidson, T. L., Chan, K., Jarrard, L. E., Kanoski, S. E., Clegg, D. J., & Benoit, S. C. (2009). Contributions of the hippocampus and medial prefrontal cortex to energy and body weight regulation. *Hippocampus*, 19, 235–252.

Davidson, T. L., Hargrave, S. L., Swithers, S. E., Sample, C. H., Fu, X., Kinzig, K. P., & Zheng, W. (2013). Inter-relationships among diet, obesity and hippocampal-dependent cognitive function. *Neuroscience*, 253, 110–122.

Davidson, T. L., & Jarrard, L. E. (1993). A role for hippocampus in the utilization of hunger signals. *Behavioral & Neural biology*, 59, 167–171.

Davidson, T. L., Monnot, A., Neal, A. U., Martin, A. A., Horton, J. J., & Zheng, W. (2012). The effects of a high-energy diet on hippocampal-dependent discrimination performance and blood-brain barrier integrity differ for diet-induced obese and diet-resistant rats. *Physiology & Behavior*, 107, 26–33.

Davis, C. (2017). A commentary on the associations among 'food addiction', binge eating disorder, and obesity: Overlapping conditions with idiosyncratic clinical features. *Appetite*, 115, 3–8.

394 References

Davis, C., Patte, J., Levitan, R., Reid, C., Tweed, S., & Curtis, C. (2007). From motivation to behavior: A model of reward sensitivity, overeating, and food preferences in the risk profile for obesity. *Appetite*, 48, 12–19.

Davis, T. Z., Lee, S. T., & Collett, M. G. (2015). Toxicity of white snakeroot (*Ageratina altissima*) and chemical extracts of white snakeroot in goats. *Journal of Agricultural & Food Chemistry*, 63, 2092–2097.

de Benoist, B., Andersson, M., Takkouche, B., & Egli, I. (2003). Prevalence of iodine deficiency worldwide. *The Lancet*, 362, 1859–1860.

de Cabo, R., & Mattson, M. P. (2019). Effects of intermittent fasting on health, aging, and disease. *New England Journal of Medicine*, 381, 2541–2551.

de Escobar, G. M., Obregon, M. J., & del Rey, F. E. (2004a). Maternal thyroid hormones early in pregnancy and fetal brain development. *Best Practice and Research Clinical Endocrinology & Metabolism*, 18, 225–248.

(2004b). Role of thyroid hormone during early brain development. *European Journal of Endocrinology*, 151, U25–U37.

De Filippis, F., Pellegrini, N., Vannini, L., Jeffery, I. B., La Storia, A., Laghi, L., & Lazzi, C. (2016). High-level adherence to a Mediterranean diet beneficially impacts the gut microbiota and associated metabolome. *Gut*, 65, 1812–1821.

de Jager, C. A., Dye, L., de Bruin, E. A., Butler, L., Fletcher, J., Lamport, D. J., Latulippe, M. E., Spencer, P. E., & Wesnes, K. (2014). Criteria for validation and selection of cognitive tests for investigation and the effects of food and nutrients. *Nutrition Reviews*, 72, 162–179.

de la Torre, R., de Sola, S., Hernandez, G., Farre, M., Pujol, J., & Rodriguez, J. (2016). Safety and efficacy of cognitive training plus epigallocatechin-3-gallate in young adults with Down's syndrome (TESDAD): A double-blind, randomised, placebo-controlled, phase 2 trial. *The Lancet Neurology*, 15, 801–810.

De Lau, L., Bornebroek, M., Witteman, J., Hofman, A., Koudstaal, P., & Breteler, M. (2005). Dietary fatty acids and the risk of Parkinson disease: The Rotterdam study. *Neurology*, 64, 2040–2045.

de Oliveira Alves, A., Bortalto, T., & Filho, F. B. (2017). Pellagra. *Journal of Emergency Medicine*, 54, 238–240.

de Paula, J., Farah, A. (2019). Caffeine consumption through coffee: Content in the beverage, metabolism, health benefits and risks. *Beverages*, 5, 37.

Defeyter, M. A., & Russo, R. (2013). The effect of breakfast cereal consumption on adolescents' cognitive performance and mood. *Frontiers in Human Neuroscience*, 7, 789.

Deijen, J. B., van der Beck, E. J., Orlebeke, J. F., & van den Berg, H. (1992). Vitamin B-6 supplementation in elderly men: Effects on mood, memory, performance and mental effort. *Psychopharmacology*, 109, 489–496.

Deitrich, R., Zimatkin, S., & Pronko, S. (2006). Oxidation of ethanol in the brain and its consequences. *Alcohol, Research & Health*, 29, 266–273.

Dekker, L. H., Boer, J. M., Stricker, M. D., Busschers, W. B., Snijder, M. B., Nicolaou, M., & Verschuren, W. M. (2013). Dietary patterns within a population are more reproducible than those of individuals. *Journal of Nutrition*, 143, 1728–1735.

Del Parigi, A., Gautier, J. -F., & Chen, K. (2002). Mapping the brain responses to hunger and satiation in humans using positron emission tomography. *Annals of the New York Academy of Sciences*, 967, 387–397.

Delange, F. (1994). The disorders induced by iodine deficiency. *Thyroid*, 4, 107–128.

Delcourt, N., Claudepierre, T., Maignien, T., Arnich, N., & Mattei, C. (2018). Cellular and molecular aspects of the β-N-methylamino-L-alanine (BMAA) mode of action within the neurodegenerative pathway: Facts of controversy. *Toxins*, 10, 1–15.

Deng-Bryant, Y., Prins, M. L., Hovda, D. A., & Harris, N. G. (2011). Ketogenic diet prevents alterations in brain metabolism in young but not adult rats after traumatic brain injury. *Journal of Neurotrauma*, 28, 1813–1825.

DeNinno, M. P. (1998). Chapter 11: Adenosine. *Annual Reports in Medicinal Chemistry*, 33, 111–120.

Deoni, S. C. L., Dean, D. C., Piryatinsky, I., O'Muircheartaigh, J., Waskiewicz, N., Lehman, K., & Dirks, H. (2013). Breastfeeding and early white matter development: A cross-sectional study. *Neuroimage*, 82, 77–86.

Der, G., Batty, G. D., & Deary, I. J. (2006). Effect of breast feeding on. intelligence in children: Prospective study, sibling pairs analysis, and meta-analysis. *British Medical Journal*, 333, 945–948a.

Derr, R. L., Ye, X., Islas, M. U., Desideri, S., Saudek, C. D., & Grossman, S. A. (2009). Association between hyperglycemia and survival in patients with newly diagnosed glioblastoma. *Journal of Clinical Oncology*, 27, 1082–1086.

Desrumaux, C. M., Mansuy, M., & Lemaire, S. (2018). Brain vitamin E deficiency during development is associated with increased glutamate levels and anxiety in adult mice. *Frontiers in Behavioral Neuroscience*, 12, 310.

Dettling, A., Grass, H., & Schuff, A. (2004). Absinthe: Attention performance and mood under the influence of thujone. *Journal of Studies on Alcohol*, 65, 573–581.

Devathasan, G., & Koh, C. (1982). Wernicke's encephalopathy in prolonged fasting. *The Lancet*, 2, 1108–1109.

Devkota, S., Wang, Y., Musch, M. W., Leone, V., Fehlner-Peach, H., Nadimpalli, A., & Chang, E. B. (2012). Dietary-fat-induced taurocholic acid promotes pathobiont expansion and colitis in Il10-/- mice. *Nature*, 487, 104–108.

Devore, E. E., Kang, J. H., Breteler, M. M. B., & Grodstein, F. (2012). Dietary intakes of berries and flavonoids in relation to cognitive decline. *Annals of Neurology*, 72, 135–143.

Devore, E. E., Stampfer, M. J., Breteler, M. M., Rosner, B., Kang, J. H., Okereke, O., & Grodstein, F. (2009). Dietary fat intake and cognitive decline in women with type 2 diabetes. *Diabetes Care*, 32, 635–640.

Dhir, S., Tarasenko, M., Napoli, E., & Giulivi, C. (2019). Neurological, psychiatric, and biochemical aspects of thiamine deficiency in children and adults. *Frontiers in Psychiatry*, 10, 207.

Dias, G. P., Cavegn, N., Nix, A., do Nascimento Bevilaqua, M. C., Stangl, D., Zainuddin, M. S., & Thuret, S. (2012). The role of dietary polyphenols on adult hippocampal neurogenesis: Molecular mechanisms and behavioural effects on depression and anxiety. *Oxidative Medicine & Cellular Longevity*, 2012, 541971.

Dick, D. M., & Beirut, L. J. (2006). The genetics of alcohol dependence. *Current Psychiatry Reports*, 8, 151–157.

Dick, D. M., Smith, G., Olausson, P., Mitchell, S. H., Leeman, R. F., O'Malley, S. S., & Sher, K. (2010). Understanding the construct of impulsivity and its relationship to alcohol use disorders. *Addiction Biology*, 15, 217–226.

Dickey, R. W., & Plakas, S. M. (2010). Ciguatera: A public health perspective. *Toxicon*, 56, 123–136.

Diethelm, K., Remer, T., Jilani, H., Kunz, C., & Buyken, A. E. (2011). Associations between the macronutrient composition of the evening meal and average daily sleep duration in early childhood. *Clinical Nutrition*, 30, 640–646.

Dietler, M. (2006). Alcohol: Anthropological/archaeological perspectives. *Annual Review of Anthropology*, 35, 229–249.

Dinan, T. G., Stanton, C., Long-Smith, C., Kennedy, P., Cryan, J. F., Cowan, C. S., & Sanz, Y. (2019). Feeding melancholic microbes: MyNewGut recommendations on diet and mood. *Clinical Nutrition*, 38, 1995–2001.

Dinh, Q. N., Drummond, G. R., Sobey, C. G., & Chrissobolis, S. (2014). Roles of inflammation, oxidative stress, and vascular dysfunction in hypertension. *Biomedical Research International*, Article 406960.

Dixit, S., Bernardo, A., & Walker, J. M. (2015). Vitamin C deficiency in the brain impairs cognition, increases amyloid accumulation and deposition, and oxidative stress in APP/PSEN1 and normally aging mice. *ACS Chemical Neuroscience*, 6, 570–581.

Dobo, M., & Czeizel, A. E. (1998). Long-term somatic and mental development of children after periconceptional multivitamin supplementation. *European Journal of Pediatrics*, 157, 719–723.

Dobrovolny, J., Smrcka, M., & Bienertova-Vasku, J. (2018). Therapeutic potential of vitamin E and its derivatives in traumatic brain injury-associated dementia. *Neurological Sciences*, 39, 989–998.

Dolan, L. C., Matulka, R. A., & Burdock, G. A. (2010). Naturally occurring food toxins. Toxins, 2, 2289–2332.

Donald, K. A., Eastman, E., Howells, F. M., Adnams, C., Riley, E. P., Woods, R. P., Narr, R. L., & Stein, D. J. (2015). Neuroimaging effects of prenatal alcohol exposure on the developing brain: A magnetic resonance imaging review. *Acta Neuropsychiatrica*, 27, 251–269.

Doniger, G. M., Simon, E. S., & Zivotofsky, A. Z. (2006). Comprehensive computerised assessment of cognitive sequelae of a complete 12–16 hour fast. *Behavioral Neuroscience*, 120, 804–816.

Donoso, F., Egerton, S., Bastiaanssen, T. F., Fitzgerald, P., Gite, S., Fouhy, F., & Cryan, J. F. (2020). Polyphenols selectively reverse early-life stress-induced behavioural, neurochemical and microbiota changes in the rat. *Psychoneuroendocrinology*, 116, 104673.

Dooling, E. C., Schoene, W. C., & Richardson, E. P. (1974). Hallervorden-Spatz syndrome. *Archives of Neurology*, 30, 70–83.

Doweiko, H. E. (2009). *Concepts of Chemical Dependency*. Belmont, CA: Brooks/Cole.

Dowjat, W. K., Adayev, T., Kuchna, I., Nowicki, K., Palminiello, S., Hwang, Y. W., & Wegiel, J. (2007). Trisomy-driven overexpression of DYRK1A kinase in the brain of subjects with Down syndrome. *Neuroscience Letters*, 413, 77–81.

Drenick, E. J., Swendseid, M. E., Blahd, W. H., & Tuttle, S. G. (1964). Prolonged starvation as treatment for severe obesity. *Journal of the American Medical Association*, 187, 100–105.

Drewnowski, A., & Rehm, C. D. (2014). Consumption of added sugars among US children and adults by food purchase location and food source. *American Journal of Clinical Nutrition*, 100, 901–907.

Driver, H. S., Shulman, I., Baker, F. C., & Buffenstein, R. (1999). Energy content of the evening meal alters nocturnal body temperature but not sleep. *Physiology & Behavior*, 68, 17–23.

Drover, J. R., Felius, J., Hoffman, D. R., Castaneda, Y. S., Garfield, S., Wheaton, D. H., & Birch, E. E. (2012). A randomized trial of DHA intake during infancy: School readiness and receptive vocabulary at 2–3.5 years of age. *Early Human Development*, 88, 885–891.

Duclos, M., Bouchet, M., Vettier, A., & Richard, D. (2005). Genetic differences in hypothalamic-pituitary-adrenal axis activity and food restriction-induced hyperactivity in three inbred strains of rats. *Journal of Neuroendocrinology*, 17, 740–752.

Duke, A. A., Bégue, L., Bell, R., & Eisenlohr-Moul, T. (2013). Revisiting the serotonin-aggression relation in humans: A meta-analysis. *Psychological Bulletin*, 139, 1148–1172.

Dumetz, F., Buré, C., & Alfos, S.(2020). Normalization of hippocampal retinoic acid level corrects age-related memory deficits in rats. *Neurobiology of Aging*, 85, 1–10.

Duncan, G. G., Jenson, W. K., Fraser, R. I., & Cristofori, F. C. (1962). Correction and control of intractable obesity. *Journal of the American Medical Association*, 181, 309–312.

Duvanel, C. B., Fawer, C. L., Cotting, J., Hohlfeld, P., & Matthieu, J. M. (1999). Long-term effects of neonatal hypoglycemia on brain growth and psychomotor development in small-for-gestational-age preterm infants. *Journal of Pediatrics*, 134, 492–498.

Dyall, S. C. (2015). Long-chain omega-3 fatty acids and the brain: A review of the independent and shared effects of EPA, DPA, and DHA. *Frontiers in Aging Neuroscience*, 7, 52.

Dye, L., Boyle, N. B., Champ, C., & Lawton, C. (2017). The relationship between obesity and cognitive health and decline. *Proceedings of the Nutrition Society*, 76, 443–454.

East, P., Delker, E., Lozoff, B., Delva, J., Castillo, M., & Gahagan, S. (2018). Associations among infant iron deficiency, childhood emotion and attention regulation, and adolescent problem behaviors. *Child Development*, 89, 593–608.

East, P., Lozoff, B., Blanco, E., Delker, E., Delva, J., Encina, P., & Gahagan, S. (2017). Infant iron deficiency, child affect, and maternal unresponsiveness: Testing the long-term effects of functional isolation. *Developmental Psychology*, 53, 2233–2244.

Eckardt, M. J., File, S. E., Gessa, G. L., Grant, K. A., Guerri, C., Hoffman, P. L., Kalant, H., Koob, G. F., Li, T. -K., & Tabakoff, B. (1998). Effects of moderate alcohol consumption on the central nervous system. *Alcoholism: Clinical and Experimental Research*, 22, 998–1040.

Eckert, E. D., Gottesman, I. J., Swigart, S. E., & Casper, R. C. (2018). A 57-year follow-up investigation and review of the Minnesota study on human starvation and its relevance to eating disorders. *Archives of Psychology*, 2, 1–19.

Edefonti, V., Bravi, F., & Ferraroni, M. (2017). Breakfast and behaviour in morning tasks: Facts or fads? *Journal of Affective Disorders*, 224, 16–26.

Edefonti, V., Rosato, V., & Parpinel, M. (2014). The effect of breakfast composition and energy contribution on cognitive and academic performance: A systematic review. *American Journal of Clinical Nutrition*, 100, 626–656.

Edington, J., & Kon, P. (1997). Prevalence of malnutrition in the community. *Nutrition*, 13, 238–240.

Edlow, A. (2017). Maternal obesity and neurodevelopmental and psychiatric disorders in offspring. *Prenatal Diagnosis*, 37, 95–110.

Edwards, L. M., Murray, A. J., Holloway, C. J., Carter, E. E., Kemp, G. J., Codreanu, I., & Clarke, K. (2011). Short-term consumption of a high-fat diet impairs whole-body efficiency and cognitive function in sedentary men. *FASEB Journal*, 25, 1088–1096.

Eilander, A., Gera, T., Sacdev, H., Transler, C., van der Knaap, H., Kok, F., & Osendarp, S. (2010). Multiple micronutrient supplementation for improving cognitive performance in children: Systematic review of randomized controlled trials. *American Journal of Clinical Nutrition*, 91, 115–130.

Ekino, S., Susa, M., Ninomiya, T., Imamura, K., & Kitamura, T. (2007). Minamata disease revisited: An update on the acute and chronic manifestations of methyl mercury poisoning. *Journal of the Neurological Sciences*, 262, 131–144.

Elgen, I., Sommerfelt, K., & Ellertsen, B. (2003). Cognitive performance in a low birth weight cohort at 5 and 11 years of age. *Pediatric Neurology*, 29, 111–116.

El-Rashidy, O., El-Baz, F., El-Gendy, Y., Khalaf, R., Reda, D., & Saad, K. (2017). Ketogenic diet versus gluten free casein free diet in autistic children: A case-control study. *Metabolic Brain Disease*, 32, 1935–1941.

Ely, A. V., Winter, S., & Lowe, M. R. (2013). The generation and inhibition of hedonically-driven food intake: Behavioral and neurophysiological determinants in healthy weight individuals. *Physiology & Behavior*, 121, 25–34. p

Erol, A., & Karpyak, V. M. (2015). Sex and gender-related differences in alcohol use and its consequences: Contemporary knowledge and future research considerations. *Drug & Alcohol Dependence*, 156, 1–13.

Eschleman, M. M. (1996). *Introductory Nutrition and Nutrition Therapy*. Philadelphia, PA: Lippincott-Raven Publishers.

Escudero-Lourdes, C. (2016). Toxicity mechanisms of arsenic that are shared with neurodegenerative diseases and cognitive impairment: Role of oxidative stress and inflammatory responses. *NeuroToxicology*, 53, 223–235.

Esgate, A., Groome, D., & Baker, K. (2005). *An Introduction to Applied Cognitive Psychology*. Madrid, ESP: Psychology Press.

Estruch, R. (2010). Anti-inflammatory effects of the Mediterranean diet: The experience of the PREDIMED study. *Proceedings of the Nutrition Society*, 69, 333–340.

Estruch, R., Ros, E., Salas-Salvado, J., Covas, M. I., Corella, D., & Aros, F. (2018). Primary prevention of cardiovascular disease with a Mediterranean diet supplemented with extra-virgin olive oil or nuts. *New England Journal of Medicine*, 378, e34.

European Food Safety Authority. (2010). Scientific opinion on dietary reference values for fats, including saturated fatty acids, polyunsaturated fatty acids, monounsaturated fatty acids, *trans* fatty acids, and cholesterol. *EFSA Journal*, 8, 1461.

Evangeliou, A., Vlachonikolis, I., Mihailidou, H., Spilioti, M., Skarpalezou, A., Makaronas, N., & Smeitink, J. (2003). Application of a ketogenic diet in children with autistic behavior: Pilot study. *Journal of Child Neurology*, 18, 113–118.

Eveleigh, E. R., Coneyworth, L. J., Avery, A., & Welham, S. J. M. (2020). Vegans, vegetarian, and omnivores: How does dietary choice influence iodine intake? A systematic review. *Nutrients*, 12, 1606.

Evenhouse, E., & Reilly, S. (2005). Improved estimates of the benefits of breastfeeding using sibling comparisons to reduce selection bias. *Health Services Research*, 40, 1781–1802.

Exley, C. (2017). Aluminum should now be considered a primary etiological factor in Alzheimer's disease. *Journal of Alzheimer's Disease Reports*, 1, 23–25.

Exon, J. H. (2006). A review of the toxicology of acrylamide. *Journal of Toxicology and Environmental Health*, 9, 397–412.

Fagerberg, C. R., Taylor, A., & Distelmaier, F. (2020). Choline transporter-like I deficiency causes a new type of childhood-onset neurodegeneration. *Brain*, 143, 94–111.

Fanelli, D. (2018). Is science really facing a reproducibility crisis, and do we need it to? *Proceedings of the National Academy of Sciences of the United States of America*, 115, 2628–2631.

Farez, M. F., Fiol, M. P., Gaitán, M. I., Quintana, F. J., & Correale, J. (2015). Sodium intake is associated with increased disease activity in multiple sclerosis. *Journal of Neurology, Neurosurgery & Psychiatry*, 86, 26–31.

Farhat, G., Lees, E., Macdonald-Clarke, C., & Amirabdollahian, F. (2019). Inadequacies of micronutrient intake in normal weight and overweight young adults aged 18-25 years: A cross-sectional study. *Public Health*, 167, 70–77.

Farquharson, J., Cockburn, F., Patrick, W. A., Jamieson, E. C., & Logan, R. W. (1992). Infant cerebral cortex phospholipid fatty-acid composition and diet. *The Lancet*, 340, 810–813.

Fattal, I., Friedmann, N., & Fattal-Valevski, A. (2011). The crucial role of thiamine in the development of syntax and lexical retrieval: A study of infantile thiamine deficiency. *Brain*, 134, 1720–1739.

Faulkner, P., & Deakin, J. F. W. (2014). The role of serotonin in reward, punishment, and behavioural inhibition in humans: Insights from studies with acute tryptophan depletion. *Neuroscience & Biobehavioral Reviews*, 46, 365–378.

Favaro, A., Rodella, F. C., & Santonastaso, P. (2000). Binge eating and eating attitudes among Nazi concentration camp survivors. *Psychological Medicine*, 30, 463–466.

Fávaro-Moreira, N. C., Krausch-Hofmann, S., & Matthys, C. (2016). Risk factors for malnutrition in older adults: A systematic review of the literature based on longitudinal data. *Advances in Nutrition*, 7, 507–522.

Fejzo, M., Poursharif, B., Korst, L., Munch, S., MacGibbon, K., Romero, R., & Goodwin, T. (2009). Symptoms and pregnancy outcomes associated with extreme weight loss among women with Hyperemesis Gravidarum. *Journal of Women's Health*, 18, 1981–1987.

Feldman, R. S., Meyer, J. S., & Quenzer, L. F. (1997). *Principles of Neuropsychopharmacology*. Sunderland, MA: Sinauer Associates, Inc., Publishers.

Ferguson, S. A., Berry, K. J., Hansen, D. K., Wall, K. S., White, G., & Antony, A. C. (2005). Behavioral effects of prenatal folate deficiency in mice. *Birth Defects Research A: Clinical and Molecular Teratology*, 73, 249–252.

Ferland, G. (2012). Vitamin K, an emerging nutrient in brain function. *BioFactors*, 38, 151–157.

Ferland, G., Feart, C., & Presse, N. (2016). Vitamin K antagonists and cognitive function in older adults: The Three-City Cohort Study. *Journals of Gerontology*, 71, 1356–1362.

Fernandez-Aranda, F., Karwautz, A., & Treasure, J. (2018). Food addiction: A transdiagnostic construct of increasing interest. *European Eating Disorders Review*, 26, 536–540.

Fernstrom, J. D. (2013). Large neutral amino acids: Dietary effects on brain neurochemistry and function. *Amino Acids*, 45, 419–430.

Fernstrom, J. D., & Wurtman, R. J. (1971). Brain serotonin content: Increase following ingestion of carbohydrate diet. *Science*, 174, 1023–1025.

Ferré, S. (2016). Mechanisms of the psychostimulant effects of caffeine: Implications for substance use disorders. *Psychopharmacology*, 233 1963–1979.

Fessler, D. M. T. (2003). The implications of starvation induced psychological changes for the ethical treatment of hunger strikers. *Psychiatric Ethics*, 29, 243–247.

Fichter, M., Pirke, K., & Holsboer, F. (1986). Weight loss causes neuroendocrine disturbances: Experimental study in healthy starving subjects. *Psychiatry Research*, 17, 61–72.

Finkelstein, Y., Markowitz, M. E., & Rosen, J. F. (1998). Low-level lead-induced neurotoxicity in children: An update on central nervous system effects. *Brain Research Reviews*, 27, 168–176.

Fiocco, A. J., Shatenstein, B., Ferland, G., Payette, H., Belleville, S., Kergoat, M. J., & Greenwood, C. E. (2012). Sodium intake and physical activity impact cognitive maintenance in older adults: The NuAge Study. *Neurobiology of Aging*, 33, e821–828.

Fishman, J. B., Rubin, J. B., Handrahan, J. V., Connor, J. R., & Fine, R. E. (1987). Receptor-mediated transcytosis of transferrin across the blood-brain barrier. *Journal of Neuroscience Research*, 18, 299–304.

Fisler, J. S., & Drenick, E. J. (1987). Starvation and semistarvation diets in the management of obesity. *Annual Review of Nutrition*, 7, 465–484.

Fitzgerald, K. C., Tyry, T., Salter, A., Cofield, S. S., Cutter, G., Fox, R., & Marrie, R. A. (2018). Diet quality is associated with disability and symptom severity in multiple sclerosis. *Neurology*, 90, e1–e11.

Flint, R. W., & Turek, C. (2003). Glucose effects on a continuous performance test of attention in adults. *Behavioural Brain Research*, 142, 217–228.

Food and Drug Administration. (2012). Bad Bug Book https://www.fda.gov/ food/foodborne-pathogens/bad-bug-book-second-edition

Ford, A. H., & Almeida, O. P. (2019). Effect of vitamin B supplementation on cognitive function in the elderly: A systematic review and meta-analysis. *Drugs & Aging*, 36, 419–434.

Förstera, B., Castro, P. A., Moraga-Cid, G., & Aguayo, L. G. (2016). Potentiation of gamma aminobutyric acid receptors (GABA$_A$R) by ethanol: How are inhibitory receptors affected? *Frontiers in Cellular Neuroscience*, 10, e00114.

Forzano, L. B., Chelonis, J. J., Casey, C., Forward, M., Stachowiak, J. A., & Wood, J. (2010). Self-control and impulsiveness in nondieting adult human females: Effects of visual food cues and food deprivation. *The Psychological Record*, 60, 587–608.

Foster, G. D., Wadden, T. A., Peterson, F. J., Letizia, K. A., Bartlett, S. J., & Conill, A. M. (1992). A controlled comparison of three very-low-calorie diets: Effects on weight, body composition, and symptoms. *The American Journal of Clinical Nutrition*, 55, 811–817.

Foster, J. K., Lidder, P. G., Sunram, S. I. (1998). Glucose and memory: Fractionation of enhancement effects? *Psychopharmacology*, 137, 259–270.

Franca, T. F., & Monserrat, J. M. (2018). Reproducibility crisis in science or unrealistic expectations? *EMBO Reports*, 19, e46008.

Francis, H. M., & Stevenson, R. J. (2011). Higher reported saturated fat and refined sugar intake is associated with reduced hippocampal-dependent memory and sensitivity to interoceptive signals. *Behavioral Neuroscience*, 125, 943–955.

Frank, G. K., Bailer, U. F., Henry, S., Wagner, A., & Kaye, W. H. (2004). Neuroimaging studies in eating disorders. *CNS Spectrums*, 9, 539–548.

Frank, S., Veit, R., & Sauer, H. (2016). Dopamine depletion reduces food-related reward activity independent of BMI. *Neuropsychopharmacology*, 41, 1551–1559.

Freeland-Graves, J. H., Sachdev, P. K., Binderberger, A. Z., & Sosanya, M. E. (2020). Global diversity of dietary intakes and standards for zinc, iron, and copper. *Journal of Trace Elements in Medicine & Biology*, 61, 126515.

Fretham, S. J. B., Carlson, E. S., & Georgieff, M. K. (2011). The role of iron in learning and memory. *Advances in Nutrition*, 2, 112–121.

Friedli, N., Stanga, Z., & Sobotka, L. (2017). Revisiting the refeeding syndrome: Results of a systematic review. *Nutrition*, 35, 151–160.

Fries, E., Green, P., & Bowen, D. J. (1995). What did I eat yesterday? Determinants of accuracy in 24-hour food memories. *Applied Cognitive Psychology*, 9, 143–155.

Frisardi, V., Panza, F., Seripa, D., Imbimbo, B. P., Vendemiale, G., Pilotto, A., & Solfrizzi, V. (2010a). Nutraceutical properties of Mediterranean diet and cognitive decline: Possible underlying mechanisms. *Journal of Alzheimer's Disease*, 22, 715–740.

Frisardi, V., Solfrizzi, V., & Capurso, C. (2010b). Aluminum in the diet and Alzheimer's disease: From current epidemiology to possible disease-modifying treatment. *Journal of Alzheimer's Disease*, 20, 17–30.

Frodl, T., & O'Keane, V. (2013). How does the brain deal with cumulative stress? A review with focus on developmental stress, HPA axis function and hippocampal structure in humans. *Neurobiology of Disease*, 52, 24–37.

Frydman-Marom, A., Levin, A., Farfara, D., Benromano, T., Scherzer-Attali, R., Peled, S., & Ovadia, M. (2011). Orally administered cinnamon extract reduces beta-amyloid oligomerization and corrects cognitive impairment in Alzheimer's disease animal models. *PLoS One*, 6, e16564.

Fuglset, T. S., Endestad, T., Landrø, N. I., & Rø, O. (2015). Brain structure alterations associated with weight changes in young females with anorexia nervosa: A case series. *Neurocase*, 21, 169–177.

Fukui, K., Nakamura, K., & Shirai, M. (2015). Long-term vitamin E-deficient mice exhibit cognitive dysfunction via elevation of brain oxidation. *Journal of Nutritional Neuroscience & Vitaminology*, 61, 362–368.

Fukui, K., Omoi, N.-O., Hayasaka, T., Shinnkai, T., Suzuki, S., Abe, K., & Urano, S. (2002). Cognitive impairment of rats caused by oxidative stress and aging, and its prevention by vitamin E. *Annals of the New York Academy of Sciences*, 959, 275–284.

Fusar-Poli, L., Gabbiadini, A., Ciancio, A., Vozza, L., Signorelli, M. S., & Aguglia, E. (2021). The effect of cocoa-rich products on depression, anxiety, and mood: A systematic review and meta-analysis. *Critical Reviews in Food Science & Nutrition*, 1–13.

Gabbai, Lisbonne, & Pourquier. (1951). Ergot poisoning at Pont St. Esprit. *British Medical Journal*, 2, 650–651.

Gailiot, M. T., & Baumeister, R. F. (2007). The physiology of willpower: Linking blood glucose to self-control. *Personality & Social Psychology Review*, 11, 303–327

Gailliot, M. T., Baumeister, R. F., & DeWall, C. N. (2007). Self-control relies on glucose as a limited energy source: Willpower is more than a metaphor. *Journal of Personality & Social Psychology*, 92, 325–336.

Galioto, R., & Spitznagel, M. B. (2016). The effects of breakfast and breakfast composition on cognition in adults. *Advances in Nutrition*, 7, 567S–589S.

Gano, L. B., Patel, M., & Rho, J. M. (2014). Ketogenic diets, mitochondria, and neurological diseases. *Journal of Lipid Research*, 55, 2211–2228.

Gao, X., Chen, H., Fung, T. T., Logroscino, G., Schwarzschild, M. A., Hu, F. B., & Ascherio, A. (2007). Prospective study of dietary pattern and risk of Parkinson disease. *American Journal of Clinical Nutrition*, 86, 1486–1494.

Gao, Y., Sheng, C., Xie, R. H., Sun, W., Asztalos, E., Moddemann, D., & Wen, S. W. (2016). New perspective on impact of folic acid supplementation during pregnancy on neurodevelopment/autism in the offspring children – A systematic review. *PLoS One*, 11, e0165626.

Garcia-Aloy, M., Rabassa, M., Casas-Agustench, p., Hidalgo-Liberona, N., Llorach, R., & Andres-Lacueva, C. (2017). Novel strategies for improving dietary exposure assessment: Multiple-data fusion is a more accurate measure than the traditional single-biomarker approach. *Trends in Food Science & Technology*, 69, 220–229.

Gashu, D., Stoecker, B. J., & Bougma, K. (2016). Stunting, selenium deficiency and anemia are associated with poor cognitive performance in preschool children from rural Ethiopia. *Nutrition Journal*, 15, 38.

Gasior, M., Rogawski, M. A., & Hartman, A. L. (2006). Neuroprotective and disease-modifying effects of the ketogenic diet. *Behavioural Pharmacology*, 17, 431–439.

Gasperi, V., Sibilano, M., Savini, I., & Catani, M. V. (2019). Niacin in the central nervous system: An update of biological aspects and clinical applications. *International Journal of Molecular Sciences*, 20, 974.

Ge, Q., Wang, Z., Wu, Y., Huo, Q., Qian, Z., Tian, Z., & Han, J. (2017). High salt diet impairs memory-related synaptic plasticity via increased oxidative stress and suppressed synaptic protein expression. *Molecular Nutrition & Food Research*, 61, Article 1700134.

Gearhardt, A. H., Corbin, W. R., & Brownell, K. D. (2009). Preliminary validation of the Yale Food Addiction Scale. *Appetite*, 52, 430–436.

Gearhardt, A. N., Yokum, S., Orr, P. T., Stice, E., Corbin, W. R., & Bronwell, K. D. (2011). Neural correlates of food addiction. *Archives of General Psychiatry*, 68, 808–816.

Gemming, L., Utter, J., & Mhurchu, C. N. (2015). Image-assisted dietary assessment: A systematic review of the evidence. *Journal of the Academy of Nutrition & Dietetics*, 115, 64–77.

Geng, F. J., Mai, X. Q., Zhan, J. Y., Xu, L., Zhao, Z. Y., Georgieff, M., & Lozoff, B. (2015). Impact of fetal-neonatal iron deficiency on recognition memory at 2 months of age. *Journal of Pediatrics*, 167, 1226–1232.

Georgieff, M. K. (2017). Iron assessment to protect the developing brain. *American Journal of Clinical Nutrition*, 106, 1588s–1593s.

Georgieff, M. K., Brunette, K. E., & Tran, P. V. (2015). Early life nutrition and neural plasticity. *Development & Psychopathology*, 27, 411–423.

Ghassabian, A., & Trasande, L. (2018). Disruption in thyroid signalling pathway: A mechanism for the effect of endocrine-disrupting chemicals on child neurodevelopment. *Frontiers in Endocrinology*, 9, 204.

Gibbs, M. E., & Summers, R. J. (2002). Effects of glucose and 2-deoxyglucose on memory formation in the chick: Interaction with beta(3)-adrenoceptor agonists. *Neuroscience*, 114, 69–79.

Gietzen, D. W., & Aja, S. M. (2012). The brain's response to an essential amino acid-deficient diet and the circuitous route to a better meal. *Molecular Neurobiology*, 46, 332–348.

Gietzen, D. W., Hao, S., & Anthony, T. G. (2007). Mechanisms of food intake repression in indispensable amino acid deficiency. *Annual Review of Nutrition*, 27, 63–78.

Gietzen, D. W., & Rogers, Q. R. (2006). Nutritional homeostasis and indispensable amino acid sensing: A new solution to an old puzzle. *Trends in Neurosciences*, 29, 91–99.

Gilbert, J., & Burger, K. (2016). Neuroadaptive processes associated with palatable food intake: Present data and future directions. *Current Opinion in Behavioral Sciences*, 9, 91–96.

Giles, G. E., Avanzato, B. F., Mora, B., Jurdak, N. A., & Kanarek, R. B. (2018). Sugar intake and expectation effects on cognition and mood. *Experimental and Clinical Psychopharmacology*, 26, 302–309.

Giles, G. E., Mahoney, C. R., & Caruso, C., (2019). Two days of calorie deprivation impairs high level cognitive processes, mood, and self-reported exertion during aerobic exercise: A randomized double-blind, placebo-controlled study. *Brain & Cognition*, 132, 33–40.

Gill, O. N., Spencer, Y., & Richard-Loendt, A., (2013). Prevalent abnormal prion protein in human appendixes after bovine spongiform encephalopathy epizootic: Large scale survey. *British Medical Journal*, 347, 1–12.

Giriko, C. A., Andreoli, C. A., Mennitti, L. V., Hosoume, L. F., Souto Tdos, S., Silva, A. V., & Mendes-da-Silva, C. (2013). Delayed physical and neurobehavioral development and increased aggressive and depression-like behaviors in the rat offspring of dams fed a high-fat diet. *International Journal of Developmental Neuroscience,* 31, 731–739.

Global Burden of Disease 2016 Alcohol Collaborators. (2018). Alcohol use and burden for 195 countries and territories, 1990-2016: A systematic analysis for the Global Burden of Disease Study 2016. *The Lancet,* 392, 1015–1035.

Goedert, M., Clavaguera, F., & Tolnay, M. (2010). The propagation of prion-like protein inclusions in neurodegenerative diseases. *Trends in Neurosciences,* 33, 317–325.

Gold, P. E. (1986). Glucose modulation of memory storage processing. *Behavioral & Neural Biology,* 45, 342–349.

(1995). Role of glucose in regulating the brain and cognition. *American Journal of Clinical Nutrition,* 61, 987S–995S.

(2014). Regulation of memory – From the adrenal medulla to liver to astrocytes to neurons. *Brain Research Bulletin,* 105, 25–35.

Goldstone, A. P., Prechtl de Hermandez, C. G., & Beaver, J. D. (2009). Fasting biases brain reward systems toward high-calorie foods. *European Journal of Neuroscience,* 30, 1625–1635.

Goodlett, C. R., & Horn, K. H. (2001). Mechanisms of alcohol-induced damage to the developing nervous system. *Alcohol Research & Health,* 25, 175–184.

Gordon, E. L., Ariel-Donges, A. H., Bauman, V., & Merlo, L. J. (2018). What is the evidence for 'food addiction'? *A systematic review. Nutrients,* 10, 477.

Gorgolewski, K. J., & Poldrack, R. A. (2016). A practical guide for improving transparency and reproducibility in neuroimaging research. *PLoS Biology,* 14, e1002506.

Gosselin, R. D. (2020). Statistical analysis must improve to address the reproducibility crisis: The ACcess to transparent statistics (ACTS) call to action. *BioEssays,* 42, e1900189.

Gould, E., & Tanapat, P. (1999). Stress and hippocampal neurogenesis. *Biological Psychiatry,* 46, 1472–1479.

Gowda, U., Mutowo, M. P., Smith, B. J., Wlulka, A., & Renzaho, A. M. N. (2015). Vitamin D supplementation to reduce depression in adults: Meta-analysis of randomized controlled trials. *Nutrition,* 31, 421–429.

Grandjean, P., Weihe, P., & Jørgensen, P. J. (1992). Impact of maternal seafood diet on fetal exposure to mercury, selenium, and lead. *Archives of Environmental & Occupational Health,* 47, 185–195.

Granholm, A. C., Bimonte-Nelson, H. A., Moore, A. B., Nelson, M. E., Freeman, L. R., & Sambamurti, K. (2008). Effects of a saturated fat and high cholesterol diet on memory and hippocampal morphology in the middle-aged rat. *Journal of Alzheimer's Disease,* 14, 133–145.

Grant, C. L., Dorrian, J., & Coates, A. M.(2017). The impact of meal timing on performance, sleepiness, gastric upset, and hunger during simulated night shift. *Industrial Health,* 55, 423–436.

Grantham-McGregor, S., Cheung, Y., Cueto, S., Glewwe, P., Richter, L., Strupp, B., & the International Child Development Group. (2007). Developmental potential in the first 5 years for children in developing countries. *The Lancet,* 369, 60–70.

Gratwicke, J., Jahanshahi, M., & Foltynie, T. (2015). Parkinson's disease dementia: A neural networks perspective. *Brain,* 138, 1454–1476.

Green, M. W., Elliman, N. A., & Kretsch, M. J. (2005). Weight loss strategies, stress, and cognitive function: Supervised versus unsupervised dieting, *Psychoneuroendocrinology,* 30, 908–918.

Green, M. W., Elliman, N. A., & Rogers, P. J. (1997). Impaired cognitive processing in dieters: Failure of attention focus or resource capacity limitation? *British Journal of Health Psychology,* 2, 259–267.

Green, M. W., & Rogers, P. J. (1995). Impaired cognitive functioning during spontaneous dieting. *Psychological Medicine,* 25, 1003–1010.

(1998). Impairments in working memory associated with spontaneous dieting behaviour. *Psychological Medicine,* 28, 1063–1070.

Green, M. W., Rogers, P. J., & Elliman, N. A. (2000). Dietary restraint and addictive behaviors: The generalizability of Tiffany's Cue Reactivity Model. *International Journal of Eating Disorders,* 27, 419–427.

Green, M. W., Rogers, P. J., Elliman, N. A., & Gatenby, S. J. (1994). Impairment of cognitive processing associated with dieting and high levels of dietary restraint. *Physiology & Behavior,* 55, 447–452.

Green, M. W., Taylor, M. A., Elliman, N. A., & Rhodes, O. (2001). Placebo expectancy effects in the relationship between glucose and cognition. *British Journal of Nutrition,* 86, 173–179.

Green, R., Allen, L. H., & Bjørke-Monsen, A. -L.(2017). Vitamin B12 deficiency. *Nature Reviews Disease Primers,* 3, 17040.

Greenwood, C. E., & Winocur, G. (1990). Learning and memory impairment in rats fed a high saturated fat diet. *Behavioral & Neural Biology,* 53, 74–87.

(1996). Cognitive impairment in rats fed high-fat diets: A specific effect of saturated fatty-acid intake. *Behavioral Neuroscience,* 110, 451–459.

Greminger, A. R., Lee, D. L., Shrager, P., & Mayer-Proschel, M. (2014). Gestational iron deficiency differentially alters the structure and function of white and gray matter brain regions of developing rats. *Journal of Nutrition,* 144, 1058–1066.

Grimm, P. (2010). Social desirability bias. In J. Sheth & N. Malhotra (Eds.) *Wiley International Encyclopedia of Marketing.* London: Wiley. https://doi .org/10.1002/9781444316568.wiem02057

Grosso, G., Godos, J., Galvano, F., & Giovannucci, E. L. (2017). Coffee, caffeine, and health outcomes: An umbrella review. *Annual Review of Nutrition,* 37, 131–156.

Grosso, G., Pajak, A., Marventano, S., Castellano, S., Galvano, F., Bucolo, C., & Caraci, F. (2014). Role of omega-3 fatty acids in the treatment of depressive disorders: A comprehensive meta-analysis of randomized clinical trials. *PLoS One,* 9, Article 9605.

Growdon, J. H., Melamed, E., Logue, M., Hefti, F., & Wurtman, R. J. (1982). Effects of oral L-tyrosine administration of CSF tyrosine and homovanillic acid levels in patients with Parkinson's disease. *Life Sciences*, 30, 827–832.

Gu, Y., Brickman, A. M., Stern, Y., Habeck, C. G., Razlighi, Q. R., Luchsinger, J. A., & Scarmeas, N. (2015). Mediterranean diet and brain structure in a multiethnic elderly cohort. *Neurology*, 85, 1744–1751.

Gu, Y., Nieves, J. W., Stern, Y., Luchsinger, J. A., & Scarmeas, N. (2010). Food combination and Alzheimer disease risk: A protective diet. *Archives of Neurology*, 67, 699–706.

Guilarte, T. R. (1993). Vitamin B6 and cognitive development: Recent research findings from human and animal studies. *Nutrition Reviews*, 51, 193–198.

Guisinger, S. (2003). Adapted to flee famine: Adding and evolutionary perspective on anorexia nervosa. *Psychological Review*, 110, 745–761.

Gunduz, A., Turedi, S., Russell, R. M., & Ayaz, F. A. (2008). Clinical review of grayanotoxin/mad honey poisoning past and present. *Clinical Toxicology*, 46, 437–442.

Guo, C. P., Wei, Z., Huang, F., Qin, M., Li, X., Wang, Y. M., & Wang, X. C. (2017). High salt induced hypertension leads to cognitive defect. *Oncotarget*, 8, 95780–95790.

Gupta, A., & Lutsenko, S. (2009). Human copper transporters: Mechanism, role in human disease and therapeutic potential. *Future Medicinal Chemistry*, 1, 1125–1142.

Gupta, C. C., Dorrian, J., & Grant, C. L. (2017). It's not just what you eat but when: The impact of eating a meal during simulated shift work on driving performance. *Chronobiology International*, 34, 66–77.

Gupta, L., Gupta, R. K., & Gupta, P. K. (2016). Assessment of brain cognitive functions in patients with vitamin B12 deficiency using resting state functional MRI: A longitudinal study. *Magnetic Resonance Imagery*, 34, 191–196.

Gutiérrez, A., González-Gross, M., Delgado, M., & Castillo, M. J. (2001). Three days fast in sportsmen decreases physical work capacity but not strength or perception-reaction time. *International Journal of Sport Nutrition & Exercise Metabolism*, 11, 420–429.

Guzmán-Gerónimo, H.-G. A.-M., Meza-Alvarado, E., Vargas-Moreno, I., & Herrera-Meza, S. Effect of blackberry juice (*Rubus fruticosus* L.) on anxiety-like behaviour in Wistar rats. *International Journal of Food Science & Nutrition*, 70, 856–867.

Hadgkiss, E. J., Jelinek, G. A., Weiland, T. J., Pereira, N. G., Marck, C. H., & van der Meer, D. M. (2015). The association of diet with quality of life, disability, and relapse rate in an international sample of people with multiple sclerosis. *Nutritioinal Neuroscience*, 18, 125–136.

Hafermann, G. (1955). School fatigue and blood sugar change. *Öffentlicher Gesundheitsdienst*, 17, 1.

Hagger, M. S., Wood, C., Stiff, C., & Chatzisarantis, N. L. D. (2010). Ego depletion and the strength model of self-control: A meta-analysis. *Psychological Bulletin*, 136, 495–525.

Hagmeyer, S., Haderspeck, J. C., & Grabrucker, A. M. (2015). Behavioral impairments in animal models for zinc deficiency. *Frontiers in Behavioral Medicine*, 8, 443.

Hales, C., & Barker, D. (1992). Type 2 diabetes mellitus: The thrifty phenotype hypothesis. *Diabetologia*, 35, 595–601.

Hall, J. L., Gonder-Frederick, L. A., Chewning, W. W., Silveira, J., & Gold, P. E. (1989). Glucose enhancement of performance of memory tests in young and aged humans. *Neuropsychologia*, 27, 1129–1138.

Hallberg, L. (2001). Perspectives on nutritional iron deficiency. *Annual Review of Nutrition*, 21, 1–21.

Hallström, H., & Thuvander, A. (1997). Toxicological evaluation of myristicin. *Natural Toxins*, 5, 186–192.

Hamer, M., & Steptoe, A. (2012). Cortisol responses to mental stress and incident hypertension in healthy men and women. *Journal of Clinical Endocrinology & Metabolism*, 97, E29–34.

Hansen, N., Chaieb, L., Derner, M., Hampel, K., Elger, C., Surges, R., Staresina, B., Axmacher, N., & Fell, J. (2018). Memory encoding-related anterior hippocampal potentials are modulated by deep brain stimulation of the entorhinal area. *Hippocampus*, 28, 12–17.

Hansen, S. N., Tveden-Nyborg, P., & Lykkesfeldt, J. (2014). Does vitamin C deficiency affect cognitive development and function? *Nutrients*, 6, 3818–3846.

Hantson, P., Duprez, T., & Mahieu, P. (1997). Neurotoxicity to the basal ganglia shown by magnetic resonance imaging (MRI) following poisoning by methanol and other substances. *Journal of Toxicology: Clinical Toxicology*, 35, 151–161.

Hao, S., Avraham, Y. Mechoulam, R., & Berry, E. M. (2000). Low dose anandamide affects food intake, cognitive function, neurotransmitter and corticosterone levels in diet-restricted mice. *European Journal of Pharmacology*, 392, 147–156.

Haque, A. M., Hashimoto, M., Katakura, M., Hara, Y., & Shido, O. (2008). Green tea catechins prevent cognitive deficits caused by A beta(1-40) in rats. *Journal of Nutritional Biochemistry*, 19, 619–626.

Harada, M. (1995). Minamata disease: Methylmercury poisoning in Japan caused by environmental pollution. *Critical Reviews in Toxicology*, 25, 1–24.

Hardman, C. A., Rogers, P. J., Dallas, R., Scott, J., Ruddock, H. K., & Robinson, E. (2015). 'Food addiction is real'. The effects of exposure to this message on self-diagnosed food addiction and eating behaviour. *Appetite*, 91, 179–184.

Hargrave, S. L., Davidson, T. L., Zheng, W., & Kinzig, K. P. (2016). Western diets induce blood-brain barrier leakage and alter spatial strategies in rats. *Behavioral Neuroscience*, 130, 123–135.

Hargrave, S. L., Jones, S., & Davidson, T. L. (2016). The outward spiral: A vicious cycle model of obesity and cognitive dysfunction. *Current Opinion in Behavioral Sciences*, 9, 40–46.

Haring, B., Wu, C., Coker, L. H., Seth, A., Snetselaar, L., Manson, J. E., & Wassertheil-Smoller, S. (2016). Hypertension, dietary sodium, and cognitive decline: Results from the women's health initiative memory study. *American Journal of Hypertension*, 29, 202–216.

Harrison, N. L., Skelly, M. J., Grosserode, E. K., Lowes, D. C., Zeric, T., Phister, S., & Salling, M. C. (2017). Effects of acute alcohol on excitability in the CNS. *Neuropharmacology*, 122, 36–45.

Harvie, M. N., Pegington, M., & Mattson, M. P. (2011). The effects of intermittent or continuous energy restriction on weight loss and metabolic disease risk markers: A randomised trial in young overweight women. *International Journal of Obesity*, 35, 714–727.

Harvie, M., Wright, C., & Pegington, M.(2013). The effect of intermittent energy and carbohydrate restriction v. daily energy restriction on weight loss and metabolic disease risk markers in overweight women. *British Journal of Nutrition*, 110, 1534–1547.

Hase, A., Jung, S. E., & aan het Rot, M. (2015). Behavioral and cognitive effects of tyrosine intake in healthy human adults. *Pharmacology Biochemistry & Behavior*, 113, 1–6.

Haslam, D. W., & James, W. P. T. (2005). Obesity. *The Lancet*, 366, 1197–1209

Hassan, A. M., Mancano, G., Kashofer, K., Frohlich, E. E., Matak, A., Mayerhofer, R., & Holzer, P. (2019). High-fat diet induces depression-like behaviour in mice associated with changes in microbiome, neuropeptide Y, and brain metabolome. *Nutritional Neuroscience*, 22, 877–893.

Hassing, L., Wahlin, A., Winblad, B., & Backman, L. (1999). Further evidence on the effects of vitamin B-12 and folate levels on episodic memory functioning: A population-based study of healthy very old adults. *Biological Psychiatry*, 45, 1472–1480.

Hasz, L. A., & Lamport, M. A. (2012). Breakfast and adolescent academic performance: An analytical review of recent research. *European Journal of Business & Social Sciences*, 1, 61–79.

Hauck, C., Cook, B., & Ellrott, T. (2020). Food addiction, eating addiction and eating disorders. *Proceedings of the Nutrition Society*, 79, 103–112.

Hausser, J., Stahlecker, C., Mojzisch, A., Leder, A., Van Lange, P., & Faber, N. (2019). Acute hunger does not always undermine prosociality. *Nature Communications*, 10, 4733.

Hawkins, R. A., O'Kane, R. L., Simpson, I. A., & Viña, J. R. (2006). Structure of the blood-brain barrier and its role in the transport of amino acids. *Journal of Nutrition*, 136, 218S–226S.

Hawks, S. R., Madanat, H. N., & Christley, H. S. (2008). Behavioral and biological associations of dietary restraint: A review of the literature. *Ecology of Food & Nutrition*, 47, 415–449.

Hay, P. J., & Sachdev, P. (2011). Brain dysfunction in anorexia nervosa: Cause or consequence of under-nutrition? *Current Opinion in Psychiatry*, 24, 251–256.

Hayden, K. E., Sandle, L. N., & Berry, J. L. (2015). Ethnicity and social deprivation contribute to vitamin D deficiency in an urban UK population. *Journal of Steroid Biochemistry & Molecular Biology*, 148, 253–255.

He, Q., Xiao, L., Xue, G., Wong, S., Ames, S. L., Schembre, S. M., & Bechara, A. (2014). Poor ability to resist tempting calorie rich food is linked to altered balance between neural systems involved in urge and self-control. *Nutrition Journal*, 13, 92.

Health.gov. (2015). Australia's Youth: Nutrition. www.aihw.gov.au/reports/children-youth/nutrition

Healy-Stoffel, M., & Levant, B. (2018). N-3 (Omega-3) fatty acids: Effects on brain dopamine systems and potential role in the etiology and treatment of neuropsychiatric disorders. *CNS & Neurological Disorders-Drug Targets*, 17, 216–232.

Heaney, J. L., Phillips, A. C., & Carroll, D. (2012). Aging, health behaviors, and the diurnal rhythm and awakening response of salivary cortisol. *Experimental Aging Research*, 38, 295–314.

Heath, C. A., Cooper, S. A., & Murray, K. (2010). Validation of diagnostic criteria for variant Creutzfeldt-Jakob disease. *Annals of Neurology*, 67, 761–770.

Hebben, N., Corkin, S., Eichenbaum, H., & Shedlack, K. (1985). Diminished ability to interpret and report internal states after bilateral medial temporal resection: Case H.M. *Behavioral Neuroscience*, 99, 1031–1039.

Heeley, N., & Blouet, C. (2016). Central amino acid sensing in the control of feeding behavior. *Frontiers in Endocrinology*, 7, 148.

Heiderstadt, K. M., McLaughlin, R. M., Wright, D. C., Walker, S. E., & Gomez-Sanchez, C. E. (2000). The effect of chronic food and water restriction on open-field behaviour and serum corticosterone levels in rats. *Laboratory Animals*, 34, 20–28.

Heikkila, K., Sacker, A., Kelly, Y., Renfrew, M. J., & Quigley, M. A. (2011). Breast feeding and child behaviour in the Millennium Cohort Study. *Archives of Diseases of Childhood*, 96, 635–642.

Heinrichs, S. C. (2010). Dietary omega-3 fatty acid supplementation for optimizing neuronal structure and function. *Molecular Nutrition & Food Research*, 54, 447–456.

Heinz, A. J., Beck, A., Meyer-Lindenberg, A., Sterzer, P., & Heinz, A. (2011). Cognitive and neurobiological mechanisms of alcohol-related aggression. *Nature Reviews Neuroscience*, 12, 400–413.

Hellenbrand, W., Seidler, A., Boeing, H., Robra, B. P., Vieregge, P., Nischan, P., & Ulm, G. (1996). Diet and Parkinson's disease. I: A possible role for the past intake of specific foods and food groups. Results from a self-administered food-frequency questionnaire in a case-control study. *Neurology*, 47, 636–643.

Henderson, S. T., Vogel, J. L., Barr, L. J., Garvin, F., Jones, J. J., & Costantini, L. C. (2009). Study of the ketogenic agent AC-1202 in mild to moderate Alzheimer's disease: A randomized, double-blind, placebo-controlled, multicenter trial. *Nutrition Metabolism*, 6, 31.

Heni, M., Kullmann, S., Preissl, H., Fritsche, A., & Häring, H. (2015). Impaired insulin action in the human brain: Causes and metabolic consequences. *Nature Reviews Endocrinology*, 11, 701–711.

Hentze, H., & Ibsen, E. (2019). Abstract 90: The 'reproducibility crisis' of animal studies in oncology – How did we get here, and how can we resolve it? *Proceedings of the American Association for Cancer Research Annual Meeting* 2019, 79.

Herbert, V. (1961). Experimental nutritional folate deficiency in man. *Transactions of the Association of American Physicians*, 75, 307–320.

Herman, J. P., McKlveen, J. M., Ghosal, S., Kopp, B., Wulsin, A., Makinson, R., & Myers, B. (2016). Regulation of the hypothalamic-pituitary-adrenocortical stress response. *Comparative Physiology*, 6, 603–621.

Herman, J. P., Ostrander, M. M., Mueller, N. K., & Figueiredo, H. (2005). Limbic system mechanisms of stress regulation: Hypothalamo-pituitary-adrenocortical axis. *Progress in Neuropsychopharmacology & Biological Psychiatry*, 29, 1201–1213.

Herrick, C. (2009). Shifting blame/selling health: Corporate social responsibility in the age of obesity. *Sociology of Health & Illness*, 31 51–65.

Hewlett, P., Smith, A., & Lucas, E. (2009). Grazing, cognitive performance, and mood. *Appetite*, 52, 245–248.

Heymsfield, S., Thomas, D., Nguyen, A., Peng, J., Martin, C., Shen, W., Strauss, B., Bosy-Westphal, A., & Muller, M. (2010). Voluntary weight loss: Systematic review of early phase body composition changes. *Obesity Reviews*, 12, e348–e361.

Heywood, A., Oppenheimer, S., Heywood, P., & Jolley, D. (1989). Behavioral effects of iron supplementation in infants in Madang, Papua New Guinea. *American Journal of Clinical Nutrition*, 50, 630–637.

Hiffler, L., Rakotoambinina, B., Lafferty, N., & Garcia, D. M. (2016). Thiamine deficiency in tropical pediatrics: New insights into a neglected but vital metabolic challenge. *Frontiers in Neuroscience*, 3, 16.

Higgs, S., & Donohoe, J. E. (2011). Focusing on food during lunch enhances lunch memory and decreases later snack intake. *Appetite*, 57, 202–206.

Higgs, S., Williamson, A. C., & Attwood, A. S. (2008). Recall of recent lunch and its effect on subsequent snack intake. *Physiology & Behavior*, 94, 454–462.

Hildebrandt, M. A., Hoffmann, C., Sherrill-Mix, S. A., Keilbaugh, S. A., Hamady, M., Chen, Y. Y., & Wu, G. D. (2009). High-fat diet determines the composition of the murine gut microbiome independently of obesity. *Gastroenterology*, 137, 1716–1724.

Hill, A. B. (1965). The environment and disease: Association or causation? *Proceedings of the Royal Society of Medicine*, 58, 295–300.

Hill, A. F., Desbruslais, M., & Joiner, S. (1997). The same prion strain causes vCJD and BSE. *Nature*, 389, 448–450.

Hill, A. J., & Heaton-Brown, L. (1994). The experience of food craving: A prospective investigation in healthy women. *Journal of Psychosomatic Research*, 38, 801–814.

Hindmarch, T., Hotopf, M., & Owen, G. (2013). Depression and decision-making capacity for treatment or research: A systematic review. *BMC Medical Ethics*, 14, 54.

Hinterberger, M., & Fischer, P. (2013). Folate and Alzheimer: When time matters. *Journal of Neural Transmission*, 120, 211–224.

Hipgrave, D. B., Chang, S., Li, X., & Wu, Y. (2016). Salt and sodium intake in China. *Journal of the American Medical Association*, 315, 703–705.

Hipólito-Reis, J., Pereira, P. A., Andrade, J. P., & Cardoso, A. (2013). Prolonged protein deprivation differentially affects calretinin- and parvalbumin-containing interneurons in the hippocampal dentate gyrus of adult rats. *Neuroscience Letters*, 555, 154–158.

Hirohata, M., Hasegawa, K., Tsutsumi-Yasuhara, S., Ohhashi, Y., Ookoshi, T., Ono, K., & Naiki, H. (2007). The anti-amyloidogenic effect is exerted against Alzheimer's beta-amyloid fibrils in vitro by preferential and reversible binding of flavonoids to the amyloid fibril structure. *Biochemistry*, 46, 1888–1899.

Hise, M. A., Sullivan, D. K., Jacobsen, D. J., Johnson, S. L., & Donnelly, J. E. (2002). Validation of energy intake measurements determined from observer-recorded food records and recall methods compared with the doubly labelled water method in overweight and obese individuals. *American Journal of Clinical Nutrition*, 75, 263–267.

Hoddinott, J., Malussio, J., Behrman, J., Flores, R., & Martorell, R. (2008). Effect of a nutrition intervention during early childhood on economic productivity in Guatemalan adults. *The Lancet*, 371, 411–416.

Holloway, C. J., Cochlin, L. E., Emmanuel, Y., Murray, A., Codreanu, I., Edwards, L. M., & Clarke, K. (2011). A high-fat diet impairs cardiac high-energy phosphate metabolism and cognitive function in healthy human subjects. *American Journal of Clinical Nutrition*, 93, 748–755.

Holmes, G. L., Yang, Y., Liu, Z., Cermak, J. M., Sarkisian, M. R., Stafstrom, C. E., & Blusztajn, J. K. (2002). Seizure-induced memory impairment is reduced by choline supplementation before or after status epilepticus. *Epilepsy Research*, 48, 3–13.

Holmes, M. C., French, K. L., & Secki, J. R. (1997). Dysregulation of diurnal rhythms of serotonin 5-HT_{2C} and corticosteroid receptor gene expression in the hippocampus with food restriction and glucocorticoids. *Journal of Neuroscience*, 17, 4056–4065.

Holmes, P., James, K. A., & Levy, L. S. (2009). Is low-level environmental mercury exposure of concern to human health? *Science of the Total Environment*, 408, 171–182.

Holt, N. R., & Nickson, C. P. (2018). Severe methanol poisoning with neurological sequalae: Implications for diagnosis and management. *Internal Medicine Journal*, 48, 335–339.

Hone-Blanchet, A., & Fecteau, S. (2014). Overlap of food addiction and substance use disorders definitions: Analysis of animal and human studies. *Neuropharmacology*, 85, 81–90.

Hooijmans, C. R., Van der Zee, C. E., Dederen, P. J., Brouwer, K. M., Reijmer, Y. D., van Groen, T., & Kiliaan, A. J. (2009). DHA and cholesterol containing diets influence Alzheimer-like pathology, cognition and cerebral vasculature in APPswe/PS1dE9 mice. *Neurobiology of Disease*, 33, 482–498.

Hopkins, L. C., Sattler, M., Steeves, E. A., Jones-Smith, J. C., & Gittelsohn, J. (2017). Breakfast consumption frequency and its relationship to overall diet quality, using healthy eating index 2010, and body mass index among adolescence in a low-income urban setting. *Ecology of Food & Nutrition*, 56, 297–311.

Hoppe, J. B., Coradini, K., Frozza, R. L., Oliveira, C. M., Meneghetti, A. B., Bernardi, A., & Salbego, C. G. (2013). Free and nanoencapsulated curcumin suppress beta-amyloid-induced cognitive impairments in rats: Involvement of BDNF and Akt/GSK-3 beta signaling pathway. *Neurobiology of Learning & Memory*, 106, 134–144.

Horsager, C., Færk, E., Lauritsen, M. B., & Østergaard, S. D. (2020). Validation of the Yale Food Addiction Scale 2.0 and estimation of the population prevalence of food addiction. *Clinical Nutrition*, 39, 2917–2928.

Horvath, A., Lukasik, J., & Szajewska, H. (2017). Omega-3 fatty acid supplementation does not affect autism spectrum disorder in children: A systematic review and meta-analysis. *Journal of Nutrition*, 147, 367–376.

Hosking, D. E., Eramudugolla, R., Cherbuin, N., & Anstey, K. J. (2019). MIND not Mediterranean diet related to 12-year incidence of cognitive impairment in an Australian longitudinal cohort study. *Alzheimers Dement*, 15, 581–589.

Hoyland, A., Dye, L., & Lawton, C. L. (2009). A systematic review of the effect of breakfast on the cognitive performance of children and adolescents. *Nutrition Research Reviews*, 22, 220–243.

Hoyland, A., Lawton, C. L., & Dye, L. (2008). Acute effects of macronutrient manipulations on cognitive test performance in healthy young adults: A systematic research review. *Neuroscience & Biobehavioral Reviews*, 32, 72–85.

Hsu, T., & Kanoski, S. (2014). Blood-brain barrier disruption: Mechanistic links between Western diet consumption and dementia. *Frontiers in Aging Neuroscience*, 6, 88.

Hu, Z. G., Wang, H. D., Qiao, L., Yan, W., Tan, Q. F., & Yin, H. X. (2009). The protective effect of the ketogenic diet on traumatic brain injury-induced cell death in juvenile rats. *Brain Injury*, 23, 459–465.

Hucke, S., Wiendl, H., & Klotz, L. (2016). Implications of dietary salt intake for multiple sclerosis pathogenesis. *Multiple Sclerosis*, 22, 133–139.

Hughes, C. A., Ward, M., & Tracey, F. (2017). B-vitamin intake and biomarker status in relation to cognitive decline in healthy older adults in a 4-year follow-up study. *Nutrients*, 9, 53.

Hulsken, S., Märtin, A., Mohajeri, M. H., & Homberg, J. R. (2013). Food-derived serotonergic modulators: Effects on mood and cognition. *Nutrition Research Reviews*, 26, 223–234.

Hunt, C. D., & Id so, J. P. (1995). Moderate copper deprivation during gestation and lactation affects dentate gyrus and hippocampal maturation in immature male rats. *Journal of Nutrition*, 125, 2700–2710.

Hurley, S. W., & Johnson, A. K. (2015). The biopsychology of salt hunger and sodium deficiency. *Pflügers Archive: European Journal of Physiology*, 467, 445–456.

Hussin, N. M., Shahar, S., Teng, N. I., Ngah, W. Z., & Das, S. K. (2013). Efficacy of fasting and calorie restriction (FCR) on mood and depression among ageing men. *The Journal of Nutrition, Health and Aging*, 17, 674–680.

Idjradinata, P., & Pollitt, E. (1993). Reversal of developmental delays in iron-deficient anaemic infants treated with iron. *The Lancet*, 341, 1–4.

Inan-Eroglu, E., & Ayaz, A. (2018). Is aluminium exposure a risk factor for neurological disorders? *Journal of Research in Medical Sciences*, 23, 1–7.

Irwin, C., Khalesi, S., Desbrow, B., & McCartney, D. (2020). Effects of acute caffeine consumption following sleep loss on cognitive, physical, occupational and driving performance: A systematic review and meta-analysis. *Neuroscience & Biobehavioral Reviews*, 108, 877–888.

Isaacs, E. B., Fischl, B. R., Quinn, B. T., Chong, W. K., Gadian, D. G., & Lucas, A. (2010). Impact of breast milk on intelligence quotient, brain size, and white matter development. *Pediatric Research*, 67, 357–362.

Islam, M. R., Ali, S., & Karmoker, J. R. (2020). Evaluation of serum amino acids and non-enzymatic antioxidants in drug-naïve first-episode major depressive disorder. *BMC Psychiatry*, 20, 333.

Ize-Ludlow, D., Ragone, S., Bruck, I. S., Bernstein, J. N., Duchowny, M., & Peña, B. M. (2004). Neurotoxicities in infants seen with the consumption of star anise tea. *Pediatrics*, 114, e653–e656.

Jack, R., Rabin, P. L., & McKinney, T. D. (1983). Dialysis encephalopathy: A review. *The International Journal of Psychiatry in Medicine*, 13, 309–326.

Jacka, F. N., Cherbuin, N., Anstey, K. J., Sachdev, P., & Butterworth, P. (2015). Western diet is associated with a smaller hippocampus: A longitudinal investigation. *BMC Medicine*, 13. Article 215.

Jacka, F. N., O'Neil, A., Opie, R., Itsiopoulos, C., Cotton, S., Mohebbi, M., & Berk, M. (2017). A randomised controlled trial of dietary improvement for adults with major depression (the 'SMILES' trial). *BMC Medicine*, 15, 23.

Jacka, F. N., Pasco, J. A., Mykletun, A., Williams, L. J., Hodge, A. M., O'Reilly, S. L., & Berk, M. (2010). Association of Western and traditional diets with depression and anxiety in women. *American Journal of Psychiatry*, 167, 305–311.

Jackson, A. C. (2018). Chronic neurological disease due to methylmercury poisoning. *Canadian Journal of Neurological Sciences*, 45, 620–623.

Jackson, A., Forsyth, C. B., Shaikh, M., Voigt, R. M., Engen, P. A., Ramirez, V., & Keshavarzian, A. (2019). Diet in Parkinson's disease: Critical role for the microbiome. *Frontiers in Neurology*, 10, 1245.

Jacobson, K. A., Gao, Z. -G., Matricon, P., Eddy, M. T., & Carlsson, J. (2020). Adenosine A$_{2A}$ receptor antagonists: From caffeine to selective non-xanthines. *British Journal of Pharmacology*, 14, 3496–3511.

Jaeger, B., & Bosch, A. M. (2016). Clinical presentation and outcome of riboflavin transporter deficiency: Mini review after five years of experience. *Journal of Inherited Metabolic Disease*, 39, 559–564.

Jahng, J. W., Kim, J. G., & Kim, H. J. (2007). Chronic food restriction in young rats results in depression- and anxiety-like behaviors with decreased expression of serotonin reuptake transporter. *Brain Research*, 1150, 100–107.

Jahng, J. W., Lee, J. Y., & Yoo, S. B. (2005). Refeeding-induced expression of neuronal nitric oxide synthase in the rat paraventricular nucleus. *Brain Research*, 1048, 185–192.

Jahromi, S. R., Toghae, M., Jahromi, M. J., & Aloosh, M. (2012). Dietary pattern and risk of multiple sclerosis. *Iranian Journal of Neurology*, 11, 47–53.

James, J. E. (2014). Caffeine and cognitive performance: Persistent methodological challenges in caffeine research. *Pharmacology, Biochemistry and Behavior*, 124, 117–122.

James, S., Montgomery, P., & Williams, K. (2011). Omega-3 fatty acids supplementation for autism spectrum disorders (ASD). *Cochrane Database of Systematic Reviews*, 11, CD007992.

Jankowsky, J. L., & Patterson, P. H. (1999). Cytokine and growth factor involvement in long-term potentiation. *Molecular & Cellular Neuroscience*, 14, 273–286.

Janthakhin, Y., Rincel, M., Costa, A. M., Darnaudery, M., & Ferreira, G. (2017). Maternal high-fat diet leads to hippocampal and amygdala dendritic remodeling in adult male offspring. *Psychoneuroendocrinology*, 83, 49–57.

Jaques, J. A., Doleski, P. H., Castilhos, L. G., da Rosa, M. M., Souza Vdo, C., Carvalho, F. B., & Leal, D. B. (2013). Free and nanoencapsulated curcumin prevents cigarette smoke-induced cognitive impairment and redox imbalance. *Neurobiology of Learning & Memory*, 100, 98–107.

Jaques, J. A., Rezer, J. F., Carvalho, F. B., da Rosa, M. M., Gutierres, J. M., Goncalves, J. F., & Leal, D. B. (2012). Curcumin protects against cigarette smoke-induced cognitive impairment and increased acetylcholinesterase activity in rats. *Physiology & Behavior*, 106, 664–669.

Jasani, B., Simmer, K., Patole, S. K., & Rao, S. C. (2017). Long chain polyunsaturated fatty acid supplementation in infants born at term. *Cochrane Database Systematic Reviews*, 3, CD000376.

Jazayeri, S., Tehrani-Doost, M., Keshavarz, S. A., Hosseini, M., Djazayery, A., Amini, H., & Peet, M. (2008). Comparison of therapeutic effects of omega-3 fatty acid eicosapentaenoic acid and fluoxetine, separately and in combination, in major depressive disorder. *Australian & New Zealand Journal of Psychiatry*, 42, 192–198.

Jenkins, D. J., & Josse, A. R. (2008). Fish oil and omega-3 fatty acids. *CMAJ*, 178, 150.

Jenkins, T. A., Nguyen, J. C. D., Polglaze, K. E., & Bertrand, P. P. (2016). Influence of tryptophan and serotonin on mood and cognition with a possible role of the gut-brain axis. *Nutrients*, 8, Article 56.

Jeong, M. Y., Jang, H. M., & Kim, D. H. (2019). High-fat diet causes psychiatric disorders in mice by increasing Proteobacteria population. *Neuroscience Letters*, 698, 51–57.

Jia, W., Li, Y., Qu, R., Baranowski, T., Burke, L. E., Zhang, H., Bai, Y., Mancino, J. M., Xu, G., Mao, Z. -H., & Sun, M. (2019). Automatic food detection in egocentric images using artificial intelligence technology. *Public Health Nutrition*, 22, 1168–1179.

Jia, X., McNeill, G., & Avenell, A. (2008). Does taking vitamin, mineral and fatty acid supplements prevent cognitive decline? A systematic review of randomized controlled trials. *Journal of Human Nutrition & Dietetics*, 21, 317–336.

Jiang, W., Ju, C., Jiang, H., & Zhang, D. (2014). Dairy foods intake and risk of Parkinson's disease: A dose-response meta-analysis of prospective cohort studies. *European Journal of Epidemiology*, 29, 613–619.

Jiang, Z., Guo, M., Shi, C., Wang, H., Yao, L., Liu, L., & Lin, Z. (2015). Protection against cognitive impairment and modification of epileptogenesis with curcumin in a post-status epilepticus model of temporal lobe epilepsy. *Neuroscience*, 310, 362–371.

Job, V., Walton, G. M., Bernecker, K., & Dweck, C. S. (2013). Beliefs about willpower determine the impact of glucose on self-control. *Proceedings of the National Academy of Sciences of the United States of America*, 110, 14837–14842.

Johnson, C. C., Gorell, J. M., Rybicki, B. A., Sanders, K., & Peterson, E. L. (1999). Adult nutrient intake as a risk factor for Parkinson's disease. *International Journal of Epidemiology*, 28, 1102–1109.

Johnson, C., Praveen, D., Pope, A., Raj, T. S., Pillai, R. N., Land, M. A., & Neal, B. (2017). Mean population salt consumption in India: A systematic review. *Journal of Hypertension*, 35, 3–9.

Johnson, J. B., Summer, W., & Cutler, R. G. (2007). Alternate day calorie restriction improves clinical findings and reduces markers of oxidative stress and inflammation in overweight adults with moderate stamina. *Free Radical Biology & Medicine*, 42, 665–674.

Johnson, M. A., Kuo, Y. M., & Westaway, S. K. (2004). Mitochondrial localization of human PANK2 and hypotheses of secondary iron accumulation in pantothenate kinase-associated neurodegeneration. *Annals of the New York Academy of Sciences*, 1012, 282–298.

Johnstone, A. M. (2007). Fasting: The ultimate diet? *Obesity Reviews*, 8, 211–222.

Jones, E. K., Sunram-Lea, S. I., & Wesnes, K. A. (2012). Acute ingestion of different macronutrients differentially enhances aspects of memory and attention in healthy young adults. *Biological Psychology*, 89, 477–486.

Jones, N., & Rogers, P. J. (2003). Preoccupation, food, and failure: An investigation of cognitive performance deficits in dieters. *International Journal of Eating Disorders*, 33, 185–192.

Jongkees, B. J., Hommel, B., Kühn, S., & Colzato, L. S. (2015). Effect of tyrosine supplementation on clinical and healthy populations under stress or cognitive demands – A review. *Journal of Psychiatric Research*, 70, 50–57.

Jorgenson, L. A., Sun, M., O'Connor, M., & Georgieff, M. K. (2005). Fetal iron deficiency disrupts the maturation of synaptic function and efficacy in area CA1 of the developing rat hippocampus. *Hippocampus*, 15, 1094–1102.

Judelson, D. A., Preston, A. G., Miller, D. L., Muñoz, C. X., Kellogg, M. D., & Lieberman, H. R. (2013). Effects of theobromine and caffeine on mood and vigilance. *Journal of Clinical Psychopharmacology*, 33, 499–506.

Julvez, J., Fortuny, J., Mendez, M., Torrent, M., Ribas-Fito, N., & Sunyer, J. (2009). Maternal use of folic acid supplements during pregnancy and four-year-old neurodevelopment in a population-based birth cohort. *Paediatric and Perinatal Epidemiology*, 23, 199–206.

Julvez, J., Guxens, M., Carsin, A. E., Forns, J., Mendez, M., Turner, M. C., & Sunyer, J. (2014). A cohort study on full breastfeeding and child neuropsychological development: The role of maternal social, psychological, and nutritional factors. *Developmental Medicine & Child Neurology*, 56, 148–156.

Julvez, J., Ribas-Fito, N., Forns, M., Garcia-Esteban, R., Torrent, M., & Sunyer, J. (2007). Attention behaviour and hyperactivity at age 4 and duration of breast-feeding. *Acta Paediatrica*, 96, 842–847.

Jung, H. Y., Kim, D. W., & Nam, S. M.(2017). Pyridoxine improves hippocampal cognitive function via increases of serotonin turnover and tyrosine hydroxylase, and its association with CB1 cannabinoid receptor-interacting protein and the CB1 cannabinoid receptor pathway. *BBA General Subjects*, 1861, 3142–3153.

Juul, F., Martinez-Steele, E., Parekh, N., Monteiro, C. A., & Chang, V. W. (2018). Ultra-processed food consumption and excess weight among US adults. *British Journal of Nutrition*, 120, 90–100.

Kadri, N., Tilane, A., & El Batal, M. (2000). Irritability during the month of Ramadan. *Psychosomatic Medicine*, 62, 280–285.

Kafouri, S., Kramer, M., Leonard, G., Perron, M., Pike, B., Richer, L., & Paus, T. (2013). Breastfeeding and brain structure in adolescence. *International Journal of Epidemiology*, 42, 150–159.

Kalk, W. J., Felix, M., Snoey, E. R., & Yeriawa, Y. (1993). Voluntary total fasting in political prisoners: Clinical and biochemical observations. *South African Medical Journal*, 83, 391–394.

Kalmijn, S., Launer, L. J., Ott, A., Witteman, J. C., Hofman, A., & Breteler, M. M. (1997). Dietary fat intake and the risk of incident dementia in the Rotterdam Study. *Annals of Neurology*, 42, 776–782.

Kalmijn, S., van Boxtel, M. P., Ocke, M., Verschuren, W. M., Kromhout, D., & Launer, L. J. (2004). Dietary intake of fatty acids and fish in relation to cognitive performance at middle age. *Neurology*, 62, 275–280.

Kamata, S., Yamamoto, J., & Kamijo, K. (2014). Dietary deprivation of each essential amino acid induces differential systemic adaptive responses in mice. *Molecular Nutrition & Food Research*, 58, 1309–1321.

414

Kanarek, R. B. (1997). Psychological effects of snacks and altered meal frequency. *British Journal of Nutrition*, 77, S105–S120.

Kanarek, R. B., & Swinney, D. (1990). Effects of food snacks on cognitive performance in male college students. *Appetite*, 14, 15–27.

Kandimalla, R., Vallamkondu, J., Corgiat, E. B., & Gill, K. D. (2016). Understanding aspects of aluminium exposure in Alzheimer's disease development. *Brain Pathology*, 26, 139–154.

Kang, S., Hong, Y., Choi, N., & Lee, K. (2017). The relationship between breastfeeding duration and preschooler problem behavior: The mediating role of cognitive development. *Korean Journal of Child Studies*, 38, 63–77.

Kanoski, S. E., & Davidson, T. L. (2010). Different patterns of memory impairments accompany short- and longer-term maintenance on a high-energy diet. *Journal of Experimental Psychology-Animal Behavioral Processes*, 36, 313–319.

Kanoski, S. E., Meisel, R. L., Mullins, A. J., & Davidson, T. L. (2007). The effects of energy-rich diets on discrimination reversal learning and on BDNF in the hippocampus and prefrontal cortex of the rat. *Behavioral Brain Research*, 182, 57–66.

Kanoski, S. E., Zhang, Y. S., Zheng, W., & Davidson, T. L. (2010). The effects of a high-energy diet on hippocampal function and blood-brain barrier integrity in the rat. *Journal of Alzheimer's Disease*, 21, 207–219.

Kant, A. K., (1996). Indexes of overall diet quality: A review. *Journal of the American Dietetic Association*, 96, 875–791.

Kaplan, R. J., & Greenwood, C. E. (1998). Dietary saturated fatty acids and brain function. *Neurochemistry Research*, 23, 615–626.

Kaplan, R. J., Greenwood, C. E., Winocur, G., & Wolever, T. M. S. (2000). Cognitive performance is associated with glucose regulation in healthy elderly persons and can be enhanced with glucose and dietary carbohydrates. *American Journal of Clinician Nutrition*, 72, 825–836.

(2001). Dietary protein, carbohydrate, and fat enhance memory in the healthy elderly. *American Journal of Clinical Nutrition*, 74, 687–693.

Karakonstantis, S., Galani, D., & Korela, D. (2020). Missing the early signs of thiamine deficiency: A case associated with a liquid-only diet. *Nutritional Neuroscience*, 23, 384–386.

Karamyan, V. T., & Speth, R. C. (2008). Animal models of BMAA neurotoxicity: A critical review. *Life Sciences*, 82, 233–246.

Karl, J. P., Thompson, L. A., & Niro, P. J. (2015). Transient decrements in mood during energy deficit are independent of dietary protein-to-carbohydrate ratio. *Physiology & Behavior*, 139, 524–531.

Kashala-Abotnes, E., Okitundu, D., & Mumba, D. (2019). Konzo: A distinct neurological disease associated with food (cassava) cyanogenic poisoning. *Brain Research Bulletin*, 145, 87–91.

Kassa, R. M., Kasensa, N. L., & Monterroso, V. H. (2011). On the biomarkers and mechanisms of konzo, a distinct upper motor neuron disease associated with food (cassava) cyanogenic exposure. *Food & Chemical Toxicology*, 49, 571–578.

Kaur, H., Agarwal, S., Agarwal, M., Agarwal, V., & Singh, M. (2020). Therapeutic and preventive role of functional foods in process of neurodegeneration. *International Journal of Pharmaceutical Sciences & Research*, 11, 2882–2891.

Kaur, H., Bal, A., & Sandhir, R. (2014). Curcumin supplementation improves mitochondrial and behavioral deficits in experimental model of chronic epilepsy. *Pharmacology Biochemistry & Behavior*, 125, 55–64.

Kaur, H., Patro, I., Tikoo, K., & Sandhir, R. (2015). Curcumin attenuates inflammatory response and cognitive deficits in experimental model of chronic epilepsy. *Neurochemistry International*, 89, 40–50.

Kaye, W. H., Fudge, J. L., & Paulus, M. (2009). New insights into symptoms and neurocircuit function of anorexia nervosa. *Nature Reviews Neuroscience*, 10, 573–584.

Ke, X., Schober, M. E., McKnight, R. A., O'Grady, S., Caprau, D., Yu, X., & Lane, R. H. (2010). Intrauterine growth retardation affects expression and epigenetic characteristics of the rat hippocampal glucocorticoid receptor gene. *Physiological Genomics*, 42, 177–189.

Ke, X., Xing, B., Yu, B., Yu, X., Majnik, A., Cohen, S., & Joss-Moore, L. (2014). IUGR disrupts the PPARgamma-Setd8-H4K20me(1) and Wnt signaling pathways in the juvenile rat hippocampus. *International Journal of Developmental Neuroscience*, 38, 59–67.

Kelly, G. S. (2011). Pantothenic acid. *Alternative Medicine Review*, 16, 263–274.

Kemps, E., & Tiggemann, M. (2005). Working memory performance and preoccupying thoughts in female dieters: Evidence for a selective central executive impairment. *British Journal of Clinical Psychology*, 44, 357–366.

Kemps, E., Tiggemann, M., & Marshall, K. (2005). Relationship between dieting to lose weight and the functioning of the central executive. *Appetite*, 45, 287–294.

Kendig, M. D. (2014). Cognitive and behavioural effects of sugar consumption in rodents. A review. *Appetite*, 80, 41–54.

Kendig, M. D., Leigh, S. J., & Morris, M. J. (2021). Unravelling the impacts of western-style diets on brain, gut microbiota and cognition. *Neuroscience & Biobehavioral Reviews*, 128, 233–243.

Kendig, M. D., & Morris, M. J. (2019). Reviewing the effects of dietary salt on cognition: Mechanisms and future directions. *Asia Pacific Journal of Clinical Nutrition*, 28, 6–14.

Kendig, M. D., Rooney, K. B., Corbit, L. H., & Boakes, R. A. (2014). Persisting adiposity following chronic consumption of 10% sucrose solution: Strain differences and behavioural effects. *Physiology & Behavior*, 130, 54–65.

Kendler, K. S. (1996). Major depression and generalised anxiety disorder. Same genes, (partly)different environments – revisited. *British Journal of Psychiatry*, S30, 68–75.

Kennedy, D. O. (2016). B vitamins and the brain: Mechanisms, dose and efficacy: A review. *Nutrients*, 8, 68.

Kennedy, D. O., & Scholey, A. B. (2000). Glucose administration, heart rate and cognitive performance: Effects of increasing mental effort. *Psychopharmacology*, 149, 63–71.

Kenny, P. J. (2011). Common cellular and molecular mechanisms in obesity and drug addiction. *Nature Reviews Neuroscience*, 12, 638–651.

Kent, K., Charlton, K., Roodenrys, S., Batterham, M., Potter, J., Traynor, V., & Richards, R. (2017). Consumption of anthocyanin-rich cherry juice for 12 weeks improves memory and cognition in older adults with mild-to-moderate dementia. *European Journal of Nutrition*, 56, 333–341.

Kerndt, P. R., Naughton, J. L., Driscoll, C. E., & Loxterkamp, D. A. (1982). Fasting: The history, pathophysiology and complications. *Western Journal of Medicine*, 137, 379–399.

Kesse-Guyot, E., Fezeu, L., Andreeva, V. A., Touvier, M., Scalbert, A., Hercberg, S., & Galan, P. (2012). Total and specific polyphenol intakes in midlife are associated with cognitive function measured 13 years later. *Journal of Nutrition*, 142, 76–83.

Kessler, R. C., Chiu, W. T., Demler, O., Merikangas, K. R., & Walters, E. E. (2005). Prevalence, severity, and comorbidity of 12-month DSM-IV disorders in the National Comorbidity Survey Replication. *Archives of General Psychiatry*, 62, 617–627.

Keys, A. (1946). Human starvation and its consequences. *Journal of the American Dietetic Association*, 22, 582–587.

Keys, A., Brožek, J., Henschel, A., Mickelsen, O., & Taylor, H. L. (1950). *The Biology of Human Starvation* (Vol. 2). Minneapolis, MN: University of Minnesota Press.

Keys, A., Menotti, A., Karvonen, M. J., Aravanis, C., Blackburn, H., & Buzina, R. (1986). The diet and 15-year death rate in the seven countries study. *American Journal of Epidemiology*, 124, 903–915.

Khayyatzadeh, S. S., Mehramiz, M., Mirmousavi, S. J., Mazidi, M., Ziaee, A., Kazemi-Bajestani, S. M. R., & Ghayour-Mobarhan, M. (2018). Adherence to a Dash-style diet in relation to depression and aggression in adolescent girls. *Psychiatry Research*, 259, 104–109.

Khedr, E. H. M., Farghaly, W. M. A., Amry, S. E., & Osman, A. A. A. (2004). Neural maturation of breastfed and formula-fed infants. *Acta Paediatrica*, 93, 734–738.

Khedr, E., Hamed, S. A., & Elbeih, E. (2008). Iron states and cognitive abilities in young adults: Neuropsychological and neurophysiological assessment. *European Archives of Psychiatry & Clinical Neuroscience*, 258, 489–496.

Khurana, S., Venkataraman, K., Hollingsworth, A., Piche, M., & Tai, T. C. (2013). Polyphenols: Benefits to the cardiovascular system in health and in aging. *Nutrients*, 5, 3779–3827.

Kiecolt-Glaser, J. K., Belury, M. A., Andridge, R., Malarkey, W. B., & Glaser, R. (2011). Omega-3 supplementation lowers inflammation and anxiety in medical students: A randomized controlled trial. *Brain Behavior & Immunity*, 25, 1725–1734.

Kiernan, M. C., Isbister, G. K., Lin, C. S., Burke, D., & Bostock, H. (2005). Acute tetrodotoxin-induced neurotoxicity after ingestion of puffer fish. *Annals of Neurology*, 57, 339–348.

Killin, L. O., Starr, J. M., Shiue, I. J., & Russ, T. C. (2016). Environmental risk factors for dementia: A systematic review. *BioMed Central Geriatrics*, 16, 1–28.

Killinger, B. A., & Labrie, V. (2017). Vertebrate food products as a potential source of prion-like α-synuclein. *NPJ Parkinson's Disease*, 3, 1–11.

Kim, J. H., Lee, K. J., & Suzuki, T. (2009). Identification of tetramine, a toxin in whelks, as the cause of a poisoning incident in Korea and the distribution of tetramine in fresh and boiled whelk. *Journal of Food Protection*, 72, 1935–1940.

Kim, Y. M., Lee, J. Y., Choi, S. H., Kim, D. G., & Jahng, J. W. (2004). RU486 blocks fasting-induced decrease of neuronal nitric oxide synthase in the rat paraventricular nucleus. *Brain Research*, 1018, 221–226.

Kim, Y. -S., Kwak, S. M., & Myung, S. -K. (2015). Caffeine intake from coffee or tea and cognitive disorders: A meta-analysis of observational studies. *Neuroepidemiology*, 44, 51–63.

Kim do, Y., Hao, J., Liu, R., Turner, G., Shi, F. D., & Rho, J. M. (2012). Inflammation-mediated memory dysfunction and effects of a ketogenic diet in a murine model of multiple sclerosis. *PLoS One*, 7, e35476.

King, G. A., Polivy, J., & Herman, C. P. (1991). Cognitive aspects of dietary restraint: Effects on person memory. *International Journal of Eating Disorders*, 10, 313–321.

Kirk, J. M., & Logue, A. W. (1997). Effects of deprivation level on humans' self-control for food reinforces. *Appetite*, 28, 215–226.

Kleinewietfeld, M., Manzel, A., Titze, J., Kvakan, H., Yosef, N., Linker, R. A., & Hafler, D. A. (2013). Sodium chloride drives autoimmune disease by the induction of pathogenic TH17 cells. *Nature*, 496, 518–522.

Klem, M. L., Wing, R. R., McGuire, M. T., Seagle, H. M., & Hill, J. O. (1998). Psychological symptoms in individuals successful at long-term maintenance of weight loss. *Health Psychology*, 17, 336–345.

Klevay, L. M. (2011). Is the Western diet adequate in copper? *Journal of Trace Elements in Medicine & Biology*, 25, 204–212.

Kloss, O., Eskin, M., & Suh, M. (2018). Thiamine deficiency on fetal brain development with and without prenatal alcohol exposure. *Biochemistry & Cell Biology*, 96, 169–177.

Klotz, J. L. (2015). Activities and effects of ergot alkaloids on livestock physiology and production. *Toxins*, 7, 2801–2821.

Koh, T. H. H. G., Eyre, J. A., Tarbit, M., & Aynsleygreen, A. (1988). Neurophysiological dysfunction in relation to the concentration of glucose in the blood. *Early Human Development*, 17, 287–287.

Kohlmeier, M., da Costa, K. -M., Fischer, L. M., & Zeisel, S. H. (2005). Genetic variation of folate-mediated one-carbon transfer pathway predicts susceptibility to choline deficiency in humans. *Proceedings of the National Academy of Sciences of the United States of America*, 102, 16025–16030.

Kohnen-Johannsen, K. L., & Kayser, O. (2019). Tropane alkaloids: Chemistry, pharmacology, biosynthesis and production. *Molecules*, 24, 1–23.

Kolahdouzan, M., & Hamadeh, M. J. (2017). The neuroprotective effects of caffeine in neurodegenerative diseases. *CNS Neuroscience & Therapeutics*, 23, 272–290.

Koletzko, B., Agostoni, C., Carlson, S. E., Clandinin, T., Hornstra, G., Neuringer, M., & Willatts, P. (2001). Long chain polyunsaturated fatty acids (LC-PUFA) and perinatal development. *Acta Paediatrica*, 90, 460–464.

Koleva, I. I., van Beek, T. A., Soffers, A. E., Dusemund, B., & Rietjens, I. M. (2012). Alkaloids in the humans food chain – Natural occurrence and possible adverse effects. *Molecular Nutrition & Food Research*, 56, 30–52.

Kopf, S. R., Buchholzer, M. L., Hilgert, M., Löffelholz, K., & Klein, J. (2001). Glucose plus choline improve passive avoidance behaviour and increase hippocampal acetylcholine release in mice. *Neuroscience*, 103, 365–371.

Korn, T., Bettelli, E., Oukka, M., & Kuchroo, V. K. (2009). IL-17 and Th17 cells. *Annual Review of Immunology*, 27, 485–517.

Korogi, Y., Takahashi, M., Okajima, T., & Eto, K. (1998). MR findings of Minamata disease – Organic mercury poisoning. *Journal of Magnetic Resonance Imaging*, 8, 308–316.

Korsmo, H. W., Jiang, X., & Caudill, M. A. (2019). Choline: Exploring the growing science on its benefits for moms and babies. *Nutrients*, 11, 1823.

Koszucka, A., Nowak, A., Nowak, I., & Motyl, I. (2019). Acrylamide in human diet, its metabolism, toxicity, inactivation and the associated European Union legal regulations in food industry. *Critical Reviews in Food Science & Nutrition*, 60, 1677–1692.

Kramer, M. S., Aboud, F., Mironova, E., Vanilovich, I., Platt, R. W., Matush, L., & Interventi, P. B. (2008). Breastfeeding and child cognitive development – New evidence from a large randomized trial. *Archives of General Psychiatry*, 65, 578–584.

Krikorian, R., Boespflug, E. L., Fleck, D. E., Stein, A. L., Wightman, J. D., Shidler, M. D., & Sadat-Hossieny, S. (2012). Concord grape juice supplementation and neurocognitive function in human aging. *Journal of Agricultural & Food Chemistry*, 60, 5736–5742.

Krikorian, R., Shidler, M. D., Dangelo, K., Couch, S. C., Benoit, S. C., & Clegg, D. J. (2012). Dietary ketosis enhances memory in mild cognitive impairment. *Neurobiology of Aging*, 33, 425.

Krska, R & Crews, C. (2008). Significance, chemistry and determination of ergot alkaloids: A review. *Food Additives & Contaminants: Part A: Chemistry, Analysis, Control, Exposure & Risk Assessment*, 25, 722–731.

Kruman, I. I., Mouton, P. R., Emokpae, R., Cutler, R. G., & Mattson, M. P. (2005). Folate deficiency inhibits proliferation of adult hippocampal progenitors. *Neuroreport*, 16, 1055–1059.

Kuhad, A., & Chopra, K. (2007). Curcumin attenuates diabetic encephalopathy in rats: Behavioral and biochemical evidences. *European Journal of Pharmacology*, 576, 34–42.

Kurihara, K., Homma, T., & Kobayashi, S.(2019). Ascorbic acid insufficiency impairs spatial memory formation in juvenile AKR1A-knockout mice. *Journal of Clinical Biochemistry & Nutrition*, 65, 209–216.

Kurland, L. T. (1988). Amyotrophic lateral sclerosis and Parkinson's disease complex on Guam linked to an environmental neurotoxin. *Trends in Neurosciences*, 11, 51–54.

Kussmann, M., Krause, L., & Siffert, W. (2010). Nutrigenomics: Where are we with genetic and epigenetic markers for disposition and susceptibility? *Nutrition Reviews*, 68, S38–S47.

Kuzawa, C. W. (1998). Adipose tissue in human infancy and childhood: An evolutionary perspective. *Yearbook of Physical Anthropology*, 41, 177–209.

LaBar, K. S., & Cabeza, R. (2006). Cognitive neuroscience of emotional memory. *Nature Reviews Neuroscience*, 7, 54–64.

Lachenmeier, D. W., Walch, S. G., Padosch, S. A., & Kröner, L. U. (2006). Absinthe – A review. *Critical Reviews in Food Science & Nutrition*, 46, 365–377.

Lafay, L., Thomas, F., Mennen, L., Charles, M. A., Eschwege, E., Borys, J. M., Basdevant, A., & Fleurbaix Laventie Ville Santé Study Group. (2001). Gender differences in the relation between food cravings and mood in an adult community: Results from the Fleurbaix Laventie Ville Santé study. *The International Journal of Eating Disorders*, 29, 195–204.

Lagercrantz, H. (2016). Origins of the mind and basic contruction of the brain. In H. Lagercrantz (Ed.), *Infant Brain Development* (pp. 1–14). Sweden: Springer.

Lai, J. S., Hiles, S., Bisquera, A., Hure, A. J., McEvoy, M., & Attia, J. (2014). A systematic review and meta-analysis of dietary patterns and depression in community-dwelling adults. *American Journal of Clinical Nutrition*, 99, 181–197.

Laird, D. A., DeLand, D., Drexel, H., & Riemer, K. (1936). A study of a dietary cause and possible elimination of early afternoon sluggishness. *Journal of American Dietetic Association*, 1, 411–421.

Lamanna, J., Sulpizio, S., & Ferro, M. (2019). Behavioral assessment of activity-based-anorexia: How cognition can become the drive wheel. *Physiology & Behavior*, 202, 1–7.

Lambrechts, D. A., de Kinderen, R. J., Vles, J. S., de Louw, A. J., Aldenkamp, A. P., & Majoie, H. J. (2016). A randomized controlled trial of the ketogenic diet in refractory childhood epilepsy. *Acta Neurologica Scandanivca*, 135, 231–239.

Lambrechts, D. A., Wielders, L. H., Aldenkamp, A. P., Kessels, F. G., de Kinderen, R. J., & Majoie, M. J. (2012). The ketogenic diet as a treatment option in adults with chronic refractory epilepsy: Efficacy and tolerability in clinical practice. *Epilepsy & Behavior*, 23, 310–314.

Lamport, D. J., Dye, J. D., Wightman, J. D., & Lawton, C. L. (2012). The effects of flavonoid and other polyphenol consumption on cognitive performance: A systematic research review of human experimental and epidemiological studies. *Nutrition & Aging*, 1, 5–25.

Lamport, D. J., Lawton, C. L., Mansfield, M. W., & Dye, L. (2009). Impairments in glucose tolerance can have a negative impact on cognitive function: A systematic research review. *Neuroscience & Biobehavioral Reviews*, 33, 394–413.

Lamport, D. J., Lawton, C. L., Merat, N., Jamson, H., Myrissa, K., Hofman, D., & Dye, L. (2016). Concord grape juice, cognitive function, and driving performance: A 12-wk, placebo-controlled, randomized crossover trial in mothers of preteen children. *American Journal of Clinical Nutrition*, 103, 775–783.

Lamport, D. J., Pal, D., Moutsiana, C., Field, D. T., Williams, C. M., Spencer, J. P., & Butler, L. T. (2015). The effect of flavanol-rich cocoa on cerebral perfusion in healthy older adults during conscious resting state: A placebo controlled, crossover, acute trial. *Psychopharmacology*, 232, 3227–3234.

Land, M.-A., Neal, B. C., Johnson, C., Nowson, C. A., Margerison, C., & Petersen, K. S. (2018). Salt consumption by Australian adults: A systematic review and meta-analysis. *Medical Journal of Australia*, 208, 75–81.

Lang, K. Roberts, M., & Harrison, A. (2016). Central coherence in eating disorders: A synthesis of studies using the Rey Osterrieth Complex Figure Test. *PLoS One*, 11, e0165467.

Langohr, H. D., Petruch, F., & Schrom, G. (1981). Vitamin-B2 and vitamin-B6 deficiency in neurological disorders. *Journal of Neurology*, 225, 95–108.

Lapp, J. E. (1981). Effects of glycemic alterations and noun imagery on the learning of paired associates. *Journal of Learning Disabilities*, 14, 35–38.

Lardner, A. L. (2014). Neurobiological effects of the green tea constituent theanine and its potential role in the treatment of psychiatric and neurodegenerative disorders. *Nutritional Neuroscience*, 17, 145–155.

Larsen, B., Bourque, J., & Moore, T. M. (2020). Longitudinal development of brain iron is linked to cognition in youth. *Journal of Neuroscience*, 40, 1810–1818.

Larson, L., & Yousafzai, A. (2016). A meta-analysis of nutrition interventions on mental development of children under two and low and middle-income countries. *Maternal & Child Nutrition*, 13, e12229.

Laus, M., Vales, L., Costa, T., & Almeida, S. (2011). Early post-natal protein-calorie malnutrition and cognition: A review of human and animal studies. *International Journal of Environmental Research & Public Health*, 8, 590–612.

Lautrup, S., Sinclair, D. A., Mattson, M. P., & Fang, E. F. (2019). NAD$^+$ in brain aging and neurodegenerative disorders. *Cell Metabolism*, 30, 630–655.

Laviano, A., Inui, A., & Marks, D. L. (2008). Neural control of the anorexia-cachexia syndrome. *American Journal of Physiology*, 295, E1000–E1008.

Laviano, A., Meguid, M. M., Inui, A., Muscaritoli, M., & Rossi, F. F. (2005). Therapy insight: Cancer anorexia-cachexia syndrome – When all you can eat is yourself. *Nature Clinical Practice Oncology*, 2, 158–165.

Lavita, S. I., Aro, R., Kiss, B., Manto, M., & Duez, P. (2016). The role of β-carboline alkaloids in the pathogenesis of essential tremor. *Cerebellum*, 15, 276–284.

Lazartigues, A., Thomas, M., & Banas, D. (2013). Accumulation and half-lives of 13 pesticides in muscle tissue of freshwater fishes through food exposure. *Chemosphere*, 91, 530–535.

Lazarus, S. A., Hammerstone, J. F., & Schmitz, H. H. (1999). Chocolate contains additional flavonoids not found in tea. *The Lancet*, 354, 1825.

Leach, P. T., & Gould, T. J. (2015). Thyroid hormone signalling: Contribution to neural function, cognition, and relationship to nicotine. *Neuroscience & Biobehavioral Reviews*, 57, 252–263.

Lebel, C., Roussotte, F., & Sowell, E. R. (2011). Imaging the impact of prenatal alcohol exposure on the structure of the developing human brain. *Neuropsychology Review*, 21, 102–118.

Leckie, R. L., Lehman, D. E., Gianaros, P. J., Erickson, K. I., Sereika, S. M., Kuan, D. C. H., & Muldoon, M. F. (2020). The effects of omega-3 fatty acids on neuropsychological functioning and brain morphology in mid-life adults: A randomized clinical trial. *Psychological Medicine*, 50, 2425–2434.

Leclerc, E., Trevizol, A. P., & Grigolon, R. B. (2020). The effect of caloric restriction on working memory in healthy non-obese adults. *CNS Spectrums*, 25, 2–8.

Lee, M. (2012). The use of ketogenic diet in special situations: Expanding use in intractable epilepsy and other neurologic disorders. *Korean Journal of Pediatrics*, 55, 316–321.

Lee, P., & Ulatowski, L. M. (2019). Vitamin E: Mechanisms of transport and regulation in the CNS. *IUBMB Life*, 71, 424–429.

Lee, R. W. Y., Corley, M. J., Pang, A., Arakaki, G., Abbott, L., Nishimoto, M., & Wong, M. (2018). A modified ketogenic gluten-free diet with MCT improves behavior in children with autism spectrum disorder. *Physiology & Behavior*, 188, 205–211.

Lee, W. L., & Klip, A. (2012). Shuttling glucose across brain microvessels, with a little help from GLUT1 and AMP kinase. Focus on "AMP kinase regulation of sugar transport in brain capillary endothelial cells during acute metabolic stress." *American Journal of Physiology*, 303, C803–C805.

Lehnert, H., Reinstein, D. K., Strowbridge, B. W., & Wurtman, R. J. (1984). Neurochemical and behavioral consequences of acute, uncontrollable stress: Effects of dietary tyrosine. *Brain Research*, 303, 215–223.

Lehrskov, L. L., Dorph, E., & Widmer, A. M. (2018). The role of IL-1 in postprandial fatigue. *Molecular Metabolism*, 12, 107–112.

Leigh, S. J., Kaakoush, N. O., Bertoldo, M. J., Westbrook, R. F., & Morris, M. J. (2020). Intermittent cafeteria diet identifies fecal microbiome changes as a predictor of spatial recognition memory impairment in female rats. *Translational Psychiatry*, 10, 36.

Leon, G. R., Butcher, J. N., Kleinman, M., Goldberg, A., & Almagor, M. (1981). Survivors of the Holocaust and their children: Current status and adjustment. *Journal of Personality & Social Psychology*, 41, 503–516.

Leon-Del-Rio, A. (2019). Biotin in metabolism, gene expression, and human disease. *Journal of Inherited Metabolic Disease*, 42, 647–654.

Levitsky, D., & Strupp, B. (1995). Malnutrition and the brain: Changing concepts, changing concerns. *Journal of Nutrition*, 125, 2212S–2220S.

Leyton, G. (1946). Effects of slow starvation. *The Lancet*, 2, 73–79.

Lezak, M. D., Howieson, D. B., Bigler, E., D., & Tranel, D. (2012). *Neuropsychological Assessment* (5th ed). Oxford: Oxford University Press.

Li, B., Lv, J., Wang, W., & Zhang, D. (2017). Dietary magnesium and calcium intake and risk of depression in the general population: A meta-analysis. *Australian & New Zealand Journal of Psychiatry*, 51, 219–229.

Li, C., Zeng, L., Wang, D., Yang, W., Dang, S., Zhou, J., & Yan, H. (2015). Prenatal micronutrient supplementation is not associated with intellectual development of young school-aged children. *Journal of Nutrition*, 145, 1844–1849.

Li, Q., Yan, H., Zeng, L., Cheng, Y., Liang, W., Dang, S., & Tsuji, I. (2009). Effects of maternal multimicronutrient supplementation on the mental development of infants in rural western China: Follow-up evaluation of a double-blind, randomized, controlled trial. *Pediatrics*, 123, e685–692.

Li, Z., Fang, F., Wang, Y. Y., & Wang, L. C. (2016). Resveratrol protects CA1 neurons against focal cerebral ischemic reperfusion-induced damage via the ERK-CREB signaling pathway in rats. *Pharmacology Biochemistry & Behavior*, 146, 21–27.

Lian, Q. W., Nie, Y. S., Zhang, X. Y., Tan, B., Cao, H. Y., Chen, W. L., & Huang, P. (2016). Effects of grape seed proanthocyanidin on Alzheimer's disease in vitro and in vivo. *Experimental & Therapeutic Medicine*, 12, 1681–1692.

Liao, Y., Xie, B., Zhang, H., He, Q., Guo, L., Subramanieapillai, M., & McIntyre, R. S. (2019). Efficacy of omega-3 PUFAs in depression: A meta-analysis. *Translational Psychiatry*, 9, 190.

Lidsky, T. I., & Schneider, J. S. (2003). Lead neurotoxicity in children: Basic mechanisms and clinical correlates. *Brain*, 126, 5–19.

Lieberman, H. R. (2007). Achieving scientific consensus in nutrition and behaviour research. *Nutrition Bulletin*, 32, 100–106.

Lieberman, H. R., Bukhari, A. S., & Caldwell, J. A. (2017). Two days of calorie deprivation induced by underfeeding and aerobic exercise degrades mood and lowers interstitial glucose but does not impair cognitive function in young adults. *Journal of Nutrition*, 147, 110–116.

Lieberman, H. R., Caruso, C. M., & Niro, P. J. (2008). A double-blind, placebo-controlled test of 2 d of calorie deprivation: Effects on cognition, activity, sleep, and interstitial glucose concentrations. *American Journal of Clinical Nutrition*, 88, 667–676.

Lien, E. L., Richard, C., & Hoffman, D. R. (2018). DHA and ARA addition to infant formula: Current status and future research directions. *Prostaglandins Leukotrienes & Essential Fatty Acids*, 128, 26–40.

Lin, M. T., & Beal, M. F. (2006). Mitochondrial dysfunction and oxidative stress in neurodegenerative diseases. *Nature*, 443, 787–795.

Lind, J. N., Li, R., Perrine, C. G., & Schieve, L. A. (2014). Breastfeeding and later psychosocial development of children at 6 years of age. *Pediatrics*, 134, S36–S41.

Lioret, S., Betoko, A., Forhan, A., Charles, M. -A., Heude, B., de Lauzon-Guillain, B., and The EDEN Mother-Child Cohort Study Group. (2015). Dietary patterns track from infancy to preschool age: Cross-sectional and longitudinal perspectives. *Journal of Nutrition*, 145, 775–782.

Lipscomb, F. (1945). Medical aspects of Belsen concentration camp. *The Lancet*, 2, 313–315.

Liu, D. X., Ke, Z. J., & Luo, J. (2017). Thiamine deficiency and neurodegeneration: The interplay among oxidative stress, endoplasmic reticulum stress, and autophagy. *Molecular Neurobiology*, 54, 5440–5448.

Liu, D., Zhang, Q., Gu, J., Wang, X., Xie, K., Xian, X., & Wang, Z. (2014). Resveratrol prevents impaired cognition induced by chronic unpredictable mild stress in rats. *Progress in Neuropsychopharmacology & Biological Psychiatry*, 49, 21–29.

Liu, H. C., & Jia, Y. (2017). Ergot alkaloids: Synthetic approaches to lysergic acid and clavine alkaloids. *Natural Product Reports*, 34, 411–432.

Liu, J. H., Leung, P., & Yang, A. (2014). Breastfeeding and active bonding protects against children's internalizing behavior problems. *Nutrients*, 6, 76–89.

Liu, J., Zhao, S., & Reyes, T. (2015). Neurological and epigenetic implications of nutritional deficienies on psychopathology: Conceptualization and review of evidence. *International Journal of Molecular Sciences*, 16, 18129–18148.

Liu, Y. Z., Chen, J. K., Li, Z. P., Zhao, T., Ni, M., Li, D. J., & Shen, F. M. (2014). High-salt diet enhances hippocampal oxidative stress and cognitive impairment in mice. *Neurobiology of Learning & Memory*, 114, 10–15.

Livingstone, M. B. E., & Black, A. E. (2003). Markers of the validity of reported energy intake. *Journal of Nutrition*, 133, S895S–S920.

Llorach, R., Garcia-Aloy, M., Tulipani, S., Vazquez-Fresno, R., & Andres-Lacueva, C. (2012). Nutrimetabolomic strategies to develop new biomarkers of intake and health effects. *Journal of Agricultural & Food Chemistry*, 60, 8797–8808.

Llorens, J., Soler-Martín, C., & Saldaña-Ruíz, S. (2011). A new unifying hypothesis for lathyrism, konzo and tropical ataxic neuropathy: Nitriles are the causative agents. *Food & Chemical Toxicology*, 49, 563–570.

Logroscino, G., Marder, K., Cote, L., Tang, M. X., Shea, S., & Mayeux, R. (1996). Dietary lipids and antioxidants in Parkinson's disease: A population-based, case-control study. *Annals of Neurology*, 39, 89–94.

Logue, A. W. (2015). *The Psychology of Eating and Drinking* (4th ed). New York, NY: Routledge.

Long, C. G., Blundell, J. E., & Finlayson, G. (2015). A systematic review of the application and correlates of YFAS-diagnosed 'food addiction' in humans: Are eating-related 'addictions' a cause for concern or empty concepts? *Obesity Facts*, 8, 386–401.

Longenbaker, S. N. (2017). *Mader's Understanding Human Anatomy & Physiology* (9th ed). New York: McGraw-Hill Education.

Lopez-Legarrea, P., Fuller, N. R., Zulet, M. A., Martinez, J. A., & Caterson, I. D. (2014). The influence of Mediterranean, carbohydrate and high protein diets on gut microbiota composition in the treatment of obesity and associated inflammatory state. *Asia Pacific Journal of Clinical Nutrition*, 23, 360–368.

Louis, E. D. (2008). Environmental epidemiology of essential tremor. *Neuroepidemiology*, 31, 139–149.

Louis, E. D., & Zheng, W. (2010). β-carboline alkaloids and essential tremor: Exploring the environmental determinants of one of the most prevalent neurological diseases. *The Scientific World Journal*, 10, 1783–1794.

Louis, E. D., Zheng, W., Applegate, L., Shi, L., & Factor-Litvak, P. (2005). Blood harmane concentrations and dietary protein consumption in essential tremor. *Neurology*, 65, 391–396.

Lowden, A., Moreno, C., Holmbäck, U., Lennernäs, M., & Tucker, P. (2010). Eating and shift work – Effects on habits, metabolism, and performance. *Scandinavian Journal of Work, Environment & Health*, 36, 150–162.

Lowell, B. B. (2019). New neuroscience of homeostasis and drives for food, water, and salt. *The New English Journal of Medicine*, 380, 459–471.

Lozoff, B. (1989). Nutrition and behavior. *American Psychologist* 44, 231–236.
(2007). Iron deficiency and child development. *Food & Nutrition Bulletin*, 28, S560–S571.

Lozoff, B., Brittenham, G. M., Viteri, F. E., Wolf, A. W., & Urrutia, J. J. (1982). The effects of short-term oral iron therapy on developmental deficits in iron-deficient anemic infants. *Journal of Pediatrics*, 100, 351–357.

Lozoff, B., Clark, K. M., Jing, Y., Armony-Sivan, R., Angelilli, M. L., & Jacobson, S. W. (2008). Dose-response relationships between iron deficiency with or without anemia and infant social-emotional behavior. *Journal of Pediatrics*, 152, 696–702.

Lozoff, B., Smith, J. B., Kaciroti, N., Clark, K. M., Guevara, S., & Jimenez, E. (2013). Functional significance of early-life iron deficiency: Outcomes at 25 years. *Journal of Pediatrics*, 163, 1260–1266.

Lucas, A., Morley, R., & Cole, T. J. (1988). Adverse neurodevelopmental outcome of moderate neonatal hypoglycemia. *British Medical Journal*, 297, 1304–1308.

Ludolph, A. C., Hugon, J., Dwivedi, M. P., Schaumburg, H. H., & Spencer, P. S. (1987). Studies on the aetiology and pathogenesis of motor neuron disease. 1. Lathyrism: Clinical findings in established cases. *Brain*, 110, 149–165.

Lukowski, A. F., Koss, M., Burden, M. J., Jonides, J., Nelson, C. A., Kaciroti, N., & Lozoff, B. (2010). Iron deficiency in infancy and neurocognitive functioning at 19 years: Evidence of long-term deficits in executive function and recognition memory. *Nutritional Neuroscience*, 13, 54–70.

Lukoyanov, N. V., & Andrade, J. P. (2000). Behavioral effects of protein deprivation and rehabilitation in adult rats: Relevance to morphological alterations in the hippocampal formation. *Behavioural Brain Research*, 112, 85–97.

Lundh, A., Lexchin, J., Mintzes, B., Schroll, J. B., & Bero, L. (2018). Industry sponsorship and research outcome: Systematic review with meta-analysis. *Intensive Care Medicine*, 44, 1603–1612.

Luppino, F. S., de Wit, L. M., Bouvy, P. F., Stijnen, T., Cuijpers, P., Penninx, B. W., & Zitman, F. G. (2010). Overweight, obesity, and depression: A systematic review and meta-analysis of longitudinal studies. *Archives of General Psychiatry*, 67, 220–229.

Lustig, R. H., Schmidt, L. A., & Brindis, C. D. (2012). Public health: The toxic truth about sugar. *Nature*, 482, 27–29.

Lv, Y. B., Yin, Z. X., Chei, C. L., Brasher, M. S., Zhang, J., Kraus, V. B., & Zeng, Y. (2016). Serum cholesterol levels within the high normal range are associated with better cognitive performance among Chinese elderly. *Journal of Nutrition Health & Aging*, 20, 280–287.

Lyons, P. M., & Truswell, S. A. (1988). Serotonin precursor influenced by type of carbohydrate meal in healthy adults. *American Journal of Clinical Nutrition*, 47, 433–439.

Ma, F., Wu, T., & Zhao, J. (2017). Plasma homocysteine and serum folate and vitamin B-12 levels in mild cognitive impairment and Alzheimer's disease: A case-control study. *Nutrients*, 9, 725.

MacCormack, J., & Lindquist, K. (2019). Feeling 'hangry': When hunger is conceptualized as emotion. *Emotion*, 19, 301–319.

Macpherson, H., Robertson, B., Sünram-Lea, S., Stough, C., Kennedy, D., & Scholey, A. (2015). Glucose administration and cognitive function: Differential effects of age and effort during a dual task paradigm in younger and older adults. *Psychopharmacology*, 232, 1135–1142.

Macready, A. L., Kennedy, O. B., Ellis, J. A., Williams, C. M., Spencer, J. P. E., & Butler, L. T. (2009). Flavonoids and cognitive function: A review of human randomized controlled trial studies and recommendations for future studies. *Genes & Nutrition*, 4, 227–242.

Madhavadas, S., Kapgal, V. K., Kutty, B. M., & Subramanian, S. (2016). The neuroprotective effect of dark chocolate in monosodium glutamate-induced nontransgenic Alzheimer disease model rats: Biochemical, behavioral, and histological studies. *Journal of Dietary Supplements*, 13, 449–460.

Madhusudanan, M., Menon, M. K., Ummer, K., & Radhakrishnanan, K. (2008). Clinical and etiological profile of tropical ataxic neuropathy in Kerala, South India. *European Neurology*, 60, 21–26.

Madsen, E., & Gitlin, J. D. (2007). Copper and iron disorders of the brain. *Annual Review of Neuroscience*, 30, 317–337.

Mahoney, C. R., Taylor, H. A., & Kanarek, R. B. (2007). Effect of an afternoon confectionary snack on cognitive processes critical to learning. *Physiology & Behavior*, 90, 344–352.

Maizey, L., & Tzavella, L. (2019). Barriers and solutions for early career researchers in tackling the reproducibility crisis in cognitive neuroscience. *Cortex*, 113, 357–359.

Majumder, S., & Banik, P. (2019). Geographical variation of arsenic distribution in paddy soil, rice, and rice-based products: A meta-analytic approach and implications to human health. *Journal of Environmental Management*, 233, 184–199.

Makimura, H., Mizuno, T. M., & Isoda, F. (2003). Role of glucocorticoids in mediating effects of fasting and diabetes on hypothalamic gene expression. *BMC Physiology*, 3, 5.

MAL-ED Network. (2018). Early childhood cognitive development is affected by interactions among illness, diet, enteropathogens and the home environment: Findings from the MAL-ED birth cohort study. *BMJ Global Health*, 3, e000752.

Mallick, R., Basak, S., & Duttaroy, A. K. (2019). Docosahexaenoic acid, 22:6n-3: Its roles in the structure and function of the brain. *International Journal of Developmental Neuroscience*, 79, 21–31.

Manara, R., D'Agata, L., & Rocco, M. C. (2017a). Neuroimaging changes in Menkes disease, Part 1. *American Journal of Neuroradiology*, 38, 1850–1857.

Manara, R., Rocco, M. C., & D'Agata, L. (2017b). Neuroimaging changes in Menkes disease, Part 2. *American Journal of Neuroradiology*, 38, 1858–1865.

Manderino, L., Carroll, I., Azcarate-Peril, M. A., Rochette, A., Heinberg, L., Peat, C., & Gunstad, J. (2017). Preliminary evidence for an association between the composition of the gut microbiome and cognitive function in neurologically healthy older adults. *Journal of the International Neuropsychological Society*, 23, 700–705.

Manna, P. K., Mohanta, G. P, Valliappan, K., & Manavalan, R. (1999). Lathyrus and lathyrism: A review. *International Journal of Food Properties*, 2, 197–203.

Manning, C. A., Parsons, M. W., Cotter, E. M., & Gold, P. E. (1997). Glucose effects on declarative and nondeclarative memory in healthy elderly and young adults. *Psychobiology*, 25, 103–108.

Manning, C. A., Ragozzino, M. E., & Gold, P. E. (1993). Glucose enhancement of memory in patients with probable senile dementia of Alzheimer's type. *Neurobiology of Aging*, 14, 523–528.

Manole, A., Jaunmuktane, Z., & Hargreaves, I. (2017). Clinical, pathological and functional characterization of riboflavin-responsive neuropathy. *Brain*, 140, 2820–2837.

Manzetti, S., Zhang, J., & van der Spoel, D. (2014). Thiamine function, metabolism, uptake, and transport. *Biochemistry*, 53, 821–835.

Maran, T., Sachse, P., Martini, M., & Furtner, M. (2017). Benefits of a hungry mind: When hungry, exposure to food facilitates proactive interference resolution. *Appetite*, 108, 343–352.

Marashly, E. T., & Bohlega, S. A. (2017). Riboflavin has neuroprotective potential: Focus on Parkinson's disease and migraine. *Frontiers in Neurology*, 8, 333.

Marder, K., Gu, Y., Eberly, S., Tanner, C. M., Scarmeas, N., Oakes, D., & The Huntington Study Group. (2013). Relationship of Mediterranean diet and caloric intake to phenoconversion in Huntington disease. *JAMA Neurology*, 70, 1382–1388.

Markus, C. R., Rogers, P. J., Brouns, F., & Schepers, R. (2017). Eating dependence and weight gain; no human evidence for a 'sugar-addition' model of overweight. *Appetite*, 114, 64–72.

Marlatt, K. L., Redman, L. M., Burton, J. H., Martin, C. K., & Ravussin, E. (2017). Persistence of weight loss and acquired behaviors 2 y after 2-y calorie restriction intervention. *American Journal of Clinical Nutrition*, 105, 928–935.

Martin, A. J., Dhillon, H. M., & Vardy, J. L. (2019). Neurocognitive function and quality of life outcomes in the ONTRAC study for skin cancer chemoprevention by nicotinamide. *Geriatrics*, 4, 31.

Martin, C. K., Bhapkar, M., & Pittas, A. (2016). Effect of calorie restriction on mood, quality of life, sleep, and sexual function in healthy nonobese adults: The CALERIE 2 randomised clinical trial. *JAMA Internal Medicine*, 176, 743–752.

Martin, C. K., Bhapkar, M., Pittas, A. G., Pieper, C. F., Das, S. K., Williamson, D. A., Scott, T., Redman, L. M., Stein, R., Gilhooly, C. H., Stewart, T., Robinson, L., & Roberts, S. B. (2016). Comprehensive assessment of long-term effects of reducing intake of energy (CALERIE) Phase 2 study group. Effect of calorie restriction on mood, quality of life, sleep, and sexual function in healthy nonobese adults: The CALERIE 2 randomized clinical trial. *JAMA Internal Medicine*, 176, 743–752.

Martin, C. K., McClernon, J., Chellino, A., & Correa, J. B. (2011). Chapter 49. Food cravings: A central construct in food intake behavior, weight loss, and the neurobiology of appetitive behavior. In V. R. Preedy (Ed.) *Handbook of Behavior, Food & Nutrition* (pp. 741–755). Berlin, DE: Springer.

Martin, P. Y., & Benton, D. (1999). The influence of a glucose drink on a demanding working memory task. *Physiology & Behavior*, 67, 69–74.

Martinez-Lapiscina, E. H., Clavero, P., Toledo, E., Estruch, R., Salas-Salvado, J., San Julian, B., & Martinez-Gonzalez, M. A. (2013). Mediterranean diet improves cognition: The PREDIMED-NAVARRA randomised trial. *Journal of Neurology Neurosurgery & Psychiatry*, 84, 1318–1325.

Martinez-Lapiscina, E. H., Galbete, C., Corella, D., Toledo, E., Buil-Cosiales, P., Salas-Salvado, J., & Martinez-Gonzalez, M. A. (2014). Genotype patterns at CLU, CR1, PICALM and APOE, cognition and Mediterranean diet: The PREDIMED-NAVARRA trial. *Genes & Nutrition*, 9, 393.

Martinowich, K., Manji, H., & Lu, B. (2007). New insights into BDNF function in depression and anxiety. *Nature Neuroscience*, 10, 1089–1093.

Martins, D., Mehta, M. A., & Prata, D. (2017). The "highs and lows" of the human brain on dopaminergics: Evidence from neuropharmacology. *Neuroscience & Biobehavioral Reviews*, 80, 351–371.

Marx, W., Lane, M., Hockey, M., Aslam, H., Berk, M., Walder, K., & Jacka, F. N. (2021). Diet and depression: Exploring the biological mechanisms of action. *Molecular Psychiatry*, 26, 134–150.

Marx, W., Moseley, G., Berk, M., & Jacka, F. (2017). Nutritional psychiatry: The present state of the evidence. *Proceedings of the Nutrition Society*, 76, 427–436.

Masana, M. F., Tyrovolas, S., Kolia, N., Chrysohoou, C., Skoumas, J., Haro, J. M., & Panagiotakos, D. B. (2019). Dietary patterns and their association with anxiety symptoms among older adults: The ATTICA study. *Nutrients*, 11, Article 1250.

Mason, L. H., Harp, J. P., & Han, D. Y. (2014). Pb neurotoxicity: Neuropsychological effects of lead toxicity. *BioMed Research International*, 2014, 1–8.

Massey, K. A., Blakeslee, C. H., & Pitkow, H. S. (1998). A review of physiological and metabolic effects of essential amino acids. *Amino Acids*, 14, 271–300.

Matsumoto, K., & Fukuda, H. (1982). Anisatin modulation of GABA- and pentobarbital-induced enhancement of diazepam binding in a rat brain. *Neuroscience Letters*, 32, 175–179.

Matthews, D. C., Davies, M., Murray, J., Williams, S., Tsui, W. H., Li, Y., & Mosconi, L. (2014). Physical activity, Mediterranean diet and biomarkers-assessed risk of Alzheimer's: A multi-modality brain imaging study. *Advances in Molecular Imaging*, 4, 43–57.

Mattison, J. A., Roth, G. S., & Beasley, T. M. (2012). Impact of caloric restriction on health and survival in rhesus monkeys: The NIA study. *Nature*, 489, 318–321.

Mattson, M. P. (2005). Energy intake, meal frequency, and health: A neurobiological perspective. *Annual Review of Nutrition*, 25, 237–260.

Mattson, M. P., Moehl, K., Ghena, N., Schmaedick, M., & Cheng, A. (2018). Intermittent metabolic switching, neuroplasticity and brain health. *Nature Reviews Neuroscience*, 19, 81–94.

Mattson, S. N., Crocker, N., & Nguyen, T. T. (2011). Fetal alcohol spectrum disorders: Neuropsychology and behavioural features. *Neuropsychology Reviews*, 21, 81–101.

Maylor, E. A., Simpson, E. E. A., & Secker, D. L. (2006). Effects of zinc supplementation on cognitive function in healthy middle-aged and older adults: The ZENITH study. *British Journal of Nutrition*, 96, 752–760.

McCann, J. C., & Ames, B. N. (2008). Is there convincing biological or behavioral evidence linking vitamin D deficiency to brain dysfunction? *FASEB Journal*, 22, 982–1001.

McCann, J. C., Hudes, M., & Ames, B. N. (2006). An overview of evidence for a causal relationship between dietary availability of choline during development and cognitive function in offspring. *Neuroscience & Biobehavioral Reviews*, 30, 696–712.

McCarty, M. F., & Lerner, A. (2012). The second phase of brain trauma can be controlled by nutraceuticals that suppress DAMP-medicated microglial activation. *Expert Review of Neurotherapeutics*, 21, 559–570.

McCurdy, S. A. (1994). Epidemiology of disaster: The Donner Party [1846-1847]. *Western Journal of Medicine*, 160, 338–342.

McDonald, T. J. W., & Cervenka, M. C. (2018). The expanding role of ketogenic diets in adult neurological disorders. *Brain Sciences*, 8, Article 148.

McEchron, M. D., Alexander, D. N., Gilmartin, M. R., & Paronish, M. D. (2008). Perinatal nutritional iron deficiency impairs hippocampus-dependent trace eyeblink conditioning in rats. *Developmental Neuroscience*, 30, 243–254.

McEwen, B. S. (2007). Physiology and neurobiology of stress and adaptation: Central role of the brain. *Physiological Reviews*, 87, 873–904.

McFarlane, O., Kozakiewicz, M., Kedziora-Kornatowska, K., Gebka, D., Szybalska, A., Szwed, M., & Klich-Raczka, A. (2020). Blood lipids and cognitive performance of aging polish adults: A case-control study based on the PolSenior project. *Frontiers in Aging Neuroscience*, 12, 590546.

McHill, A. W., Melanson, E. L., & Higgins, J. (2014). Impact of circadian misalignment on energy metabolism during simulated nightshift work. *Proceedings of the National Academy of Sciences of the United States of America*, 111, 17302–17307.

McLean, A., Rubinsztein, J. S., Robbins, T. W., & Sahakian, B. J. (2004). The effects of tyrosine depletion in normal healthy volunteers: Implications for unipolar depression. *Psychopharmacology*, 171, 286–297.

McLean, E., Cogswell, M., Egli, I., Woidyla, D., & de Benoist, B. (2009). Worldwide prevalence of anaemia, WHO Vitamin and Mineral Nutrition Information System, 1993-2005. *Public Health Nutrition*, 12, 444–454.

McLellan, T. M., Caldwell, J. A., & Lieberman, H. R. (2016). A review of caffeine's effects on cognitive, physical and occupational performance. *Neuroscience & Biobehavioral Reviews*, 71, 294–312.

McMillan, L., Owen, L., Kras, M., & Scholey, A. (2011). Behavioural effects of a 10-day Mediterranean diet. Results from a pilot study evaluating mood and cognitive performance. *Appetite*, 56, 143–147.

McNamara, A. E., Walon, J., Flynn, A., Nugent, A. P., McNulty, B. A., & Brennan, L. (2021). The potential of multi-biomarker panels in nutrition research: Total fruit intake as an example. *Frontiers in Nutrition*, 7, e577720.

McNay, E. C., Fries, T. M., & Gold, P. E. (2000). Decreases in rat extracellular hippocampal glucose concentration associated with cognitive demand during a spatial task. *Proceedings of the National Academy of Sciences of the United States of America*, 97, 2881–2885.

McNay, E. C., & Gold, P. E. (2002). Food for thought: Fluctuations in brain extracellular glucose provide insight into the mechanisms of memory modulation. *Behavioral & Cognitive Neuroscience Reviews*, 1, 264–280.

References

McNulty, B., Pentieva, K., Marshall, B., Ward, M., Molloy, A. M., Scott, J. M., & McNulty, H. (2011). Women's compliance with current folic acid recommendations and achievement of optimal vitamin status for preventing neural tube defects. *Human Reproduction*, 26, 1530–1536.

McTavish, S. F. B., Mannie, Z. N., Harmer, C. J., & Cowen, P. J. (2005). Lack of effect of tyrosine depletion on mood in recovered depressed women. *Neuropsychopharmacology*, 30, 786–791.

Meadway, C., George, S., & Braithwaite, R. (1998). Opiate concentrations following the ingestion of poppy seed products – Evidence for 'the poppy seed defence.' *Forensic Science International*, 96, 29–38.

Mehla, J., Reeta, K. H., Gupta, P., & Gupta, Y. K. (2010). Protective effect of curcumin against seizures and cognitive impairment in a pentylenetetrazole-kindled epileptic rat model. *Life Sciences*, 87, 596–603.

Melo, H. M., Santos, L. E., & Ferreira, S. T. (2019). Diet-derived fatty acids, brain inflammation, and mental health. *Frontiers in Neuroscience*, 13, 265.

Mendelsohn, D., Riedel, W. J., & Sambeth, A. (2009). Effects of acute tryptophan depletion on memory, attention, and executive functions: A systematic review. *Neuroscience & Biobehavioral Reviews*, 33, 926–952.

Meng, L., Chen, D., Yang, Y., Zheng, Y., & Hui, R. (2012). Depression increases the risk of hypertension incidence: A meta-analysis of prospective cohort studies. *Journal of Hypertension*, 30, 842–851.

Meng, Q., Ying, Z., Noble, E., Zhao, Y., Agrawal, R., Mikhail, A., Zhuang, Y., Tyagi, E., Zhang, Q., Lee, J. -H., Morselli, M., Orozco, L., Guo, W., Kilts, T. M., Zhu, J., Zhang, B., Pellegrini, M., Xiao, X., & Young, M. F. (2016). Systems nutrigenomics reveals brain gene networks linking metabolic and brain disorders. *EBioMedicine*, 7, 157–166.

Mercer, M. E., & Holder, M. D. (1997). Food cravings, endogenous opioid peptides, and food intake: A review. *Appetite*, 29, 325–352.

Meredith, S. E., Juliano, L. M., Hughes, J. R., & Griffiths, R. R. (2013). Caffeine use disorder: A comprehensive review and research agenda. *Journal of Caffeine Research*, 3, 114–130.

Merrill, D. A., Siddarth, P., Raji, C. A., Emerson, N. D., Rueda, F., Ercoli, L. M., & Small, G. W. (2016). Modifiable risk factors and brain positron emission tomography measures of amyloid and tau in nondemented adults with memory complaints. *American Journal of Geriatric Psychiatry*, 24, 729–737.

Messier, C. (2004). Glucose improvement of memory: A review. *European Journal of Pharmacology*, 490, 33–57.

Messier, C., Gagnon, M., & Knott, V. (1997). Effect of glucose and peripheral glucose regulation on memory in the elderly. *Neurobiology of Aging*, 18, 297–304.

Messier, C., Pierre, J., Desrochers, A., & Gravel, M. (1998). Dose-dependent action of glucose on memory processes in women: Effect on serial position and recall priority. *Cognitive Brain Research*, 7, 221–233.

Messier, C., Tsiakas, M., Gagnon, M., Desrochers, A., & Awad, N. (2003). Effect of age and glucoregulation on cognitive performance. *Neurobiology of Aging*, 24, 985–1003.

Messier, C., Whately, K., Liang, J., Du, L., & Puissant, D. (2007). The effects of a high-fat, high-fructose, and combination diet on learning, weight, and glucose regulation in C57BL/6 mice. *Behavioral Brain Research*, 178, 139–145.

Messier, C., & White, N. M. (1984). Contingent and non-contingent actions of sucrose and saccharin reinforcers Effects on taste preference and memory. *Physiology & Behavior*, 32, 195–203.

Metges, C. C., Petzke, K. J., & Young, V. R. (1999). Dietary requirements for indispensable amino acids in adult humans: New concepts, methods of estimation, uncertainties and challenges. *Nutrition & Metabolism*, 43, 267–276.

Metzger, M. M. (2000). Glucose enhancement of a facial recognition task in young adults. *Physiology & Behavior*, 68, 549–553.

Meule, A. (2016). Dieting and food cue-related working memory performance. *Frontiers in Psychology*, 7, 1944.

Meule, A., Gearhardt, A. N. (2014). Food addiction in the light of DSM-5. *Nutrients*, 6, 3653–3671.

Middaugh, L. D., Grover, T. A., Blackwell, L. A., & Zemp, J. W. (1976). Neurochemical and behavioral effects of diet related perinatal folic acid restriction. *Pharmacology Biochemistry & Behavior*, 5, 129–134.

Milder, J. B., Liang, L. P., & Patel, M. (2010). Acute oxidative stress and systemic Nrf2 activation by the ketogenic diet. *Neurobiology of Disease*, 40, 238–244.

Miller, C. (2009). Updates on pediatric feeding and swallowing problems. *Current Opinion in Otolaryngology Head & Neck Surgery*, 17, 194–199.

Miller, H. C., Struyf, D., Baptist, P., Dalile, B., Van Oudenhove, L., & Van Diest, I. (2018). A mind cleared by walnut oil: The effects of polyunsaturated and saturated fat on extinction learning. *Appetite*, 126, 147–155.

Miller, J. W. (2004). Folate, cognition, and depression in the era of folic acid fortification. *Journal of Food Science*, 69, S61–S64.

Miller, R., Benelam, B., Stanner, S. A., & Buttriss, J. L. (2013). Is snacking good or bad for health: An overview. *Nutrition Bulletin*, 38, 302–332.

Millet, Y., Jouglard, J., & Steinmetz, M. D. (1981). Toxicity of some essential plant oils. *Clinical and experimental study*. *Clinical Toxicology*, 18, 1485–1498.

Millour, S., Noël, L., & Kadar, A. (2011). Pb, Hg, Cd, As, Sb, and Al levels in foodstuffs from the 2nd French total diet study. *Food Chemistry*, 126, 1787–1799.

Mills, J. D., Bailes, J. E., Sedney, C. L., Hutchins, H., & Sears, B. (2011). Omega-3 fatty acid supplementation and reduction of traumatic axonal injury in a rodent head injury model: Laboratory investigation. *Journal of Neurosurgery*, 114, 77–84.

Mills, J. D., Hadley, K., & Bailes, J. E. (2011). Dietary supplementation with the omega-3 fatty acid docosahexaenoic acid in traumatic brain injury. *Neurosurgery,* 68, 474–481.

Milner, S. E., Brunton, N. P., & Jones, P. W. (2011). Bioactivities of glycoalkaloids and their aglycones from Solanum species. *Journal of Agricultural & Food Chemistry,* 59, 3454–3484.

Mischley, L. K., Lau, R. C., & Bennett, R. D. (2017). Role of diet and nutritional supplements in Parkinson's disease progression. *Oxidative Medicine & Cellular Longevity,* 6405278.

Misner, D. L., Jacobs, S., & Shimizu, Y. (2001). Vitamin A deprivation results in reversible loss of hippocampal long-term synaptic plasticity. *Proceedings of the National Academy of Sciences of the United States of America,* 98, 11714–11719.

Mizoroki, T., Meshitsuka, S., & Maeda, S. (2007). Aluminium induces tau aggregation in vitro but not in vivo. *Journal of Alzheimer's Disease,* 11, 419–427.

Mocking, R. J. T., Harmsen, I., Assies, J., Koeter, M. W. J., Ruhe, H. G., & Schene, A. H. (2016). Meta-analysis and meta-regression of omega-3 polyunsaturated fatty acid supplementation for major depressive disorder. *Translational Psychiatry,* 6, e756.

Modabbernia, A., Velthorst, E., & Reichenberg, A. (2017). Environmental risk factors for autism: An evidence-based review of systematic reviews and meta-analyses. *Molecular Autism,* 8, 13.

Mogg, K., Bradley, B. P., Hyare, H., & Lee, S. (1998). Selective attention to food-related stimuli in hunger: Are attentional biases specific to emotional and psychopathological states, or are they also found in normal drive states? *Behaviour Research & Therapy,* 36, 227–237.

Mogi, M., Tsukuda, K., Li, J. M., Iwanami, J., Min, L. J., Sakata, A., & Horiuchi, M. (2007). Inhibition of cognitive decline in mice fed a high-salt and cholesterol diet by the angiotensin receptor blocker, Olmesartan. *Neuropharmacology,* 53, 899–905.

Mohan, D., Yap, K. H., Reidpath, D., Soh, Y. C., McGrattan, A., Stephan, B. C. M., & De, P. E. C. t. (2020). Link between dietary sodium intake, cognitive function, and dementia risk in middle-aged and older adults: A systematic review. *Journal of Alzheimer's Disease,* 76, 1347–1373.

Molden, D. C., Hui, C. M., & Scholer, A. A.(2012). Motivational versus metabolic effects of carbohydrates on self-control. *Psychological Science,* 23, 1137–1144.

Molendijk, M., Molero, P., Ortuno Sanchez-Pedreno, F., Van der Does, W., & Angel Martinez-Gonzalez, M. (2018). Diet quality and depression risk: A systematic review and dose-response meta-analysis of prospective studies. *Journal of Affective Disorders,* 226, 346–354.

Molfino, A., Iannace, A., & Colaiacomo, M. C. (2017). Cancer anorexia: Hypothalamic activity and its association with inflammation and appetite-regulating peptides in lung cancer. *Journal of Cachexia, Sarcopenia & Muscle*, 8, 40–47.

Mollison, P. L. (1946). Observations on cases of starvation at Belsen. *British Medical Journal*, 1, 4–8.

Molteni, R., Barnard, R. J., Ying, Z., Roberts, C. K., & Gomez-Pinilla, F. (2002). A high-fat, refined sugar diet reduces hippocampal brain-derived neurotrophic factor, neuronal plasticity, and learning. *Neuroscience*, 112, 803–814.

Monk, C., Georgieff, M. K., Xu, D., Hao, X., Bansal, R., Gustafsson, H., & Peterson, B. S. (2016). Maternal prenatal iron status and tissue organization in the neonatal brain. *Pediatric Research*, 79, 482–488.

Monteiro, J., Alves, M. G., Oliveira, P. F., & Silva, B. M. (2019). Pharmacological potential of methylxanthines: Retrospective analysis and future expectations. *Critical Reviews in Food Science & Nutrition*, 59, 2597–2625.

Montgomery, A. J., McTavish, S. F. B., Cowen, P. J., & Grasby, P. M. (2003). Reductions of brain dopamine concentration with dietary tyrosine plus phenylalanine depletion: An [¹¹C]raclopride PET study. *American Journal of Psychiatry*, 160, 1887–1889.

Moodie, R., Stuckler, D., Monteiro, C., Sheron, N., Neal, B., Thamarangsi, T., Lincoln, P., Casswell, S., & Lancet NCD Action Group. (2013). Profits and pandemics: Prevention of harmful effects of tobacco, alcohol, and ultra-processed food and drink industries. *The Lancet*, 381, 670–679.

Moody, L., Chen, H., & Pan, Y. X. (2017). Early-life nutritional programming of cognition-The fundamental role of epigenetic mechanisms in mediating the relation between early-life environment and learning and memory process. *Advances in Nutrition*, 8, 337–350.

Moog, N. K., Entringer, S., & Heim, C. (2017). Influence of maternal thyroid hormones during gestation on fetal brain development. *Neuroscience*, 342, 68–100.

Moore, E. M., Ames, D., & Mander, A. G. (2014). Among vitamin B12 deficient older people, high folate levels are associated with worse cognitive function: Combined data from three cohorts. *Journal of Alzheimer's Disease*, 39, 661–668.

Moore, S. A., Yoder, E., Murphy, S., Dutton, G. R., & Spector, A. A. (1991). Astrocytes, not neurons, produce docosahexaenoic acid (22:6 omega-3) and arachidonic acid (20:4 omega-6). *Journal of Neurochemistry*, 56, 518–524.

Morell-Hart, S. (2012). Foodways and resilience under apocalyptic conditions. *Journal of Culture and Agriculture*, 34, 161–171.

Moreno, F. A., Parkinson, D., & Palmer, C. (2010). CSF neurochemicals during tryptophan depletion in individuals with remitted depression and healthy controls. *European Neueropsychopharmacology*, 20, 18–24.

Moreton, E., Baron, P., Tiplady, S., McCall, S., Clifford, B., Langley-Evans, S. C., & Voigt, J. P. (2019). Impact of early exposure to a cafeteria diet on prefrontal cortex monoamines and novel object recognition in adolescent rats. *Behavioural Brain Research,* 363, 191–198.

Morgane, P. J., Austin-LaFrance, R. J., & Bronzino, J. D. (1993). Prenatal malnutrition and development of the brain. *Neuroscience & Biobehavioral Reviews,* 17, 91–128.

Morgane, P. J., Miller, M., & Kemper, T. (1978). The effects of protein malnutrition on the developing central nervous system in the rat. *Neuroscience & Biobehavioral Reviews,* 2, 137–230.

Morgane, P., Mokler, D., & Galler, J. (2002). Effects of prenatal protein malnutrition on the hippocampal formation. *Neuroscience & Biobehavioral Reviews,* 26, 471–483.

Morgese, M. G., & Trabace, L. (2016). Maternal malnutrition in the etiopathogenesis of psychiatric diseases: Role of polyunsaturated fatty acids. *Brain Sciences,* 6, 24.

Morris, G., Puri, B. K., & Frye, R. E. (2017). The putative role of environmental aluminium in the developmental of chronic neuropathology in adults and children. How strong is the evidence and what could be the mechanisms involved? *Metabolic Brain Disease,* 32, 1335–1355.

Morris, J. S., & Dolan, R. J. (2001). Involvement of human amygdala and orbitofrontal cortex in hunger-enhanced memory for food stimuli. *Journal of Neuroscience,* 21, 5304–5310.

Morris, M. C., Evans, D. A., Bienias, J. L., Tangney, C. C., Bennett, D. A., Aggarwal, N., & Wilson, R. S. (2003). Dietary fats and the risk of incident Alzheimer disease. *Archives of Neurology,* 60, 194–200.

Morris, M. C., Evans, D. A., Bienias, J. L., Tangney, C. C., & Wilson, R. S. (2004). Dietary fat intake and 6-year cognitive change in an older biracial community population. *Neurology,* 62, 1573–1579.

Morris, M. C., Tangney, C. C., Wang, Y., Sacks, F. M., Barnes, L. L., Bennett, D. A., & Aggarwal, N. T. (2015). MIND diet slows cognitive decline with aging. *Alzheimers Dementia,* 11, 1015–1022.

Morris, M. C., Tangney, C. C., Wang, Y., Sacks, F. M., Bennett, D. A., & Aggarwal, N. T. (2015). MIND diet associated with reduced incidence of Alzheimer's disease. *Alzheimers Dementia,* 11, 1007–1014.

Morris, M. S., Selhub, J., & Jacques, P. F. (2012). Vitamin B-12 and folate status in relation to decline in scores on the Mini-Mental State Examination in the Framingham Heart Study. *Journal of the American Geriatrics Society,* 60, 1457–1464.

Mosconi, L., Murray, J., Tsui, W. H., Li, Y., Davies, M., Williams, S., & de Leon, M. J. (2014). Mediterranean diet and magnetic resonance imaging-assessed brain atrophy in cognitively normal individuals at risk for Alzheimer's disease. *Journal of Prevention of Alzheimers Disease,* 1, 23–32.

Mosegaard, S., Dipace, G., & Bross, P. (2020). Riboflavin deficiency: Implications for general human health and inborn errors of metabolism. *International Journal of Molecular Sciences,* 21, 3847.

Mosek, A., Natour, H., Neufeld, M. Y., Shiff, Y., & Vaisman, N. (2009). Ketogenic diet treatment in adults with refractory epilepsy: A prospective pilot study. *Seizure-European Journal of Epilepsy*, 18, 30–33.

Most, J., Tosti, V., Redman, L. M., & Fontana, L. (2017). Calorie restriction in humans: An update. *Ageing Research Reviews*, 39, 36–45.

Moubarac, J. -C., Parra, D. C., Cannon, G., & Monteiro, C. A. (2014). Food classification systems based on food processing: Significance and implications for policies and actions: A systematic literature review and assessment. *Current Obesity Reports*, 3, 256–272.

Moulton, C. D., Costafreda, S. G., Horton, P., Ismail, K., & Fu, C. H. Y. (2015). Meta-analysis of structural regional cerebral effects in type 1 and type 2 diabetes. *Brain Imaging and Behavior*, 9, 651–662.

MRC Vitamin Study Research Group. (1991). Prevention of neural tube defects: Results of the Medical Research Council Vitamin Study. *The Lancet*, 338, 131–137.

Muller, D. P. R. (2010). Vitamin E and neurological function. *Molecular Nutrition & Food Research*, 54, 710–718.

Müller, K., Libuda, L., Terschlüsen, A. M., & Kersting, M. (2013). A review of the effects of lunch on adults' short-term cognitive functioning. *Canadian Journal of Dietetic Practice & Research*, 74, 181–188.

Muraven, M., & Baumeister, R. F. (2000). Self-regulation and depletion of limited resources: Does self-control resemble a muscle? *Psychological Bulletin*, 126, 247–259.

Murch, S. J., Cox, P. A., & Banack, S. A. (2004). A mechanism for slow release of biomagnified cyanobacterial neurotoxins and neurodegenerative disease in Guam. *Proceedings of the National Academy of Sciences of the United States of America*, 101, 12228–12231.

Murphy, T., Dias, G. P., & Thuret, S. (2014). Effects of diet on brain plasticity in animal and human studies: Mind the gap. *Neural Plasticity*, 2014, 1–32.

Nabb, S., & Benton, D. (2006). The influence on cognition of the interaction between the macro-nutrient content of breakfast and glucose tolerance. *Physiology & Behavior*, 87, 16–23.

Nagano-Saito, A., Cisek, P., & Perna, A. S. (2012). From anticipation to action, the role of dopamine in perceptual decision making: An fMRI-tyrosine depletion study. *Journal of Neurophysiology*, 108, 501–512.

Najafabadi, M. G., Nikoukar, L. R., Memari, A., Ekhtiari, H., & Beygi, S. (2015). Does Ramadan fasting adversely affect cognitive function in young females? *Scientifica*, 2015, 432428.

Natarajan, C., & Bright, J. J. (2002). Curcumin inhibits experimental allergic encephalomyelitis by blocking IL-12 signaling through Janus kinase-STAT pathway in T lymphocytes. *Journal of Immunology*, 168, 6506–6513.

National CJD Research and Surveillance Unit. (2017). 2017 annual report. https://www.cjd.ed.ac.uk/sites/default/files/report26.pdf (last accessed 21 February 2020).

Naughton, M., Dinan, T. G., & Scott, L. V. (2014). Corticotropin-releasing hormone and the hypothalamic–pituitary–adrenal axis in psychiatric disease. *Handbook of Clinical Neurology*, 124, 69–91.

Nazir, M., Lone, R., & Charoo, B. A. (2019). Infantile thiamine deficiency: New insights into an old disease. *Indian Pediatrics*, 56, 673–681.

Neale, C., Camfield, D., Reay, J., Stough, C., & Scholey, A. (2012). Cognitive effects of two nutraceuticals ginseng and bacopa benchmarked against modafinil: A review and comparison of effect sizes. *British Journal of Clinical Pharmacology*, 75, 728–737.

Nehlig, A. (2016). Effects of coffee/caffeine on brain health and disease: What should I tell my patients? *Practical Neurology*, 16, 89–95.

Nelson, K. M., Dahlin, J. L., Bisson, J., Graham , J., Pauli, G. F., & Walters, M. A. (2017). Curcumin may (not) defy science. *SCD Medical Chemistry Letters*, 8, 467–470.

Nemets, B., Stahl, Z., & Belmaker, R. H. (2002). Addition of omega-3 fatty acid to maintenance medication treatment for recurrent unipolar depressive disorder. *American Journal of Psychiatry*, 159, 477–479.

Nettle, D. (2017). Does hunger contribute to socioeconomic gradients in behavior? *Frontiers in Psychology*, 8, 358.

Netto, A. B., Netto, C. M., Mahadevan, A., Taly, A. B., & Agadi, J. B. (2016). Tropical ataxic neuropathy – A century old enigma. *Neurology India*, 64, 1151–1159.

Newby, P. K., & Tucker, K. L. (2004). Empirically derived eating patterns using factor or cluster analysis: A review. *Nutrition Reviews*, 62, 177–203.

Newby, P. K., Weismayer, C., Akesson, A., Tucker, K. L., & Wolk, A. (2006). Long-term stability of food patterns identified by use of factor analysis among Swedish women. *Journal of Nutrition*, 136, 626–633.

Ng, F., Berk, M., Dean, O., & Bush, A. I. (2008). Oxidative stress in psychiatric disorders: Evidence base and therapeutic implications. *International Journal of Neuropsychopharmacology*, 11, 851–876.

Nguyen, P. H., Gonzalez-Casanova, I., Young, M. F., Truong, T. V., Hoang, H., Nguyen, H., & Ramakrishnan, U. (2017). Preconception micronutrient supplementation with iron and folic acid compared with folic acid alone affects linear growth and fine motor development at 2 years of age: A randomized controlled trial in Vietnam. *Journal of Nutrition*, 147, 1593–1601.

Nicolas, J., Hendriksen, P. J. M., Gerssen, A., Bovee, T. F., & Rietjens, I. M. (2014). Marine neurotoxins: State of the art, bottlenecks, and perspectives for mode of action based on methods of detection in seafood. *Molecular Nutrition & Food Research*, 58, 87–100.

Niculescu, M. D., Craciunescu, C. N., & Zeisel, S. H. (2006). Dietary choline deficiency alters global and gene-specific DNA methylation in the developing hippocampus of mouse fetal brains. *FASEB Journal*, 20, 43–49.

Niederhofer, R. E. (1985). The milk sickness. Drake on medical interpretation. *Journal of the American Medical Association*, 254, 2123–2125.

Nielsen, T., & Powell, R. A. (2015). Dreams of the Rarebit Fiend: Food and diet as instigators of bizarre and disturbing dreams. *Frontiers in Psychology*, 6, article 47.

Nikanorova, M., Miranda, M. J., Atkins, M., & Sahlholdt, L. (2009). Ketogenic diet in the treatment of refractory continuous spikes and waves during slow sleep. *Epilepsia*, 50, 1127–1131.

Nishimune, T., Watanabe, Y., Okazaki, H., & Akai, H. (2000). Thiamine is decomposed due to Anaphe spp. Entomophagy in seasonal ataxia patients in Nigeria. *Journal of Nutrition*, 130, 1625–1628.

Nishizawa, S., Benkelfat, C., & Young, S. N. (1997). Differences between males and females in rates of serotonin synthesis in human brain. *Proceedings of the National Academy of Sciences of the United States of America*, 94, 5308–5313.

Nowak, K. L., Fried, L., Jovanovich, A., Ix, J., Yaffe, K., You, Z., & Chonchol, M. (2018). Dietary sodium/potassium intake does not affect cognitive function or brain imaging indices. *American Journal of Nephrology*, 47, 57–65.

Nyaradi, A., Li, J., Hickling, S., Foster, J., & Oddy, W. (2013). The role of nutrition in children's neurocognitive development, from pregnancy through childhood. *Frontiers in Human Neuroscience*, 7, Article 97.

Nzwalo, H., & Cliff, J. (2011). Konzo: From poverty, cassava, and cyanogen intake to toxico-nutritional neurological disease. *PLOS Neglected Tropical Diseases*, 5, 1–8.

O'Brien, P. D., Hinder, L. M., Callaghan, B. C., & Feldman, E. L. (2017). Neurological consequences of obesity. *The Lancet Neurology*, 16, 465–477.

O'Leary, F., Allman-Farinelli, M., & Samman, S. (2012). Vitamin B-12 status, cognitive decline and dementia: A systematic review of prospective cohort studies. *British Journal of Nutrition*, 108, 1948–1961.

O'Neil, A., Quirk, S. E., Housden, S., Brennan, S. L., Williams, L. J., Pasco, J. A., & Jacka, F. N. (2014). Relationship between diet and mental health in children and adolescents: A systematic review. *American Journal of Public Health*, 104, e31–e42.

O'Neil, P. M., & Jarrell, M. P. (1992). Psychological aspects of obesity and very-low-calorie diets. *American Journal of Clinical Nutrition*, 56, S185–S189.

Oddy, W. H., Kendall, G. E., Li, J., Jacoby, P., Robinson, M., de Klerk, N. H., & Stanley, F. J. (2010). The long-term effects of breastfeeding on child and adolescent mental health: A pregnancy cohort study followed for 14 years. *Journal of Pediatrics*, 156, 568–574.

Oguri, T., Hattori, M., & Yamawaki, T. (2012). Neurological deficits in a patient with selenium deficiency due to long-term total parenteral nutrition. *Journal of Neurology*, 259, 1734–1735.

Okereke, O. I., Reynolds, C. F., & Mischoulon, D. (2020). Effect of long-term vitamin D3 supplementation vs placebo on risk of depression or clinically relevant depressive symptoms and on change in mood scores: A randomized clinical trial. *Journal of the American Medical Association*, 324, 471–480.

Okereke, O. I., Rosner, B. A., Kim, D. H., Kang, J. H., Cook, N. R., Manson, J. E., & Grodstein, F. (2012). Dietary fat types and 4-year cognitive change in community-dwelling older women. *Annals of Neurology, 72*, 124–134.

Okubo, H., Miyake, Y., Sasaki, S., Murakami, K., Tanaka, K., Fukushima, W., & Fukuoka Kinki Parkinson's Disease Study Group. (2012). Dietary patterns and risk of Parkinson's disease: A case-control study in Japan. *European Journal of Neurology, 19*, 681–688.

Olanow, C. W., & Brundin, P. (2013). Parkinson's disease and alpha synuclein: Is Parkinson's disease a prion-like disorder? *Movement Disorders, 28*, 31–40.

Olivares, M., & Uauy, R. (1996). Copper as an essential nutrient. *American Journal of Clinical Nutrition, 63*, S791–S796.

Olivo, G., Solstrand Dahlberg, L., & Wiemerslage, L. (2017). Atypical anorexia is not related to brain structural changes in newly diagnosed adolescent patients. *International Journal of Eating Disorders, 51*, 39–45.

Olson, C. M., Bove, C. F., & Miller, E. O. (2007). Growing up poor: Long-term implications for eating patterns and body weight. *Appetite, 49*, 198–207.

Olson, C. R., & Mello, C. V. (2010). Significance of vitamin A to brain function, behavior and learning. *Molecular Nutrition and Food Research, 54*, 489–495.

Omran, M. L., & Morley, J. E. (2000). Assessment of protein energy malnutrition in older persons, Part i: History, examination, body composition, and screening tools. *Nutrition, 16*, 50–63.

Ono, K., Condron, M. M., Ho, L., Wang, J., Zhao, W., Pasinetti, G. M., & Teplow, D. B. (2008). Effects of grape seed-derived polyphenols on amyloid beta-protein self-assembly and cytotoxicity. *Journal of Biological Chemistry, 283*, 32176–32187.

Orquin, J. L., & Kurzban, R. (2016). A meta-analysis of blood glucose effects on human decision making. *Psychological Bulletin, 142*, 546–567.

Oscar-Berman, M., & Marinkovic, K. (2007). Alcohol: Effects on neurobehavioral functions and the brain. *Neuropsychology Review, 17*, 239–257.

Overeem, K., Eyles, D. W., McGrath, J. J., & Burne, T. H. J. (2016). The impact of vitamin D deficiency on behaviour and brain function in rodents. *Current Opinion in Behavioral Sciences, 7*, 47–52.

Owens, D. S., & Benton, D. (1994). The impact of raising blood glucose on reaction time. *Neuropsychobiology, 30*, 106–113.

Pachucki, M. A. (2012). Food pattern analysis over time: Unhealthful eating trajectories predict obesity. *International Journal of Obesity, 36*, 686–694.

Paidi, M. D., Schjoldager, J. G., Lykkesfeldt, J., & Tveden-Nyborg, P. (2014). Chronic vitamin C deficiency promotes redox imbalance in the brain but does not alter sodium-dependent vitamin C transporter 2 expression. *Nutrients, 6*, 1809–1822.

Pan, W., Chang, Y., & Yeh, W. (2012). Co-occurrence of anemia, marginal vitamin B-6, and folate status and depressive symptoms in older adults. *Journal of Geriatric Psychiatry & Neurology, 25*, 170–178.

Pandit, R., Mercer, J. G., Overduin, J., la Fleur, S. E., & Adan, R. A. (2012). Dietary factors affect food reward and motivation to eat. *Obesity Facts, 5*, 221–242.

Panter, K. E., & James, L. F. (1990). Natural plant toxicants in milk: A review. *Journal of Animal Science*, 68, 892–904.

Pardridge, W. M. (2007). Blood-brain barrier delivery. *Drug Discovery Today*, 12, 54–61.

Parent, M. B., Krebs-Kraft, D. L., Ryan, J. P., Wilson, J. S., Harenski, C., & Hamann, S. (2011). Glucose administration enhances fMRI brain activation and connectivity related to episodic memory encoding for neutral and emotional stimuli. *Neuropsychologia*, 49, 1052–1066.

Parent, M. B., Varnhagen, C., & Gold, P. E. (1999). A memory-enhancing emotionally arousing narrative increases blood glucose levels in human subjects. *Psychobiology*, 27, 386–396.

Pariera Dinkins, C. L., & Peterson, R. K. (2008). A human dietary risk assessment associated with glycoalkaloid responses of potato to Colorado potato beetle defoliation. *Food & Chemical Toxicology*, 46, 2837–2840.

Parkes, M., & White, K. G. (2000). Glucose attenuation of memory impairments. *Behavioral Neuroscience*, 114, 307–319.

Parletta, N., Zarnowiecki, D., Cho, J., Wilson, A., Bogomolova, S., Villani, A., ... O'Dea, K. (2019). A Mediterranean-style dietary intervention supplemented with fish oil improves diet quality and mental health in people with depression: A randomized controlled trial (HELFIMED). *Nutritional Neuroscience*, 22, 474–487.

Parsons, A. G., Zhou, S. J., Spurrier, N. J., & Makrides, M. (2008). Effect of iron supplementation during pregnancy on the behaviour of children at early school age: Long-term follow-up of a randomised controlled trial. *British Journal of Nutrition*, 99, 1133–1139.

Parsons, M. W., & Gold, P. E. (1992). Glucose enhancement of memory in elderly humans: An inverted-U dose-response curve. *Neurobiology of Aging*, 13, 401–404.

Pase, M. P., Scholey, A. B., Pipingas, A., Kras, M., Nolidin, K., Gibbs, A., & Stough, C. (2013). Cocoa polyphenols enhance positive mood states but not cognitive performance: A randomized, placebo-controlled trial. *Journal of Psychopharmacology*, 27, 451–458.

Patel, P. S., Sharp, S. J., Jansen, E., Luben, R. N., Khaw. K. -T., Wareham, N. J., & Forouhi, N. G. (2010). Fatty acids measured in plasma and erythrocyte-membrane phospholipids and deprived by food-frequency questionnaire and the risk of new-onset type 2 diabetes: A pilot study in the European Prospective Investigation into Cancer and Nutrition (EPIC)-Norfolk cohort. *American Journal of Clinical Nutrition*, 92, 1214–1222.

Patočka, J., & Plucar, B. (2003). Pharmacology and toxicology of absinthe. *Journal of Applied Biomedicine*, 1, 199–205.

Patra, J., Bakker, R., Irving, H., Jaddoe, V. W., Malini, S., & Rehm, J. (2011). Dose-response relationship between alcohol consumption before and during pregnancy and the risks of low birthweight, preterm birth and small for gestational age (SGA): A systematic review and meta-analysis. *British Journal of Obstetrics & Gynaecology*, 118, 1441–1421.

Paula-Barbosa, M. M., Andrade, J. P., Azevedo, F. P., Madeira, M. D., & Alves, M. C. (1988). Lengthy administration of low-protein diet to adult rats induces cell loss in the hippocampal formation but not in the medial prefrontal cortex. *Society for Neuroscience Abstracts*, 14, 368.

Paula-Barbosa, M. M., Andrade, J. P., & Castedo, J. L. (1989). Cell loss in the cerebellum and hippocampal formation of adult rats after long-term low-protein diet. *Experimental Neurology*, 103, 186–193.

Peacock, A., Leung, J., Larney, S., College, S., Hickman, M., Rehm, J., Giovino, G. A., West, R., Hall, W., Griffiths, P., Ali, R., Gowing, L., Marsden, J., Ferrari, A. J., Grebely, J., Farrell, M., & Degenhardt, L. (2018). Global statistics on alcohol, tobacco and illicit drug use: 2017 status report. *Addiction*, 113, 1905–1926.

Pearson-Leary, J., Jahagirdar, V., Sage, J., & McNay, E. C. (2018). Insulin modulates hippocampally-mediated spatial working memory via glucose transporter-4. *Behavioural Brain Research*, 338, 32–39.

Pedditizi, E., Peters, R., & Beckett, N. (2016). The risk of overweight/obesity in mid-life and late life for the development of dementia: A systematic review and meta-analysis of longitudinal studies. *Age & Ageing*, 45, 14–21.

Peet, M., & Horrobin, D. F. (2002). A dose-ranging study of the, effects of ethyl-eicosapentaenoate in patients with ongoing depression despite apparently adequate treatment with standard drugs. *Archives of General Psychiatry*, 59, 913–919.

Pelchat, M. L., Johnson, A., Chan, R., Valdez, J., & Ragland, J. D. (2004). Images of desire: Food-craving activation during fMRI. *NeuroImage*, 23, 1486–1493.

Pelsser, L. M., Frankena, K., Toorman, J., & Rodrigues Pereira, R. (2017). Diet and ADHD, reviewing the evidence: A systematic review of meta-analyses of double-blind placebo-controlled trials evaluating the efficacy of diet interventions on the behavior of children with ADHD. *PLoS One*, 12, e0169277.

Pender, S., Gilbert, S. J., & Serpell, L. (2014). The neuropsychology of starvation: Set-shifting and central coherence in a fasted nonclinical sample. *PLoS One*, 9, e110743.

Penland, J. G. (2000). Behavioral data and methodology issues in studies of zinc nutrition in humans. *Journal of Nutrition*, 130, S361–S364.

Pentieva, K., McGarel, C., McNulty, B., Ward, M., Elliott, N., Strain, J. J., & McNulty, H. (2012). Effect of folic acid supplementation during pregnancy on growth and cognitive development of the offspring: A pilot follow-up investigation of children of FASSTT study participants. *Proceedings of the Nutrition Society*, 71, E139–E139.

Perez-Cornago, A., de la Iglesia, R., Lopez-Legarrea, P., Abete, I., Navas-Carretero, S., Lacunza, C. I., & Zulet, M. A. (2014). A decline in inflammation is associated with less depressive symptoms after a dietary intervention in metabolic syndrome patients: A longitudinal study. *Nutrition Journal*, 13, Article 36.

Perez-Cornago, A., Sanchez-Villegas, A., Bes-Rastrollo, M., Gea, A., Molero, P., Lahortiga-Ramos, F., & Martinez-Gonzalez, M. Á. (2017). Relationship between adherence to dietary approaches to stop hypertension (DASH) diet indices and incidence of depression during up to 8 years of follow-up. *Public Health Nutrition*, 20, 2383–2392.

Perkins, A. J., Hendrie, H. C., Callahan, C. M., Gao, S., Unverzagt, F. W., Xu, Y., & Hui, S. L. (1999). Association of antioxidants with memory in a multiethnic elderly sample using the Third National Health and Nutrition Examination Survey. *American Journal of Epidemiology*, 150, 37–44.

Perkins, J., Rockli, K., Krishna, A., McGovern, M., Aguayo, M., & Subramanian, S. (2017). Understanding the association between stunting and child development in low and middle income countries: Next steps for research and intervention. *Social Science & Medicine*, 193, 101–109.

Perlis, R. H., Perlis, C. S., Wu, Y., Hwang, C., Joseph, M., & Nierenberg, A. A. (2005). Industry sponsorship and financial conflict of interest in the reporting of clinical trials in psychiatry. *American Journal of Psychiatry*, 162, 1957–1960.

Pervin, M., Hasnat, M. A., Lee, Y. M., Kim, D. H., Jo, J. E., & Lim, B. O. (2014). Antioxidant activity and acetylcholinesterase inhibition of grape skin anthocyanin (GSA). *Molecules*, 19, 9403–9418.

Petersen, M., Aaroe, L., Jensen, N., & Curry, O. (2014). Social welfare and the psychology of food sharing: Short-term hunger increases support for social welfare. *Political Psychology*, 35, 757–773.

Petersson, S. D., & Philippou, E. (2016). Mediterranean diet, cognitive function, and dementia: A systematic review of the evidence. *Advances in Nutrition*, 7, 889–904.

Peuhkuri, K., Sihvola, N., & Korpela, R. (2012). Diet promotes sleep duration and quality. *Nutrition Research*, 32, 309–319.

Pfisterer, K. J., Sharrat, M. T., Heckman, G. G., & Keller, H. H. (2016). Vitamin B-12 status in older adults living in Ontario long-term care homes: Prevalence and incidence of deficiency with supplementation as a protective factor. *Applied Physiology Nutrition & Metabolism*, 41, 219–222.

Philippou, E., & Constantinou, M. (2014). The influence of glycemic index on cognitive functioning: A systematic review of the evidence. *Advances in Nutrition*, 5, 119–130.

Phillips, F., Chen, C. N., & Crisp, A. H. (1975). Isocaloric diet changes and electroencephalographic sleep. *The Lancet*, 2, 723–725.

Piech, R. M., Hampshire, A., Owen, A. M., & Parkinson, J. A. (2009). Modulation of cognitive flexibility by hunger and desire. *Cognition & Emotion*, 23, 528–540.

Piech, R. M., Pastorino, M. T., & Zald, D. H. (2010). All I saw was the cake: Hunger effects on attentional capture by visual food cues. *Appetite*, 54, 579–582.

Pifferi, F., & Aujard, F. (2019). Caloric restriction, longevity and aging: Recent contributions from human and non-human primate studies. *Progress in Neuropsychopharmacology & Biological Psychiatry*, 95, 109702.

Pinelli, J., Saigal, S., & Atkinson, S. A. (2003). Effect of breastmilk consumption on neurodevelopmental outcomes at 6 and 12 months of age in VLBW infants. *Advances in Neonatal Care*, 3, 76–87.

Pino, J. M. V., Nishiduka, E. S., & da Luz, M. H. M. (2020). Iron-deficient diet induces distinct protein profile related to energy metabolism in the striatum and hippocampus of adult rats. *Nutritional Neuroscience*, 25, 207–218.

Pistell, P. J., Morrison, C. D., Gupta, S., Knight, A. G., Keller, J. N., Ingram, D. K., & Bruce-Keller, A. J. (2010). Cognitive impairment following high fat diet consumption is associated with brain inflammation. *Journal of Neuroimmunology*, 219, 25–32.

Pittenger, C., & Duman, R. S. (2008). Stress, depression, and neuroplasticity: A convergence of mechanisms. *Neuropsychopharmacology*, 33, 88–109.

Polivy, J. (1996). Psychological consequences of food restriction. *Journal of the American Dietetic Association*, 96, 589–592.

Polivy, J., Zeitlin, S. B., Herman, C. P., & Beal, A. L. (1994). Food restriction and binge eating: A study of former prisoners of war. *Journal of Abnormal Psychology*, 103, 409–411.

Pomponi, M., Loria, G., Salvati, S., Di Biase, A., Conte, G., Villella, C., La Torre, G. (2014). DHA effects in Parkinson disease depression. *Basal Ganglia*, 4, 61–66.

Pomytkin, I., Costa-Nunes, J. P., & Kasatkin, V. (2018). Insulin receptor in the brain: Mechanisms of activation and the role in the CNS pathology and treatment. *CNS Neuroscience & Therapeutics*, 24, 763–774.

Popova, S., Lange, S., Probst, C., Gmel, G., & Rehn, J. (2017). Estimation of national, regional, and global prevalence of alcohol use during pregnancy and fetal alcohol syndrome: A systematic review and meta-analysis. *The Lancet Global Health*, 4, e290–e299.

Power, A. J., Keegan, B. F., & Nolan, K. (2002). The seasonality and role of neurotoxin tetramine in the salivary glands of the red whelk *Neptunea antiqua* (L.). *Toxicon*, 40, 419–425.

Power, M. L., & Schulkin, J. (2008). Anticipatory physiological regulation in feeding biology: Cephalic phase responses. *Appetite*, 50, 194–206.

Powers, H. J. (2003). Riboflavin (vitamin B-2) and health. *American Journal of Clinical Nutrition*, 77, 1352–1360.

Prado, E., & Dewey, K. (2014). Nutrition and brain development in early life. *Nutrition Reviews*, 72, 267–284.

Prasad, A. N., Levin, S., Rupar, C. A., & Prasad, C. (2011). Menkes disease and infantile epilepsy. *Brain & Development*, 33, 866–876.

Prehn, K., Jumpertz von Schwartzenberg, R. J., & Mai, K. (2017). Caloric restriction in older adults: Differential effects of weight loss and reduced weight on brain structure and function. *Cerebral Cortex*, 27, 1765–1778.

Prentice, A. M. (2005). Starvation in humans: Evolutionary background and contemporary implications. *Mechanisms of Ageing & Development*, 126, 976–981.

Prins, M. L., Fujima, L. S., & Hovda, D. A. (2005). Age-dependent reduction of cortical contusion volume by ketones after traumatic brain injury. *Journal of Neuroscience Research*, 82, 413–420.

Prinz, R. J., Roberts, W. A., & Hantman, E. (1980). Dietary correlates of hyperactive behavior in children. *Journal of Consulting & Clinical Psychology*, 48, 760–769.

Prusiner, S. B. (1997). Prion diseases and the BSE crisis. *Science*, 278, 245–251.

Prust, M., Meijer, J., & Westerink, R. (2020). The plastic brain: Neurotoxicity of micro- and nanoplastics. *Particle & Fibre Toxicology*, 17, Article 24.

Pu, H., Guo, Y., Zhang, W., Huang, L., Wang, G., Liou, A. K., & Wang, Y. (2013). Omega-3 polyunsaturated fatty acid supplementation improves neurologic recovery and attenuates white matter injury after experimental traumatic brain injury. *Journal of Cerebral Blood Flow & Metabolism*, 33, 1474–1484.

Pursey, K. M., Stanwell, P., Gearhardt, A. N., Collins, C. E., & Burrows, T. L. (2014). The prevalence of food addiction as assessed by the Yale Food Addiction Scale: A systematic review. *Nutrients*, 6, 4552–4590.

Qin, B., Xun, P., & Jacobs, D. R. (2017). Intake of niacin, folate, vitamin B-6, and vitamin B-12 through young adulthood and cognitive function in midlife: The Coronary Artery Risk Development in Young Adults (CARDIA) Study. *American Journal of Clinical Nutrition*, 106, 1032–1040.

Qiu, G., Liu, S., & So, K. -F. (2010). Dietary restriction and brain health. *Neuroscience Bulletin*, 26, 55–65.

Quigley, M., Embleton, N. D., & McGuire, W. (2018). Formula versus donor breast milk for feeding preterm or low birth weight infants. *Cochrane Database of Systematic Reviews*(6). doi: 10.1002/14651858.CD002971.pub3

Raab, K., Kirsch, P., & Mier, D. (2016). Understanding the impact of 5-HTTLPR, antidepressants, and acute tryptophan depletion on brain activation during facial emotion processing: A review of the imaging literature. *Neuroscience & Biobehavioral Reviews*, 71, 176–197.

Rabassa, M., Cherubini, A., Zamora-Ros, R., Urpi-Sarda, M., Bandinelli, S., Ferrucci, L., & Andres-Lacueva, C. (2015). Low levels of a urinary biomarker of dietary polyphenol are associated with substantial cognitive decline over a 3-year period in older adults: The Invecchiare in Chianti Study. *Journal of the American Geriatric Society*, 63, 938–946.

Ragozzino, M. E., Unick, K. E., & Gold, P. E. (1996). Hippocampal acetylcholine release during memory testing in rats: Augmentation by glucose. *Proceedings of the National Academy of Sciences of the United States of America*, 93, 4693–4698.

Rainey-Smith, S. R., Brown, B. M., Sohrabi, H. R., Shah, T., Goozee, K. G., Gupta, V. B., & Martins, R. N. (2016). Curcumin and cognition: A randomised, placebo-controlled, double-blind study of community-dwelling older adults. *British Journal of Nutrition*, 115, 2106–2113.

Rajakumar, K. (2000). Pellagra in the United States: A historical perspective. *Southern Medical Journal*, 93, 272–277.

Ralph-Nearman, C., Achee, M., Lapidus, R., Stewart, J. L., & Filik, R. (2019). A systematic and methodological review of attentional biases in eating disorders: Food, body, and perfectionism. *Brain & Behavior*, 9, e01458.

Ramirez, M. R., Izquierdo, I., Raseira, M. D. B., Zuanazzi, J. A., Barros, D., & Henriques, A. T. (2005). Effect of lyophilised Vaccinium berries on memory, anxiety and locomotion in adult rats. *Pharmacological Research*, 52, 457–462.

Ramm-Pettersen, A., Stabell, K. E., Nakken, K. O., & Selmer, K. K. (2014). Does ketogenic diet improve cognitive function in patients with GLUT1-DS? A 6- to 17-month follow-up study. *Epilepsy & Behavior*, 39, 111–115.

Ramos, M. I., Allen, L. H., & Mungas, D. M. (2005). Low folate status is associated with impaired cognitive function and dementia in the Sacramento Area Latino Study on Aging. *American Journal of Clinical Nutrition*, 82, 1346–1352.

Rana, S., Kumar, S., Rathore, N., Padwad, Y., & Bhushan, S. (2016). Nutrigenomics and its impact on life-style associated metabolic diseases. *Current Genomics*, 17, 261–278.

Randolph, T. G. (1956). The descriptive features of food addiction. *Addictive Eating & Drinking*, 17, 198–224.

Rawat, K., Singh, N., Kumari, P., & Saha, L. (2021). A review on preventive role of ketogenic diet (KD) in CNS disorders from the gut microbiota perspective. *Reviews in the Neurosciences*, 32, 143–157.

Raynor, H. A., & Epstein, L. H. (2003). The relative-reinforcing value of food under differing levels of food deprivation and restriction. *Appetite*, 40, 15–24.

Reboul, E. (2018). Vitamin E intestinal absorption: Regulation of membrane transport across the enterocyte. *IUBMB Life*, 71, 416–423.

Reeds, P. J. (2000). Dispensable and indispensable amino acids for humans. *Journal of Nutrition*, 130, S1835–S1840.

Reedy, J., & Krebs-Smith, S. M. (2010). Dietary sources of energy, solid fats, and added sugars among children and adolescents in the United States. *Journal of the American Dietetic Association*, 110, 1477–1484.

Reeta, K. H., Mehla, J., Pahuja, M., & Gupta, Y. K. (2011). Pharmacokinetic and pharmacodynamic interactions of valproate, phenytoin, phenobarbitone and carbamazepine with curcumin in experimental models of epilepsy in rats. *Pharmacology Biochemistry & Behavior*, 99, 399–407.

Reger, M. A., Henderson, S. T., Hale, C., Cholerton, B., Baker, L. D., Watson, G. S., & Craft, S. (2004). Effects of beta-hydroxybutyrate on cognition in memory-impaired adults. *Neurobiology of Aging*, 25, 311–314.

Rehm, J., Hasan, O. S., Black, S. R., Shield, K. D., & Schwarzinger, M. (2019). Alcohol use and dementia: A systematic scoping review. *Alzheimer's Research & Therapy*, 11, Article 1.

Reichelt, A. C., Killcross, S., Hambly, L. D., Morris, M. J., & Westbrook, R. F. (2015). Impact of adolescent sucrose access on cognitive control, recognition memory, and parvalbumin immunoreactivity. *Learning & Memory*, 22, 215–224.

Reichelt, A. C., Loughman, A., Bernard, A., Raipuria, M., Abbott, K. N., Dachtler, J., & Moore, R. J. (2020). An intermittent hypercaloric diet alters gut microbiota, prefrontal cortical gene expression and social behaviours in rats. *Nutritional Neuroscience, 23*, 613–627.

Reijmer, Y. D., van den Berg, E., Ruis, C., Kappelle, L. J., & Biessels, G. J. (2010). Cognitive dysfunction in patients with type 2 diabetes. *Diabetes Metabolism Research & Reviews, 26*, 507–519.

Reitz, C., & Mayeux, R. (2014). Alzheimer disease: Epidemiology, diagnostic criteria, risk factors and biomarkers. *Biochemical Pharmacology, 88*, 640–651.

Rennie, G., Chen, A. C., Dhillon, H., Vardy, J., & Damian, D. L. (2015). Nicotinamide and neurocognitive function. *Nutritional Neuroscience, 18*, 193–200.

Ribeiro, J. A., & Sebastião, A. M. (2010). Caffeine and adenosine. *Journal of Alzheimer's Disease, 20*, S3–S15.

Riby, L. M. (2004). The impact of age and task domain on cognitive performance: A meta-analytic review of the glucose facilitation effect. *Brain Impairment, 5*, 145–165.

Ricciarelli, R., Argellati, F., Pronzato, M. A., & Domenicotti, C. (2007). Vitamin E and neurodegenerative diseases. *Molecular Aspects of Medicine, 28*, 591–606.

Rice, D., & Barone, S. (2000). Critical periods of vulnerability for the developing nervous system: Evidence from humans and animal models. *Environmental Health Perspectives, 108*, 511–533.

Rieger, J., Bähr, O., Maurer, G. D., Hattingen, E., Franz, K., Brucker, D., & Steinbach, J. P. (2014). ERGO: A pilot study of ketogenic diet in recurrent glioblastoma Erratum in /ijo/45/6/2605. *International Journal of Oncology, 44*, 1843–1852.

Rijnsburger, M., Unmehopa, U., Eggels, L., Serlie, M., & La Fleur, S. (2019). One-week exposure to a free choice high-fat high-sugar diet does not disrupt blood-brain barrier permeability in fed or overnight fasted rats. *Nutritional Neuroscience, 22*, 541–550.

Rincel, M., Lepinay, A. L., Janthakhin, Y., Soudain, G., Yvon, S., Da Silva, S., & Darnaudery, M. (2018). Maternal high-fat diet and early life stress differentially modulate spine density and dendritic morphology in the medial prefrontal cortex of juvenile and adult rats. *Brain Structure & Function, 223*, 883–895.

Rivadeneyra, J., Cubo, E., Gil, C., Calvo, S., Mariscal, N., & Martinez, A. (2016). Factors associated with Mediterranean diet adherence in Huntington's disease. *Clinical Nutrition ESPEN, 12*, e7–e13.

Rizza, R., Haymond, M., Cryer, P., & Gerich, J. (1979). Differential effects of epinephrine on glucose production and disposal in man. *American Journal of Physiology, 237*, E356–E362.

Rizzo, T., Metzger, B., Dooley, S., & Cho, N. (1997). Early malnutrition and child neurobehavioral development: Insights from the study of children of diabetic mothers. *Child Development, 68*, 26–38.

Robinson, E., Aveyard, P., Daley, A., Jolly, K., Lewis, A., Lycett, D., & Higgs, S. (2013). Eating attentively: A systematic review and meta-analysis of the effect of food intake memory and awareness on eating. *American Journal of Clinical Nutrition*, 97, 728–742.

Rogers, P. J. (2017). Food and drug addictions: Similarities and differences. *Pharmacology, Biochemistry & Behavior*, 153, 182–190.

Rogers, P. J., Ferriday, D., Jebb, S. A., & Brunstrom, J. M. (2016). Connecting biology with psychology to make sense of appetite control. *Nutrition Bulletin*, 41, 344–352.

Ropacki, S. A., Patel, S. M., & Hartman, R. E. (2013). Pomegranate supplementation protects against memory dysfunction after heart surgery: A pilot study. *Evidence Based Complementary & Alternative Medicine*, 2013, Article 932401.

Rosas, L. G., & Eskenazi, B. (2008). Pesticides and child neurodevelopment. *Current Opinion in Pediatrics*, 20, 191–197.

Rose, W. C. (1968). The sequence of events leading to the establishment of the amino acid needs of man. *American Journal of Public Health*, 58, 2020–2027.

Rose, W. C., Haines, W. J., & Warner, D. T. (1954). The amino acid requirements of man: The role of lysine, arginine and tryptophan. *Journal of Biological Chemistry*, 206, 421–430.

Rosko, L., Smith, V. N., Yamazaki, R., & Huang, J. K. (2019). Oligodendrocyte bioenergetics in health and disease. *The Neuroscientist*, 25, 334–343.

Roth, C., Magnus, P., Schjolberg, S., Stoltenberg, C., Suren, P., McKeague, I. W., & Susser, E. (2011). Folic acid supplements in pregnancy and severe language delay in children. *Journal of the American Medical Association*, 306, 1566–1573.

Rothstein, D. S. (2013). Breastfeeding and children's early cognitive outcomes. *Review of Economics and Statistics*, 95, 919–931.

Rotstein, D. L., Cortese, M., Fung, T. T., Chitnis, T., Ascherio, A., & Munger, K. L. (2019). Diet quality and risk of multiple sclerosis in two cohorts of US women. *Multiple Sclerosis*, 25, 1773–1780.

Roytio, H., Mokkala, K., Vahlberg, T., & Laitinen, K. (2017). Dietary intake of fat and fibre according to reference values relates to higher gut microbiota richness in overweight pregnant women. *British Journal of Nutrition*, 118, 343–352.

Roza, S. J., van Batenburg-Eddes, T., Steegers, E. A., Jaddoe, V. W., Mackenbach, J. P., Hofman, A., & Tiemeier, H. (2010). Maternal folic acid supplement use in early pregnancy and child behavioural problems: The Generation R Study. *British Journal of Nutrition*, 103, 445–452.

Rozin, P., Dow, S., Moscovitch, M., & Rajaram, S. (1998). What causes humans to begin and end a meal? A role for memory for what has been eaten, as evidenced by a study of multiple meal eating in amnesic patients. *Psychological Science*, 9, 392–396.

Ruddock, H. K., Christiansen, P., Halford, J., & Hardman, C. A. (2017). The development and validation of the Addiction-like Eating Behaviour Scale. *International Journal of Obesity*, 41, 1710–1717.

Rude, R. K. (1998). Magnesium deficiency: A cause of heterogenous disease in humans. *Journal of Bone & Mineral Research*, 13, 749–758.

Rudell, J. B., Rechs, A. J., & Kelman, T. J. (2011). The anterior piriform cortex is sufficient for detecting depletion of an indispensable amino acid, showing independent cortical sensory function. *Journal of Neuroscience*, 31, 1583–1590.

Ruhé, H. G., Mason, N. S., & Schene, A. H. (2007). Mood is indirectly related to serotonin, norepinephrine, and dopamine levels in humans: A meta-analysis of monoamine depletion studies. *Molecular Psychiatry*, 12, 331–359.

Rutkowsky, J. M., Lee, L. L., Puchowicz, M., Golub, M. S., Befroy, D. E., & Wilson, D. W. (2018). Reduced cognitive function, increased blood-brain-barrier transport and inflammatory responses, and altered brain metabolites in LDLr -/-and C57BL/6 mice fed a western diet. *PLoS One*, 13, e0191909.

Sadeghi, O., Keshteli, A. H., Afshar, H., Esmaillzadeh, A., & Adibi, P. (2021). Adherence to Mediterranean dietary pattern is inversely associated with depression, anxiety and psychological distress. *Nutritional Neuroscience*, 24, 248–259.

Saito, Y. (2020). Selenoprotein P as an *in vivo* redox regulator: Disorders related to its deficiency and excess. *Journal of Clinical Biochemistry & Nutrition*, 66, 1–7.

Sakurai, T., Kitadate, K., Nishioka, H., Fujii, H., Ogasawara, J., Kizaki, T., & Ohno, H. (2013). Oligomerised lychee fruit-derived polyphenol attenuates cognitive impairment in senescence-accelerated mice and endoplasmic reticulum stress in neuronal cells. *British Journal of Nutrition*, 110, 1549–1558.

Salzman, M. (2006). Methanol neurotoxicity. *Clinical Toxicology*, 44, 89–90.

Sample, C. H., Jones, S., Hargrave, S. L., Jarrard, L. E., & Davidson, T. L. (2016). Western diet and the weakening of the interoceptive stimulus control of appetitive behavior. *Behavioral Brain Research*, 312, 219–230.

Sánchez-Lara, K., Arrieta, O., & Pasaye, E. (2013). Brain activity correlated with food preferences: A functional study comparing advanced non-small cell lung cancer patients with and without anorexia. *Nutrition*, 29, 1013–1019.

Sánchez-Lozada, L. G., Le, M.. Segal, M., & Johnson, R. J. (2008). How safe is fructose for persons with or without diabetes? *American Journal of Clinical Nutrition*, 88, 1189–1890.

Sanchez-Villegas, A., Delgado-Rodriguez, M., Alonso, A., Schlatter, J., Lahortiga, F., Serra Majem, L., & Martinez-Gonzalez, M. A. (2009). Association of the Mediterranean dietary pattern with the incidence of depression: The Seguimiento Universidad de Navarra/University of Navarra follow-up (SUN) cohort. *Archives of General Psychiatry*, 66, 1090–1098.

Sánchez-Villegas, A., Galbete, C., Martinez-González, M. Á., Martinez, J. A., Razquin, C., Salas-Salvadó, J., & Martí, A. (2011). The effect of the

Mediterranean diet on plasma brain-derived neurotrophic factor (BDNF) levels: The PREDIMED-NAVARRA randomized trial. *Nutritional Neuroscience,* 14, 195–201.

Sandhu, K. V., Sherwin, E., Schellekens, H., Stanton, C., Dinan, T. G., & Cryan, J. F. (2017). Feeding the microbiota-gut-brain axis: Diet, microbiome, and neuropsychiatry. *Translational Research,* 179, 223–244.

Sandstead, H. H. (2000). Causes of iron and zinc deficiencies and their effects on brain. *Journal of Nutrition,* 130, S347–S349.

(2003). Zinc is essential for brain development and function. *Journal of Trace Elements in Experimental Medicine,* 16, 165–173.

Sanfeliu, C., Sebastià, J., Cristòfol, R., & Rodrìguez-Farrê, E. (2003). Neurotoxicity of organomercurial compounds. *Neurotoxicity Research,* 5, 283–306.

Sarkar, T., Patro, N., & Patro, I. (2019). Cumulative multiple early life hits – A potent threat leading to neurological disorders. *Brain Research Bulletin,* 147, 58–68.

Sato, K. (2018). Why is vitamin B6 effective in alleviating the symptoms of autism? *Medical Hypotheses,* 115, 103–106.

Sato, S., Nakagawasai, O., & Tan-No, K. (2011). Executive function of post-weaning protein malnutrition in mice. *Biological & Pharmaceutical Bulletin,* 34, 1413–1417.

Saunders, J., Degenhardt, L., Reed, G., & Poznyak, V. (2019). Alcohol use disorders in ICD-11: Past, present and future. *Alcohol: Clinical and Experimental Research,* 43, 1617–1631.

Sayette, M. A. (2016). The role of craving in substance use disorders: Theoretical and methodological issues. *Annual Review of Clinical Psychology,* 12, 407–433.

Scally, M. C., Ulus, I., & Wurtman, R. J. (1977). Brain tyrosine level controls striatal dopamine synthesis in haloperidol-treated rats. *Journal of Neural Transmission,* 41, 1–6.

Scalzo, S. J., Bowden, S. C., Ambrose, M. L., Whelan, G., & Cook, M. J. (2015). Wernicke-Korsakoff syndrome not related to alcohol use: A systematic review. *Journal of Neurology, Neurosurgery and Psychiatry,* 86, 1362–1368.

Scarmeas, N., Luchsinger, J. A., Stern, Y., Gu, Y., He, J., DeCarli, C., & Brickman, A. M. (2011). Mediterranean diet and magnetic resonance imaging-assessed cerebrovascular disease. *Annals of Neurology,* 69, 257–268.

Schacht, J. P., Anton, R. F., & Myrick, H. (2012). Functional neuroimaging studies of alcohol cue reactivity: A quantitative meta-analysis and systematic review. *Addiction Biology,* 18, 121–133.

Scheiber, I. F., Mercer, J. F. B., & Dringen, R. (2014). Metabolism and functions of copper in brain. *Progress in Neurobiology,* 116, 33–57.

Schmatz, R., Mazzanti, C. M., Spanevello, R., Stefanello, N., Gutierres, J., Correa, M., .& Morsch, V. M. (2009). Resveratrol prevents memory deficits and the increase in acetylcholinesterase activity in streptozotocin-induced diabetic rats. *European Journal of Pharmacology,* 610, 42–48.

Schmidt, R. J., Hansen, R. L., Hartiala, J., Allayee, H., Schmidt, L. C., Tancredi, D. J., & Hertz-Picciotto, I. (2011). Prenatal vitamins, one-carbon metabolism gene variants, and risk for autism. *Epidemiology*, 22, 476–485.

Schmidt, R. J., Tancredi, D. J., Ozonoff, S., Hansen, R. L., Hartiala, J., Allayee, H., & Hertz-Picciotto, I. (2012). Maternal periconceptional folic acid intake and risk of autism spectrum disorders and developmental delay in the CHARGE (CHildhood Autism Risks from Genetics and Environment) case-control study. *American Journal of Clinical Nutrition*, 96, 80–89.

Schneider, M. L., Moore, C. F., & Adkins, M. M. (2011). The effects of prenatal alcohol exposure on behavior: Rodent and primate studies. *Neuropsychology Review*, 21, 186–203.

Schoeller, D. A. (1995). Limitations in the assessment of dietary energy intake by self-report. *Metabolism*, 44, 18–22.

Scholey, A. B., Macpherson, H., Sünram-Lea, S., Elliott, J., Stough, C., & Kennedy, D. (2013). Glucose enhancement of recognition memory: Differential effects on effortful processing but not aspects of 'remember-know' responses. *Neuropharmacology*, 64, 544–549.

Scholey, A. B., Sünram-Lea, S. I., Greer, J., Elliott, J., & Kennedy, D. O. (2009). Glucose administration prior to a divided attention task improves tracking performance but not word recognition: Evidence against differential memory enhancement? *Psychopharmacology*, 202, 549–558.

Schroder, M., Muller, K., Falkenstein, M., Stehl, P., Kersting, M., & Libuda, L. (2015). Short-term effects of lunch on children's executive cognitive functioning: The randomised crossover Cognition Intervention Study Dortmund PLUS (CogniDo PLUS). *Physiology & Behavior*, 152, 307–314.

(2016). Lunch at school and children's cognitive functioning in the early afternoon: Results from the Cognition Intervention Study Dortmund Continued (CoCo). *British Journal of Nutrition*, 116, 1298–1305.

Schroeder, J. P., & Packard, M. G. (2003). Systemic or intra-amygdala injections of glucose facilitate memory consolidation for extinction of drug-induced conditioned reward. *European Journal of Neuroscience*, 17, 1482–1488.

Schuckit, M. A. (2009). Alcohol-use disorders. *The Lancet*, 373, 492–501.

Schuler, R., Seebeck, N., Osterhoff, M. A., Witte, V., Floel, A., Busjahn, A., & Pfeiffer, A. F. H. (2018). VEGF and GLUT1 are highly heritable, inversely correlated and affected by dietary fat intake: Consequences for cognitive function in humans. *Molecular Metabolism*, 11, 129–136.

Schulte, E. M., Avena, N. M., & Gearhardt, A. N. (2015). Which foods may be addictive? The roles of processing, fat content, and glycemic load. *PLoS One*, 10, e0117959.

Schulte, E. M., & Gearhardt, A. N. (2017). Development of the Modified Yale Food Addiction Scale Version 2.0. *European Eating Disorders Review*, 25, 302–308.

Schulz, J. B., Cookson, M. R., & Hausmann, L. (2016). The impact of fraudulent and irresponsible data to the translational research crisis – Solutions and implementation. *Journal of Neurochemistry*, 139, 253–270.

Schuster, J., & Mitchell, E. S. (2019). More than just caffeine: Psychopharmacology of methylxanthine interactions with plant-derived phytochemicals. *Progress in Neuropsychopharmacology & Biological Psychiatry*, 89, 263–274.

Schwartz, K., Chang, H. T., Nikolai, M., Pernicone, J., Rhee, S., Olson, K., & Noel, M. (2015). Treatment of glioma patients with ketogenic diets: Report of two cases treated with an IRB-approved energy-restricted ketogenic diet protocol and review of the literature. *Cancer & Metabolism*, 3, 3.

Scott, S. P., & Murray-Kolb, L. E. (2016). Iron status is associated with performance on executive functioning. *Journal of Nutrition*, 146, 30–37.

Scrimshaw, N. S. (1987). The phenomenon of famine. *Annual Review of Nutrition*, 7, 1–21.

Sedaghat, F., Jessri, M., Behrooz, M., Mirghotbi, M., & Rashidkhani, B. (2016). Mediterranean diet adherence and risk of multiple sclerosis: A case-control study. *Asia Pacific Journal of Clinical Nutrition*, 25, 377–384.

Sedighiyan, M., Djafarian, K., Dabiri, S., Abdolahi, M., & Shab-Bidar, S. (2019). The Effects of omega-3 supplementation on the expanded disability status scale and inflammatory cytokines in multiple sclerosis patients: A systematic review and meta-analysis. *CNS & Neurological Disorders – Drug Targets*, 18, 523–529.

Sembulingam, K., & Sembulingam, P. (2016). *Essentials of Medical Physiology (7th ed)*. New Delhi, India: Jaypee Brothers.

Serdaru, M., Hausser-Hauw, C., & LaPlane, D. (1998). The clinical spectrum of alcoholic pellagra encephalopathy. *Brain*, 111, 829–842.

Serra-Majem, L., Roman, B., & Estruch, R. (2006). Scientific evidence of interventions using the Mediterranean diet: A systematic review. *Nutrition Reviews*, 64, S27–S47.

Sevy, S., Hassoun, Y., & Bechara, A. (2006). Emotion-based decision-making in healthy subjects: Short-term effects of reducing dopamine levels. *Psychopharmacology*, 188, 228–235.

Shafiei, F., Salari-Moghaddam, A., Larijani, B., & Esmaillzadeh, A. (2019). Adherence to the Mediterranean diet and risk of depression: A systematic review and updated meta-analysis of observational studies. *Nutrition Reviews*, 77, 230–239.

Shakersain, B., Santoni, G., Larsson, S. C., Faxen-Irving, G., Fastbom, J., Fratiglioni, L., & Xu, W. (2016). Prudent diet may attenuate the adverse effects of Western diet on cognitive decline. *Alzheimers Dementia*, 12, 100–109.

Shanley, D. P., & Kirkwood, T. B. L. (2006). Calorie restriction does not enhance longevity in all species and is unlikely to do so in humans. *Biogerontology*, 7, 165–168.

Sharma, S., Ying, Z., & Gomez-Pinilla, F. (2010). A pyrazole curcumin derivative restores membrane homeostasis disrupted after brain trauma. *Experimental Neurology*, 226, 191–199.

Sharma, S., Zhuang, Y., Ying, Z., Wu, A., & Gomez-Pinilla, F. (2009). Dietary curcumin supplementation counteracts reduction in levels of molecules involved in energy homeostasis after brain trauma. *Neuroscience,* 161, 1037–1044.

Sharp, T., Bramwell, S. R., & Grahame-Smith, D. G. (1992). Effect of acute administration of L-tryptophan on the release of 5-HT in rat hippocampus in relation to serotoninergic neuronal activity: an in vivo microdialysis study. *Life Sciences,* 50, 1215–1223.

Sharrief, A. Z., Raffel, J., & Zee, D. S. (2012). Vitamin B-12 deficiency with bilateral globus pallidus abnormalities. *Archives of Neurology,* 69, 769–772.

Shearer, K. D., Stoney, P. N., Morgan, P. J., & McCaffery, P. J. (2012). A vitamin for the brain. *Trends in Neuroscience,* 35, 733–741.

Shen, Q., Li, Z. Q., Sun, Y., Wang, T., Wan, C. L., Li, X. W., & Yu, L. (2008). The role of pro-inflammatory factors in mediating the effects on the fetus of prenatal undernutrition: Implications for schizophrenia. *Schizophrenia Research,* 99, 48–55.

Sher, K. J., Grekin, E. R., & Williams, N. A. (2005). The development of alcohol use disorders. *Annual Review of Clinical Psychology,* 1, 493–523.

Sherbaf, F. G., Aarabi, M. H., Yazdi, M. H., & Haghshomar, M. (2019). White matter microstructure in fetal alcohol spectrum disorders: A systematic review of diffusion tensor imaging studies. *Human Brain Mapping,* 40, 1017–1036.

Shi, H., Yu, Y., Lin, D., Zheng, P., Zhang, P., Hu, M., & Huang, X. F. (2020). Beta-glucan attenuates cognitive impairment via the gut-brain axis in diet-induced obese mice. *Microbiome,* 8, 143.

Shie, F. S., Jin, L. W., Cook, D. G., Leverenz, J. B., & LeBoeuf, R. C. (2002). Diet-induced hypercholesterolemia enhances brain A beta accumulation in transgenic mice. *Neuroreport,* 13, 455–459.

Shrivastava, A., Kumar, A., & Thomas, J. D. (2017). Association of acute toxic encephalopathy with litchi consumption in an outbreak in Muzaffarpur, India, 2014: A case-control study. *The Lancet Global Health,* 5, e458–e466.

Shukitt-Hale, B., Askew, E. W., & Lieberman, H. R. (1997). Effects of 30 days of undernutrition on reaction time, moods, and symptoms. *Physiology & Behavior,* 62, 783–789.

Shulkin, M., Pimpin, L., Bellinger, D., Kranz, S., Fawzi, W., Duggan, C., & Mozaffarian, D. (2018). n-3 fatty acid supplementation in mothers, preterm infants, and term infants and childhood psychomotor and visual development: A systematic review and meta-analysis. *Journal of Nutrition,* 148, 409–418.

Siddappa, A. M., Georgieff, M. K., Wewerka, S., Worwa, C., Nelson, C. A., & Deregnier, R. A. (2004). Iron deficiency alters auditory recognition memory in newborn infants of diabetic mothers. *Pediatric Research,* 55, 1034–1041.

Siddappa, A. M., Rao, R., Long, J. D., Widness, J. A., & Georgieff, M. K. (2007). The assessment of newborn iron stores at birth: A review of the literature and standards for ferritin concentrations. *Neonatology,* 92, 73–82.

Sidhu, G. K., Singh, S., & Kumar, V. (2019). Toxicity, monitoring and biodegradation of organophosphate pesticides: A review. *Critical Reviews in Environmental Science & Technology,* 49, 1135–1187.

Sidorova, Y. S., Petrov, N. A., Shipelin, V. A., Zorin, S. N., Kochetkova, A. A., & Mazo, V. K. (2019). The impact of bilberry leaves' polyphenols on the anxiety level, spatial learning and memory of db/db mice. *Voprosy Pitaniia,* 88, 53–62.

Siega-Riz, A. M., Popkin, B. M., & Carson, T. (1998). Trends in breakfast consumption for children in the United States from 1965-1991. *American Journal of Clinical Nutrition,* 67, 748S–756S.

Siervo, M., Arnold, R., & Wells, J. C. K. (2011). Intentional weight loss in overweight and obese individuals and cognitive function: A systematic review and meta-analysis. *Obesity Reviews,* 12, 968–983.

Siesjo, B. K. (1978). *Brain Energy Metabolism,* New York: Wiley & Sons.

Sigurdson, C. J., Bartz, J. C., & Glatzel, M. (2019). Cellular and molecular mechanisms of prion disease. *Annual Reviews of Pathology: Mechanisms of Disease,* 14. 497–516.

Sikalidis, A. K. (2019). From food for survival to food for personalised optimal health: A historical perspective of how food and nutrition gave rise to nutrigenomics. *Journal of the American College of Nutrition,* 38, 84–95.

Silber, B. Y., & Schmitt, J. A. J. (2010). Effects of tryptophan loading on human cognition, mood, and sleep. *Neuroscience & Biobehavioral Reviews,* 34, 387–407.

Silverstone, J. T., Stark, J. E., & Buckle, R. M. (1966). Hunger during total starvation. *The Lancet,* 7451, 1343–1344.

Simopoulos, A. P. (1991). Omega-3-fatty-acids in health and disease and in growth and development. *American Journal of Clinical Nutrition,* 54, 438–463.

(1999). Essential fatty acids in health and chronic disease. *American Journal of Clinical Nutrition,* 70, 560s–569s.

Sindler, A. J., Wellman, N. S., & Stier, O. B. (2004). Holocaust survivors report long-term effects on attitudes toward food. *Journal of Nutrition Education & Behavior,* 36, 189–196.

Singh, B., Parsaik, A. K., Mielke, M. M., Erwin, P. J., Knopman, D. S., Petersen, R. C., & Roberts, R. O. (2014). Association of Mediterranean diet with mild cognitive impairment and Alzheimer's disease: A systematic review and meta-analysis. *Journal of Alzheimer's Disease,* 39, 271–282.

Singh, G. K., Kogan, M. D., & Dee, D. L. (2007). Nativity/immigrant status, race/ethnicity, and socioeconomic determinants of breastfeeding initiation and duration in the United States, 2003. *Pediatrics,* 119, S38–S46.

Sirven, J., Whedon, B., Caplan, D., Liporace, J., Glosser, D., O'Dwyer, J., & Sperling, M. R. (1999). The ketogenic diet for intractable epilepsy in adults: Preliminary results. *Epilepsia,* 40, 1721–1726.

Small, D. M., & DiFeliceantonio, A. G. (2019). Processed foods and food reward. *Science,* 363, 346–347.

Small, D. M., Jones-Gotman, M., & Dagher, A. (2003). Feeding-induced dopamine release in dorsal striatum correlates with meal pleasantness ratings in healthy human volunteers. *NeuroImage*, 19, 1709–1715.

Smeets, P. A. M., Erkner, A., & de Graaf, C. (2010). Cephalic phase responses and appetite. *Nutrition Reviews*, 68, 643–655.

Smith, A., Kendrick, A., Maben, A., & Salmon, J. (1994). Effects of breakfast and caffeine on cognitive performance, mood, and cardiovascular functioning. *Appetite*, 22, 39–55.

Smith, A., Leekam, S., Ralph, A., & McNeill, G. (1988). The influence of meal composition on post-lunch changes in performance efficiency and mood. *Appetite*, 10, 195–203.

Smith, A., Maben, A., & Brockman, P. (1994). Effects of evening meals and caffeine on cognitive performance, mood, and cardiovascular functioning. *Appetite*, 22, 57–65.

Smith, A., & Miles, C. (1986). The effects of lunch on cognitive vigilance tasks. *Ergonomics*, 29, 1251–1261.

Smith, A., Ralph, A., & McNeill, G. (1991). Influences of meal size on post-lunch changes in performance efficiency, mood, and cardiovascular function. *Appetite*, 16, 85–91.

Smith, A. D., Smith, S. M., & de Jager, C. A. (2010). Homocysteine-lowering by B vitamins slows the rate of accelerated brain atrophy in mild cognitive impairment: A randomized controlled trial. *PLoS One*, 5, e12244.

Smith, A. F. (1993). Cognitive psychological issues of relevance to the validity of dietary reports. *European Journal of Clinical Nutrition*, 47, S6–S18.

Smith, B., & Reyes, T. (2017). Offspring neuroimmune consequences of maternal malnutrition: Potential mechanism for behavioral impairments that underlie metabolic and neurodevelopmental disorders. *Frontiers in Neuroendocrinology*, 47, 109–122.

Smith, C., & Richards, R. (2008). Dietary intake, overweight status, and perceptions of food insecurity among homeless Minnesotan youth. *American Journal of Human Biology*, 20, 550–563.

Smith, K. E., Mason, T. B., Johnson, J. S., Lavender, J. M., & Wonderlich, S. A. (2018). A systematic review of reviews of neurocognitive functioning in eating disorders: The state-of-the-literature and future directions. *International Journal of Eating Disorders*, 51, 798–821.

Smith, M. A., Riby, L. M., van Eekelen, J. A. M., & Foster, J. K. (2011). Glucose enhancement of human memory: A comprehensive research review of the glucose memory facilitation effect. *Neuroscience & Biobehavioral Reviews*, 35, 770–783.

Smith, P. J., Blumenthal, J. A., Babyak, M. A., Craighead, L., Welsh-Bohmer, K. A., Browndyke, J. N., & Sherwood, A. (2010). Effects of the dietary approaches to stop hypertension diet, exercise, and caloric restriction on neurocognition in overweight adults with high blood pressure. *Hypertension*, 55, 1331–1338.

458 *References*

Soares, E., Prediger, R. D., Nunes, S., Castro, A. A., Viana, S. D., Lemos, C., & Pereira, F. C. (2013). Spatial memory impairments in a prediabetic rat model. *Neuroscience,* 250, 565–577.

Sofi, F., Macchi, C., & Casini, A. (2013). Mediterranean diet and minimizing neurodegeneration. *Current Nutrition Reports,* 2, 75–80.

Soh, N. L., & Walter, G. (2011). Tryptophan and depression: Can diet alone be the answer? *Acta Neuropsychiatrica,* 23, 3–11.

Soldevila-Domenech, N., Boronat, A., Langohr, K., & de la Torre, R. (2019). N-of-1 clinical trials in nutritional interventions directed at improving cognitive functions. *Frontiers in Nutrition,* 6, e00110.

Solfrizzi, V., Agosti, P., & Lozupone, M. (2018). Nutritional intervention as a preventative approach for cognitive-related outcomes in cognitively healthy older adults: A systematic review. *Journal of Alzheimer's Disease,* 64, S229–S254.

Solianik, R., & Sujeta, A. (2018). Two-day fasting evokes stress, but does not affect mood, brain activity, and cognitive, psychomotor, and motor performance in overweight women. *Behavioural Brain Research,* 338, 166–172.

Solianik, R., Sujeta, A., & Čekanauskaite, A. (2018). Effects of 2-day calorie restriction on cardiovascular autonomic response, mood, and cognitive and motor functions in obese young adult women. *Experimental Brain Research,* 236, 2299–2308.

Solianik, R., Sujeta, A., Terentjevienė, A., & Skurvydas, A. (2016). Effect of 48 h fasting on autonomic function, brain activity, cognition, and mood in amateur weight-lifters. *BioMed Research International,* 2016, 1503956.

Song, S. B., Park, J. S., Chung, G. J., Lee, I. H., & Hwang, E. S. (2019). Diverse therapeutic efficacies and more diverse mechanisms of nicotinamide. *Metabolomics,* 15, 137.

Sonmez, U., Sonmez, A., Erbil, G., Tekmen, I., & Baykara, B. (2007). Neuroprotective effects of resveratrol against traumatic brain injury in immature rats. *Neuroscience Letters,* 420, 133–137.

Sonnenburg, E. D., Smits, S. A., Tikhonov, M., Higginbottom, S. K., Wingreen, N. S., & Sonnenburg, J. L. (2016). Diet-induced extinctions in the gut microbiota compound over generations. *Nature,* 529, 212–215.

Souchet, B., Duchon, A., Gu, Y., Dairou, J., Chevalier, C., Daubigney, F., & Delabar, J. M. (2019). Prenatal treatment with EGCG enriched green tea extract rescues GAD67 related developmental and cognitive defects in Down syndrome mouse models. *Science Reports,* 9, 3914.

Soutif-Veillon, A., Ferland, G., & Rolland, Y. (2016). Increased dietary vitamin K intake is associated with less severe subjective memory complaint among older adults. *Maturitas,* 93, 131–136.

Souza, C. G., Moreira, J. D., Siqueira, I. R., Pereira, A. G., Rieger, D. K., Souza, D. O., & Perry, M. L. (2007). Highly palatable diet consumption increases protein oxidation in rat frontal cortex and anxiety-like behavior. *Life Sciences,* 81, 198–203.

References 459

Spear, L. P. (2018). Effects of adolescent alcohol consumption on the brain and behaviour. *Nature Reviews Neuroscience*, 19, 197–214.
Speed, N., Engdahl, B., Schwartz, J., & Eberly, R. (1989). Posttraumatic stress disorder as a consequence of the POW experience. *Journal of Nervous & Mental Disease*, 177, 147–153.
Spence, C. (2017). Breakfast: The most important meal of the day? *International Journal of Gastronomy & Food Science*, 8, 1–6.
Spencer, P. S., Ludolph, A. C., & Kisby, G. E. (1993). Neurologic diseases associated with use of plant components with toxic potential. *Environmental Research*, 62, 106–113.
Spencer, P. S., & Palmer, V. S. (2012). Interrelationships of undernutrition and neurotoxicity: Food for thought and research attention. *NeuroToxicology*, 33, 605–616.
(2017). The enigma of litchi toxicity: An emerging health concern in southern Asia. *The Lancet Global Health*, 5, e383–e384.
Spencer, P. S., Roy, D. N., & Ludolph, A. (1986). Lathyrism: Evidence for role of the neuroexcitatory amino acid BOAA. *The Lancet*, 8515, 1066–1067.
Sperling, R., Chua, E., Cocchiarella, A., Rand-Giovannetti, E., Poldrack, R., Schacter, D. L., & Albert, M. (2003). Putting names to faces: Successful encoding of associative memories activates the anterior hippocampal formation. *Neuroimage*, 20, 1400–1410.
Spinneker, A., Sola, R., & Lemmen, V.(2007). Vitamin B6 status, deficiency and its consequences: An overview. *Nutrición Hospitalaria*, 22, 7–24.
St Clair, D., Xu, M., Wang, P., Yu, Y., Fang, Y., Zhang, F., & He, L. (2005). Rates of adult schizophrenia following prenatal exposure to the Chinese famine of 1959-1961. *Journal of the American Medical Association*, 294, 557–562.
Stabler, S. P. (2013). Vitamin B12 deficiency. *New England Journal of Medicine*, 368, 149–160.
Stahl, T., Falk, S., Taschan, H., Boschek, B., & Brunn, H. (2018). Evaluation of human exposure to aluminium from food and food contact materials. *European Food Research & Technology*, 244, 2077–2084.
Ståhle, L., Ståhle, E. L., & Granström, E. (2011). Effects of sleep or food deprivation during civilian survival training on cognition, blood glucose and 3-OH-butyrate. *Wilderness & Environmental Medicine*, 22, 202–210.
Stalmach, A., Edwards, C. A., Wightman, J. D., & Crozier, A. (2011). Identification of (poly)phenolic compounds in concord grape juice and their metabolites in human plasma and urine after juice consumption. *Journal of Agricultural & Food Chemistry*, 59, 9512–9522.
Staubo, S. C., Aakre, J. A., Vemuri, P., Syrjanen, J. A., Mielke, M. M., Geda, Y. E., & Roberts, R. O. (2017). Mediterranean diet, micronutrients and macronutrients, and MRI measures of cortical thickness. *Alzheimers Dementia*, 13, 168–177.
Stavric, B. (1988). Methylxanthines: Toxicity to humans. 3. Theobromine, para-xanthine and the combined effects of methylxanthines. *Food & Chemical Toxicology*, 26, 725–733.

Steenbergen, L., Jongkees, B. J., Sellaro, R., & Colzato, L. S. (2016). Tryptophan supplementation modulates social behaviour: A review. *Neuroscience & Biobehavioral Reviews*, 64, 346–358.

Steenbergen, L., Sellaro, R., & Colzato, L. S. (2014). Tryptophan promotes charitable donating. *Frontiers in Psychology*, 5, article 1451.

Steenweg-de Graaff, J., Roza, S. J., Steegers, E. A., Hofman, A., Verhulst, F. C., Jaddoe, V. W., & Tiemeier, H. (2012). Maternal folate status in early pregnancy and child emotional and behavioral problems: The Generation R Study. *American Journal of Clinical Nutrition*, 95, 1413–1421.

Stefani, M. R., Nicholson, G. M., & Gold, P. E. (1999). ATP-sensitive potassium channel blockade enhances spontaneous alternation performance in the rat: A potential mechanism for glucose-mediated memory enhancement. *Neuroscience*, 93, 557–563.

Stefurak, T. L., & van der Kooy, D. (1992). Saccharin's rewarding, conditioned reinforcing, and memory-improving properties: Mediation by isomorphic or independent processes? *Behavioral Neuroscience*, 106, 125–139.

Stein, U., Greyer, H., & Hentschel, H. (2001). Nutmeg (myristicin) poisoning – Report on a fatal case and a series of cases recorded by a poison information centre. *Forensic Science International*, 118, 87–90.

Stein, Z., & Susser, M. (1975). The Dutch famine, 1944–1945, and the reproductive process. I. Effects on six indices at birth. *Pediatric Research*, 9, 70–76.

Stevenson, R. J., & Francis, H. M. (2017). The hippocampus and the regulation of human food intake. *Psychological Bulletin*, 143, 1011–1032.

Stevenson, R. J., Francis, H. M., Attuquayefio, T., Gupta, D., Yeomans, M. R., Oaten, M. J., & Davidson, T. (2020). Hippocampal-dependent appetitive control is impaired by experimental exposure to a Western-style diet. *Royal Society Open Science*, 7, 191338.

Stevenson, R. J., Mahmut, M., & Rooney, K. (2015). Individual differences in the interoceptive states of hunger, fullness and thirst. *Appetite*, 95, 44–57.

Stewart, G. R, Zorumski, C. F., Price, M. T., & Olney, J. W. (1990). Domoic acid: A dementia-inducing excitotoxic food poison with kainic acid receptor specificity. *Experimental Neurology*, 110, 127–138.

Stice, E., Yokum, S., Burger, K. S., Epstein, L. H., & Small, D. M. (2011). Youth at risk for obesity show greater activation of striatal and somatosensory regions to food. *Journal of Neuroscience*, 31, 4360–4366.

Stockburger, J., Schmälzle, R., Flaisch, T., Bublatzky, F., & Schupp, H. T. (2009). The impact of hunger on food cue processing: An event-related brain potential study. *NeuroImage*, 47, 1819–1829.

Stockwell, T., Zhao, J., Panwar, S., Roemer, A., Naimi, T., & Chikritzhs, T. (2016). Do "moderate" drinkers have reduced mortality risk? A systematic review and meta-analysis of alcohol consumption and all-cause mortality. *Journal of Studies on Alcohol & Drugs*, 77, 185–198.

Stollery, B., & Christian, L. (2013). Glucose and memory: The influence of drink, expectancy, and beliefs. *Psychopharmacology*, 228, 685–697.

(2015). Glucose, relational memory, and the hippocampus. *Psychopharmacology*, 232, 2113–2125.

Stone, S. W., Thermenos, H. W., Tarbox, S. I., Poldrack, R. A., & Seidman, L. J. (2005). Medial temporal and prefrontal lobe activation during verbal encoding following glucose ingestion in schizophrenia: A pilot fMRI study. *Neurobiology of Learning & Memory*, 83, 54–64.

Stough, C., Pipingas, A., Camfield, D., Nolidin, K., Savage, K., Deleuil, S., & Scholey, A. (2019). Increases in total cholesterol and low density lipoprotein associated with decreased cognitive performance in healthy elderly adults. *Metabolic Brain Disease*, 34, 477–484.

Strahler, J., & Nater, U. M. (2018). Differential effects of eating and drinking on wellbeing-an ecological ambulatory assessment study. *Biological Psychology*, 131, 72–88.

Stranahan, A. M., Norman, E. D., Lee, K., Cutler, R. G., Telljohann, R. S., Egan, J. M., & Mattson, M. P. (2008). Diet-induced insulin resistance impairs hippocampal synaptic plasticity and cognition in middle-aged rats. *Hippocampus*, 18, 1085–1088.

Strazzullo, P., D'Elia, L., Kandala, N. B., & Cappuccio, F. P. (2009). Salt intake, stroke, and cardiovascular disease: Meta-analysis of prospective studies. *British Medical Journal*, 339, 4567.

Stubbs, R., & Turicchi, J. (2020). From famine to therapeutic weight loss: Hunger, psychological responses, and energy balance-related behaviors. *Obesity Reviews*, 22, e13191.

Stumbo, P. J. (2013). New technology in dietary assessment: A review of digital methods in improving food record accuracy. *Proceedings of the Nutrition Society*, 72, 70–76.

Stunkard, A. J., & Messick, S. (1985). The three-factor eating questionnaire to measure dietary restraint, disinhibition, and hunger. *Journal of Psychosomatic Research*, 29, 71–83.

Su, K.-P., Tseng, P.-T., Lin, P.-Y., Okubo, R., Chen, T.-Y., Chen, Y.-W., & Matsuoka, Y. J. (2018). Association of use of omega-3 polyunsaturated fatty acids with changes in severity of anxiety symptoms: A systematic review and meta-analysis. *JAMA Network Open*, 1, e182327–e182327.

Suh, S. W., Kim, H. S., & Han, J. H. (2020). Efficacy of vitamins on cognitive function of non-demented people: A systematic review and meta-analysis. *Nutrients*, 12, 1168.

Sullivan, P. G., Rippy, N. A., Dorenbos, K., Concepcion, R. C., Agarwal, A. K., & Rho, J. M. (2004). The ketogenic diet increases mitochondrial uncoupling protein levels and activity. *Annals of Neurology*, 55, 576–580.

Sultan, A., Yang, K. S., & Isaev, D. (2017). Thujone inhibits the function of α_7-nicotinic acetylcholine receptors and impairs nicotine-induced memory enhancement in one-trial passive avoidance paradigm. *Toxicology*, 384, 23–32.

Sünram-Lea, S. I., Foster, J. K., Durlach, P., & Perez, C. (2001). Glucose facilitation of cognitive performance in healthy young adults: Examination of the influence of fast-duration, time of day and pre-consumption plasma glucose levels. *Psychopharmacology*, 157, 46–54.

Sünram-Lea, S. I., & Owen, L. (2017). The impact of diet-based glycaemic response and glucose regulation on cognition: Evidence across the lifespan. *Proceedings of the Nutrition Society*, 76, 466–477.

Sünram-Lea, S. I., Owen, L., Finnegan, Y., & Hu, H. (2011). Dose-response investigation into glucose facilitation of memory performance and mood in healthy young adults. *Journal of Psychopharmacology*, 25, 1076–1087.

Suren, P., Roth, C., Bresnahan, M., Haugen, M., Hornig, M., Hirtz, D., & Stoltenberg, C. (2013). Association between maternal use of folic acid supplements and risk of autism spectrum disorders in children. *Journal of the American Medical Association*, 309, 570–577.

Susser, E., Neugebauer, R., Hoek, H. W., Brown, A. S., Lin, S., Labovitz, D., & Gorman, J. M. (1996). Schizophrenia after prenatal famine. Further evidence. *Archives of General Psychiatry*, 53, 25–31.

Swank, R. L., Lerstad, O., Strøm, A., & Backer, J. (1952). Multiple sclerosis in rural Norway: Its geographic and occupational incidence in relation to nutrition. *New England Journal of Medicine*, 246, 721–728.

Szenczi-Cseh, J., & Ambrus, Á. (2017). Uncertainty of exposure assessment of consumer to pesticide residues derived from food consumed. *Journal of Environmental Science & Health*, 52, 658–670.

Szewczyk, B., Kubera, M., & Kowak, G. (2011). The role of zinc in neurodegenerative inflammatory pathways in depression. *Progress in Neuro-Psychopharmacology & Biological Psychiatry*, 35, 693–701.

Szucs, D., & Ioannidis, J. P. (2017). Empirical assessment of published effect sizes and power in the recent cognitive neuroscience and psychology literature. *PLoS Biology*, 15, e3001151.

Tabarki, B., Al-Shafi, S., & Al-Shahwan, S. (2013). Biotin-responsive basal ganglia disease revisited. *Neurology*, 80, 261–267.

Taghizadeh, M., Tamtaji, O. R., Dadgostar, E., Kakhaki, R. D., Bahmani, F., Abolhassani, J., & Asemi, Z. (2017). The effects of omega-3 fatty acids and vitamin E co-supplementation on clinical and metabolic status in patients with Parkinson's disease: A randomized, double-blind, placebo-controlled trial. *Neurochemistry International*, 108, 183–189.

Tahvonen, R. (1996). Contents of lead and cadmium in foods and diets. *Food Reviews International*, 12, 1–70.

Takase, K., Tsuneoka, Y., Oda, S., Kuroda, M., & Funato, H. (2016). High-fat diet feeding alters olfactory-, social-, and reward-related behaviors of mice independent of obesity. *Obesity (Silver Spring)*, 24, 886–894.

Takeda, A. (2001). Zinc homeostasis and functions of zinc in the brain. *Biometals*, 14, 343–351.

Takeda, A., & Tamano, H. (2009). Insight into zinc signalling from dietary zinc deficiency. *Brain Research Reviews*, 62, 33–44.

Takeuchi, H., Taki, Y., & Nouchi, R.(2019). Association of copper levels in the hair with gray matter volume, mean diffusivity, and cognitive functions. *Brain Structure & Function,* 224, 1203–1217.

Talebi, M., Kakouri, E., Talebi, M., Tarantilis, P. A., Farkhondeh, T., İlgün, S., Pourbagher-Shahri, A. M., & Samarghandian, S. (2021). Nutraceuticals-based therapeutic approach: Recent advances to combat pathogenesis of Alzheimer's disease. *Expert Review of Neurotherapeutics,* 21, 625–642.

Tamadon-Nejad, S., Ouliass, B., Rochford, J., & Ferland, G. (2018). Vitamin K deficiency induced by Warfarin is associated with cognitive and behavioral perturbations, and alterations in brain sphingolipids in rats. *Frontiers in Aging Neuroscience,* 10, 213.

Tamgüney, G., & Korczyn, A. D. (2018). A critical review of the prion hypothesis of human synucleinopathies. *Cell & Tissue Research,* 373, 213–220.

Tamura, B., Bell, C., Masaki, K., & Amella, E. (2013). Factors associated with weight loss, low BMI, and malnutrition among nursing home patients: A systematic review of the literature. *Journal of the American Medical Directors Association,* 14, 649–655.

Tan, K. W., Graf, B. A., Mitra, S. R., & Stephen, I. A. (2015). Daily consumption of a fruit and vegetable smoothie alters facial skin color. *PLoS One,* 10, e0133445.

Tang, H., Lu, D., Pan, R., Qin, X., Xiong, H., & Dong, J. (2009). Curcumin improves spatial memory impairment induced by human immunodeficiency virus type 1 glycoprotein 120 V3 loop peptide in rats. *Life Sciences,* 85, 1–10.

Tangney, C. C., Aggarwal, N. T., & Li, H. (2011). Vitamin B12, cognition, and brain MRI measures: A cross-sectional examination. *Neurology,* 77, 1276–1282.

Tangney, C. C., Li, H., Wang, Y. M., Barnes, L., Schneider, J. A., Bennett, D. A., & Morris, M. C. (2014). Relation of DASH- and Mediterranean-like dietary patterns to cognitive decline in older persons. *Neurology,* 83, 1410–1416.

Tao, L., Liu, K., & Chen, S. (2019). Dietary intake of riboflavin and unsaturated fatty acid can improve the multi-domain cognitive function in middle-aged and elderly populations: A 2-year prospective cohort study. *Frontiers in Aging Neuroscience,* 11, 226.

Tappy, L. (2012). 'Toxic' effects of sugar: Should we be afraid of fructose? *BMC Biology,* 10, 42.

Tasevska, N., Runswick, S. A., McTaggart, A., & Bingham, S. A. (2005). Urinary sucrose and fructose as biomarkers for sugar consumption. *Cancer Epidemiology, Biomarkers & Prevention,* 5, 1287–1294.

Tassebehji, N. M., Corniola, R. S., Alshingiti, A., & Levenson, C. W. (2008). Zinc deficiency induces depression-like symptoms in adult rats. *Physiology & Behavior,* 95, 365–369.

Tayebati, S. K., & Amenta, F. (2013). Choline-containing phospholipids: Relevance to brain functional pathways. *Clinical Chemistry & Laboratory Medicine,* 51, 513–521.

Taylor, R., Fealy, S., Bisquera, A., Smith, R., Collins, C., Evans, T., & Hure, A. (2017). Effects of nutritional interventions during pregnancy on infant and child cognitive outcomes: A systematic review and meta-analysis. *Nutrients*, 9, Article 1265.

Telle-Hansen, V. H., Holven, K. B., & Ulven, S. M. (2018). Impact of a healthy dietary pattern on gut microbiota and systemic inflammation in humans. *Nutrients*, 10, 1783.

Tellez, L. A., Medina, S., Han, W., Ferreira, J. G., Licona-Limòn, P., Ren, X., Lam, T., T., Schwartz, G. J., & de Araujo, I. E. (2013). A gut lipid messenger links excess dietary fat to dopamine deficiency. *Science*, 341, 800–802.

Temple, J. L., Bernard, C., Lipshultz, S. E., Czachor, J. D., Westphal, J. A., & Mestre, M. A. (2017). The safety of ingested caffeine: A comprehensive review. *Frontiers in Psychiatry*, 8, 80.

Tey, S. L., Brown, R. C., Gray, A. R., Chisholm, A. W., & Delahunty, C. M. (2012). Long-term consumption of high energy-dense snack foods on sensory-specific satiety and intake. *American Journal of Clinical Neuropsychology*, 95, 1038–1047.

Thompson, F. E., & Byers, T. (1994). Dietary assessment resource manual. *Journal of Nutrition*, 124, S2245–S2317.

Thomson, T. J., Runcie, J., & Miller, V. (1966). Treatment of obesity by total fasting for up to 249 days. *The Lancet*, 7471, 992–996.

Tian, H. -H., Aziz, A. -R., & Png, W. (2011). Effects of fasting during Ramadan month on cognitive function in Muslim athletes. *Asian Journal of Sports Medicine*, 2, 145–153.

Tiani, K., Stover, P., & Field, M. (2019). The role of brain barriers in maintaining brain vitamin levels. *Annual Review of Nutrition*, 39, 147–173.

Timmermans, S., Bogie, J. F., Vanmierlo, T., Lütjohann, D., Stinissen, P., Hellings, N., & Hendriks, J. J. (2014). High fat diet exacerbates neuroinflammation in an animal model of multiple sclerosis by activation of the Renin Angiotensin system. *Journal of Neuroimmune Pharmacology*, 9, 209–217.

Tojo, R., Suarez, A., Clemente, M. G., de los Reyes-Gavilan, C. G., Margolles, A., Gueimonde, M., & Ruas-Madiedo, P. (2014). Intestinal microbiota in health and disease: Role of bifidobacteria in gut homeostasis. *World Journal of Gastroenterology*, 20, 15163–15176.

Tom, G., & Rucker, M. (1975). Fat, full, and happy: Effects of food deprivation, external cues, and obesity on preference ratings, consumption, and buying intentions. *Journal of Personality & Social Psychology*, 32, 761–766.

Tong, J., Satyanarayanana, S. K., & Su, H. (2020). Nutraceuticals and probiotics in the management of psychiatric and neurological disorders: A focus on microbiota-gut-brain-immune axis. *Brain, Behavior & Immunity*, 80, 403–419.

Tooze, J. A., Subar, A. F., Thompson, F. E., Troiano, R, Schatzkin, A., & Kipnis, V. (2004). Psychosocial predictors of energy underreporting in a large doubly labelled water study. *American Journal of Clinical Nutrition*, 79, 795–804.

Tou, J. C., Jaczynski, J., & Chen, Y. C. (2007). Krill for human consumption: Nutritional value and potential health benefits. *Nutrition Reviews*, 65, 63–77.

Traber, M. G. (2014). Vitamin E inadequacy in humans: Causes and consequences. *Advances in Nutrition*, 5, 503–514.

Tran, D. M. D., & Westbrook, R. F. (2017). A high-fat high-sugar diet-induced impairment in place-recognition memory is reversible and training-dependent. *Appetite*, 110, 61–71.

Traversy, G., & Chaput, J. (2015). Alcohol consumption and obesity: An update. *Current Obesity Reports*, 4, 122–130.

Travica, N., Ried, K., & Sali, A. (2017). Vitamin C status and cognitive function: A systematic review. *Nutrients*, 9, 960.

(2019). Plasma vitamin C concentrations and cognitive function: A cross-sectional study. *Frontiers in Aging Neuroscience*, 11, 72.

Trevizol, A. P., Brietzke, E., & Grigolon, R. B. (2019). Peripheral interleukin-6 levels and working memory in non-obese adults: A post-hoc analysis from the CALERIE study. *Nutrition*, 58, 18–22.

Truitt, E. B., Callaway, E., Braude, M. C., & Krtantz, J. C. (1961). The pharmacology of myristicin. A contribution to the psychopharmacology of nutmeg. *Journal of Neuropsychiatry*, 2, 205–210.

Tsilioni, I., Taliou, A., Francis, K., & Theoharides, T. C. (2015). Children with autism spectrum disorders, who improved with a luteolin-containing dietary formulation, show reduced serum levels of TNF and IL-6. *Translational Psychiatry*, 5, e647.

Turnbaugh, P. J., Ridaura, V. K., Faith, J. J., Rey, F. E., Knight, R., & Gordon, J. I. (2009). The effect of diet on the human gut microbiome: A metagenomic analysis in humanized gnotobiotic mice. *Science Translational Medicine*, 1, 14.

Tveden-Nyborg, P., Johansen, L. K., & Raida, Z. (2009). Vitamin C deficiency in early postnatal life impairs spatial memory and reduces the number of hippocampal neurons in guinea pigs. *American Journal of Clinical Nutrition*, 90, 540–546.

Tyler, C. R., & Allan, A. M. (2014). The effects of arsenic exposure on neurological and cognitive dysfunction in human and rodent studies: A review. *Current Environmental Health Reports*, 1, 132–147.

U.S. Food & Drug Administration. Center for Food Safety & Applied Nutrition. (2012). Bad Bug Book – Tetrodotoxin. www.fda.gov/files/food/published/Bad-Bug-Book-2nd-Edition-%28PDF%29.pdf

Uher, R., Treasure, J., Heining, M., Brammer, M. J., & Campbell, L. C. (2006). Cerebral processing of food-related stimuli: Effects of fasting and gender. *Behavioural Brain Research*, 169, 111–119.

Ulatowski, L. M., & Manor, D. (2015). Vitamin E and neurodegeneration. *Neurobiology of Disease*, 84, 78–83.

Vahidnia, A., van der Voet, G. B., & de Wolff, F. A. (2007). Arsenic neurotoxicity – A review. *Human & Experimental Toxicology*, 26, 823–832.

Vairo, F. P., Chwal, B. C., & Perini, S. (2019). A systematic review and evidence-based guideline for diagnosis and treatment of Menkes disease. *Molecular Genetics & Metabolism,* 126, 6–13.

Valdes, A. M., Walter, J., Segal, E., & Spector, T. D. (2018). Role of the gut microbiota in nutrition and health. *British Medical Journal,* 361, 2179.

Valipour, G., Esmaillzadeh, A., Azadbakht, L., Afshar, H., Hassanzadeh, A., & Adibi, P. (2017). Adherence to the DASH diet in relation to psychological profile of Iranian adults. *European Journal of Nutrition,* 56, 309–320.

Valls-Pedret, C., Lamuela-Raventos, R. M., Medina-Remon, A., Quintana, M., Corella, D., Pinto, X., & Ros, E. (2012). Polyphenol-rich foods in the Mediterranean diet are associated with better cognitive function in elderly subjects at high cardiovascular risk. *Journal of Alzheimer's Disease,* 29, 773–782.

Valls-Pedret, C., Sala-Vila, A., Serra-Mir, M., Corella, D., de la Torre, R., Martinez-Gonzalez, M. A., & Ros, E. (2015). Mediterranean diet and age-related cognitive decline: A randomized clinical trial. *JAMA Internal Medicine,* 175, 1094–1103.

van de Rest, O., Bloemendaal, M., de Heus, R., & Aarts, E. (2017). Dose-dependent effects of oral tyrosine administration on plasma tyrosine levels and cognition in aging. *Nutrients,* 9, 1279.

van de Rest, O., Van Hooijdonk, L., & Doets, E. (2012). B vitamins and n-3 fatty acids for brain development and function: Review of human studies. *Annals of Nutrition & Metabolism,* 60, 272–292.

van den Kommer, T. N., Dik, M. G., Comijs, H. C., Fassbender, K., Lutjohann, D., & Jonker, C. (2009). Total cholesterol and oxysterols: Early markers for cognitive decline in elderly? *Neurobiology of Aging,* 30, 534–545.

van der Laan, L. N., de Ridder, D. T. D., Viergever, M. A., & Smeets, P. A. M. (2011). The first taste is always with the eyes: A meta-analysis on the neural correlates of processing visual food cues. *NeuroImage,* 55, 296–303.

van der Zwaluw, N. L., Brouwer-Brolsma, E. M., & van de Rest, O. (2017). Folate and vitamin B12-related biomarkers in relation to brain volumes. *Nutrients,* 9, 8.

van der Zwaluw, N. L., van de Rest, O., Kessels, R. P. C., & de Groot, L. C. P. G. M. (2015). Effects of glucose load on cognitive functions in elderly people. *Nutrition Reviews,* 73, 92–105.

Van Dolah, F. M. (2000). Marine algal toxins: Origins, health effects, and their increased occurrence. *Environmental Health Perspectives,* 108, 133–141.

van Donkelaar, E. L., Blokland, A., Ferrington, L., Kelly, P. A. T., Steinbusch, H. W. M., & Prickaerts, J. (2011). Mechanism of acute tryptophan depletion: Is it only serotonin? *Molecular Psychiatry,* 16, 695–713.

Van Moorhem, M., Lambein, F., & Leybaert, L. (2011). Unraveling the mechanism of β-N-oxalyl-a, β-diaminopropionic acid (β-ODAP) induced excitotoxicity and oxidative stress, relevance for neurolathyrism prevention. *Food & Chemical Toxicology,* 49, 550–555.

van Onselen, R., & Downing, T. G. (2018). BMAA-protein interactions: A possible new mechanism of toxicity. *Toxicon*, 143, 74–80.

van Rossem, L., Oenema, A., Steegers, E. A. P., Moll, H. A., Jaddoe, V. W. V., Hofman, A., & Raat, H. (2009). Are starting and continuing breastfeeding related to educational background? The Generation R Study. *Pediatrics*, 123, E1017–E1027.

van Ruitenbeek, P., Sambeth, A., Vermeeren, A., Young, S. N., & Riedel, W. J. (2009). Effects of L-histidine depletion and L-tyrosine/L-phenylalanine depletion on sensory and motor process in healthy volunteers. *British Journal of Pharmacology*, 157, 92–103.

van Ruitenbeek, P., Vermeeren, A., & Riedel, W. J. (2010). Cognitive domains affected by histamine H_1-antagonism in humans: A literature review. *Brain Research Reviews*, 64, 263–282.

Vandereycken, W., & van Deth, R. (1994). *From Fasting Saints to Anorexic Girls*. London: The Athlone Press.

Vauzour, D. (2017). Polyphenols and brain health. *OCL*, 24, A202.

Veena, S., Gale, C., Krishnaveni, G., Kehoe, S., Srinivasan, K., & Fall, C. (2016). Association between maternal nutritional status in pregnancy and offspring cognitive function during childhood and adolescence: A systematic review. *BMC Pregnancy & Childbirth*, 16, Article 220.

Veena, S. R., Krishnaveni, G. V., Srinivasan, K., Wills, A. K., Muthayya, S., Kurpad, A. V., & Fall, C. H. (2010). Higher maternal plasma folate but not vitamin B-12 concentrations during pregnancy are associated with better cognitive function scores in 9- to 10- year-old children in South India. *Journal of Nutrition*, 140, 1014–1022.

Veggiotti, P., Teutonico, F., Alfei, E., Nardocci, N., Zorzi, G., Tagliabue, A., & Balottin, U. (2010). Glucose transporter type 1 deficiency: Ketogenic diet in three patients with atypical phenotype. *Brain Development*, 32, 404–408.

Vengeliene, V., Bilbao, A., Molander, A., & Spanagel, R. (2008). Neuropharmacology of alcohol addiction. *British Journal of Pharmacology*, 154, 299–315.

Veniaminova, E., Cespuglio, R., Cheung, C. W., Umriukhin, A., Markova, N., Shevtsova, E., & Strekalova, T. (2017). Autism-like behaviours and memory deficits result from a Western diet in mice. *Neural Plasticity*, 2017, 9498247.

Veniaminova, E., Cespuglio, R., Markova, N., Mortimer, N., Cheung, C. W., Steinbusch, H. W., & Strekalova, T. (2016). Behavioral features of mice fed with a cholesterol-enriched diet: Deficient novelty exploration and unaltered aggressive behavior. *Translational Neuroscience & Clinics*, 2, 87–95.

Veniaminova, E., Oplatchikova, M., Bettendorff, L., Kotenkova, E., Lysko, A., Vasilevskaya, E., & Strekalova, T. (2020). Prefrontal cortex inflammation and liver pathologies accompany cognitive and motor deficits following Western diet consumption in non-obese female mice. *Life Sciences*, 241, 117163.

Vergeres, G. (2013). Nutrigenomics – Linking food to human metabolism. *Trends in Food Science & Technology*, 31, 6–12.

Veronese, N., Facchini, S., & Stubbs, B. (2017). Weight loss is associated with improvements in cognitive function among overweight and obese people: A systematic review and meta-analysis. *Neuroscience & Biobehavioral Reviews*, 72, 87–94.

Vetrani, C., Costabile, G., Di Marino, L., & Rivellese, A. A. (2013). Nutrition and oxidative stress: A systematic review of human studies. *International Journey of Food Science & Nutrition*, 64, 312–326.

Vignes, M., Maurice, T., Lanté, F., Nedjar, M., Thethi, K., Guiramand, J., & Récasens, M. (2006). Anxiolytic properties of green tea polyphenol (-)-epigallocatechin gallate (EGCG). *Brain Research*, 1110, 102–115.

Villain, N., Picq, J. -L. Aujard, F., & Pifferi, F. (2016). Body mass loss correlates with cognitive performance in primates under acute caloric restriction conditions. *Behavioural Brain Research*, 305, 157–163.

Villamor, E., Rifas-Shiman, S. L., Gillman, M. W., & Oken, E. (2012). Maternal intake of methyl-donor nutrients and child cognition at 3 years of age. *Paediatrics & Perinatal Epidemiology*, 26, 328–335.

Virmani, A., Pinto, L., Binienda, Z., & Ali, S. (2013). Food, nutrigenomics, and neurodegeneration – Neuroprotection by what you eat! *Molecular Biology*, 48, 353–362.

Visek, W. J. (1984). An update of concepts of essential amino acids. *Annual Review of Nutrition*, 4, 137–155.

Vitousek, K. M., Manke, F. P., Gray, J. A., & Vitousek, M. N. (2004). Caloric restriction for longevity: II – The systematic neglect of behavioural and psychological outcomes in animal research. *European Eating Disorders Review*, 12, 338–360.

Vogel, T., Dali-Youcef, N., Kaltenbach, G., & Andres, E. (2009). Homocysteine, vitamin B-12, folate and cognitive functions: A systematic and critical review of the literature. *International Journal of Clinical Practice*, 63, 1061–1067.

von Deneen, K. M., Gold, M. S., & Liu, Y. (2009). Food addiction and cues in Prader-Willi syndrome. *Journal of Addiction Medicine*, 3, 19–25

Vu, T., Lin, F., Alshurafa, N., & Xu, W. (2017). Wearable food intake monitoring technologies: A comprehensive review. *Computers*, 6, e6010004.

Vyas, A., Mitra, R., Rao, B., & Chattarji, S. (2002). Chronic stress induces contrasting patterns of dendritic remodelling in hippocampal and amygdaloid neurons. *Journal of Neuroscience*, 22, 6810–6818.

Walford, R. L., Mock, D., MacCallum, T., & Laseter, J. L. (1999). Physiologic changes in humans subjected to severe, selective calorie restriction for two years in Biosphere 2: Health, aging, and toxicological perspectives. *Toxicological Sciences*, 52, 61–65.

Walter, T., Kovalskys, J., & Stekel, A. (1983). Effect of mild iron deficiency on infant mental development scores. *Journal of Pediatrics*, 102, 519–522.

Wang, B. Z., Zailan, F. Z., Wong, B. Y. X., Ng, K. P., & Kandiah, N. (2020). Identification of novel candidate autoantibodies in Alzheimer's disease. *European Journal of Neurology*, 27, 2292–2296.

Wang, D. (2008). Neurotoxins from marine dingoflagellates: A brief review. *Marine Drugs*, 6, 349–371.

Wang, J., Ho, L., Zhao, Z., Seror, I., Humala, N., Dickstein, D. L., & Pasinetti, G. M. (2006). Moderate consumption of Cabernet Sauvignon attenuates A beta neuropathology in a mouse model of Alzheimer's disease. *Faseb Journal*, 20, 2313–2320.

Warburg, O., Wind, F., & Negelein, E. (1927). The metabolism of tumors in the body. *Journal of General Physiology*, 8, 519.

Wardle, J., Rogers, P., Judd, P., Taylor, M. A., Rapoport, L., Green, M., & Nicholson Perry, K. (2000). Randomized trial of the effects of cholesterol-lowering dietary treatment on psychological function. *American Journal of Medicine*, 108, 547–553.

Warren, M. A., Freestone, T., & Thomas, A. J. (1989). Undernutrition during early adult life significantly affects neuronal connectivity in rat visual cortex. *Experimental Neurology*, 103, 290–292.

Warthon-Medina, M., Moran, V. H., & Stammers, A.-L. (2015). Zinc intake, status and indices of cognitive function in adults and children: A systematic review and meta-analysis. *European Journal of Clinical Nutrition*, 69, 649–661.

Wasim, M., Awan, F. R., & Khan, H. N. (2018). Aminoacidopathies: Prevalence, etiology, screening, and treatment options. *Biochemical Genetics*, 56, 7–21.

Waylen, A., Ford, T., Goodman, R., Samara, M., & Wolke, D. (2009). Can early intake of dietary omega-3 predict childhood externalizing behaviour? *Acta Paediatrica*, 98, 1805–1808.

Weed, J. L., Lane, M. A., Roth, G. S., Speer, D. L., & Ingram, D. K. (1997). Activity measures in rhesus monkeys on long-term calorie restriction. *Physiology & Behavior*, 62, 97–103.

Wengreen, H., Munger, R. G., Cutler, A., Quach, A., Bowles, A., Corcoran, C., & Welsh-Bohmer, K. A. (2013). Prospective study of dietary approaches to stop hypertension- and Mediterranean-style dietary patterns and age-related cognitive change: The Cache County Study on Memory, Health and Aging. *American Journal of Clinical Nutrition*, 98, 1263–1271.

Wesensten, N. J. (2014). Legitimacy of concerns about caffeine and energy drink consumption. *Nutrition Reviews*, 72, 78–86.

Westwater, M. K., Fletcher, P. C., & Ziauddeen, H. (2016). Sugar addiction: The state of the science. *European Journal of Nutrition*, 55, S55–S69.

Weyer, C., Walford, R. L., & Harper, I. T. (2000). Energy metabolism after 2 years of energy restriction: The Biosphere 2 experiment. *American Journal of Clinical Nutrition*, 72, 946–953.

Whang, R., Hampton, E. M., & Whang, D. D. (1994). Magnesium homeostasis and clinical disorders of magnesium deficiency. *Annals of Pharmacotherapy*, 28, 220–226.

Whanger, P. D. (2001). Selenium and the brain: A review. *Nutritional Neuroscience*, 4, 81–97.

White, C. L., Pistell, P. J., Purpera, M. N., Gupta, S., Fernandez-Kim, S. O., Hise, T. L., & Bruce-Keller, A. J. (2009). Effects of high fat diet on Morris maze performance, oxidative stress, and inflammation in rats: Contributions of maternal diet. *Neurobiology of Disease*, 35, 3–13.

White, N. (1989). Reward or reinforcement: What's the difference? *Neuroscience & Biobehavioral Reviews*, 13, 181–186.

White, N. M. (1991). Peripheral and central memory-enhancing actions of glucose. In R. C. A. Frederickson, J. L. McGaugh, & D. L. Felten (Eds.), *Neuronal Control of Bodily Function: Basic and Clinical aspects, Vol. 6. Peripheral Signalling of the Brain: Role in Neural-Immune Interactions and Learning and Memory* (pp. 421–441). Ashland, OH: Hogrefe & Huber Publishers.

Whitfield, J. T., Pako, W. H., Collinge, J., & Alpers, M. P. (2017). Cultural factors that affected the spatial and temporal epidemiology of kuru. *Royal Society Open Science*, 4, 1–13.

Whitfield, K. C., Bourassa, M. W., & Adamolekun, B. (2018). Thiamine deficiency disorders: Diagnosis, prevalence, and a roadmap for global control programs. *Annals of the New York Academy of Sciences*, 1430, 3–43.

Wieckowska-Gacek, A., Mietelska-Porowska, A., Wydrych, M., & Wojda, U. (2021). Western diet as a trigger of Alzheimer's disease: From metabolic syndrome and systemic inflammation to neuroinflammation and neurodegeneration. *Ageing Research Review*, 70, 101397.

Wiehl, D., & Reed, R. (1960). Development of new or improved dietary methods for epidemiological investigations. *American Journal of Public Health*, 50, 824–828.

Wight, N., Marinelli, K. A., & Med, A. B. (2014). ABM clinical protocol #1: Guidelines for blood glucose monitoring and treatment of hypoglycemia in term and late-preterm neonates, revised 2014. *Breastfeeding Medicine*, 9, 173–179.

Wilder, R. M. (1921). The effects of ketonemia on the course of epilepsy. *Mayo Clinical Proceedings*, 2, 307–308.

Wilken, M., Bartmann, P., Dovey, T., & Bagci, S. (2018). Characteristics of feeding tube dependency with respect to food aversive behaviour and growth. *Appetite*, 123, 1–6.

Willett, W. C. (1994). Diet and health: What should we eat? *Science*, 264, 532–537.

Willett, W. C., Sampson, L., Stampfer, M. J., Rosner, B., Bain, C., Witschi, J., Hennekens, C. H., & Speizer, F. E. (1985). Reproducibility and validity of a semiquantitative food frequency questionnaire. *American Journal of Epidemiology*, 122, 51–65.

Williams, P. G. (2014). The benefits of breakfast cereal consumption: A systematic review of the evidence base. *Advances in Nutrition*, 5, 636S–673S.

Williams, R. J., Mohanakumar, K. P., & Beart, P. M. (2015). Neuro-nutraceuticals: The path to brain health via nourishment is not so distant. *Neurochemistry International*, 89, 1–6.

(2016). Neuroscience-nutraceuticals: Further insights into their promise for brain health. *Neurochemistry International*, 95, 1–3.

Williamson, D. A., Martin, C. K., & Anton, S. D. (2008). Is caloric restriction associated with development of eating-disorder symptoms? Results from the CALERIE Trial. *Health Psychology*, 27, S32–S42.

Willis, N. D., Lloyd, A. J., Xie, L., Stiegler, M., Tailliart, K., Garcia-Perez, I., Chambers, E. S., Beckmann, M., Draper, J., & Mathers, J. C. (2020). Design and characterisation of a randomized food intervention that mimics exposure to a typical UK diet to provide urine samples for identification and validation of metabolite biomarkers of food intake. *Frontiers in Nutrition*, 7, e561010.

Wing, R. R., Epstein, L. H., Marcus, M. D., & Kupfer, D. J. (1984). Mood changes in behavioral weight loss programs. *Journal of Psychosomatic Research*, 28, 189–196.

Wirdefeldt, K., Adami, H. O., Cole, P., Trichopoulos, D., & Mandel, J. (2011). Epidemiology and etiology of Parkinson's disease: A review of the evidence. *European Journal of Epidemiology*, 26, S1–S58.

Wiss, D. A., Avena, N., & Rada, P. (2018). Sugar addiction: From evolution to revolution. *Frontiers in Psychiatry*, 9, 545.

Witte, A. V., Fobker, M., Gellner, R., Knecht, S., & Flöel, A. (2009). Caloric restriction improves memory in elderly humans. *Proceedings of the National Academy of Sciences of the United States of America*, 106, 1255–1260.

Witte, A. V., Kerti, L., Margulies, D. S., & Floel, A. (2014). Effects of resveratrol on memory performance, hippocampal functional connectivity, and glucose metabolism in healthy older adults. *Journal of Neuroscience*, 34, 7862–7870.

Wolf, B. (2011). The neurology of biotinidase deficiency. *Molecular Genetics & Metabolism*, 104, 27–34.

Wolraich, M. L., Wilson, D. B., & White, J. W. (1995). The effect of sugar on behavior or cognition in children. A meta-analysis. *Journal of the American Medical Association*, 274, 1617–1621.

Woods, S. E., & Seeley, R. J. (2000). Adiposity signals and the control of energy homeostasis. *Nutrition*, 16, 894–902.

Woolf, E. C., & Scheck, A. C. (2015). The ketogenic diet for the treatment of malignant glioma. *Journal of Lipid Research*, 56, 5–10.

World Health Organization. (2021). Malnutrition. https://who.int/news-room/fact-sheets/detail/malnutrition (last accessed 18 June 2021).

Wu, A., Ying, Z., & Gomez-Pinilla, F. (2004a). Dietary omega-3 fatty acids normalize BDNF levels, reduce oxidative damage, and counteract learning disability after traumatic brain injury in rats. *Journal of Neurotrauma*, 21, 1457–1467.

(2004b). The interplay between oxidative stress and brain-derived neurotrophic factor modulates the outcome of a saturated fat diet on synaptic plasticity and cognition. *European Journal of Neuroscience*, 19, 1699–1707.

(2006). Dietary curcumin counteracts the outcome of traumatic brain injury on oxidative stress, synaptic plasticity, and cognition. *Experimental Neurology*, 197, 309–317.

(2007). Omega-3 fatty acids supplementation restores mechanisms that maintain brain homeostasis in traumatic brain injury. *Journal of Neurotrauma*, 24, 1587–1595.

Wu, L., & Sun, D. (2017). Adherence to Mediterranean diet and risk of developing cognitive disorders: An updated systematic review and meta-analysis of prospective cohort studies. *Scientific Reports*, 7, 41317.

Wurtman, R. J., Hefti, F., & Melamed, E. (1980). Precursor control of neurotransmitter synthesis. *Pharmacological Reviews*, 32, 315–335.

Wurtman, R. J., Wurtman, J. J., Regan, M. M., McDermott, J. M., Tsay, R. H., & Breu, J. J. (2003). Effects of normal meals rich in carbohydrates or proteins on plasma tryptophan and tyrosine ratios. *American Journal of Clinical Nutrition*, 77, 128–132.

Xiao, S., Hansen, D. K., Horsley, E. T., Tang, Y. S., Khan, R. A., Stabler, S. P., & Antony, A. C. (2005). Maternal folate deficiency results in selective upregulation of folate receptors and heterogeneous nuclear ribonucleoprotein-E1 associated with multiple subtle aberrations in fetal tissues. *Birth Defects Research A: Clinical and Molecular Teratology*, 73, 6–28.

Xie, L., Li, X. K., Funeshima-Fuji, N., Kimura, H., Matsumoto, Y., Isaka, Y., & Takahara, S. (2009). Amelioration of experimental autoimmune encephalomyelitis by curcumin treatment through inhibition of IL-17 production. *International Immunopharmacology*, 9, 575–581.

Xu, K., Sun, X. Y., Eroku, B. O., Tsipis, C. P., Puchowicz, M. A., & La Manna, J. C. (2010). Diet-induced ketosis improves cognitive performance in aged rats. *Oxygen Transport to Tissue*, 662, 71–75.

Xu, M. Q., Sun, W. S., Liu, B. X., Feng, G. Y., Yu, L., Yang, L., & He, L. (2009). Prenatal malnutrition and adult schizophrenia: Further evidence from the 1959–1961 Chinese famine. *Schizophrenia Bulletin*, 35, 568–576.

Xu, Q., Liu, F., Chen, P., Jez, J. M., & Krishnan, H. B. (2017). β-N-Oxalyl-L-α, β-diaminopropionic acid (β-ODAP) content in lathyrus sativus: The integration of nitrogen and sulfur metabolism through β-cyanoalanine synthase. *International Journal of Molecular Sciences*, 18, 526.

Xu, Y., Lin, D., Li, S., Li, G., Shyamala, S. G., Barish, P. A., & Ogle, W. O. (2009). Curcumin reverses impaired cognition and neuronal plasticity induced by chronic stress. *Neuropharmacology*, 57, 463–471.

Yanai, S., Okaichi, H., & Sugioka, K. (2008). Dietary restriction inhibits spatial learning ability and hippocampal cell proliferation in rats. *Japanese Psychological Research*, 50, 36–48.

Yasin, W. M., Khattak, M. M. A. K., Mamat, N. M., & Bakar, W. A. M. A. (2013). Does religious fasting affect cognitive performance? *Nutrition & Food Science*, 43, 483–489.

Ye, F., Li, X.-J., Jiang, W.-L., Sun, H.-B., & Liu, J. (2015). Efficacy of and patient compliance with a ketogenic diet in adults with intractable epilepsy: A meta-analysis. *Journal of Clinical Neurology*, 11, 26–31.

Yehuda, S., Rabinovitz, S., & Mostofsky, D. I. (2005). Mixture of essential fatty acids lowers test anxiety. *Nutritional Neuroscience*, 8, 265–267.

Yip, R. (2002). Prevention and control of iron deficiency: Policy and strategy issues. *Journal of Nutrition*, 132, 802s–805s.

Yokel, R. A., Hicks, C. L., & Florence, R. L. (2008). Aluminum bioavailability from basic sodium aluminum phosphate, an approved food additive emulsifying agent, incorporated in cheese. *Food & Chemical Toxicology*, 46, 2261–2266.

Yoon, J.-H., & Baek, S. J. (2005). Molecular targets of dietary polyphenols with anti-inflammatory properties. *Yonsei Medical Journal*, 46, 585–596.

Young, S. N. (1996). Behavioral effects of dietary neurotransmitter precursors: Basic and clinical aspects. *Neuroscience & Biobehavioral Reviews*, 20, 313–323.

(2013). Acute tryptophan depletion in humans: A review of theoretical, practical and ethical aspects. *Journal of Psychiatry & Neuroscience*, 38, 294–305.

Ysart, G., Miller, P., & Croasdale, M., (2000). 1997 UK total diet study – Dietary exposures to aluminium, arsenic, cadmium, chromium, copper, lead, mercury, nickel, selenium, tin and zinc. *Food Additives & Contaminants*, 17, 775–786.

Yu, Y., Wang, Q., & Huang, X. F. (2009). Energy-restricted pair-feeding normalizes low levels of brain-derived neurotrophic factor/tyrosine kinase B mRNA expression in the hippocampus, but not ventromedial hypothalamic nucleus, in diet-induced obese mice. *Neuroscience*, 160, 295–306.

Yucel, F., Warren, M. A., & Gumusburun, E. (1994). The effects of undernutrition on connectivity in the cerebellar cortex of adult rats. *Journal of Anatomy*, 184, 59–64.

Zafra, M. A., Molina, F., & Puerto, A. (2006). The neural/cephalic phase reflexes in the physiology of nutrition. *Neuroscience & Biobehavioural Reviews*, 30, 1032–1044.

Zahr, N. M., Kaufman, K. L., & Harer, C. G. (2011). Clinical and pathological features of alcohol-related brain damage. *Nature Reviews Neurology*, 7, 284–294.

Zahr, N. M., & Pfefferbaum, A. (2017). Alcohol's effects on the brain: Neuroimaging results in humans and animal models. *Alcohol Research*, 38, 183–206.

Zakhari, S. (2006). Overview: How is alcohol metabolized by the body? *Alcohol Research and Health*, 29, 245–254.

Żarnowska, I., Chrapko, B., Gwizda, G., Nocuń, A., Mitosek-Szewczyk, K., & Gasior, M. (2018). Therapeutic use of carbohydrate-restricted diets in an autistic child; a case report of clinical and 18FDG PET findings. *Metabolic Brain Disorders*, 33, 1187–1192.

Zatta, P., & Frank, A. (2007). Copper deficiency and neurological disorders in man and animals. *Brain Research Reviews*, 54, 19–33.

Zeisel, S. H. (2006). Choline: Critical role during fetal development and dietary requirements in adults. *Annual Review of Nutrition*, 26, 229–250.

Zempleni, J., Wijeratne, S. S. K., & Hassan, Y. I. (2009). Biotin. *Biofactors*, 35, 36–46.

Zhang, L., Zhu, J. -H., Zhang, X., & Cheng, W. -H. (2019). The thioredoxin-like family of selenoproteins: Implications in aging and age-related degeneration. *Biological Trace Element Research*, 188, 189–195.

Zhang, X., Dong, F., Ren, J., Driscoll, M. J., & Culver, B. (2005). High dietary fat induces NADPH oxidase-associated oxidative stress and inflammation in rat cerebral cortex. *Experimental Neurology*, 191, 318–325.

Zhang, Y.-P., Miao, R., Li, Q., Wu, T., & Ma, F. (2017). Effects of DHA supplementation on hippocampal volume and cognitive function in older adults with mild cognitive impairment: A 12-month randomized, double-blind, placebo-controlled trial. *Journal of Alzheimer's Disease*, 55, 497–507.

Zhao, X., Xu, X., Li, X., Yang, Y., & Zhu, S. (2021). Emerging trends of technology-based dietary assessment: A perspective study. *European Journal of Clinical Nutrition*, 75, 582–587.

Zhou, S. J., Gibson, R. A., Crowther, C. A., Baghurst, P., & Makrides, M. (2006). Effect of iron supplementation during pregnancy on the intelligence quotient and behavior of children at 4 years of age: Long-term follow-up of a randomized controlled trial. *American Journal of Clinical Nutrition*, 83, 1112–1117.

Zhu, C., Sawrey-Kubicek, L., Beals, E., Rhodes, C. H., Houts, H. E., Sacchi, R., & Zivkovic, A. M. (2020). Human gut microbiome composition and tryptophan metabolites were changed differently by fast food and Mediterranean diet in 4 days: A pilot study. *Nutrition Research*, 77, 62–72.

Zhu, X., Krasnow, S. M., & Roth-Carter, Q. R. (2012). Hypothalamic signalling in anorexia induced by indispensable amino acid deficiency. *American Journal of Physiology -Endocrinology and Metabolism*, 303, E1446–E1458.

Ziauddeen, H., Farooqi, I. S., & Fletcher, P. C. (2012). Obesity and the brain: How convincing is the addiction model? *Nature Reviews Neuroscience*, 13, 279–286.

Zilberter, T., & Zilberter, E. Y. (2013). Breakfast and cognition: Sixteen effects in nine populations, no single recipe. *Frontiers in Human Neuroscience*, 7, article 631.

Zimmerman, M. B. (2009). Iodine deficiency. *Endocrine Reviews*, 30, 376–408.

Zimmerman, M. B., & Boelaert, K. (2015). Iodine deficiency and thyroid disorders. *The Lancet Diabetes & Endocrinology*, 3, 286–295.

Zohar, A. H., Giladi, L., & Givati, T. (2007). Holocaust exposure and disordered eating: A study of multi-generational transmission. *European Eating Disorders Review*, 15, 50–57.

Zuccoli, G., Marcello, N., Pisanello, A., Servadei, F., Vaccaro, S., Mukherjee, P., & Seyfried, T. N. (2010). Metabolic management of glioblastoma multiforme using standard therapy together with a restricted ketogenic diet: Case report. *Nutrition & Metabolism*, 7, 1–7.

Index